W9-AAV-645

Chasteen's
ESSENTIALS OF
Clinical Dental Assisting

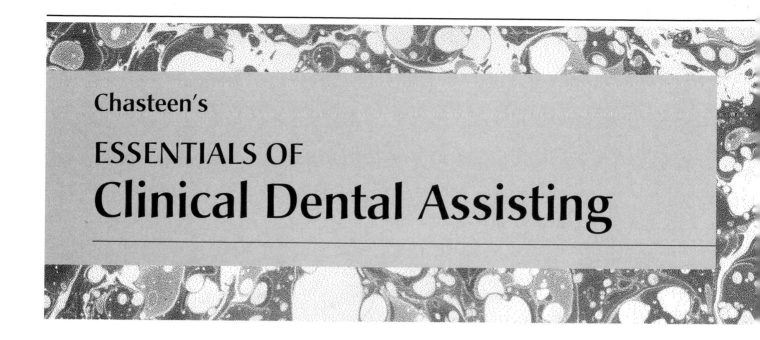

Chasteen's

ESSENTIALS OF
Clinical Dental Assisting

CARA M. MIYASAKI-CHING, RDH, MS

Director, Dental Assisting Program and Dental Hygiene Program
Foothill College
Los Altos Hills, California

FIFTH EDITION

With 1007 *illustrations*

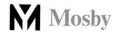 Mosby

St. Louis Baltimore Boston
Carlsbad Chicago Naples New York Philadelphia Portland
London Madrid Mexico City Singapore Sydney Tokyo Toronto Wiesbaden

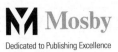
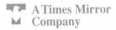

Vice President and Publisher: Don E. Ladig
Executive Editor: Linda L. Duncan
Managing Editor: Penny Rudolph
Project Manager: Patricia Tannian
Production Editor: Melissa Mraz
Book Design Manager: Gail Morey Hudson
Manufacturing Supervisor: Karen Lewis
Editing and Production: Top Graphics
Cover Designer: Teresa Breckwoldt

FIFTH EDITION
Copyright © 1997 by Mosby-Year Book, Inc.

Previous editions copyrighted 1975, 1980, 1984, 1989

All rights reserved. No part of this publication may be reproduced,
stored in a retrieval system, or transmitted, in any form or by any
means, electronic, mechanical, photocopying, recording, or otherwise,
without written permission of the publisher.

Permission to photocopy or reproduce solely for internal or personal
use is permitted for libraries or other users registered with the Copyright
Clearance Center, provided that the base fee of $4.00 per chapter plus $.10
per page is paid directly to the Copyright Clearance Center, 27 Congress
Street, Salem, MA 01970. This consent does not extend to other kinds
of copying, such as copying for general distribution, for advertising or
promotional purposes, for creating new collected works, or for resale.

Printed in the United States of America
Composition by Top Graphics
Printing/binding by Maple-Vail Book Mfg. Group

Mosby–Year Book, Inc.
11830 Westline Industrial Drive
St. Louis, Missouri 63146

Miyasaki-Ching, Cara M.
    Chasteen's essentials of clinical dental assisting.—5th ed./
Cara M. Miyasaki-Ching.
        p. cm.
    Rev. ed. of: Essentials of clinical dental assisting / Joseph E.
Chasteen. 4th ed. 1989.
    Includes bibliographical references and index.
    ISBN 0-8151-6211-1
    1. Dental assistants. 2. Dentistry. I. Chasteen, Joseph E.
Essentials of clinical dental assisting.   II. Title.
    [DNLM: 1. Dental Assistants. 2. Dentistry. 3. Technology.
Dental. WU 90 M685c 1996]
    RK60.5.C45 1996
    617.6—dc20
DNLM/DLC
for Library of Congress   96-30951
                                                    CIP

96 97 98 99 00 / 9 8 7 6 5 4 3 2 1

To my husband
Jeffrey Ching
for all his love and support

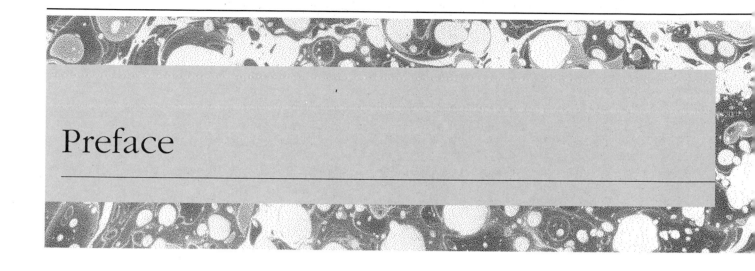

Preface

The fifth edition of *Chasteen's Essentials of Clinical Dental Assisting* was written with two goals in mind:

- To offer a source of detailed and comprehensive information concerning the clinical aspects of dental assisting in a book of reasonable size.
- To present complex information in a form that is understandable to beginning dental assistants who have little or no basic science or dental background.

Dentistry is a dynamic and evolving field. As advances in dental research are made, corresponding changes are made in the way that dentistry is practiced. Every chapter in the fifth edition of this book has been revised and updated in both format and content. Extensive revisions have been made in the areas of infection control and restorative materials to reflect the significant changes that have occurred over the last several years. Chapter 7, Infection Control in the Dental Office, contains the latest information about OSHA regulations, sterilization, and disinfection procedures. Information on restorative materials and cavity medications has also been extensively updated to highlight the many recent changes in these areas. For example, information on the newer glass ionomer cements and liners that have been increasing in popularity has been added, while discussions about cements such as zinc phosphate, zinc oxide, eugenol, and polycarboxylate, which are still in use, have been retained. Other significant updates in content include discussion of child neglect and abuse, implants, bonded amalgams, fabrication of bleaching splints, sports mouthguards, and composite resin temporaries. Step-by-step instructions for each dental procedure are outlined in boxes, with the rationale for each step provided.

In this edition great care has been taken to address the need to target the majority of our students, who are visual learners. Methods used to present material visually include the following:

- Adding 150 new illustrations/photographs to depict equipment and procedures
- Opening each chapter with a list of key terms, with each term shown in boldface type in its chapter discussion
- Highlighting important information with Key Points boxes throughout each chapter
- Providing a glossary that defines all key terms
- Adding multiple choice test questions at the end of each chapter
- Providing answers to all questions at the end of the book, along with rationales for each possible answer

INSTRUCTOR'S MANUAL

This is the first edition of *Chasteen's Essentials of Clinical Dental Assisting* to be accompanied by an Instructor's Manual. We sincerely hope that this manual meets the needs of instructors of dental assisting programs. The Instructor's Manual includes these features:

- Learning objectives for each chapter in the book
- A set of 20 enlarged illustrations to be used as transparency masters
- A total of 37 process evaluation forms to help instructors score dental assisting students on their performance of procedures routinely performed by a dental assistant
- A 310-question test bank that simulates the Dental Assisting National Board Examination (DANBE)

ACKNOWLEDGMENTS

I would like to thank Linda Duncan (Executive Editor), Penny Rudolph (Managing Editor), and Angie Reiner (Editorial Assistant), all of Mosby, for their invaluable assistance along every step of this revision. I also wish to thank Carlotta Seely of Top Graphics for her expertise during the production phase of the revision. Finally, I want my parents and my husband to know that I am forever grateful to them for their love and understanding.

Cara M. Miyasaki-Ching

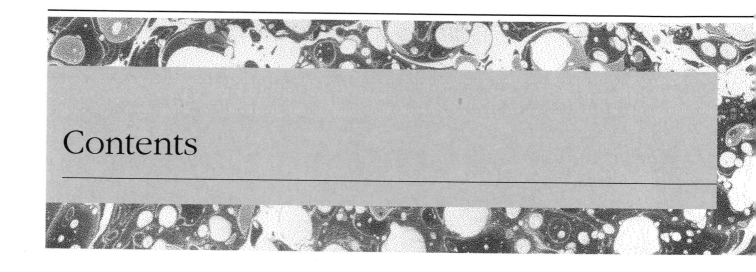

Contents

GENERAL DENTISTRY

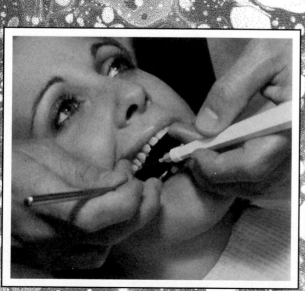

Courtesy Viadent Inc, Fort Collins, Colo.

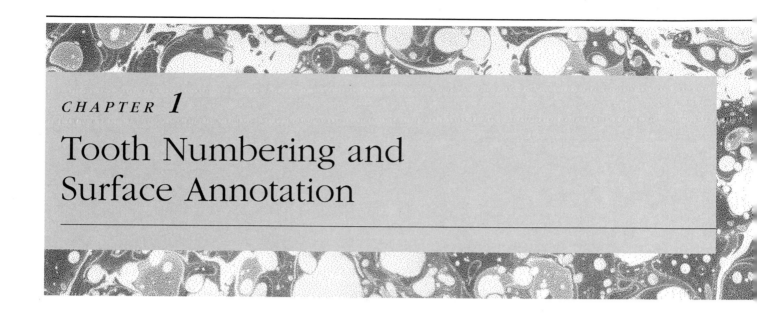

CHAPTER 1

Tooth Numbering and Surface Annotation

KEY TERMS

Buccal
Distal
Facial
Incisal
Labial
Lingual
Mesial
Occlusal
Palatal

TOOTH NUMBERING SYSTEMS

Since proper names for each tooth can be cumbersome, numbering systems have been developed to simplify identification of individual teeth. These systems are helpful in charting information on records, in verbal communication, and in correspondence such as referral letters. There are three numbering systems in common use today:

- American Dental Association sequential numbering system
- Zsigmondy-Palmer system
- Federation Dentaire Internationale system

Each of these systems has a method of numbering permanent and primary teeth.

American Dental Association Sequential Numbering System

The American Dental Association (ADA) has adopted a standard sequential numbering system for all 32 teeth in the permanent dentition. Each tooth is assigned a number to identify it. This system is sometimes called the *universal numbering system* (Box 1-1).

American Dental Association sequential numbering system for permanent teeth

Tooth #1 represents the patient's maxillary right third molar. The numbering progresses toward the anterior teeth and continues through the patient's maxillary left quadrant, where the maxillary left third molar is assigned #16. The mandibular teeth are numbered starting in the mandibular left quadrant, and the third molar is assigned #17. Numbering continues around the arch to the mandibular right third molar, which is represented as tooth #32 (Figure 1-1, *A*).

This system has widespread use in the dental profession because it is simple. It prevents confusion when reference is made to specific teeth or areas around specific teeth. It is easier to refer to tooth numbers that to cumbersome anatomical names.

American Dental Association sequential lettering system for primary teeth

The same basic system is used to identify the primary teeth, except that they are identified with the uppercase letters A through T (Figure 1-1, *B*). Tooth A represents the

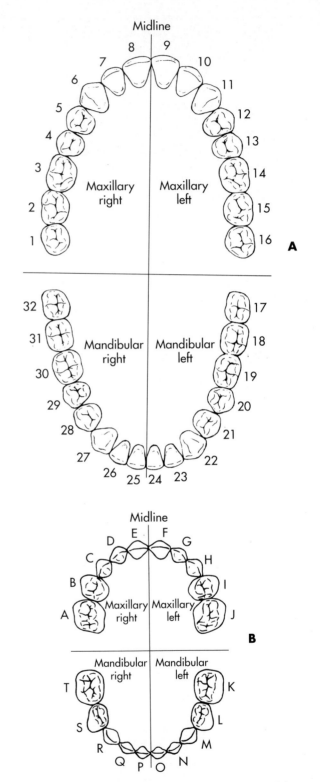

BOX 1-1

AMERICAN DENTAL ASSOCIATION SEQUENTIAL NUMBERING SYSTEM OF PERMANENT DENTITION

ADA TOOTH NUMBER	PROPER TOOTH NAME
UPPER TEETH	
1	Maxillary right third molar
2	Maxillary right second molar
3	Maxillary right first molar
4	Maxillary right second premolar (bicuspid)
5	Maxillary right first premolar (bicuspid)
6	Maxillary right canine (cuspid)
7	Maxillary right lateral incisor
8	Maxillary right central incisor
9	Maxillary left central incisor
10	Maxillary left lateral incisor
11	Maxillary left canine (cuspid)
12	Maxillary left first premolar (bicuspid)
13	Maxillary left second premolar (bicuspid)
14	Maxillary left first molar
15	Maxillary left second molar
16	Maxillary left third molar
LOWER TEETH	
17	Mandibular left third molar
18	Mandibular left second molar
19	Mandibular left first molar
20	Mandibular left second premolar (bicuspid)
21	Mandibular left first premolar (bicuspid)
22	Mandibular left canine (cuspid)
23	Mandibular left lateral incisor
24	Mandibular left central incisor
25	Mandibular right central incisor
26	Mandibular right lateral incisor
27	Mandibular right canine (cuspid)
28	Mandibular right first premolar (bicuspid)
29	Mandibular right second premolar (bicuspid)
30	Mandibular right first molar
31	Mandibular right second molar
32	Mandibular right third molar

Figure 1-1 **A,** American Dental Association sequential numbering system for permanent teeth. **B,** American Dental Association sequential lettering system for primary teeth.

primary maxillary right second molar. The lettering progresses just as in the numbering system described for permanent teeth. The use of letters instead of numbers to designate *primary* teeth prevents confusion with permanent teeth.

Zsigmondy-Palmer System

The Zsigmondy-Palmer system identifies specific teeth by using a grid system (Figure 1-2) and assigning a number (1 to 8 for a permanent tooth [Figure 1-3, *A*]) or a letter (A to E for a primary tooth [Figure l-3, *B*]) to teeth in each of the four quadrants of the mouth.

Zsigmondy-Palmer system for permanent teeth

In the permanent dentition the number 8 represents third molars and the number 1 represents central incisors. A grid system is used to identify specific teeth.

The quadrant symbols are as follows:

Symbol	Quadrant
⌐	Maxillary right
⌐	Maxillary left
⌐	Mandibular left
⌐	Mandibular right

The grid represents the patient's mouth as the operator or assistant views it. The symbol 8⌐ is used to designate the maxillary right third molar. The bracket around the number indicates the quadrant in which the tooth is located. In this example the number 8 is placed above the horizontal line, which indicates that it is a maxillary tooth. Since the number 8 is located to the left of the vertical line as it is viewed, the tooth is located in the patient's right quadrant. Hence this tooth is the maxillary right third molar.

Zsigmondy-Palmer system for primary teeth

The primary teeth can be identified by using this same basic system. The teeth in each quadrant are labeled with letters A through E. The primary second molars are assigned the letter E, and the central incisors are assigned the letter

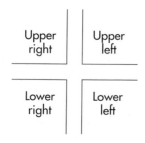

Figure 1-2   Zsigmondy-Palmer grid system.

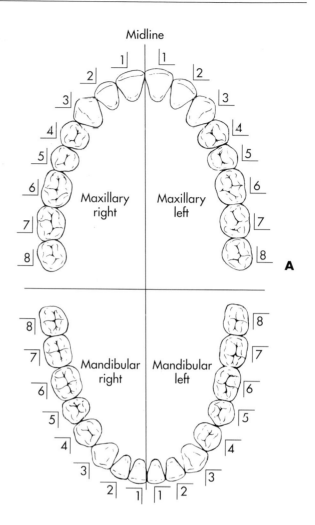

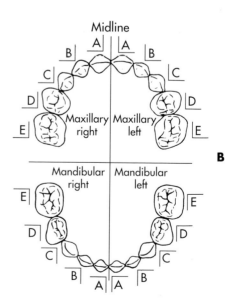

Figure 1-3   A, Zsigmondy-Palmer numbering system for permanent dentition. **B,** Zsigmondy-Palmer lettering system for primary dentition.

A. For example, the symbol C̲ would represent the primary maxillary right cuspid in the primary dentition.

This system is frequently used by orthodontists because the entire dentition can be displayed on one grid, regardless of whether the patient has a primary, mixed, or permanent dentition. The example shown in Figure 1-4 is a mixed dentition. The patient has most of the primary teeth, as indicated by letters in all quadrants, but the numbers in each quadrant indicate that some permanent teeth have erupted. Specifically, the number 6 in each bracket indicates that all four first permanent molars are present. The number 1 in each bracket of the lower arch indicates that both permanent mandibular central incisors have also erupted and have replaced the primary central incisors.

Federation Dentaire Internationale System

The Federation Dentaire Internationale (FDI) system was designed to facilitate computer storage of records, which is often used in research, as well as in some dental offices.

Federation Dentaire Internationale system for permanent teeth

The numbering system for permanent teeth uses a two-digit number to identify each tooth (Figure 1-5).

- The first digit indicates the quadrant in which the tooth is located. The quadrants are labeled 1 to 4 as follows:

Quadrant number	Quadrant identification
1	Maxillary right
2	Maxillary left
3	Mandibular left
4	Mandibular right

- The second digit identifies the specific tooth in that quadrant. The teeth are assigned numbers 1 through 8 in each quadrant. Number 1 is the central incisor, and number 8 is the third molar.

The following are random examples of the FDI tooth numbering system for the *permanent* dentition:

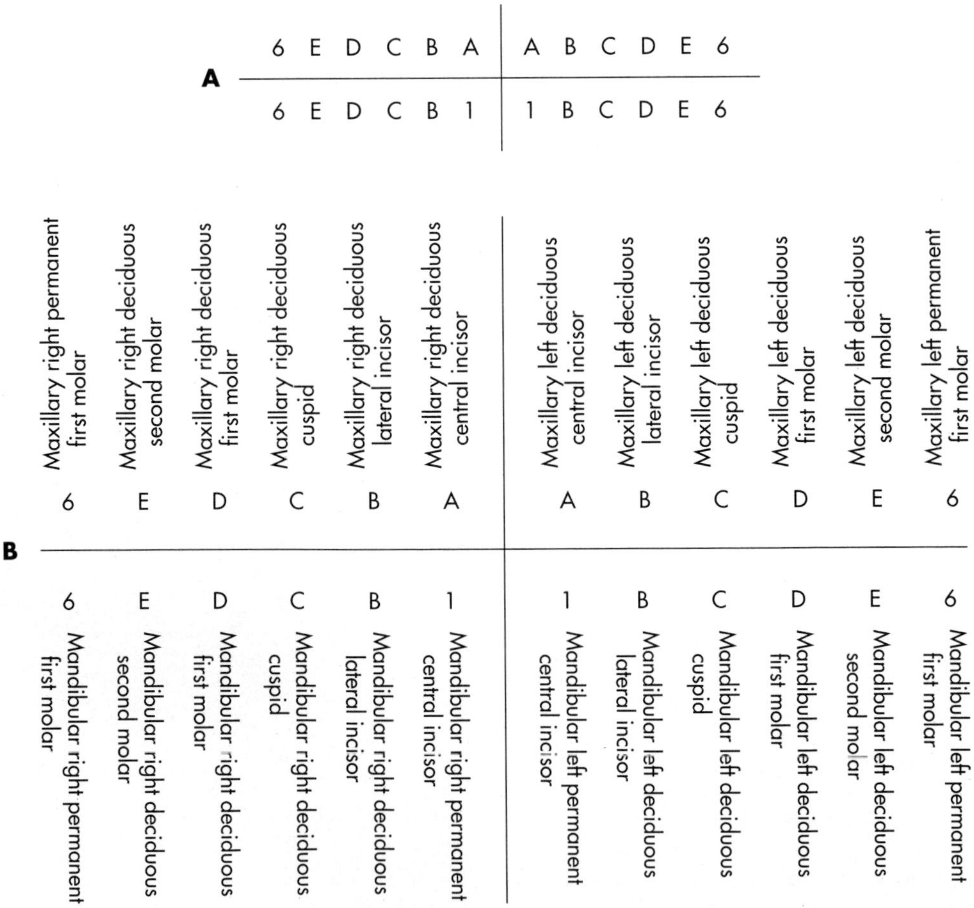

Figure 1-4 **A,** Schematic display of mixed dentition using Zsigmondy-Palmer tooth identification system. **B,** Key to display shown in **A.**

FDI number	Tooth name
15*	Maxillary right second premolar
22	Maxillary left lateral incisor
36	Mandibular left first molar
44	Mandibular right first premolar

*Pronounce digits only. For example, say "one-five," not "fifteen."

FDI system for primary teeth

The primary dentition is numbered in a similar fashion (Figure 1-6).

- The quadrants in the primary dentition are numbered as follows:

Quadrant number	Quadrant identification
5	Maxillary right
6	Maxillary left
7	Mandibular left
8	Mandibular right

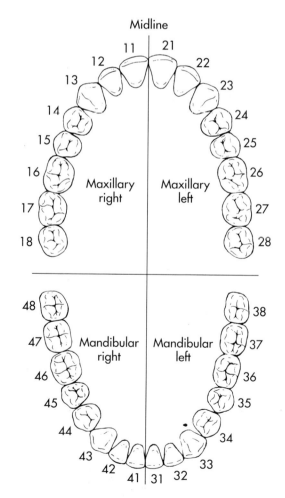

- Teeth are numbered 1 through 5 in each quadrant. Number 1 is the central incisor, and number 5 is the second molar.

The following list shows random examples of the FDI tooth numbering system for the primary dentition:

FDI number	Tooth name
54	Maxillary right first primary molar
63	Maxillary left primary cuspid
75	Mandibular left second primary molar
84	Mandibular right first primary molar

The choice of which tooth numbering system is used in a dental practice is left entirely to the dentist.

TOOTH SURFACE ANNOTATION
Tooth Surface Names

Each surface of a tooth crown is identified by a specific name, such as **buccal, distal, facial, incisal, labial, lingual, mesial, occlusal,** and **palatal.** Figure 1-7 demonstrates the various surfaces. These surface names and their abbreviations are summarized at the end of this discussion.

Tooth surface names are used in clinical dentistry to describe the location of caries, defects, or restorations in a patient's teeth. It is imperative that the dental assistant learn these surface names and where to apply them.

Tooth Surface Designations

Tooth surface numbering and lettering systems have been used for years to simplify recording of clinical information. In these systems each tooth surface is assigned a

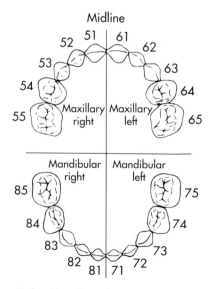

Figure 1-5 Federation Dentaire Internationale numbering system for permanent dentition.

Figure 1-6 Federation Dentaire Internationale numbering system for primary dentition.

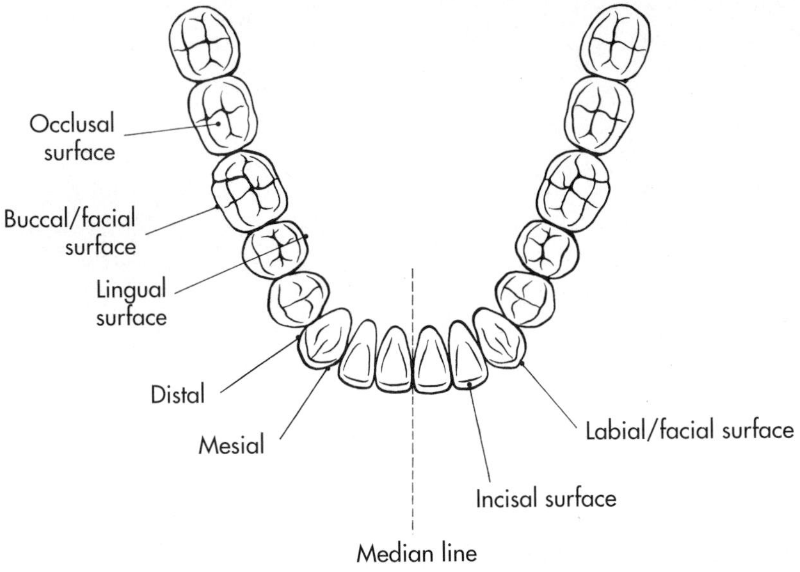

Figure 1-7 Surfaces of anterior and posterior teeth.

number or a letter so that surface names do not need to be written out on clinical records. When combined with tooth numbering systems, tooth surface designation systems create a shorthand method for recording clinical information.

The most common methods of designating tooth surfaces are as follows:

Tooth surface	Surface abbreviation
Mesial	M
Distal	D
Facial (Buccal, Labial)	F (B = Buccal, Lab = Labial)
Lingual (Palatal)	L (P = Palatal)
Occlusal (Incisal)	O (I = Incisal)

BIBLIOGRAPHY

Finkbeiner BL, Johnson CS: *Mosby's comprehensive dental assisting: a clinical approach,* St Louis, 1995, Mosby.
Brand RW, Isselhard DE: *Anatomy of orofacial structures,* St Louis, 1994, Mosby.

QUESTIONS–Chapter 1

1. The biting surface of anterior teeth is called the _____ surface.
   a. Mesial
   b. Distal
   c. Incisal
   d. Lingual
   e. Occlusal

2. The surface of the teeth closest to the tongue is called the _____ surface.
   a. Mesial
   b. Distal
   c. Incisal
   d. Lingual
   e. Occlusal

3. The surface of the tooth closest to the midline is called the _____ surface.
   a. Mesial
   b. Distal
   c. Incisal
   d. Lingual
   e. Occlusal

- Use the American Dental Association tooth numbering system to identify the teeth in questions 4 through 9.

4. Tooth #14
   a. First molar
   b. Second molar
   c. Maxillary left first molar
   d. Maxillary left permanent first molar
   e. Maxillary left permanent second molar

5. Tooth #8
   a. Third molar
   b. Central incisor
   c. Maxillary right permanent third molar
   d. Maxillary left permanent central incisor
   e. Maxillary right permanent central incisor

6. Tooth #21
   a. Mandibular left deciduous first molar
   b. Maxillary right permanent second molar
   c. Mandibular left permanent first premolar
   d. Maxillary left permanent central incisor
   e. Maxillary right deciduous lateral incisor

7. Tooth M
   a. Mandibular left deciduous cuspid
   b. Mandibular right deciduous third molar
   c. Mandibular left permanent second molar
   d. Mandibular right deciduous first premolar
   e. Mandibular left permanent central incisor

8. Maxillary right permanent cuspid
   a. 3
   b. 6
   c C
   d. 11
   e. 22

9. Mandibular right deciduous first molar
   a. S
   b. 31
   c. C
   d. 4
   e. M

- Use the Zsigmondy-Palmer tooth identification system to identify the teeth in questions 10 through 15.

10. Tooth 5⌐
    a. First premolar
    b. Second premolar
    c. Maxillary right second premolar
    d. Maxillary left first premolar
    e. Maxillary left permanent second premolar

11. Tooth B̄⌐
    a. Maxillary right second molar
    b. Mandibular left lateral incisor
    c. Mandibular left permanent second molar
    d. Maxillary right deciduous lateral incisor
    e. Mandibular right deciduous lateral incisor

12. Tooth ⌐7
    a. Maxillary left permanent second molar
    b. Mandibular right permanent first molar
    c. Mandibular left deciduous lateral incisor
    d. Maxillary left permanent lateral incisor
    e. Mandibular right deciduous central incisor

13. Maxillary right deciduous cuspid
    a. 2⌐
    b. D̄⌐
    c. 3̄⌐
    d. C̲⌐
    e. ⌐3̲

14. Mandibular right permanent central incisor
    a. 1̄⌐
    b. ⌐5̲
    c. 24
    d. 25
    e. 41

15 Maxillary left deciduous second molar
    a. 5̄⌐
    b. ⌐7̲
    c. ⌐E̲
    d. J
    e. D̲⌐

- Use the Federation Dentaire Internationale tooth numbering system to identify the teeth in questions 16 through 20.

16. Tooth #11
    a. Maxillary left permanent cuspid
    b. Maxillary right deciduous first molar
    c. Mandibular left deciduous second molar
    d. Maxillary right permanent second molar
    e. Maxillary right permanent central incisor

17. Tooth #32
    a. Mandibular right permanent third molar
    b. Mandibular left permanent second molar
    c. Mandibular right permanent second molar
    d. Mandibular left permanent lateral incisor
    e. Mandibular right permanent lateral incisor

18. Tooth #65
    a. Maxillary left deciduous second molar
    b. Maxillary left permanent second molar
    c. Maxillary left deciduous lateral incisor
    d. Mandibular right deciduous second premolar
    e. Mandibular right deciduous first premolar

19. Maxillary left permanent second molar
    a. 13
    b. 17
    c. 25
    d. 27
    e. 37

20. Mandibular right deciduous first molar
    a. 30
    b. 36
    c. 46
    d. 74
    e. 84

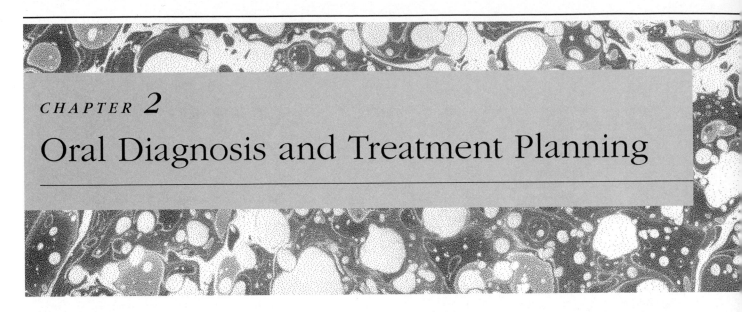

CHAPTER *2*

Oral Diagnosis and Treatment Planning

KEY TERMS

Biopsy
Diagnosis
Exfoliative cytology
Extraoral radiographs
Intraoral radiographs
Occlusion
Palpation
Percussion
Sign
Study models
Symptom
Treatment plan

The concept of all health treatment is to identify and eliminate disease. Identification of a disease is called **diagnosis.** This chapter deals with diagnosis of oral disease and systemic conditions that relate to it.

DIAGNOSTIC TOOLS
Medical–Dental History

The accuracy of diagnoses greatly depends on dentists' knowledge of anatomy and physiology and their understanding of oral and systemic disease. To diagnose a disease, dentists must know how body parts look and function normally. Identification of the "normal condition" of a patient must be determined before any abnormality is defined. Another important aspect of diagnosis is the collection and analysis of data concerning both the patient's general health and dental health. This information is obtained by an assortment of data-collecting techniques and

devices referred to as diagnostic tools. The dental assistant plays an active role in the collection and recording of the diagnostic information used in arriving at a diagnosis and formulating a plan of treatment.

> ✦ **KEY POINT**
> - The dental assistant can update the medical history at the beginning of each dental appointment by asking the patient about any changes since the last visit.

Figure 2-1 shows an example of a medical-dental history form.

Clinical Examination

Clinical examination of a patient calls for dentists to use their physical senses to aid in the diagnosis of oral disease. Sight, sound, and touch are all used during a clinical examination.

A visual inspection of the patient's hard and soft tissues can reveal changes in color, shape, and size of oral structures. Abnormal functioning can be detected by watching the patient's face, eyes, and mouth during conversation. Unusual movements of the facial muscles, tongue, and eyes are often signs of neuromuscular disease. Observing a patient's reaction to various diagnostic tests is helpful in arriving at an accurate diagnosis.

Unusual sounds are also beneficial in diagnostic procedures. Clicking of the patient's temporomandibular joint may indicate joint disease. Abnormal speech patterns may prompt the examiner to investigate possible oral causes of the abnormality, such as abnormal positioning of the teeth. Tapping on teeth with the handle of a mirror to determine tenderness is called **percussion.**

Palpation is the use of the examiner's sense of touch to reveal abnormalities. The tissues of the body all have a certain texture under normal circumstances. Often one of the first signs of disease is a change in texture of a tissue. It may be more or less firm, larger or smaller, or tender to the touch.

The medical-dental history, the clinical examination, and other diagnostic tools yet to be discussed reveal signs and symptoms of disease. Generally these two terms are used together to describe the characteristics of a disease. A **sign** is a characteristic that is observable by either the patient or the examiner. Examples of clinical signs are swelling; ulcerations; fever; and changes in the color, texture, or position of structures. A **symptom** is a characteristic of a disease that the patient feels and relates to the examiner. Examples of symptoms include pain, dizziness, nausea, bad taste, and difficulty in chewing and swallowing.

> **➥ KEY POINT**
> - The operator uses his or her fingers to examine the soft tissues of the head and oral cavity. This technique is called palpation.

Clinical examination of a patient should include a visual examination and palpation of three general areas:
1. *Extraoral structures.* The general shape of the face and head, skin texture and color, eye size, the color of the sclera (white of the eye), the temporomandibular joint, the lymph nodes surrounding the head and neck region, and the shape of the jaws should be examined.
2. *Intraoral soft tissues.* The entire oral mucosa and submucosal structures (e.g., glands, lymph nodes, and muscles) need to be examined.
3. *Intraoral hard tissues.* The intraoral portion of the jaw bones and the teeth should be examined for abnormalities.

The dental assistant records the clinical findings as they are dictated by the dentist. In some states the extraoral and intraoral examination can be delegated to the dental assistant. The armamentarium for a clinical dental examination is shown in Figure 2-2.

Dental Radiographs

Radiographs, or x-ray films, of teeth and bone are perhaps the most valuable diagnostic tool that dentists have to evaluate structures that cannot be seen by clinical observation. The information revealed by radiographs, when used with the patient history and clinical findings, constitutes a major source of diagnostic information.

The value of a radiograph depends on the quality of the picture itself and the ability of the dentist to interpret it.

Dentists today use dental auxiliaries to take radiographs. This is a great responsibility to be delegated to assistants and hygienists. Without a good-quality radiographic survey of the patient, the dentist's ability to interpret diagnostic findings is greatly limited. An auxiliary who can provide this service is an asset to a dental practice.

Two classes of radiographs are used in oral diagnostic procedures: intraoral and extraoral views. **Intraoral radiographs** are taken with the film placed in the patient's mouth. **Extraoral radiographs** are taken with the film held outside the mouth. Examples of the intraoral view by periapical and bitewing radiographs are shown in Figure 2-3, *A* and *B*.

The radiograph shown in Figure 2-3, *C*, is an example of the extraoral view called a panoramic radiograph.

> **➥ KEY POINT**
> - Intraoral radiographs are taken with the film placed inside the patient's mouth.

Intraoral radiographs are used more than extraoral radiographs. The extraoral radiograph is generally considered to be a supplemental film that is taken in special cases. A typical complete radiographic survey of a patient may include a series of 14 to 16 periapical and four bitewing radiographs. A complete radiographic survey is called a *full mouth series* and may be abbreviated as "FMX" or "FMS." Periapical views reveal discrepancies in both the crown and root portions of teeth and the surrounding supporting tissues. Bitewing views provide information primarily in the area of the crowns of teeth and the level of the surrounding bone.

> **➥ KEY POINT**
> - A periapical radiograph shows the entire tooth, including the apex.

The American Dental Association (ADA) has recommended that radiographs be taken only as deemed necessary by the dentist. Therefore there is not a set schedule for when to take a radiographic series. However, a full mouth series is usually taken every 3 to 5 years. A bitewing set of films can be taken as often as every year.

> **➥ KEY POINT**
> - A full mouth radiographic series usually consists of 14 periapical films and 4 bitewing films.

Table 2-1 demonstrates some common radiographic findings on the various views.

MEDICAL HISTORY INTERVIEW

ADA®

Date _____

Part I *(to be completed by patient or guardian)*

Name _____ Home Phone (_____) _____

Address_____ Business Phone (_____) _____

City _____ State _____ Zip Code _____

Occupation_____ Social Security No. _____

Date of Birth _____ Sex   M   F   Height _____ Weight _____ Single ____ Married ____

Name of Spouse_____ Closest Relative_____ Phone (_____) _____

If the person completing this form is other than the patient, what is his/her relationship to the patient? _____

Referred by_____

Part II *(to be completed by dentist)*

A. CHIEF COMPLAINT

_____

B. DENTAL HISTORY

Frequency of visits to dentist_____

Type of care received _____

Difficulties with past treatment _____

Adverse reactions to local anesthetics, latex gloves, rubber dam_____

Date of most recent dental radiographic exam _____

C. MEDICAL HISTORY

Are you now or have you been under the care of a physician during the past 12 months? _____

Last time at physician _____ For what purpose? _____

Physician _____ Physician's Phone No. _____

Do you have any known allergies or sensitivities?_____

Do you take any medications at the present time?_____

Females only: Do you take oral contraceptives? _____ Are you pregnant?_____

Have you noted a change in your menstrual pattern?_____

D. FAMILY HISTORY

(Have any members of your family ever been treated for the conditions listed or any other medical problems?)

Diabetes _____ High blood pressure _____ Heart problem _____ Seizures _____

Other_____

E. SOCIAL HISTORY

Smoking _____ Alcohol _____ Other _____

S-502

Figure 2-1   Sample medical–dental history form.
(Courtesy American Dental Association, Chicago.)

F. REVIEW OF SYSTEMS (Have you ever had or do you now have any of the conditions listed?)

I. Skin

Itching _____

Rash _____

Ulcers _____

Pigmentations _____

Lack or loss of body hair _____

II. Extremities

Varicose veins _____

Swollen, painful joints _____

Muscle weakness, pain _____

Bone deformity, fracture _____

Prosthetic joints _____

III. Eyes

Blurring of vision _____

Double vision _____

Drooping of eyelid _____

Glaucoma _____

IV. Ear, Nose, Throat

Earache _____

Hearing loss _____

Frequent nosebleeds _____

Sinusitis _____

Frequent sore throat _____

Hoarseness _____

V. Respiratory

Cough, blood in sputum _____

Emphysema, bronchitis _____

Wheezing, asthma _____

Tuberculosis, exposure to _____

VI. Cardiac

Shortness of breath _____

Pain, pressure in chest _____

Swelling of ankles _____

High, low blood pressure _____

Rheumatic, scarlet fever _____

Heart murmur, attack _____

Prosthetic valves/pacemakers _____

VII. Gastrointestinal

Difficulty swallowing _____

Abdominal pain, ulcers _____

Hepatitis, jaundice _____

Liver disease _____

VIII. Genitourinary

Difficulty, pain on urination _____

Blood in urine _____

Excessive urination _____

Kidney infections _____

Sexually transmitted diseases _____

IX. Endocrine

Thyroid trouble _____

Weight change _____

Diabetes _____

Excessive thirst _____

X. Hematopoietic

Easy bruising, excessive bleeding _____

Persistent lymphadenopathy _____

G6PD deficiency _____

Anemia _____

HIV infection, AIDS _____

Leukemia, problems with immune system _____

Spleen problems _____

XI. Neurologic

Frequent headaches _____

Dizziness, fainting _____

Epilepsy, fits _____

Neuritis, neuralgia _____

Paresthesias, numbness _____

Paralysis _____

XII. Psychiatric

Nervousness _____

Irritability _____

Depression, excessive worry _____

Nervous breakdown _____

XIII. Growth or Tumor

Radiotherapy/chemotherapy _____

I certify that any and all questions I had about the inquiries above have been answered to my satisfaction. I was asked all of the questions on this form and I have answered these questions truthfully and completely. I will not hold my dentist, or any other member of his/her staff, responsible for any errors or omissions that I may have made.

_____   _____
date   signature of patient

_____   _____
date   signature of guardian (where applicable)

Comments on patient interview concerning medical history: _____

Significant findings from questionnaire or oral interview: _____

Dental management considerations: _____

_____

_____   _____
(date)   (signature of dentist)

Medical History Update:

Date	Comments	Signature
_____	_____	_____
_____	_____	_____
_____	_____	_____

© 1992 AMERICAN DENTAL ASSOCIATION

Figure 2-1, cont'd   For legend, see opposite page.

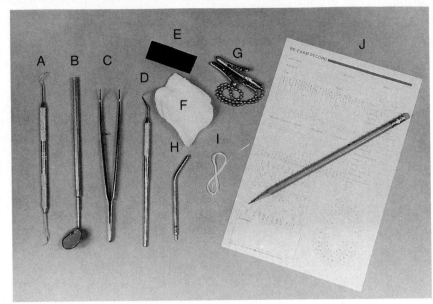

Figure 2-2 Armamentarium for clinical dental examination. *A,* Explorer; *B,* mirror; *C,* cotton pliers; *D,* periodontal probe; *E,* articulating paper; *F,* 2 × 2 gauze; *G,* napkin chain; *H,* air/water syringe tip; *I,* dental floss; *J,* chart and pencil. Optional: articulating paper holder.

(From Finkbeiner BL, Johnson CS: *Mosby's comprehensive dental assisting: a clinical approach,* St Louis, 1995, Mosby.)

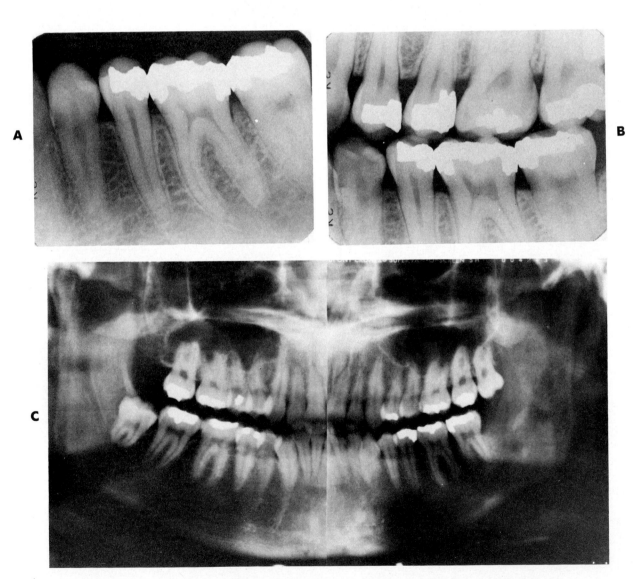

Figure 2-3 Radiographs commonly used for oral region. **A,** Periapical view. **B,** Posterior bitewing view. **C,** Panoramic radiograph (Panorex), approximately one third of normal size.

Table 2-1 Common radiographic findings

Type of radiograph	Findings
Posterior bitewing	Interproximal caries
	Restorative contour
	Integrity of cervical margins of restoration
	Pulp size and relationship to caries and restorations
	Height of alveolar crest
	Location of calculus
Periapical	Pathological changes in periapical area
	Integrity of supporting bone
	Root size and shape
	Integrity of periodontal space and lamina dura
Panorex	Entire dentition in view on one film
	Pathology in bone and the temporomandibular joint
	Development of dentition (children)
	Position of impacted teeth
	Jaw fractures
	Location of foreign bodies

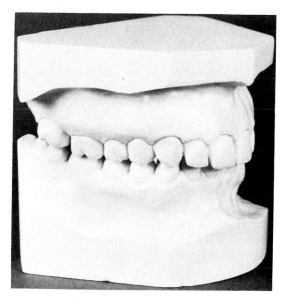

Figure 2-4　Study model.

Several excellent texts on dental radiography are available for dental auxiliaries who want to review this subject in detail.

Proper processing of x-ray films in a darkroom provides a permanent radiographic record of the patient's condition. This record is important as a future reference to determine the progress of disease or healing. Radiographs are also valuable in medicolegal suits that may be brought against the dentist. They can also assist in identifying victims of accidents or crime in which facial features are destroyed or decomposed.

Pulp Tests

The health status of a tooth's pulp can be determined by a battery of tests. These tests are discussed in detail in Chapter 22.

Plaque Disclosure

The application of a disclosing agent on the patient's teeth reveals the status of the patient's oral hygiene (see Chapter 10). The presence of dental plaque can explain oral conditions that may be damaging to the patient.

Study Models

Study models, or "casts," are plaster reproductions of the patient's teeth and surrounding tissues (Figure 2-4). They are obtained by an impression-taking procedure, described in Chapter 24, in which an alginate impression material is used. Study models give the dentist a perma-

nent, three-dimensional record of the patient's teeth and jaws. They provide information on the position, size, and shape of teeth. The size, shape, and contour of the surrounding soft tissues and jaws are also recorded on the study model.

Study models give dentists a unique opportunity to study **occlusion,** or biting relationship, in detail. They afford views of the teeth and jaws from angles that are not possible by only looking into the patient's mouth.

In addition to their diagnostic value, study models are beneficial in planning treatment for the patient. After treatment has been completed, a new set of models can be made to demonstrate the improvements obtained through treatment. Orthodontists use this before-and-after idea during and after treatment, to demonstrate the improvements in appearance and function of the teeth.

Photographs

Dentistry uses the time-honored photograph more and more in everyday practice. Color prints and slides are excellent ways to record the progress of treatment of many oral conditions. The before-and-after effect also can be accomplished with photographs.

Photographs enable dentists to consult with specialists, arrive at diagnoses, and plan treatment. The old adage that "a picture is worth a thousand words" applies in dentistry.

Manufacturers of photographic equipment have developed many easy-to-use cameras and computerized video equipment for intraoral photography. Assistants should not be surprised to find that photographing patients is a part of their daily tasks. All dental photographs should become a part of the patient's permanent record.

Bacterial Analysis

The identification of organisms that may be present in the oral cavity helps the dentist arrive at an accurate diagnosis and treatment plan. Bacterial studies are done by collecting samples of material from suspect areas in the oral cavity and placing them in sterile containers. The samples can be incubated and studied to determine what type of organism may be present and in what quantity. Three common uses of bacterial studies in dentistry are in caries prevention, periodontal disease, and treatment of infections.

Patients who have oral infections that persist after antibiotics have been administered are candidates for a bacterial analysis of the infection. The bacterial analysis reveals the organism that is the offender, and a specific drug can then be selected to eliminate it.

Vigorous caries-control measures have been developed (see Chapter 9) based on the elimination of certain *Streptococcus* and *Lactobacillus* organisms from the oral cavity. Saliva samples are taken and analyzed to determine the presence and quantity of these organisms in the saliva. If the quantity is great, a vigorous diet-control plan may be indicated.

Biopsy

Biopsy is the surgical removal of a piece of tissue from the body for examination under the microscope to help establish an accurate diagnosis. The tissue sample usually consists of both diseased and normal adjacent tissue for comparison. Common biopsy techniques are discussed in Chapter 25.

Exfoliative Cytology

Cytology is the study of cells. Exfoliation means the process of shedding—in this instance, shedding of tissue cells.

Through **exfoliative cytology** some suspected soft tissue diseases such as oral cancer can be detected by scraping the surface of the lesion with a tongue blade and examining the scrapings under a microscope for abnormal tissue cells to confirm the diagnosis.

Medical Tests and Consultations

On occasion certain medical information must be obtained through the patient's physician. Such a request is made in written form so that it can become a part of the patient's record for future reference and medicolegal reasons. An example of a form used for this purpose is shown in Figure 3-5.

Other medical information can be obtained through medical tests. These tests are used to establish a diagnosis and subsequent modifications in the treatment plan if necessary. Such tests include the following:
1. Blood pressure determination

2. Blood tests for the presence of infectious disease, bleeding time, and clotting time when indicated
3. Heart rate determination

TREATMENT PLANNING

After all the diagnostic information has been obtained and analyzed, dentists will make a diagnosis, or perhaps they will make more than one diagnosis because patients often have more than one condition at a time. It is not uncommon to see caries, periodontal disease, and a variety of other oral discrepancies at the same time in one patient.

The dentist then assembles all information available regarding the diagnosis and formulates a plan of treatment. A **treatment plan** is a carefully sequenced series of services designed to eliminate or control causative factors, repair existing damage, and create a functional and maintainable environment.* Treatment plans can vary from a single restoration to multiple treatment regimens.

Probably one of the most challenging tasks for the dentist is planning the appropriate treatment for a patient. Since treatment plans vary from simple to complex, the dentist must call on a variety of resources to formulate an acceptable treatment regimen. This stage may include consulting with dental specialists to explore all possible alternatives.

Although there is no standard format for a treatment plan, it should establish the following:
1. The proposed treatment
2. The sequence in which treatment will be done
3. A fee estimate for the service rendered
4. A consent statement giving the dentist permission to perform the procedures

A treatment plan benefits the dental staff and the patient in appointment scheduling. Since patients will know the aftereffects of treatment, they can schedule their appointments in advance around vacations, work schedules, and other personal activities. Advance scheduling helps the dental staff plan for needed dental laboratory services and treatment room preparation on the day of the appointment. A copy of the treatment plan should be given to patients to assist them in planning appointments and to prevent any misunderstanding regarding planned treatment and fees.

Factors Influencing Treatment Planning

The format of a treatment plan is influenced by several factors. These factors may alter the entire treatment plan or a portion of it, or they may simply change the sequence of treatment. Following are some of the common factors to be considered:

---

*Sturdevant CM and others: *The art and science of operative dentistry*, ed 3, St Louis, 1995, Mosby.

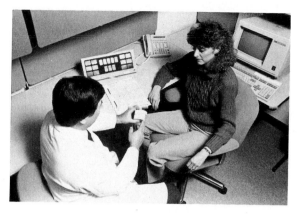

Figure 2-5 Case presentation: diagnosis, treatment, fees, and number of appointments needed are discussed with patient.

1. *Patient attitude.* The patient must have an interest in receiving care. This attitude may be influenced by the patient's personal background, oral hygiene, priorities, and fears.
2. *Economics.* The question of cost is a major factor in patients' acceptance of a proposed treatment plan. Fees are far more acceptable to patients when well-organized treatment plans are presented in an understandable way. Patients can then appreciate the time and effort that will be devoted to their well-being. This approach is called case presentation (Figure 2-5).
3. *Presence of systemic disease.* The influence of systemic disease may cause a delay of treatment or a modification of treatment; it may even make some aspects of treatment impossible because of the systemic risks involved. Terminal illnesses certainly influence the dentist's thoughts on choosing a reasonable plan.
4. *Chief complaint.* The reason the patient seeks treatment in the first place must be considered strongly in the sequence of treatment. A patient with a throbbing abscess on a lower molar is not interested in having a teeth cleaning or other treatment performed until the pain in the offending tooth is treated.
5. *Age of the patient.* Age often has a strong influence on treatment planning. A child who has a loose primary tooth with decay would be better served by extraction than by restoration, since the tooth is about to be shed anyway. An elderly patient near death poses the question of whether extensive treatment will be useful to the individual.

These factors may be present individually or in various combinations. It is not unusual for the dentist to create alternate treatment plans based on the factors just discussed. Because of unforeseen circumstances, modification of a selected treatment plan may need to be made as treatment progresses.

Format of the Treatment Plan

Before the start of dental therapy, the dentist will evaluate the patient for indications of systemic treatment such as the following:

1. Referral to a physician for systemic evaluation and treatment as indicated by the history and clinical findings.
2. Appraisal of the influence of systemic treatment on the dental treatment plan
3. Premedication with antibiotics or sedatives as indicated by the history
4. Corrective therapy for oral infection

Sturdevant and associates suggest a general outline for treatment planning that is widely used in general practice:

1. Control phase
   a. Elimination of pain (e.g., endodontics and/or extractions)
   b. Elimination of active periodontal disease, caries, or other causes of inflammation (e.g., periodontal therapy and caries removal)
   c. Removal of conditions preventing maintenance (e.g., overhang removal)
   d. Elimination of causes of disease (e.g., nutritional counseling)
   e. Initiation of preventive measures (e.g., oral hygiene instructions)
2. Holding phase
   a. Healing period from control-phase procedures
3. Definitive phase
   a. Endodontics
   b. Periodontics
   c. Orthodontics
   d. Oral surgery
   e. Operative procedures (The patient receives fixed or removable prosthodontic treatment after steps a through e are completed.)
4. Maintenance phase
   a. Regular periodontal recall
   b. Regular recall examinations
   c. Reinforcement of home care

Essentially what the format suggests is that the general well-being of patients be considered above all else. The next priority is to establish a proper foundation for restoring the mouth by eliminating pain, diseased tissue, progressive disease, and malocclusion. After the foundation is sound, restoration of the mouth with various dental restorations and prosthetic appliances can begin. After the corrective phase of treatment, patients must maintain their healthy state by proper home care procedures and routine recall examinations.

BIBLIOGRAPHY

Sturdevant CM and others: *The art and science of operative dentistry,* ed 3, St Louis, 1995, Mosby.

QUESTIONS–Chapter 2

1. All the following instruments are part of a preset examination tray *except:*
   a. Explorer
   b. Hatchet
   c. Cotton pliers
   d. Periodontal probe

2. Which of the following is the definition of percussion?
   a. Tapping on the teeth with a mirror handle
   b. Applying a disclosing agent on the patient's teeth
   c. Plaster reproduction of a patient's teeth
   d. Surgical removal of a piece of tissue from the body for examination under the microscope

3. Identification of a disease is called a:
   a. Prognosis
   b. Biopsy
   c. Treatment plan
   d. Diagnosis

4. Which of the following are not considered diagnostic tools for the treatment plan?
   a. Study models
   b. Periodontal probing
   c. Pit and fissure sealants
   d. Radiographs

5. The medical-dental history is an important diagnostic tool for all the following reasons *except:*
   a. To determine if a patient has dental insurance
   b. To provide important oral health information
   c. To provide important information about general health
   d. As a valuable legal document

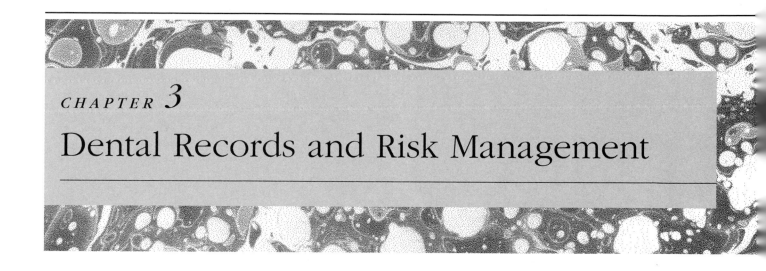

CHAPTER *3*

Dental Records and Risk Management

KEY TERMS

Incident report
Informed consent
Malpractice
Medical consultation (consult) form
Medical-dental history form
Risk management
Statute of limitations

DENTAL RECORD

Record keeping is an essential part of dental practice. A dental record is the entire collection of information obtained from a patient. In essence a dental record is a library on a patient to which the dentist and staff members refer repeatedly. Records must be complete and in order for easy reference. It is wise to preserve dental records for medicolegal reasons and to assist law enforcement agencies during forensic procedures.

Uses of the Dental Record

The dental record has the following uses:
1. Recording diagnostic findings, as described in Chapter 2
2. Documenting treatment rendered to the patient
3. Retrieving information for research purposes
4. Presenting evidence in legal proceedings
5. Justifying dental insurance claims
6. Validating tax claims during Internal Revenue Service audits
7. Identifying patients for law enforcement agencies

Contents of the Dental Record

Dental records vary in format from one office to another, yet they all contain the same elements. The specific design of the dental record is determined by each dentist, and the dental record is stored in a large envelope or folder. The elements of a typical dental record include the following:
1. Patient file envelope
2. General patient information
3. Medical-dental history
4. Medical consultation (consult) forms or letters
5. Medical laboratory test results
6. Dental specialist consultation forms or referral letters
7. Dental charts
8. Treatment plans
9. Informed consents
10. Laboratory requisitions
11. Radiographs
12. Photographs

NOTE: Financial records (accounts receivable) are not part of a patient's dental chart and are kept in a separate file.

Patient File Envelope

A dental office may choose to use either a plain envelope or a color-coded envelope. Color-coded envelopes can be used to arrange the files in alphabetical order. Group practices may use a specific colored envelope for each dentist in the practice. Envelopes can usually be labeled with the patient's name for filing purposes (Figure 3-1).

File envelopes of patients who do not return to the practice after several years should be removed and placed in storage. Small stickers are available to place on the file to indicate the year that the patient last visited the prac-

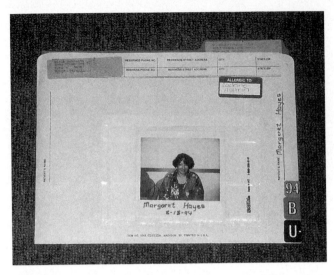

Figure 3-1 Patient file envelope with medical-alert sticker.

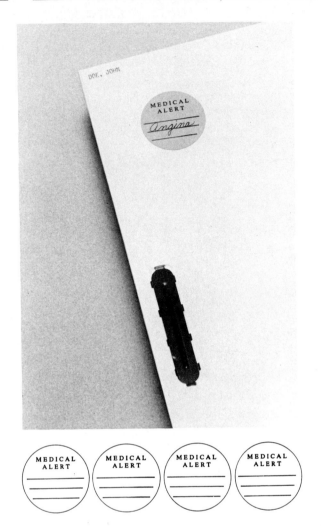

Figure 3-2 **A,** Medical-alert sticker placed on outside of dental record folder. **B,** Supply of medical-alert stickers (normally bright orange).

(Courtesy Prosystems, Brentwood, NY. Designed by Burton Pollack, DDS, JD.)

tice for ease in sorting. Medical-alert stickers can also be placed on the outside of the file to indicate conditions such as allergies, prosthetic implants, or a need for prophylactic premedication (Figure 3-2). All medical alerts should also be noted in the appointment book as a reminder to take appropriate precautions before treatment.

General Patient Information

Every business that has an appointment and billing system requires certain information about its customers to run efficiently. Dental offices are no exception. The dental staff must be able to contact patients by telephone and by mail. Dental insurance preauthorization and claim forms need to be filled out correctly, and other business procedures that require personal information about the patient must be performed. Occasionally a patient may feel faint or collapse during a dental appointment. In the event of an actual collapse an emergency contact person must be notified. The general patient information section of the dental record should contain such vital information. It must be complete and current so that business procedures can be conducted efficiently.

Some offices obtain this information in a registration form (Figure 3-3) and then type it onto a dental chart (such as the one shown in Figure 3-4, *B*). Other offices simply use the application in the patient's own handwriting as a reference. Sometimes the patient information section is combined with the medical-dental history form. Medical precautions (alerts) should be written in red ink on the dental chart to attract attention.

Medical-Dental History

The rationale for taking a medical-dental history is discussed in Chapter 2. Since this record also serves as a le-

gal document if medical complications should occur during or after dental treatment, the health questionnaire must be signed and dated by the patient or the patient's guardian to make it valid. This document should be updated at each dental visit for any medical or dental changes that the patient may have had since the last time the patient visited the dental office. Changes in the patient's health status can be documented in one of several areas, depending on the preference of the dental office:

- On the original **medical-dental history form** (see Figure 2-1)
- In the treatment progress notes (see Figure 3-4, *B)*
- On a one-page update form (Figure 3-5)

Regardless of where the update occurs in the chart, the patient should sign the update after it is documented.

A new medical-dental history form should be filled out periodically to provide complete and accurate informa-

PATIENT REGISTRATION

Patient's name _____ Birthdate _____

Name of spouse _____ Birthdate _____

Single ☐
Widowed ☐
Married ☐
Divorced ☐
Separated ☐

If a child, parent's name _____

Street address _____ Phone _____

City _____ State _____ Zip _____

Patient employed by _____ Phone _____

Business address _____

Present position _____ How long held _____

Spouse employed by _____ Phone _____

Business address _____

Present position _____ How long held _____

Purpose of this appointment _____

In case of emergency, who should be notified _____ Phone _____

Person responsible for this account _____

Social Security number _____

Drivers License number _____

Spouse's Social Security number _____

Spouse's Drivers License number _____

If using Charge Card, name _____ Card no. _____ Exp. date _____

If Welfare, your number _____ County of _____

If you have insurance, name of insured _____

Name of insurance company _____ Policy no. _____

Is policy connected with a Union Yes _____ No _____ If yes, name of Union _____

Local no. _____ Group no. _____

If spouse has insurance, name of insured _____

Name of insurance company _____ Policy no. _____

Is policy connected with a Union Yes _____ No _____ If yes, name of Union _____

Local no. _____ Group no. _____

Whom may we thank for referring you _____

Your Signature _____ **Date** _____

Comments: _____

_____

_____

_____

_____

Form 4047 • 12/89 SYCOM Madison, WI Printed in U.S.A.

Figure 3-3 Patient registration form.
(Courtesy SYCOM, Groton, Mass.)

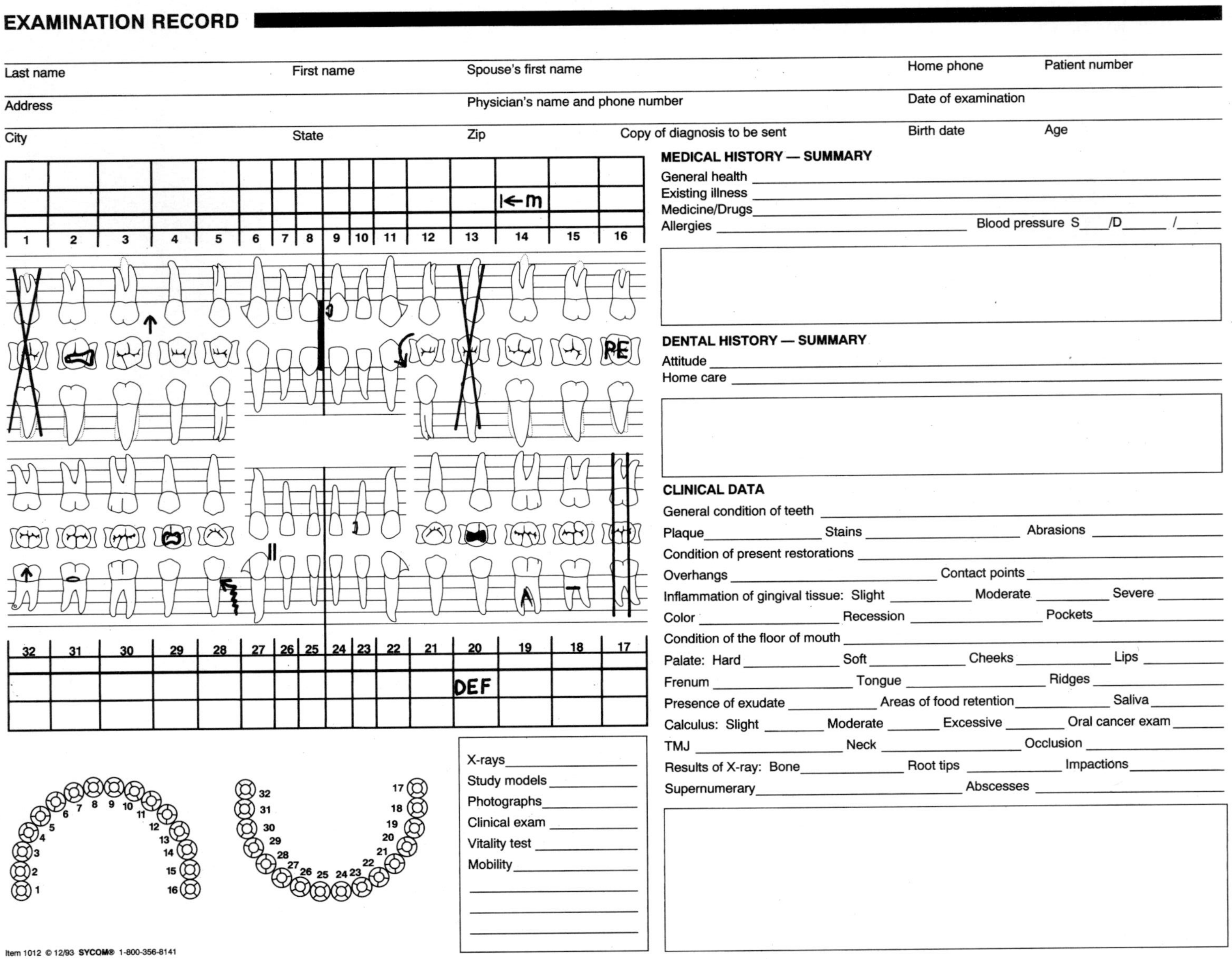

EXAMINATION RECORD

Last name _____ First name _____ Spouse's first name _____ Home phone _____ Patient number _____

Address _____

City _____ State _____ Zip _____ Physician's name and phone number _____ Date of examination _____

Copy of diagnosis to be sent _____ Birth date _____ Age _____

Blood pressure S ___ /D ___ /

MEDICAL HISTORY — SUMMARY

General health _____
Existing illness _____
Medicine/Drugs _____
Allergies _____

DENTAL HISTORY — SUMMARY

Attitude _____
Home care _____

CLINICAL DATA

General condition of teeth _____
Plaque _____ Stains _____ Abrasions _____
Condition of present restorations _____
Overhangs _____ Contact points _____
Inflammation of gingival tissue: Slight _____ Moderate _____ Severe _____
Color _____ Recession _____ Pockets _____
Condition of the floor of mouth _____
Palate: Hard _____ Soft _____ Cheeks _____ Lips _____
Frenum _____ Tongue _____ Ridges _____ Saliva _____
Presence of exudate _____ Areas of food retention _____
Calculus: Slight _____ Moderate _____ Excessive _____ Oral cancer exam _____
TMJ _____ Neck _____ Occlusion _____
Results of X-ray: Bone _____ Root tips _____ Impactions _____
Supernumerary _____ Abscesses _____

X-rays _____
Study models _____
Photographs _____
Clinical exam _____
Vitality test _____
Mobility _____

Item 1012 © 12/93 **SYCOM®** 1-800-356-8141

A

Figure 3-4 **A,** Patient examination record completed to show following charting situation: #1 is missing; #2 has mesoocclusal caries; food impaction between #3 and #4; diastema between #8 and #9; #9 has mesial caries; #12 is rotated distally; #13 is missing; #14 is shifted mesially; #15 is partially erupted; #17 needs to be extracted; #18 has beginning furcation; #19 has furcation involvement; #10 has defective distoocclusal amalgam; #23 has mesiofacial caries; between #26 and #27, there is open contact; #28 is hypersensitive; #29 has occlusal caries; #31 has cervical buccal caries; #32 is hypererupted.

(From Finkbeiner BL, Johnson CS: *Mosby's comprehensive dental assisting: a clinical approach,* St Louis, 1995, Mosby.)

PROGRESS NOTES

Name _____   Page No. _____

TS #	Date	Tooth	Treatment	Initials

B

Figure 3-4, cont'd   B, Treatment progress notes (services rendered) section of dental record.
(Courtesy Prosystems, Brentwood, NY. Designed by Burton Pollack, DDS, JD.)

tion about the patient's medical status. Some dental offices may perform this task as often as once each year. If so, the medical history form can be color coded each year to assist the dental staff when determining when a new form should be completed.

⟐ KEY POINTS
- The patient's medical history should be updated at each dental visit.
- Returning patients should fill out a new medical history periodically.

Date: *4-15-87*

I have reviewed the attached MEDICAL HISTORY. My general health status and medication has changed as follows (if no change, write "NO CHANGE"):

Pregnant, 3 months along.

Person Completing The Update: Signature *Kim Kerchner*

Print Name *Kim Kerchner*

If other than the patient, indicate relationship:

Update reviewed by Dr. *J.E. Chasteen*

Date: *11-28-87*

I have reviewed the attached MEDICAL HISTORY. My general health status and medication has changed as follows (if no change, write "NO CHANGE"):

Childbirth last month; now normal

Person Completing The Update: Signature *Kim Kerchner*

Print Name *Kim Kerchner*

If other than the patient, indicate relationship:

Update reviewed by Dr. *J.E. Chasteen*

Date: *5-18-88*

I have reviewed the attached MEDICAL HISTORY. My general health status and medication has changed as follows (if no change, write "NO CHANGE"):

No change

Person Completing The Update: Signature *Kim Kerchner*

Print Name *Kim Kerchner*

If other than the patient, indicate relationship:

Update reviewed by Dr. *J.E. Chasteen*

Date: _____

I have reviewed the attached MEDICAL HISTORY. My general health status and medication has changed as follows (if no change, write "NO CHANGE"):

_____

Person Completing The Update: Signature _____

Print Name _____

If other than the patient, indicate relationship: _____

Update reviewed by Dr. _____

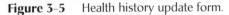

Figure 3-5   Health history update form.

(Courtesy Prosystems, Brentwood, NY. Designed by Burton Pollack, DDS, JD.)

5A

SCHOOL OF DENTISTRY
UNIVERSITY OF COLORADO
HEALTH SCIENCES CENTER

4200 EAST NINTH AVENUE
DENVER, COLORADO 80262
BOX C-284

MEDICAL CONSULTATION REQUEST

DATE: *9-10-88*

John Doe
(Name of Patient) _____ is planning to receive dental treatment at the University of Colorado Health Sciences Center School of Dentistry.

Patient relates a history of:

Placement of a prosthetic hip joint in May, 1985

Questions to be answered:

1. Is antibiotic prophylaxis necessary during routine dental cleanings and restorative procedures?
2. During an extraction of a tooth?

If prophylactic antibiotics are necessary, we will follow the most recent recommendations of the American Heart Association and the American Dental Association.

Eric Billard
Student Signature

Thomas Pollack, D.D.S.
Faculty Signature

PHYSICAL FINDINGS AND RECOMMENDATIONS

I strongly urge the use of prophylactic antibiotics during all dental treatment procedures. Use of current AHA and ADA recommendations are acceptable.

9-15-88
Consult Date

Joseph McClain, M.D.
Physician's Signature

Please keep Blue copy for patient's dental record. White and Green copy to physician. Physician to return White copy. Green copy for physician's records.

Figure 3-6   Medical consultation form for requesting and receiving medical advice from patient's physician.

(Courtesy School of Dentistry, University of Colorado, Denver.)

Medical Consultation Forms or Letters

Some patients may have medical conditions that require the advice of the patient's physician before dental treatment is begun. Figure 3-6 is an example of a **medical consultation (consult) form** used to request information from a patient's physician regarding the health status of the individual that may affect the planned treatment. A letter can be used in lieu of a form, but in either case the information should become a permanent part of the patient's record.

❖ KEY POINT
- The dental assistant or receptionist is often involved in obtaining the medical consult, especially if the medical consult is by telephone. Always obtain the name of the person you have talked to, and ask the medical office to make a notation in the patient's chart concerning the consult.

Medical Laboratory Test Results

On occasion the dentist may order medical laboratory tests to clarify the condition of a patient. Reports sent back to the dentist are stored in the record.

Dental Specialist Consultation Forms or Letters

It is not uncommon for a dentist to consult with a dental specialist to determine the appropriate treatment for a patient. Like a medical consultation form, this form or letter should be in writing and should be kept in the patient record for future reference. The same is true of referrals to specialists for treatment.

Dental Chart

The dental chart (see Figure 3-4, *A*) is a convenient form for recording clinical data acquired during oral and radiographic examinations. Although many chart designs are available, most of them contain a schematic drawing of the dentition. Some contain a "services rendered" or "treatment progress notes" section within the chart rather than on a separate document (see Figure 3-4, *B*).

A schematic drawing of the dentition helps the assistant record information quickly as it is dictated during the examination. Various charting symbols can be used to expedite the recording process (Figure 3-7). Afterward the dentist has a pictorial display of the needed treatment, which can be referred to at a glance. A dental chart helps dentists create detailed analyses of patient conditions and form plans of treatment.

There are several uses of the dental chart besides recording the planned treatment. The following list represents some information commonly found on charts.

1. *Patient information section.* Typing information from the application form into this section offers the advantage of legibility.

2. *Medical precaution section.* Whenever the medical-dental history reveals a systemic condition that the dentist must be aware of before and during treatment, the information can be written in a special area on the chart as a medical alert. Such alerts can be placed on the outside of the file as an additional precaution. Medical-alert stickers are available through dental stationery suppliers for this purpose (see Figure 3-2).

3. *Radiographic history.* A listing of patient radiographs can be displayed in this area on the chart. This helps the dental staff locate the most recent radiographs quickly. Such a listing also allows the dentist to quickly review which radiographs are available for reference.

4. *Remarks.* Every chart should have an area designated for personal notations regarding treatment or characteristics of the patient. This type of information is helpful during future appointments. If a dentist has already discussed with a patient the need for a bridge, this kind of notation prevents unnecessary repetition of information during future visits. It is also helpful to know in advance if a patient is apprehensive or uncooperative. The "remarks" section of the chart is ideal for such notations.

5. *Fee estimates.* If a dentist has discussed treatment with a patient and established a service fee, it is helpful to record this on the chart for easy reference if the patient should decide to have the treatment done in the future. The treatment plan is the primary source of information for extensive treatment to which the patient has already consented.

6. *Treatment rendered.* Opinions vary on the use of the dental chart to record treatment rendered. It is common for dentists to record this information on the back side of the chart in a "progress notes" or "services rendered" section. Other dentists choose to use separate forms for this purpose (see Figure 3-4, *B*, and Figure 3-12).

Many dentists establish a set of abbreviations used as a shorthand to describe treatment rendered. This approach often includes a set of charting symbols on a drawing of the teeth for clarification and simplification when reviewing treatment status.

Not all dentists include all items discussed here on dental charts, but charting can be done as shown in Figure 3-4, *A*. It is convenient for the entire staff to have this information available at a glance.

Another variation of dental charts is to record all existing restorations in a new patient's oral cavity on a separate examination sheet (Figure 3-8). This sheet becomes a handy reference in the future to determine what treatment was done by the patient's previous dentist. Other

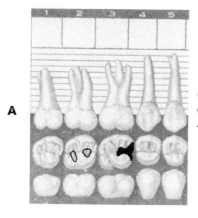

A Cavities and "watch" areas. Red sketch of outline form indicates "watch" area. Area filled in with red indicates caries.

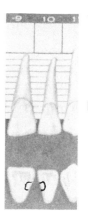

Aesthetic restorations are outlined in blue. **B**

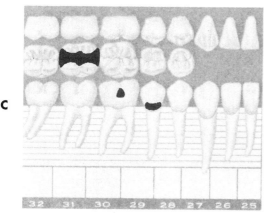

C Completed amalgam restorations. After tooth has been restored, outline of restoration is filled in with blue.

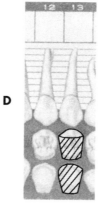

D Gold restorations can be represented by outlining surfaces covered by restoration and then drawing diagonal lines with blue pencil. Example is three-quarter crown on tooth #13.

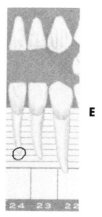

E Circle around root apex indicates endodontic periapical abscess.

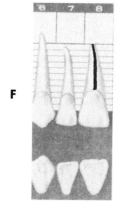

F Solid blue line through center of root indicates filled root canal. Solid red line indicates root canal to be done.

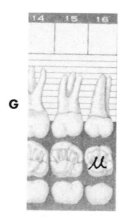

G Letter *u* on occlusal view of tooth indicates that it is *u*nerupted.

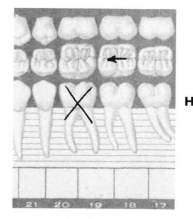

H Arrow on occlusal view indicates that tooth is malposed or drifted out of normal position in direction of arrow. X on facial view indicates missing tooth.

Figure 3-7 Colored pencils are helpful in charting to designate specific types of restorations. A suggested code is *blue* for restorations and *red* for problems. Shown are examples of symbols that can be used in charting. Each dentist has his or her own system of charting clinical information.

EXAMINATION SHEET

Case No. _____

Patient _____

Date _____

Student D.A. _____

Doctor _____

Instructor's Approval _____

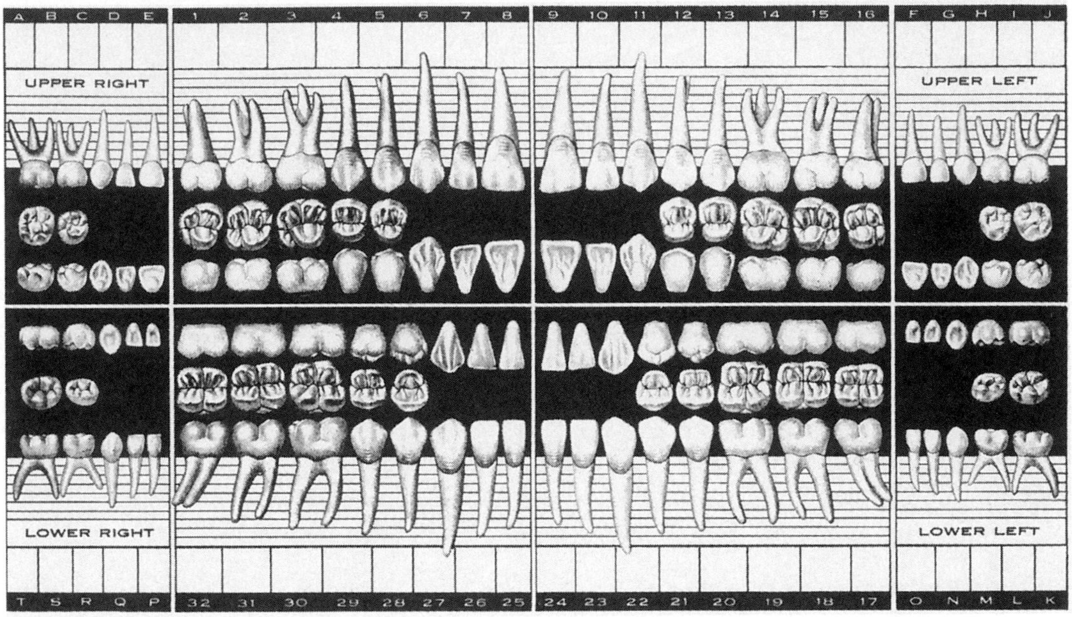

Diagnostic Findings:

Extra Oral: _____

Oral Mucosa: _____

_____

Teeth:

Missing: _____

Defective Restorations: _____

_____

Caries: _____

_____

Unerupted: _____

Other: _____

_____

T.M.J. _____

Occlusion _____

FORM C—103-D

COPYRIGHT 1968 BY PROFESSIONAL PUBLISHERS • 3980 FABIAN WAY • PALO ALTO, CALIFORNIA 94303

Figure 3-8 Examination sheet.

(Courtesy Professional Publishers, Palo Alto, Calif.)

oral findings in new patients may also be recorded and transferred to the main chart during the treatment planning process.

Treatment Plan

The purpose of the treatment plan is discussed in Chapter 2. The plan can be written on commercially available forms or typed on the dental office letterhead. Figure 3-9 shows a custom-designed treatment plan form. This example lists the treatment in the order it will be performed and includes a description of the services, fees, and the approved American Dental Association (ADA) procedure codes used for submitting dental insurance claims. It also includes a consent statement that the patient signs to give permission formally to carry out the treatment listed.

Informed Consent

Consent must be obtained from a patient for any treatment planned. Although much has been written about the concept of **informed consent,** it is essentially a process of shared decision making between the dentist and the patient. The patient is given all information regarding his or her oral health status along with treatment alternatives. Using this information, the patient then decides what treatment to accept. This decision is formalized when the patient signs and dates a statement that gives the dentist permission to proceed with treatment. Consent is not just a ritual of having the patient sign a standard form.

Since dental auxiliaries are often responsible for presenting treatment plan proposals, they should be aware of all the elements of the consent process if consent is to be truly valid. The elements of consent that should be recognized and incorporated into the consent process include the following:

1. An explanation of the patient's condition in lay terms
2. An explanation of the nature and purpose of the proposed treatment
3. An explanation of the possible risks and consequences of the proposed treatment; this element is particularly important for procedures with either a high risk of side effects or a significant risk of failure
4. Clarification of the probability of success of the procedure (although a guarantee should not be offered)
5. A presentation of the feasibility of treatment alternatives; doing nothing may in fact be a feasible alternative
6. An explanation of the risks and consequences of doing nothing
7. A statement of who will perform the treatment; this information is essential in a dental practice in which more than one provider may render the treatment

Informed consent provides patients with a complete explanation of the treatment plan proposal in terms they can understand. This information lets them make an intelligent decision regarding their health. It is advisable to document the explanation of the "significant risks and consequences" aspect of informed consent in the treatment progress notes in addition to the signed consent statement. Documentation of informed consent can also be achieved for standard procedures, such as simple extractions or periodontal surgery, by having the patient sign a prewritten form (see Figure 3-9).

Laboratory Requisitions

A copy of laboratory requisitions or prescriptions can be placed in the patient's chart for documentation of the requested laboratory work.

Radiographs

Radiographs can be stored either in the same file with the rest of the dental records or in a separate radiographic file. Individual office systems and personal preferences will determine how radiographs are filed. All radiographs should be placed in radiographic mounts and labeled with the patient's full name, the date they were taken, and the dentist's name.

Radiographs transferred to another dentist, to the patient's dental insurance company, or to another party should be documented in the patient's chart. Document the date the films were sent and to whom they were sent.

Photographs

Photographs of the patient are usually mounted in commercially available holders and can be kept in the patient record envelope (see Figure 3-1). Like radiographs, these should be labeled with the patient's name and the date they were taken.

RISK MANAGEMENT

In a society increasingly prone to filing lawsuits against health professionals, it is imperative that every effort be made to eliminate exposure to risk. Dental auxiliaries represent a major area of contact with patients. Their jobs require them to play a key role in patient relations, business office procedures, radiography, and record keeping. As a result dental auxiliaries should be aware of the fundamentals of **risk management** as they apply to the daily routine of patient care.

Patient Relations

It has often been said that a happy patient is less likely to initiate legal action than a disgruntled patient. Lawsuits are often initiated because of a lack of communication rather than as a result of inadequate dental treatment. Therefore it is essential that dental auxiliaries communicate clearly and effectively when patients voice their concerns. Special attention should be paid to the following areas:

15

INTERIM TREATMENT PLAN
UNIVERSITY OF COLORADO
SCHOOL OF DENTISTRY

PATIENT: _____ PATIENT CODE: _ _ _ _ _

STUDENT:_____ DATE: _____

CONFIRMATION THAT THE FOLLOWING PROCEDURES WERE APPROVED ON A TREATMENT
PLANNING WORKSHEET: _____

TOOTH	SURF AREA	ADA CODE	PHASE	ORDER	DESCRIPTION	FEE	BD
					ESTIMATE FEE FOR SERVICES		

I HAVE BEEN INFORMED OF THE NEED FOR THE SERVICES LISTED ABOVE AND UNDERSTAND BOTH THE
POSSIBLE SIDE EFFECTS OF ANY TREATMENT RENDERED AND THE POSSIBLE CONSEQUENCES OF NOT
RECEIVING TREATMENT IN THE NEAR FUTURE. IN CONSIDERATION FOR TREATMENT I AGREE TO PAY THE
STATED FEES IN EFFECT AT THE TIME SERVICES ARE RENDERED AND TO PRESENT MYSELF OR MINOR
CHILD FOR TREATMENT AT THE MINIMUM NUMBER OF TIMES STATED IN MY APPLICATION. I HAVE READ,
UNDERSTAND, AND HEREBY GIVE PERMISSION FOR DIAGNOSIS AND TREATMENT IN THE DENTAL CLINIC
AT THE UNIVERSITY OF COLORADO FOR MYSELF OR THE MINOR PATIENT NAMED ABOVE.

_____   _____
PATIENT (GUARDIAN) SIGNATURE   DATE

Yellow = Chart   Pink = Student   Blue = Patient   White = Clinical Affairs

Figure 3-9 Custom-designed treatment plan form.
(Courtesy School Of Dentistry, University of Colorado, Denver.)

- Warning the patient about unanticipated inconveniences
- Avoiding conflicting messages
- Explaining complications or mistakes
- Scheduling appointments appropriately

Informed consent

The risks, consequences, and outcome of a procedure must be accurately explained to the patient. Minimizing risks or giving false reassurances will only create dissatisfaction if the patient experiences a problem that was more severe than anticipated.

Warning the patient about unanticipated inconveniences

Although this step is not required for informed consent, patients are often unhappy if they are not forewarned about an inconvenience that may occur following treatment. Inconveniences such as pain, limitations in activity, and effects of local anesthetic agents or other drugs should be explained accurately, and anticipated time periods should be included.

Demonstrating a sense of caring

Avoid answering questions from patients or their families in a flippant or sarcastic manner. Months of effort to build patient rapport can be destroyed by one careless remark. Being sensitive and displaying concern demonstrate that you are truly concerned about the patient. Be sure to relate significant comments made by the patient or family, such as a request for a second opinion, immediately to the dentist.

Patients also expect dental staff members to direct their full attention to the patients' care. When rendering patient treatment, avoid talking about issues that do not pertain to the patient's care. Discussions between staff members about their weekend plans or shopping excursions will only annoy the patient.

Avoiding conflicting messages

The delivery of dental care is unique for each patient. What is done for one patient may not be the same procedure done for another patient with the same problem. This difference is due to many factors and conditions unique to each patient. Although the dental staff work closely with the dentist and can usually predict what treatment the dentist may choose, it is unwise to speculate about what the dentist may decide. Speculation about treatment before the dentist's confirmation will result in mixed messages to the patient and also will take unnecessary time and effort to explain why the speculated treatment was not desirable. Auxiliaries should also avoid narrowing treatment options by statements such as "I don't think that tooth will need a root canal"; not using such statements will avoid unnecessary concern by the patient if the tooth does indeed need a root canal.

Avoiding unprofessional comments

Patients look to the dental staff for expert advice and opinions about their dental care. Patients often ask staff their opinion about treatment received from the dentist or other dentists. Even if the auxiliary suspects that inadequate treatment was given, it is impossible to know all the details based only on the patient's account of the treatment. A careless negative remark such as "It doesn't surprise me that you had a problem, we have had many patients complain about that dentist" can result in a request to testify for a lawsuit in a patient's behalf. It is best to avoid any type of criticism or negative remarks. Responses about prior treatment can be answered in a neutral manner such as "I'm not exactly sure of all the circumstances regarding your treatment, so I can't tell you if I think it was appropriate or not."

> ➭ **KEY POINT**
> - Do not offer opinions about other dental staff members or other dental health care workers. Doing so is considered unprofessional.

Explaining complications or mistakes

Never cover up a complication or mistake. Such behavior will only solicit anger from patients and their families. Patients are much more accepting of the truth when a complication or mistake occurs. Explanations should be precise and should not include blame to other staff members if the occurrence of negligence or guilt is unclear. For example, a patient suffers a seizure after the administration of a local anesthetic agent and goes to the hospital. The family asks the auxiliary if the seizure occurred because of the local anesthetic agent. An appropriate response might be: "He had a seizure after the administration of the local anesthesia, and we do not know why it occurred. We will know better when we receive the medical report." Following a complication that implicates the auxiliary, the auxiliary should contact his or her personal liability (**malpractice**) carrier to inform the company of the complication. The liability carrier may request that the auxiliary complete an **incident report** from which the carrier will obtain information pertaining to the incident. The information on this form (Figure 3-10) is the property of the insurance carrier and is confidential between the insurance carrier and the auxiliary.

Financial arrangements

A deterrent to misunderstanding fees is the use of detailed treatment plans (described previously) that include a statement of fees. If fees are valid only for a limited time, this information should be stated in the plan. For example, "Fees quoted in this treatment plan are valid for 6

UCSF SCHOOL OF DENTISTRY

CONFIDENTIAL PATIENT INCIDENT REPORT

Instructions for Completing Form: Complete all sections as instructed, place ALL COPIES in an envelope marked "CONFIDENTIAL," and return to the Office for Clinical Services, Box 0752. The report should be completed by a dental provider. This report is a PRIVILEGED DOCUMENT, subject to attorney-client privileges. **Do not photocopy. Do not remove copies. Do not place this report in the dental record.**

Name of Patient (Print): _____

Sex: F _____   M _____

Chart Number: _____   Student Provider Number: _____

Account Number: _____   Faculty Provider Number: _____

Exact Location of Incident: _____   Date of Incident: _____

Time of Incident: _____   Date of Report: _____

Nature of Incident (Use back of this sheet if necessary):

A

_____

_____

_____

_____

Persons Familiar with Incident (Identify by Title and Dept. <u>or</u> Relationship to Patient):

_____

_____

Report Completed By: _____

Print Name: _____

Class Year or Department: _____

Supervisor's Action or Suggestion to Prevent Recurrence (Use back of this sheet if necessary):

_____

_____

_____

_____

Supervisor's Signature: _____

Print Name: _____

Title: _____

Clinic or Department: _____

2/8/90

Figure 3-10 **A,** Confidential patient incident report.
(**A** Courtesy University of California, San Francisco.)

PROTOCOL FOR USE OF THE
CONFIDENTIAL PATIENT INCIDENT REPORT

WARNING:

This report is a CONFIDENTIAL AND PRIVILEGED DOCUMENT, not available for use in litigation. To protect this privilege:

1. NEVER SHOW it to unauthorized persons.
2. NEVER MENTION it in the dental or medical record.
3. NEVER PHOTOCOPY the completed report.
4. NEVER REMOVE COPIES of the completed report.

The School of Dentistry's repository for the Confidential Patient Incident Report is the Office for Clinical Services, Room D-1000, Box 0752, Parnassus Dental Clinic Building, 707 Parnassus Avenue.

PURPOSE:

The purpose of the Confidential Patient Incident Report is to track incidents involving patients at the School of Dentistry; to monitor safety and health conditions in the clinics operated by the School of Dentistry; and to monitor the quality of patient services provided in the clinics operated by the School of Dentistry.

B

INSTRUCTIONS FOR COMPLETING THE CONFIDENTIAL INCIDENT REPORT:

The student or faculty provider will complete this report if the following occurs:

1. Conduct or circumstances that injure or could injure a patient.
2. An incident that causes a negative reaction by a patient or family member.

The student or faculty provider will complete the first two sections of the report, relaying the specifics of the incident (such as the date and location), and provide a detailed account of the incident by completing the "Nature of Incident" section. ALL COPIES OF THE REPORT should be returned to the Parnassus Office for Clinical Services (Box 0752) in an envelope marked "CONFIDENTIAL."

The Parnassus Office for Clinical Services will forward the report to the Campus Office for Risk Management. In addition, the Office for Clinical Services will provide a copy of the report to the appropriate supervisor. The supervisor should review the details of the incident and make appropriate suggestions, or take appropriate actions, to prevent a recurrence of the incident. The supervisor should complete the appropriate section of the report and return it to the Parnassus Office for Clinical Services (Box 0752) in an envelope marked "CONFIDENTIAL."

NO PORTION OF THIS REPORT SHOULD BE RETAINED BY ANY SCHOOL OF DENTISTRY PERSONNEL OTHER THAN THE DIRECTOR OF THE OFFICE FOR CLINICAL SERVICES.

2/8/90

Figure 3-10, cont'd **B,** Protocol for use of confidential patient incident report.

months from the date of this plan." If a payment plan for services rendered has been agreed on, the patient should sign a truth-in-lending agreement (Figure 3-11). Such forms are available from dental stationery suppliers or can be created on a computer.

Appointment planning

Patients in pain or discomfort should be seen as soon as possible. Appointment schedules can be arranged to allow for "buffer" time slots during the working day for this purpose. If a patient needs to be seen after hours, dentists should have someone accompany them to the office to avoid treating a patient alone. After-hours emergency patients should be told to have a friend or relative accompany them to the office if the dentist cannot provide a third party as a witness.

Patient bonding is the result of dental staff efforts to make patients feel that the dental staff cares about them. This approach is the very essence of building a practice and a powerful risk-management principle. Keeping patients waiting more than 15 minutes past their appointment time sends them a message that the dentist's time is more valuable than theirs. Patients appreciate a telephone call to inform them that the office is running behind schedule and to offer the option of coming later in the day or rescheduling the appointment for another day.

Record keeping

A detailed chronological account of all treatment rendered is an essential element of risk management. Treatment progress notes make it possible to document treatment provided and are critical pieces of medicolegal evidence in malpractice lawsuits.

The following list of basic dental rules should serve as a guide to favorable documentation of treatment in the "services rendered" section of the dental record:

1. Make all entries with nonerasable ink.
2. Label all pages with the patient's full name and a page number.
3. Make all entries legible.
4. The provider of service should initial all entries. This step is especially significant in a multiple provider practice. (Some states require the provider to place his or her dental license number next to each entry alongside his or her initials.)
5. Date entries at the time the service is rendered.
6. Cross out errors with a single line followed by the correct information. An erroneous entry should not be obliterated so that it cannot be read at a later date. Such a practice can be suspect in the eyes of a jury during a malpractice trial.
7. Do not amend progress notes by writing in the margins. If more information needs to be added regarding treatment on a given date, enter a new date

and note, "Addendum to progress notes of (date)"; then enter the additional information.
8. Progress notes should include the following:
   a. Reason for treatment (diagnosis)
   b. Type and dosage of anesthetic and/or analgesic used
   c. Specific brands of materials used, not just generic names
   d. Detailed summary of conditions during treatment, such as pulp exposures, unusual bleeding, and hematomas
   e. Specific medications and dosages administered or prescribed before, during, or after treatment
   f. Special postoperative instructions
9. Enter descriptions of any treatment instructions given over the telephone as soon as possible. Include the date and time instructions are given. Figure 3-12 is an example of a well-done set of treatment progress notes.
10. Only entries pertaining to patient treatment belong in the chart. Do not document risk prevention activities in the chart such as "Malpractice insurance company notified" or "Contacted a lawyer regarding this incident."

Confidentiality Law

Most states have laws that protect the information recorded or stored in the dental record. This information includes radiographs, health histories, progress notes, consent statements, photographs, insurance claim forms, laboratory prescriptions, medical reports, and medical consultations. Although the dentist usually owns the original elements of the dental record, confidentiality laws generally give patients the right to obtain a copy of the record contents. A reasonable cost of duplicating parts of a record can be passed on to the patient.

Before any part of a dental record is sent to patients or their designees, a written request should be obtained from the patient. Such a request can be in letter form, or a records release form can be signed by the patient (Figure 3-13). Records release forms should be stored in the dental record and an entry made in the progress notes describing the disposition of the copy of the record (e.g., 8/12/87—Patient requested copy of entire dental record. Mailed to Dr. James Smith, 300 Elm Street, Bend, Oregon). If the records are mailed, obtain a return receipt to document that the record was received. The original dental record should not be sent unless the dentist is ordered by a court to do so. If an original record is requested by a court, a copy should be made and retained, and the original record should be delivered to the court in person or by a bonded courier. A receipt should always be kept in the patient's file.

FINANCIAL AGREEMENT

Patient_____ Date_____
                         (Print Name)

Guarantor's Name (if other than patient) _____
                                            (Print Name)

I agree to pay the amount of $ _____ to the office of Dr._____

for dental services described to me on _____ .
                                       (Date)

Payment Arrangement: _____

_____

_____

_____

_____

_____

I understand that as the treatment progresses modifications may be necessary and these may affect the fee. Should this occur, I further understand that the modification of treatment and the change in fee will be discussed with me at the earliest possible time.

Signature of Patient or Guarantor _____

Signature of Office Representative_____

Figure 3-11   Truth-in-lending, or financial, agreement form.
(Courtesy Prosystems, Brentwood, NY. Designed by Burton Pollack, DDS, JD.)

PROGRESS NOTES

Name Mary Fisk   Page No. 1

TS #	Date	Tooth	Treatment	Initials
—	1/8/95		Initial exam. FMX radiographs	JB
—	1/15/95		Periodontal scaling/root planing all quadrants. Moderate subgingival calculus and plaque. Oral hygiene instructions - sulcular tooth brushing and floss. Post-op instructions: warm salt water rinses	
			Next recall: 3 mos	CM
—	1/15/95 cont		4:00pm (later same day) Patient called office and reported her teeth are sensitive to cold. Patient informed that sensitivity to cold is a normal post-op complication and the sensitivity should gradually go away.	TM
—	1/22/95	—	Case presentation. Explained risk of pulp exposure and possible need for endodontic therapy on tooth #19.	
MO	2/4/95	19	Caries, indirect pulp cap with "Dycal", IRM base, Tytin. Anesthesia given. 2% Lidocaine with 1:100,000 epinephrine, 1 cartridge total for lower left mandibular block. Pt responded well to anesthesia. Post op: Tylenol, 2 tabs, q 4h, p.r.n.	JB
—	2/9/95	—	Addendum to progress notes of 1-8-95: Panorex radiograph taken in addition to FMX.	
—	2/15/95	—	Patient broke appointment without notification	TM

Figure 3-12   Sample page of treatment progress notes.

(Courtesy Prosystems, Brentwood, NY. Designed by Burton Pollack, DDS, JD.)

REQUEST FOR RELEASE OF HEALTH INFORMATION

I, _____, hereby grant permission to
(Print Name)

_____
(Print Name of Doctor or Hospital)
to release information related to my health history, status, and treatment, and copies of my health
record, X-rays, and any test results to;

_____

At   _____

_____

Signature_____ Date _____
(If a minor, parent or guardian must sign)

Figure 3-13   Records release form.
(Courtesy Prosystems, Brentwood, NY. Designed by Burton Pollack, DDS, JD.)

Record Storage

Dental records should be kept in a safe place at least until the particular statute of limitations expires for each patient. **A statute of limitations** allows a patient a specified length of time to file a malpractice claim; the length varies from state to state. If a dental practice is sold, provision should be made for the new owner to preserve all dental records until the statute of limitations expires.

Photographs

It is not uncommon for assistants to have the responsibility of taking photographs to document treatment. If photographs are used in publications or lectures and the patient is identifiable, written permission must be obtained. Use of close-up photographs that do not reveal a patient's identity does not require written permission.

BIBLIOGRAPHY

Boyce JS: Risk management: an introduction for the dental practice, *Dental Hygiene* 61:504, 1987.
Finkbeiner BL, Finkbeiner CA: *Practice management for the dental team,* ed 4, St Louis, 1996, Mosby.
Miyasaki-Ching CM, Tennenhouse DJ: *Dental risk prevention for dental auxiliaries,* San Rafael, Calif, 1991, Tennenhouse Professional Publications.
Pollack BR: *Handbook of dental jurisprudence and risk management,* Littleton, Mass, 1987, PSG Publishing.
Rozovsky FA: *Consent to treatment: a practical guide,* Boston, 1984, Little, Brown.
Schafler NL: *Medical malpractice: handling dental cases,* Colorado Springs, Colo, 1985, Shepard's McGraw-Hill.

QUESTIONS–Chapter 3

1. At what interval should the patient be asked if there are any changes in his or her medical history?
   a. At every visit
   b. Once each year
   c. Twice each year
   d. Every 2 years

2. The process by which the dentist or auxiliary has given information to the patient regarding planned treatment and the alternatives to the treatment and obtains permission from the patient is called:
   a. The treatment plan
   b. An informed consent
   c. A medical consult
   d. Risk management

3. A patient had a gold crown placed on a tooth at another dental office. The patient has come to your office because the tooth has recurrent decay and is now bothering him. As you are taking a radiograph of the tooth, the patient asks you, "Do you think the other dentist didn't do a good job with that crown?" Which of the following would be the most appropriate reply?
   a. Say nothing.
   b. "I wouldn't be surprised, we have had many patients come to us from that office with similar problems."
   c. "Well, you wouldn't have had decay under the crown if the dentist did it right in the first place."
   d. "I don't really know all the details that were involved with your treatment of that tooth, so I wouldn't be able to give you an informed opinion."

4. The patient has a tooth with a large filling that has fractured. When you are seating the patient, he asks you if the tooth will need a crown. Which of the following would be the most appropriate reply?
   a. "It will probably need a crown or another large filling."
   b. "When people have this sort of problem, they usually need a crown."
   c. "I'm not sure. Sometimes teeth like this need to have a root canal."
   d. "I'm really not sure because we really don't have the information yet to decide."

5. The patient asks you about another dentist you know who sees many patients but does not do very good work. Which of the following would be the most appropriate reply?
   a. "I don't know anything about him."
   b. "He's not very good. I wouldn't go to him."
   c. "I know of him, and he sees many patients."
   d. "It's really not appropriate for me to say bad things about other dental professionals."

6. While you are fitting a crown, it slips and the patient swallows it. The patient's husband is a friend of your family and calls you to ask what happened. Which of the following is the most appropriate reply?
   a. "Things like this happen all the time. I'm surprised it hasn't happened before."
   b. "We've been lucky, and it's not happened before."
   c. Say nothing.
   d. "The crown fell down the patient's throat, and it was swallowed."

7. The patient will be having some extractions and asks, "Will it be painful?" Which of the following is the most appropriate reply?
   a. "There is always some degree of pain associated with this type of procedure; however, the amount will vary from person to person depending on pain tolerance."
   b. "When my sister had some extractions, it was very painful, so I would expect the same."
   c. "You will probably just feel some discomfort. We'll give you medication for it."
   d. "The oral surgeon is very good, and you probably won't feel any pain."

8. The patient calls and complains of a broken filling in the first premolar on the lower right. A note is made in the chart by the receptionist. The patient comes in, and the broken filling is in the second premolar. Which would be the most appropriate entry for the chart?
   a. "Patient reported wrong tooth bothering him. The second premolar has the broken filling."
   b. "The receptionist wrote down the wrong tooth for the broken filling. It is the second premolar."
   c. Tell the receptionist to cross out her comment on the chart, and tell her not to write statements like that in the chart.
   d. "First premolar checked and not broken filling. The second premolar has a broken filling."

9. You have explained the procedure to the patient several times already, and the patient continues to ask you questions that you have answered repeatedly. Which of the following should you say?
   a. "I've already answered that question several times. What is it you don't understand?"
   b. "Can't you understand what I am saying? I've already explained this."
   c. Answer the patient's questions patiently, and if the patient does not understand ask the patient what it is that he or she is having a difficult time understanding.
   d. "I'm not going to answer that because I've already told you."

10. The dentist gave the injection on the wrong side of the mouth; however, there was dental work that needed to be done on that side anyway. Which of the following is the most appropriate remark to the patient?
    a. Say nothing. No unnecessary harm was done to the patient.
    b. "Oops, the dentist did the wrong side by mistake."
    c. Tell the patient that the dentist was planning to do the other side but gave the injection on the wrong side; however, there was work to be done on that side.
    d. Answers *a* and *c* are both correct.

Chapter 3 questions courtesy Miyasaki-Ching CM, Tennenhouse DJ: *Dental risk prevention for dental auxiliaries,* San Rafael, Calif, 1991, Tennenhouse Professional Publications.

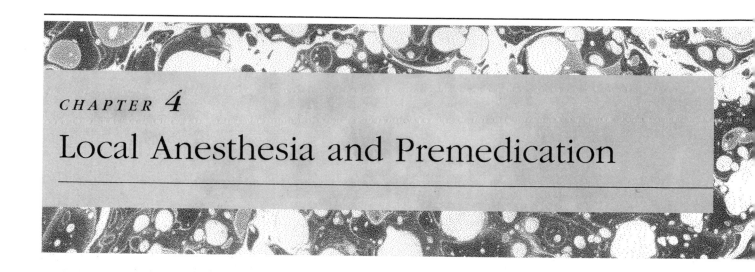

CHAPTER *4*

Local Anesthesia and Premedication

KEY TERMS
Aspiration
Field block anesthesia
General anesthesia
Infiltration anesthesia
Local anesthesia
Nerve block anesthesia
Prophylactic premedication
Subacute bacterial endocarditis
Topical anesthesia
Trieger test
Vasoconstrictors

LOCAL ANESTHESIA

Many dental procedures involve cutting or manipulation of living tissue. The painful nature of these procedures necessitates the use of anesthesia. Anesthesia is the loss of sensation or feeling in a body part. Various drugs are available that produce temporary anesthesia in the body. These drugs are classified as either general anesthetics or local anesthetics.

General anesthetics temporarily alter the central nervous system so that sensation is lost throughout the entire body. The patient is unconscious while under the influence of a general anesthetic. In dentistry **general anesthesia** is most commonly used during oral surgery procedures.

Local anesthetics temporarily prevent the conduction of sensory impulses such as pain, touch, and thermal change from a body part along nerve pathways to the brain. Thus only certain selected regions of the body lose sensation when the patient is under **local anesthesia.** Patients remain conscious while under the influence of local anesthetic agents. With the exception of certain surgical and operative procedures, local anesthesia is more commonly used than general anesthesia in dentistry.

For local anesthetics to work, they must come in direct contact with either nerve fibers that carry the sensory impulse to the brain or tiny nerve endings that pick up sensations in tissue.

A special type of local anesthetic that acts only on tiny nerve endings located in the surface of skin and mucosa is called a topical anesthetic. In **topical anesthesia** some sensation on surface tissues, such as skin and especially mucosa, is eliminated. Sunburn lotion usually contains a topical anesthetic that temporarily eliminates the discomfort of sunburn. Oral mucosa can be anesthetized by wiping a topical anesthetic on the tissue surface. This step is helpful in reducing the discomfort of dental injections and eliminating the gag reflex during impression-taking and radiographic procedures. Local anesthetic agents are available in liquid, gel, paste, and cream forms (Figure 4-1).

Local anesthetics used for operative and surgical procedures must be injected into the soft tissue so that the anesthetic agent can come in contact with sensory nerve fibers. Once an anesthetic solution surrounds a nerve, sensations cannot pass through the nerve at that point. As a result the structure that receives its innervation from the surrounded nerve can be operated on without pain. Local anesthetic agents used for injection are available in liquid form in premeasured cartridges and ampules (see Figure 4-1).

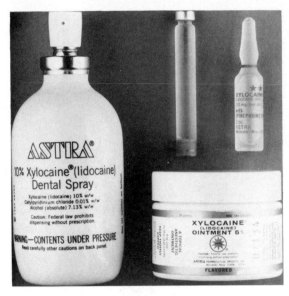

Figure 4-1 Anesthetic agents. *Left* and *bottom right,* Topical agents. *Top right,* Injectable agents.

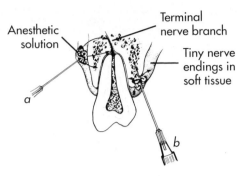

Figure 4-2 Injection needle placement for *(a)* field block anesthesia and *(b)* infiltration anesthesia.

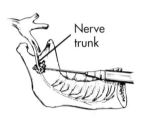

Figure 4-3 Injection needle placement for nerve block anesthesia.

Methods of Injection

The three principal injection methods used in dentistry are infiltration, field block, and nerve block.

The term **infiltration anesthesia** is often misused. Infiltration is an injection method used to deposit anesthetic solution to prevent pain impulses from being picked up by tiny terminal nerve branches located throughout living tissue. It is fairly common to infiltrate an area of soft tissue so an incision can be made without producing pain. Infiltration anesthesia can be used anywhere in the oral cavity where the soft tissue is to be operated on. This method of anesthetic administration is used in procedures such as biopsy, gingivectomy, frenectomy, and excision of abnormal tissue.

The term *infiltration anesthesia* is often used interchangeably with **field block anesthesia.** The two methods of injection are similar. The difference between infiltration and field block anesthesia centers on which nerve branches are targets of the injection procedure. Infiltration procedures are directed toward the tiny terminal branches of the nerve. Field block procedures are directed toward larger terminal nerve branches. In the oro-dental region, field blocks often accomplish infiltration anesthesia at the same time. Anesthetic solutions injected into areas near large terminal nerve branches also eliminate pain impulses from adjacent tiny nerve branches. These solutions are not selective and will anesthetize branches in any given area. Figure 4-2 demonstrates the difference in needle placement for the two procedures.

Field block anesthesia is used whenever teeth or bone is operated on in the maxillary (and sometimes the

mandibular) anterior region. Larger terminal branches of the trigeminal nerve provide innervation to teeth and bone in these areas. Field block anesthesia cannot be used successfully to anesthetize the posterior mandibular teeth. These teeth are surrounded by very dense bone that does not allow penetration of anesthetic solution to the terminal branches that innervate the teeth. Field block procedures are successful throughout the entire maxilla and in the mandibular anterior area because the bone surrounding the teeth is thinner and less dense. The anesthetic solution can penetrate this bone and contact the terminal nerve branches that innervate these teeth. Some patients can be anesthetized in the mandibular premolar region by a field block injection; however, use of this approach depends on the anatomical features of the individual patient.

Nerve block anesthesia involves deposition of anesthetic solution near a main nerve trunk. A successful nerve block prevents passage of any pain impulse past the site of injection to the brain. Therefore any structure innervated by the nerve trunk or its branches beyond the injection site away from the brain is anesthetized. Nerve blocks eliminate pain sensation from larger areas than either field blocks or infiltrations.

The most common nerve block used in dentistry is the mandibular nerve block. The inferior alveolar nerves supply all the lower teeth and the surrounding bone. To anesthetize these structures, a needle is placed near the mandibular foramen on the medial aspect of the ramus (Figure 4-3). The solution is deposited near this main nerve trunk where it enters the mandible. All the mandibular teeth and bone are anesthetized beyond this point to the patient's midline.

> **KEY POINTS**
> - Infiltration anesthesia is used primarily for soft tissue anesthesia.
> - Field block anesthesia is generally used to anesthetize maxillary teeth and mandibular anterior teeth.
> - Nerve block anesthesia is used to anesthetize mandibular teeth.

Table 4-1 summarizes the injection procedures used to anesthetize specific structures in dental procedures.

Anesthetic Agents

Although approximately 15 different anesthetics are available for dental use (Table 4-2), 2% lidocaine with a vasoconstrictor (Xylocaine) and 3% mepivacaine (Carbocaine)

are probably the most commonly used. Both agents have a rapid onset of action and provide profound local anesthesia of the dental pulp (lidocaine, 60 minutes; mepivacaine, 40 minutes).

The trend in dental practice is to do more dental procedures during longer appointments. When anesthetic agents are used with vasoconstrictors such as epinephrine, they provide a favorable working time for this type of practice.

If a short procedure is anticipated, anesthesia with a short duration can be accomplished with a 3% mepiva-

Table 4-1 Injection methods used for dental procedures

Area	Injection method
Oral soft tissue	Infiltration
Maxillary teeth and bone	Field block
Mandibular anterior teeth and bone	Field block
All mandibular teeth and bone	Nerve block

From Malamed SF: *Handbook of local anesthesia*, ed 3, St Louis, 1990, Mosby.

Table 4-2 Anesthetic agents and duration of pulpal and soft tissue anesthesia

Agent	Category	Duration (approx. minutes)	
		Pulpal	Soft tissue
SHORT DURATION			
Lidocaine 2%	Amide	5–10	60–120
Prilocaine 4% (infiltration)	Amide	5–10	90–120
Mepivacaine 3%	Amide	20–40	120–180
INTERMEDIATE DURATION			
Articaine 4%, epinephrine 1:200,000*	Amide	45	180–240
Mepivacine 2%, epinephrine 1:200,000*	Amide	45	120–240
Procaine 2%, propoxycaine 0.4%, levonordefrin 1:20,000	Ester	30–60	120–180
Lidocaine 2%, epinephrine 1:50,000	Amide	60	180–240
Lidocaine 2%, epinephrine 1:100,000	Amide	60	180–240
Mepivacaine 2%, levonordefrin 1:20,000	Amide	60	180–240
Prilocaine 4% (block)	Amide	60	120–240
Articaine 4%, epinephrine 1:100,000*	Amide	75	180–300
Prilocaine 4%, epinephrine 1:200,000	Amide	60–90	120–240
LONG DURATION			
Bupivacaine 0.5%, epinephrine 1:200,000	Amide	>90	240–540
Etidocaine 1.5%, epinephrine 1:200,000	Amide	>90	240–540

Short-duration agents provide pulpal anesthesia for 30 minutes or less; intermediate-duration agents for approximately 60 minutes; long-duration for longer than 90 minutes. The classification of duration is approximate. Variations may be noted.

Modified from Malamed SF: *Handbook of local anesthesia*, ed 3, St Louis: Mosby, 1990, p 47.
*Not available in United States of America (January 1994).

caine (Carbocaine) solution without a vasoconstrictor. In dentistry 30 minutes is considered a short duration.

Vasoconstrictors

Vasoconstrictors are drugs that cause blood vessels to constrict so that blood flow is reduced. The drugs accomplish this by stimulating certain receptors in the arterial system. When vasoconstrictors are used with local anesthetic agents, they reduce blood flow at the site of the injected solution. The effect retards absorption of the anesthetic solution into the bloodstream. This result is desirable because the anesthetic solution is kept in the injection site longer before being carried into the bloodstream. Thus the profoundness and duration of the anesthesia are increased.

Since most anesthetics are somewhat toxic to the central nervous system, vasoconstrictors increase the safety margin because smaller quantities of anesthetic can be used to obtain adequate anesthesia. In addition, the amount of anesthetic used cannot enter the bloodstream rapidly and be carried to the brain in great enough quantity to produce a toxic effect.

The most common vasoconstrictor is epinephrine. Lidocaine 2% is available without any vasoconstrictor or with epinephrine in either a 1:100,000 or a 1:50,000 concentration. A concentration of 1:50,000 means that 1 part of vasoconstrictor is diluted by 50,000 parts of nonvasoconstrictor. The 1:100,000 concentration seems to be the most favorable. Lidocaine without epinephrine produces approximately 10 minutes of anesthesia, whereas lidocaine with 1:100,000 or 1:50,000 epinephrine lasts approximately 60 minutes. The anesthetic solutions without vasoconstrictors are convenient choices for short-

acting anesthetics or in cases in which a vasoconstrictor is contraindicated.

> **KEY POINTS**
> - A local anesthetic agent with a vasoconstrictor allows the anesthetic agent to last longer.
> - The most common vasoconstrictor is epinephrine.

Armamentarium

The armamentarium needed to administer local anesthesia in the oral cavity is shown in Figure 4-4.

Syringes

Dental injection syringes vary in design (Table 4-3). The choice of syringe is a matter of personal preference. The most commonly used anesthetic syringes are the breech-loading injection syringe with harpoon and the self-aspirating syringe without harpoon.

Probably the most widely used aspirating syringe is the metal breech-loading style with a harpoon type of plunger. This type of syringe is available with a thumb ring, which helps the dentist apply back pressure on the plunger after needle placement in the tissue (Figure 4-5).

Another type of syringe that is gaining popularity is the self-aspirating syringe, which uses a thumb disk (instead of a harpoon) attached to the piston to aspirate (Figure 4-6).

As mentioned previously, all local anesthetics are potentially toxic to the central nervous system if they are

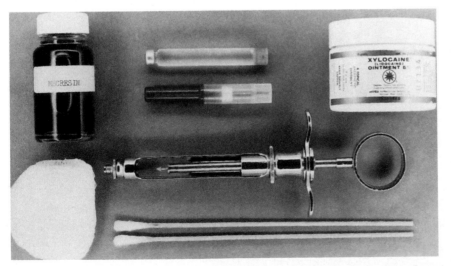

Topical antiseptic (Mecresin or Betadine)
Anesthetic cartridge
Injection needle
Topical anesthetic (optional)
Gauze sponges, 2 × 2 inch
Syringe
Cotton swabs

Figure 4-4   Local anesthetic armamentarium.

injected in sufficient quantities into the bloodstream. Toxicity can occur if a needle is inadvertently placed in a blood vessel and the solution is injected directly into the bloodstream. To prevent this accident, the dentist must apply back pressure on the thumb ring of a breech-loading syringe with harpoon after needle placement. If the needle is placed in a vessel, blood will be drawn into the anesthetic cartridge; the action of applying a negative pressure is called **aspiration.** If blood does enter the cartridge (a positive aspiration), it is recommended that the needle be removed, the cartridge replaced, and the injection started again in a different position. This procedure is a safety measure designed to protect the patient. Aspiration is not as important in field block and infiltration injections as it is in nerve blocks, since the larger vessels are located deep in the tissues near main nerve trunks.

When the aspirating type of syringe is loaded, it is im-

Table 4-3 Description of parts of syringe

Part	Use	Rationale
Thumb ring for breech-loading syringe with harpoon	Aspiration	To avoid injecting anesthetic into a blood vessel, which could burst blood vessel or quickly carry anesthetic into circulatory system, causing an overdose reaction
Thumb disk for self-aspirating syringe		
Piston	Administration of local anesthetic	Places pressure on rubber stopper of anesthetic cartridge to administer anesthetic
Harpoon	Aspiration	Engaged into rubber stopper of anesthetic cartridge, which allows operator to apply negative pressure to anesthetic cartridge
Syringe barrel	Cartridge containment	Syringe barrel holds anesthetic cartridge; window on barrel enables operator to observe for positive aspiration
Needle adaptor	Needle engagement	Allows operator to engage anesthetic needle; care must be taken to avoid accidentally removing and discarding needle adaptor when removing disposable needle

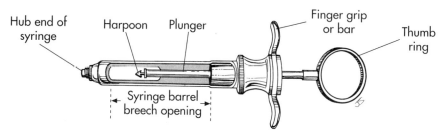

Figure 4-5   Breech-loading injection syringe.

(From Finkbeiner BL, Johnson CS: *Mosby's comprehensive dental assisting: a clinical approach,* St Louis, 1995, Mosby.)

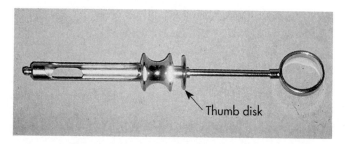

Figure 4-6   Self-aspirating syringe.

portant to drive the small harpoon on the end of the plunger into the rubber stopper in the anesthetic cartridge. The harpoon engages the rubber stopper when back pressure is applied to the plunger, allowing the aspiration to occur. Caution should be used during this procedure to avoid excessive force that could result in a shattered anesthetic cartridge.

Injection needles

The most common type of needle used for local anesthetic injections is a disposable sterile needle packaged in individual protective plastic containers (Figure 4-7).

Another common type of disposable needle has two sections to its plastic container. One section covers the syringe/cartridge penetrating end of the needle. The other section covers the shank and bevel portions of the needle (Figure 4-8).

After the syringe is loaded with an anesthetic cartridge, the syringe/cartridge penetrating end of the needle can be uncovered and screwed onto the end of the syringe. This small portion of the needle punctures the small rubber seal in the center of the metal end of the cartridge. The section of the plastic container covering the shank of the needle is left in place until the needle is used. This precaution prevents contamination of the needle.

Needles are available in different lengths. Length is measured from the hub to the tip of the needle bevel. Two common lengths are the 1-inch needle (short needle) and the 1⅝-inch needle (long needle).

It is common to use a short needle for infiltration and field blocks and a long needle for deep nerve blocks (e.g., mandibular nerve block). The choice is a matter of personal preference.

Needles are also available in different diameter openings. The gauge of a needle is the measurement of the diameter of the needle shaft. Some of the common gauges used in dentistry are 23, 25, 27, and 30. A *lower* gauge number indicates a *larger* needle shaft diameter. For example, a 30-gauge needle has a smaller diameter opening than a 25-gauge needle.

The selection of needle gauge is dictated in part by the depth of the injection and the needle length used. Generally speaking, the longer the needle length, the larger the diameter of needle used. Although small-diameter needles may cause less pain, they can be easily deflected in the tissue and miss the intended target. This problem occurs especially when long, thin needles are used for deep injections. Inadequate anesthesia is often the result of needle deviation, since the solution is deposited away from the nerve target. Fine-gauge needles, such as short-length 27- and 30-gauge needles, are recommended for shallow infiltration and field block injections.

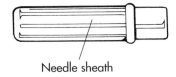

Figure 4-7 Disposable injection needle. *Top,* Covered. *Bottom,* Uncovered.

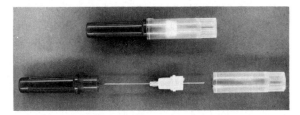

Bevel   Shank   Hub   Syringe   Syringe/cartridge
                          adapter   penetrating end

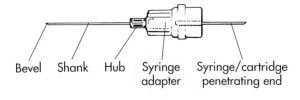

Needle sheath

Figure 4-8 Common type of disposable needle with two sections.

> **KEY POINTS**
> - Needles are available in two lengths: long (1⅝ inches) and short (1 inch).
> - The gauge of the needle indicates the diameter of the needle opening.

Anesthetic cartridges

The cartridge is a glass tube with a metal cap sealing one end. The metal cap has a rubber center into which the needle is inserted after the cartridge is loaded into the syringe. The other end of the tube is sealed with a rubber stopper. The small harpoon on the aspirating syringe is driven into this stopper after the cartridge is loaded into the syringe. The cartridge is commonly called a *carpule* (Figure 4-9).

The anesthetic cartridges contain 1.8 ml of anesthetic solution, which is an adequate dose for most dental procedures.

The anesthetic cartridges should be stored in their original containers at room temperature in a dark place. Although this step is not necessary, the rubber diaphragm can be disinfected before insertion in the anesthetic syringe by wiping it with an alcohol swab. Before inserting the cartridge into the syringe, the assistant should inspect the cartridge for the following:

1. Large bubbles
2. Extruded rubber stopper
3. Corroded cap
4. Rust on the cap
5. Cracks in the glass

If any of the above are found, the assistant should not use the cartridge and should check all remaining cartridges for similar problems.

Studies demonstrate that anesthetic cartridges should not be immersed in a disinfectant because the disinfectant can pass through the rubber diaphragm and contaminate the anesthetic solution. Likewise, cartridges should not be left uncovered in the presence of acrylic monomer that is stored in dropper bottles. It has been shown that monomer vapor passes from the rubber dropper bulb to anesthetic cartridges that are stored nearby. This phenomenon could result in inadvertent injection of contaminated anesthetic solution into a patient.

⮕ KEY POINT
- **Do not store anesthetic cartridges in a disinfecting solution.**

Auxiliary items

The auxiliary items used in administration of local anesthesia are all used to prepare the injection site before the needle is inserted into the tissue.

Item	Use
2 × 2–inch gauze sponge	A sponge is used to dry the mucosa before applications of topical anesthetic and antiseptic. It is also used to gain a firm grasp for tissue retraction if necessary.
Cotton swabs	Swabs are used to apply the topical anesthetic and antiseptic.
Topical anesthetic	Before the injection, topical anesthetic is applied to the mucosa to reduce the discomfort of the needle penetration into the tissues.
Hemostat or cotton forceps	If the needle breaks, the hemostat or cotton forceps can be used to retrieve the broken needle.

Preparation of the Injection Site With Topical Anesthetic

For a summary of the steps followed in preparation of the injection site with a topical anesthetic agent, see Box 4-1.

Preparation of the Breech-Loading Aspirating Injection Syringe

A suggested sequence of preparing a breech-loading aspirating injection syringe for use is summarized in Box 4-2.

Recapping the Needle

It is a standard recommendation in medical practices to dispose of used needles immediately in a puncture-proof sharps container without recapping. This rule does not apply in dentistry for the administration of local anes-

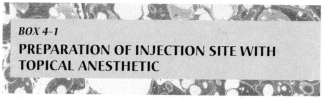

BOX 4-1

PREPARATION OF INJECTION SITE WITH TOPICAL ANESTHETIC

PROCEDURE	RATIONALE
1. Dry mucosa at injection site with 2 × 2–inch gauze sponge.	1. To clear site of saliva and other debris and for better visibility
2. Apply topical anesthetic with cotton swab. Wait 1 to 2 minutes for topical anesthetic to take effect.	2. To temporarily anesthetize surface tissue to minimize discomfort from inserting needle
3. Make injection.	3. To administer drug
4. Observe patient for any adverse effects.	4. Patient should be observed for possible reactions or problems to anesthetic
5. Record injection in patient's chart.	5. Record type of injection, side given, how much anesthetic was administered, and reactions to anesthetic

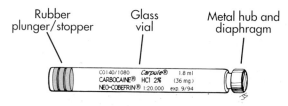

Figure 4-9   Carpule.

BOX 4-2

PREPARATION OF BREECH-LOADING ASPIRATING INJECTION SYRINGE

PROCEDURE	RATIONALE
1. Remove syringe from container; keep syringe in its sterilized packaging until ready to hold.	1. To prevent cross contamination
2. Retract piston.	2. To enable insertion of anesthetic cartridge
3. Insert cartridge by placing rubber stopper end toward harpoon.	3. To place cartridge in its proper orientation
4. Engage harpoon.	4. To allow for proper aspiration dring injection (NOTE: not necessary for self-aspirating syringes)
5. Use gentle pressure on thumb ring to engage harpoon.	5. Excessive force may break or crack glass cartridge
6. Pull back gently on thumb ring.	6. To check if harpoon is properly engaged in rubber stopper
7. Attach needle by breaking safety seal and removing white or clear plastic cap and screw into syringe.	7. To engage needle into syringe
8. Carefully remove colored plastic cap and expel a few drops of solution.	8. To determine if needle is engaged in cartridge and also to test syringe
9. Cover needle.	9. To prevent contamination until use

thetic because the local anesthetic may be injected into several areas and at different times during the appointment. Therefore state safety and health agencies recommend that the anesthetic needle be recapped immediately after it is removed from the patient's mouth. This step is also a safety measure to protect the dental assistant.

Recapping should be performed without risk of being stuck by the needle. A cap-holding device can be used to ensure safe recapping (Figure 4-10). Cotton forceps can be used in lieu of a cap-holding device (Figure 4-11). Another acceptable method for recapping a needle is to use a one-handed "scoop" technique (Figure 4-12).

Once the procedure is finished, the contaminated needle should be removed from the syringe and placed in a

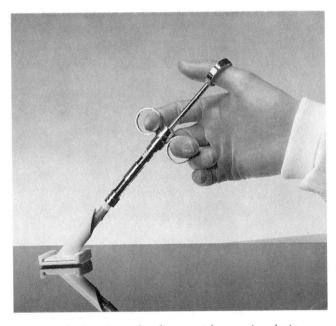

Figure 4-10   Example of approved recapping device.
(Courtesy Palco/Palermo Dental Manufacturing, Stratford, Conn.)

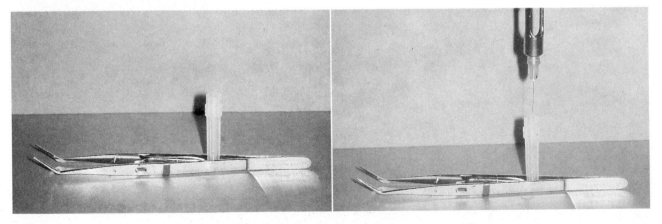

Figure 4-11   Cotton forceps used for recapping needle.

puncture-proof sharps container (Figure 4-13). The Centers for Disease Control and Prevention (CDC) recommend not bending, breaking, or otherwise manipulating a contaminated needle before throwing it away. Unnecessary manipulation of a contaminated needle may result in inadvertent puncture.

> ## ◆◆ KEY POINTS
> - Avoid recapping a used needle with one hand holding the cap and the other holding the needle. Instead, use a one-handed technique or a cap holding device.
> - Do not bend, break, or otherwise manipulate a used needle before throwing it away.

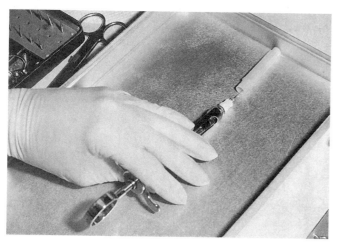

Figure 4-12 One-handed scoop technique for recapping needle.

Unloading the Breech-Loading Aspirating Syringe

Instructions on how to unload a breech-loading aspirating syringe are presented in Box 4-3. If the needle is inadvertently touched to a nonsterile surface at any time before the injection, it should be discarded and replaced with a new sterile needle.

Hidden Syringe Transfer

A technique for transferring the anesthetic syringe to the dentist out of the patient's view is discussed in Chapter 15.

Placement of Topical Anesthesia

Table 4-4 and Figure 4-14 demonstrate the correct placement of topical anesthesia.

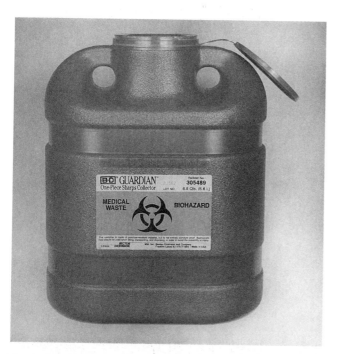

Figure 4-13 Sharps container for needles and other devices, as designated by U.S. Occupational Safety and Health Administration (OSHA) guidelines.

(Courtesy Becton-Dickinson, Franklin Lakes, N.J.)

BOX 4-3
UNLOADING OF BREECH-LOADING ASPIRATING SYRINGE

PROCEDURE	RATIONALE
1. Retract piston.	1. To allow for removal of cartridge
2. With your thumb and forefinger pull cartridge away from needle and remove cartridge.	2. To disengage cartridge from needle
3. Discard used cartridge and carefully unscrew recapped needle and dispose in an appropriate sharps container.	3. To avoid sharps injury
4. Do not bend, break, or otherwise manipulate needle before discarding.	4. Guidelines recommended by CDC; manipulation of needle more than necessary can result in inadvertent injury

Table 4-4 Topical anesthesia placement

Injections	Placement
Maxillary	
Subperiosteal "local infiltration"	In vestibule near root of tooth to be anesthetized
Posterior superior alveolar (PSA) nerve block	Behind last maxillary molar in vestibule
Middle superior alveolar (MSA) nerve block	Above maxillary second premolar in vestibule
Infraorbital nerve block (anterior superior alveolar [ASA] nerve block)	Above maxillary first premolar in vestibule NOTE: may be placed in mucobuccal fold mesial to canine eminence
Nasopalatine nerve block	Lateral to incisive papilla, at or near incisive foramen, which is behind maxillary central incisors
Greater palatine nerve block	To tissue overlying posterior palatine foramen; usually located on hard palate near apex of maxillary second molar
Mandibular	
Inferior alveolar (mandibular) nerve block	Above retromolar pad area between maxillary and mandibular teeth
Buccal nerve block	Distal and buccal to last mandibular molar
Mental/incisive nerve block	In vestibule, at or near mental foramen, usually between first and second mandibular premolars

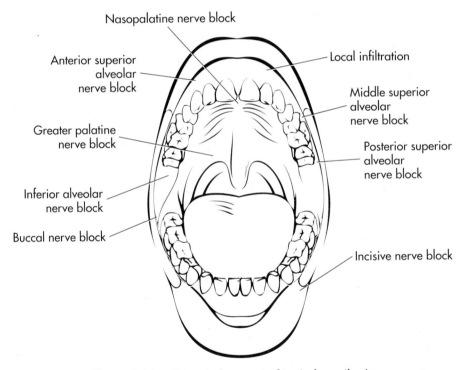

Figure 4-14   Correct placement of topical anesthesia.

Standard Injection Sites

Table 4-5 discusses the areas anesthetized by standard injection sites. The injection sites are depicted in Figure 4-14. The areas anesthetized by the standard local anesthetic injections are shown in Figure 4-15.

Supplementary injections are sometimes given to the patient when the circumstances indicate such a need (Table 4-6).

PREMEDICATION

Premedication is the administration of a drug before the actual treatment of the patient. It can also be an adjustment of the dosage of a drug that the patient is already taking routinely for a systemic disorder. Premedication is most frequently employed to control apprehension. However, it may be necessary to administer certain drugs to protect the patient from the undesirable effects of a procedure or to improve working conditions for the opera-

Table 4–5 Standard injection sites

Injection	Teeth anesthetized	Tissue anesthetized	Needle
Subperiosteal injection (local infiltration)	One or two teeth in area injected	Buccal tissue in area of injection	Short
Posterior superior alveolar (PSA) nerve block	First, second, and third maxillary molars on side injected (this injection does not anesthetize entire first molar)	Buccal tissue of maxillary molars on side injected	Short
Middle superior alveolar (MSA) nerve block	First and second maxillary premolars. A portion of first molar	Buccal tissue of maxillary premolars and part of first molar on side injected	Short
Infraorbital nerve block (anterior superior alveolar [ASA] nerve block)	Maxillary central incisor, lateral incisor, and cuspid on side injected. Maxillary premolars and part of first molar (72% of patients)	Buccal tissue in same area of side injected	Short
Nasopalatine nerve block (incisive nerve block)	Does not anesthetize teeth	Palatal tissue from cuspid to cuspid	Short
Greater palatine nerve block	Does not anesthetize teeth	Posterior potion of hard palate on side injected	Short
Inferior alveolar nerve block (mandibular block)	Mandibular teeth on side of injection	Buccal tissue for mandibular premolars, cuspids, and incisors on side injected	Long
Buccal nerve block	Does not anesthetize teeth	Buccal tissue of mandibular molars on side injected	Short
Incisive nerve block (sometimes called mental nerve block)	Mandibular premolars, cuspids, and incisors on side injected	Buccal tissue of mandibular premolars, cuspids, and incisors on side injected. Lower lip and chin	Short

Table 4–6 Supplementary injection of anesthesia

Injection	Uses	Technique
Periodontal ligament injection (intraligamentary injection)	Usually used to anesthesize single mandibular teeth	Needle inserted directly into periodontal ligament. Needle may be bent for access
Intrapulpal injection	Often used for endodontics to obtain pulpal anesthesia after pulp chamber has been exposed	Anesthesia injected directly into exposed pulp chamber or canal
Intraosseous injection	Used when there is difficulty achieving pulpal anesthesia	Incision must be made in gingiva and a small round bur used to make an opening in bone. Anesthesia deposited directly into opening in bone

tor. This section discusses some of the most common uses of premedication in general dentistry.

Agents to Control Apprehension

Even though dentistry has eliminated pain in most routine procedures, some dental patients are apprehensive about receiving dental services. If the dentist considers the patient's apprehension great enough to interfere with the proposed treatment, premedication of the patient with an antianxiety agent is indicated.

The decision to premedicate a patient for any purpose must be based on a study of a patient's general health. Such information is acquired during the medical-dental history inquiry. This information, coupled with the dentist's knowledge of the effects of drugs on vital systems of the body, leads the dentist to a decision on the advisability of premedication.

Preoperative sedation can be achieved with narcotics, barbiturates, benzodiazephines, and nitrous oxide analgesia.

Barbiturates

Barbiturates are principally sedative agents, whereas narcotics are generally analgesics. Barbiturates have become popular in dentistry for preoperative anxiety control. Short-acting barbiturates such as pentobarbital (Nembutal) and secobarbital (Seconal) are usually the drugs of choice.

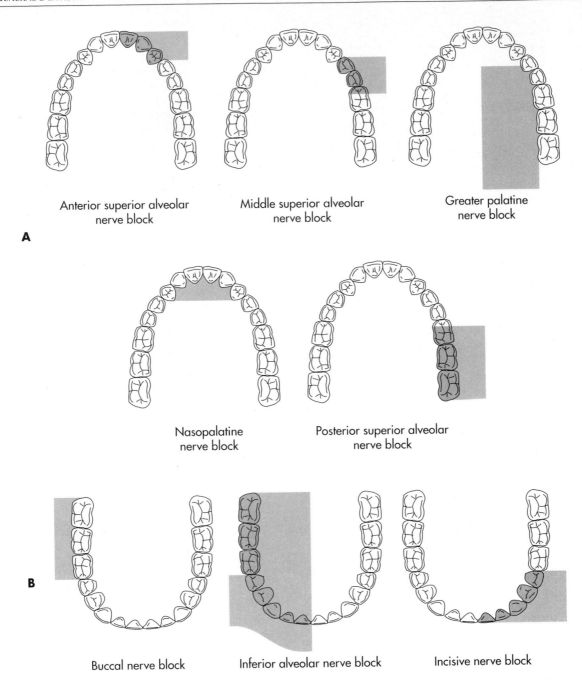

Anterior superior alveolar nerve block

Middle superior alveolar nerve block

Greater palatine nerve block

A

Nasopalatine nerve block

Posterior superior alveolar nerve block

B

Buccal nerve block

Inferior alveolar nerve block

Incisive nerve block

Figure 4-15   Areas anesthetized for standard local anesthetic injections. **A,** Mandibular. **B,** Maxillary.

Narcotic Agents

Narcotic agents are useful drugs for preoperative sedation in the presence of severe preoperative pain. They are effective for anxiety relief and even more so for pain relief (analgesia). Morphine sulfate and meperidine hydrochloride (Demerol) are examples of such narcotic agents. Use of narcotic agents for anxiety has become less popular with the development of newer sedative agents. However, narcotics are still used widely for the relief of pain.

Benzodiazepines

Benzodiazepines are useful for preoperative anxiety control. They do not produce the hangover effect often seen when barbiturates are taken, and they are considered the drug of choice for the relief of anxiety. Benzodiazepines also present less of a pharmacological risk to the patient. Probably the most common benzodiazepines are chlordiazepoxide (Librium) and diazepam (Valium). Flurazepam, temazepam, triazolam, lorazepam,

BOX 4-4

ADMINISTRATION OF NITROUS OXIDE ANALGESIA

PROCEDURE	RATIONALE	PROCEDURE	RATIONALE
1. Check medical history for contraindications.	1. Certain conditions such as claustrophobia, emphysema, bronchitis, pregnancy, or upper respiratory tract infections may preclude use of nitrous oxide analgesia	6. Recline patient in dental chair, start flow of oxygen, and place hood over patient's nose.	6. If oxygen flow is started after placement of nasal hood, patient may feel "suffocated"
2. Take and record baseline vital signs.	2. In event of emergency, vital signs taken before nitrous oxide administration will help indicate severity of emergency	7. Adjust oxygen flow according to patient comfort.	7. Oxygen flow individualized for each patient
3. Administer baseline Trieger test to patient.	3. Given before and after nitrous oxide administration to evaluate residual effects of gas	8. Authorized personnel begins administration of nitrous gas to patient, and dental treatment is started.	8. Refer to state dental practice act for authorized personnel
4. Give patient instructions: Breathe through nose at all times. Avoid excessive talking or laughing. In case of extreme discomfort do not take off nasal hood. A 100% flush system administered through nasal hood will help patient recover faster if termination of nitrous oxide is desired.	4. To prevent escape of gases into surrounding environment	9. Observe patient at all times during procedure.	9. Patient must never be left alone during nitrous oxide administration
		10. At end of procedure, terminate flow of nitrous gas, but continue flow of oxygen gas. Give patient 100% oxygen for 3 to 5 minutes.	10. To reverse action of nitrous oxide
		11. After oxygenating patient, administer postprocedural Trieger test.	11. To evaluate whether patient has recovered from effects of nitrous oxide; patient may require more time breathing 100% oxygen
5. Request that patient visit restroom if necessary.	5. To avoid interruptions during administration	12. Verbally check patient for signs of recovery.	12. Answers such as "I feel normal" are good indicators of recovery
		13. Record nitrous oxide administration in patient's chart.	

and nitrazepam are other examples of the benzodiazepine group.

Benzodiazepines are given orally approximately 1 hour before the appointment time. Caution must be exercised in prescribing any of these drugs because the effects last up to 4 hours. This effect creates a distinct disadvantage for patients because they must be escorted to and from the dental office under the influence of the drug. Another disadvantage is that the effect of the drug lasts longer than is needed in most instances. Some of the drugs used to allay anxiety and apprehension can be addictive. However, if these drugs are used properly, little danger of addiction exists with normal use.

Combinations of various sedatives are sometimes selected to achieve a sedative effect. Demerol compound is such a drug. It is a combination of meperidine (Demerol), promethazine (Phenergan), and chlorpromazine (Thorazine). Demerol is effective for use in children younger than 13 years. The dosage is calculated according to the child's body weight.

Nitrous Oxide Analgesia

Nitrous oxide analgesia, or "tranquilizing air" as it is sometimes called, can be used as a convenient preoperative sedative. Nitrous oxide is a general anesthetic that has been available since approximately 1844. Although early use of nitrous oxide gas was crude by today's standards, it was the most popular anesthetic used by dentists until local anesthesia was developed around 1905. Local anesthesia rapidly gained popularity and virtually eliminated the use of nitrous oxide as an anesthetic in dental practice.

Nitrous oxide has slowly regained popularity in dental practice, not as an anesthetic but as a means of sedating a patient and raising the pain reaction threshold while the patient remains conscious. The goal of nitrous oxide analgesia is to provide sedation for the patient immediately before the dental procedure begins. Other means of achieving sedation by the use of oral agents require that the patient take the medication well in advance of the dental appointment. Although intravenous sedatives eliminate this problem, they require an injection procedure that is often objectionable to an apprehensive patient. Nitrous oxide can be administered continually to maintain sedation throughout the dental procedure. After completion of the dental treatment, the nitrous oxide is discontinued, and the patient returns to a normal alert status and can usually drive home safely. This prompt return to alertness is not possible with oral sedatives. In short, the use of nitrous oxide is convenient for both the dentist and the patient (Box 4-4).

Since nitrous oxide is a gaseous substance, it is administered with a gas machine that mixes it with oxygen and delivers it to the patient through a nosepiece (Figure 4-16).

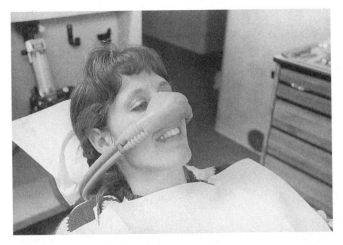

Figure 4-16 Disposable or sterilizable mask is placed securely over patient's nose to administer nitrous oxide.

(Courtesy Helen Zylman, DDS, Ann Arbor, Mich.)

The patient inhales this mixture, and sedation results. The mixture commonly used is approximately 35% nitrous oxide and 65% oxygen. The mixture is almost odorless and not unpleasant for the patient.

After the nitrous oxide enters the lungs, it is absorbed into the bloodstream and depresses the central nervous system. The degree of central nervous system depression is controlled by the mixture of gases delivered to the patient. Patients in the analgesic state created by nitrous oxide have the following characteristics:

1. They are still conscious, communicative, and cooperative.
2. They are relaxed, breathe normally, and can hold their mouth open voluntarily.
3. They have an elevated pain reaction threshold and do not react to a minor pain stimulus such as the injection of a local anesthetic.

This state of analgesia produced by nitrous oxide is very safe because the patient remains conscious, yet protective reflex mechanisms such as the cough reflex and eye blinking remain. The patient may have a feeling of profound relaxation; tingling in the fingers, toes, and tongue; and a general feeling of well-being. It is recommended that all dentists and auxiliary personnel experience nitrous oxide analgesia if it is to be used in the office. This experience will help them reassure patients about the effects of nitrous oxide.

After completion of treatment the flow of nitrous oxide is discontinued, and only oxygen is delivered through the nosepiece for approximately 3 to 5 minutes. Some patients may require more time to "clear," or completely recover. Recovery should be assessed by the following methods:

1. The patient claims to feel normal.
2. Blood pressure, pulse rate, and respiratory rate are similar to the values recorded before nitrous oxide was administered.
3. The patient successfully completes a Trieger test.

The **Trieger test** is designed to assess the psychomotor ability of the patient. The test is first given before nitrous oxide is administered and again after the patient has been cleared to provide comparative results. Both tests are conducted with the patient positioned in an upright position to standardize the test conditions. The patient is given a clipboard with a test sheet containing a pattern of dots (Figure 4-17, *A*) and is asked to connect the dots with a pencil (Figure 4-17, *B*). When the "before" and "after" tests are comparable, recovery is complete. If the tests are not comparable, the clearing time should be extended until they are.

Premedication to Protect the Patient

Sometimes patients have systemic disorders that require continued use of certain drugs to maintain their health.

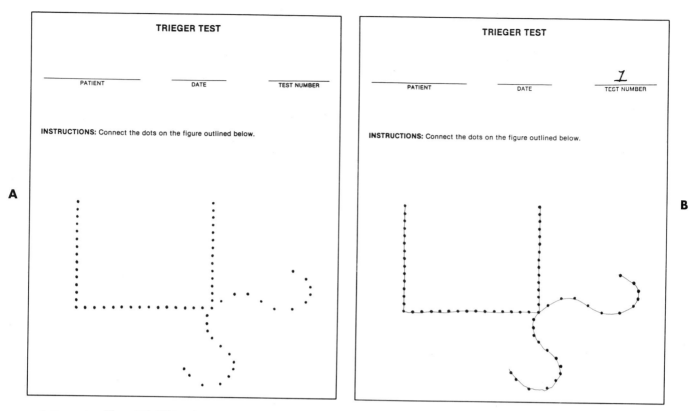

Figure 4-17   Trieger test. **A**, Sample test sheet. **B**, Initial test of ability to connect dots before administration of nitrous oxide.

Table 4-7   Recommended standard prophylactic regimen for adults and children to prevent bacterial endocarditis

Medication	Child or adult	Initial dose	Follow-up dose
Amoxicillin V* (oral)	Adult	3.0 g 1 hour before procedure	1.5 g 6 hours after initial dose
	Child	50 mg/kg of body weight 1 hour before procedure	Half of initial dose 6 hours after initial dose
Erythromycin stearate (oral)	Adult	1.0 g 2 hours before the procedure	500 mg 6 hours after initial dose
	Child	20 mg/kg of body weight 1 hour before procedure	Half of initial dose 6 hours after initial dose
Clindamycin (oral)	Adult	300 mg 1 hour before procedure	150 mg 6 hours after initial dose
	Child	10 mg/kg of body weight 1 hour before procedure	Half of initial dose 6 hours after initial dose

Modified with permission from Dajani AS and others: Prevention of bacterial endocarditis, *JAMA* 264(22):2919-2922, 1990. Copyright 1990, American Medical Association.

*Amoxicillin is now recommended because it is better absorbed and provides higher sustained serum levels. However, the use of penicillin rather than amoxicillin is rational and acceptable.

Table 4-8   Recommended antibiotic regimen for adults and children with total joint replacements

Medication	Initial dose	Follow-up dose
Cephalexin (Keflex)	2 g orally 1 hour before procedure	1 g 6 hours after initial dose
Clindamycin (Cleocin): for persons allergic to cephalexin	600 mg orally 1 hour before procedure	600 mg 6 hours after initial dose

Modified from Cioffi GA, Terezhalmy GT, Taybos GM: Total joint replacement: a consideration for antimicrobial prophylaxis, *Oral Surg Oral Med Oral Pathol* 66(1):124-129, 1988.

Examples of such conditions include diabetes, epilepsy, hypothyroidism, hypertension, coronary thrombosis, and rheumatic heart disease. The medical-dental history taken at the diagnostic appointment reveals these conditions and the medications taken to control them. Dentists often work with patients' physicians to regulate dosages of these drugs at the time dental treatment is being done. For example, patients who are taking anticoagulants (blood-thinning agents) must have the dosage carefully regulated to prevent problems of bleeding after oral surgical procedures.

Patients with rheumatic heart disease, mitral valve prolapse, or various blood diseases that make them extremely vulnerable to severe systemic infections must be premedicated with antibiotics to protect them against transient bacteremias. Taking antibiotics before dental procedures to prevent bacteremias is called **prophylactic premedication.** A transient bacteremia (bacteria in the blood) can occur as a result of the entry of organisms into the bloodstream through ruptured oral soft tissues. Not only do obvious procedures such as oral surgery allow bacteria from the oral cavity to enter the bloodstream, but also a routine cleaning of the teeth can cause bacteremia. Bacteremias can lead to a serious and life-threatening infection of the heart called **subacute bacterial endocarditis.** Table 4-7 depicts the recommended prophylactic regimen for the prevention of bacterial endocarditis.

Prophylactic antibiotics are also needed for patients who have received a total joint replacement (Table 4-8). Transient bacteremias can cause rejection of the replacement joint.

Premedication for Operator Convenience

Certainly preoperative sedative agents provide convenience for the dentist, since the apprehensive patient is rendered more cooperative; but there are other agents helpful in controlling problems such as excessive salivation, gagging, and muscle spasm, which create technical difficulties for the operating team.

Excessive salivation occurs in patients with extremely active salivary glands. It can create difficulty in isolation of the operative field. This problem is of particular significance in procedures for which a rubber dam cannot be used, such as surgery and impression-taking. Premedication with an agent such as propantheline (Pro-Banthine), atropine, or scopolamine will decrease the secretion from the salivary glands temporarily while the dental procedure is accomplished.

Gagging can be a problem during restorative, surgical, and radiographic procedures. Nitrous oxide analgesia reduces the gag reflex significantly. Simply applying a topical anesthetic to the mucosa in the posterior regions of the mouth is of temporary assistance for short procedures. A topical anesthetic is especially useful for taking radiographs of posterior regions of the mouth, when contact of the film packet with the mucosa triggers the gag reflex.

Sometimes patients appear for dental treatment when their muscles of mastication are in a state of constant contraction, or spasm. This condition is often so profound that patients cannot open their mouths wide enough for the dentist to correct the intraoral cause of the spasm. Other patients experience problems of muscle spasms or cramping during dental procedures because of fatigue caused by holding the mouth open. The dentist can often overcome this problem by prescribing skeletal muscle relaxants such as methocarbamol (Robaxin), diazepam (Valium), or orphenadrine (Norflex) preoperatively. Nitrous oxide analgesia has also been useful in circumventing this problem.

BIBLIOGRAPHY

Allen GD: *Dental anesthesia and analgesia (local and general)*, ed 2, Baltimore, 1979, Williams & Wilkins.

Chasteen JE, Hatch R, Passon JC: Contamination of local anesthetic cartridges with acrylic monomer, *JADA* 116:375, 1988.

Jastak JT, Malamed SF: Nitrous oxide and sexual phenomena, *JADA* 101:38, 1980.

Jastak JT, Paravecchio R: An analysis of 1331 sedations using inhalation, intravenous, and other techniques, *JADA* 91:1241, 1975.

Lambert C: Sexual phenomena, hypnosis, and nitrous oxide sedation, *JADA* 105:990, 1982.

Malamed SF: *Handbook of local anesthesia*, ed 3, St Louis, 1991, Mosby.

Malamed SF: *Sedation: a guide to patient management*, ed 3, St Louis, 1995, Mosby.

Requa-Clark B, Holroyd SV: *Applied pharmacology for the dental hygienist*, ed 3, St Louis, 1995, Mosby.

Shannon IL, Wescott WB: Alcohol contamination of local anesthetic cartridges, *J Acad Gen Dent* 22:20, 1974.

LOCAL ANESTHESIA PRACTICE EXAM

Assume the following:

- For composite or amalgam fillings, anesthesia is required only for the tooth.
- For gold or porcelain crowns, anesthesia is required for the tooth and the surrounding gingiva.
- For scaling and root planing, anesthesia is required only for the gingiva surrounding the teeth to be scaled.

Type of procedure	Type of injection	Long or short needle?
1. #2 MOD amalgam		
2. #2 and #3 full gold crown		
3. #2 and #3 MO amalgam		
4. #5 O amalgam		
5. #3 full gold crown		
6. #4 and #5 full gold crown		
7. #8 D composite		
8. #13 full porcelain crown		
9. #18 MOD amalgam		
10. #18, #19, and #20		
11. #19 full gold crown		
12. #22 D composite		
13. #24 full gold crown		
14. #29 MO amalgam		
15. #29 full gold crown		
16. Scale and root plane upper right quadrant		
17. Scale and root plane lower left quadrant		
18. Scale and root plane upper anterior teeth		

Note: Answers are found on p. 471.

QUESTIONS–Chapter 4

1. The type of anesthetic agent that numbs the surface of the skin or mucous membrane is called:
   a. Topical anesthetic
   b. Local anesthetic
   c. General anesthetic

2. The type of anesthesia that is used to numb a main nerve trunk is called:
   a. Infiltration anesthesia
   b. Nerve block anesthesia
   c. Field block anesthesia

3. A vasoconstrictor that is added to the local anesthetic solution will _____ the duration of the anesthetic agent.
   a. Prolong
   b. Shorten

4. The higher the gauge number for the needle, the larger the diameter of the opening of the needle is. A long needle is used for mandibular nerve block injections.
   a. Both statements are true.
   b. The first statement is true, and the second statement is false.
   c. The first statement is false, and the second statement is true.
   d. Both statements are false.

5. All the following are appropriate instructions for a patient receiving nitrous oxide analgesia *except*:
   (1) Breathe through the nose.
   (2) Avoid excessive talking.
   (3) Avoid excessive laughing.
   (4) Take off the mask if discomfort is felt.
      a. (1) and (3)
      b. (2) and (4)
      c. (1), (2), and (3)
      d. (4) only

6. Which of the following is the standard regimen for prophylactic premedication?
   a. Amoxicillin, 3 g orally 1 hour before the appointment and 1.5 g 6 hours after the initial dose
   b. Amoxicillin, 3 g orally 1 hour before the appointment and 1.5 g 6 hours after the appointment
   c. Penicillin, 3 g orally 1 hour before the appointment and 1.5 g 6 hours after the initial dose
   d. Penicillin, 3 g orally 1 hour before the appointment and 1.5 g 6 hours after the appointment

7. The anesthetic needle _____ be bent before it is discarded into a sharps container to avoid IV drug users from taking the used needles from the trash.
   a. Should
   b. Should not

8. What kind of injection anesthetizes the upper anterior teeth and the accompanying buccal tissue:
   a. Anterior superior alveolar (ASA)
   b. Middle superior alveolar (MSA)
   c. Inferior alveolar (IA) or mandibular block
   d. Nasopalatine

9. What kind of injection anesthetizes the lower anterior teeth and the buccal tissue opposite the molar teeth?
   a. Anterior superior alveolar (ASA)
   b. Middle superior alveolar (MSA)
   c. Inferior alveolar (IA) or mandibular block
   d. Nasopalatine

10. What kind of injection anesthetizes the gingiva on the hard palate anterior to the maxillary cuspids?
   a. Anterior superior alveolar (ASA)
   b. Middle superior alveolar (MSA)
   c. Inferior alveolar (IA) or mandibular block
   d. Nasopalatine

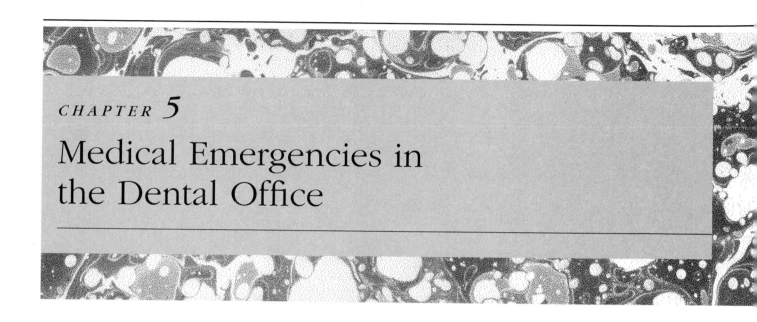

CHAPTER 5

Medical Emergencies in the Dental Office

KEY TERMS

Allergic reaction
Ambu bag (bag-valve-mask device)
Angina pectoris
Aspirate
Asthma
Cardiac arrest
Cardiopulmonary resuscitation (CPR)
Cerebrovascular accident (CVA)
Cricothyrotomy
Epilepsy
Heimlich maneuver
Hyperventilation
Hypoglycemia
Magill intubation forceps
Myocardial infarct (heart attack)
Positive-pressure oxygen
Sphygmomanometer
Supine
Syncope (fainting)
Trendelenburg position (subsupine)

Life-threatening emergencies can and do occur occasionally in the dental office. The dental team is responsible for providing emergency treatment to safeguard the lives and welfare of patients until a physician can attend to them. In many emergencies the initial treatment is most important in prevention of tragedy.

The dental team must be well prepared to handle such emergencies. Preparation includes a basic knowledge of emergency care, emergency equipment and supplies, a knowledge of the patient's medical history, and a preplanned approach to handling unexpected emergencies.

The greatest emphasis in the discussion of emergency treatments should be placed on the techniques of providing the collapsed patient with an oxygen supply to the brain. In all medical emergencies the ABCs of first aid must be remembered and exercised:

A = Airway—establish an open airway

B = Breathing—establish respiration, if needed, with resuscitative measures

C = Circulation—support circulation with external cardiac compression and cardiovascular drugs

All other treatment measures are secondary to these ABCs, which can save a life.

> ➥ **KEY POINT**
> - For all medical emergencies, the ABC rule should be followed:
>   A = Airway
>   B = Breathing
>   C = Circulation

MEDICAL HISTORY

The old saying "Know your patient" certainly applies to emergency care. This knowledge can be gained by taking a thorough medical history at the first appointment and updating it at each visit. The medical history is a useful tool for the operating team in handling emergencies. It reveals known systemic conditions that make a patient a more likely candidate for an emergency situation. Probably the greatest problem to overcome in a medical crisis is panic. If the dentist and the assistant lose control in a medical crisis, the crisis worsens. Panic is usually a product of surprise and unpreparedness. There is no excuse for being unprepared for medical emergencies. The element of surprise can be reduced by knowing the patient's medical history. This knowledge creates some degree of anticipation of a possible emergency. If a patient has a history of epilepsy, the operating team should anticipate the possibility of a convulsive episode while the patient is in the dental office. A prepared operating team is ready to handle any emergency. Even patients with a favorable medical history can surprise an operating team with an unexpected emergency.

The medical history also assists the dentist in selecting the proper treatment as quickly as possible. If a patient with a history of a heart condition such as angina pectoris complains of chest pains, nitroglycerin should be administered immediately. Time is of utmost value in many serious emergencies. Proper diagnosis and prompt treatment can save valuable time and prevent unnecessary harm to patients.

The history can also reveal allergies and medications the patient is already taking, which influences the dentist's choice of drugs for emergency treatment.

It is often the responsibility of the dental auxiliary to update the medical history. The patient is usually asked if there are any changes in his or her medical history after being seated by the dental assistant. Changes reported by the patient should be noted in permanent ink in the patient's chart and reported to the dentist. Any medications or changes in medication may affect the patient's treatment because certain medications may be contraindicated with drugs or medications given to the patient for dental treatment. Information about unfamiliar medications can be obtained from a book called *Physicians GenRx*. This reference is updated annually and provides valuable information about prescription drug products. Information is provided about a drug's manufacturer, actions, usage, contraindications, warnings, precautions, and availability (Figure 5-1).

⚬ KEY POINT
- *Physicians GenRx* is a useful guide for information about unfamiliar medications.

STANDARD EMERGENCY EQUIPMENT

A recommended emergency armamentarium includes the following items, some of which are presented in Figure 5-2:

1. Oxygen supply (**positive-pressure oxygen**)
2. Emergency drug kit (Figure 5-2, *A*)
3. Blood pressure cuff
4. Stethoscope

Oxygen Supply
Positive-pressure oxygen

An oxygen supply is an essential part of any emergency setup. Any emergency that deprives the brain of oxygen for even a short time will require an oxygen supply. Most oxygen systems are easy to use. They consist of a pressurized oxygen tank, a regulator to control the flow of oxygen, and a hose and mask to deliver oxygen to the patient (see Figure 5-2, *B*). If the patient collapses and breathing is reduced, oxygen should be used. The mask is placed over the patient's nose and mouth, and the regulator is turned on. The patient breathes a higher concentration of oxygen than would be received by breathing room air. This compensates for the decreased oxygen intake that results from suppressed respiration. Oxygen therapy should be continued until the patient recovers completely. Oxygen levels in the oxygen tanks should be *checked daily* by a member of the dental team to ensure an adequate supply of oxygen is available when necessary.

Bag-valve-mask device

Not all dental emergencies occur in an area where the positive-pressure equipment is located or where the equipment can be transported quickly. Therefore it is necessary to have a portable, self-inflating manual resuscitator (**Ambu bag**) in reserve as a backup for such an emergency (see Figure 5-2, *C*).

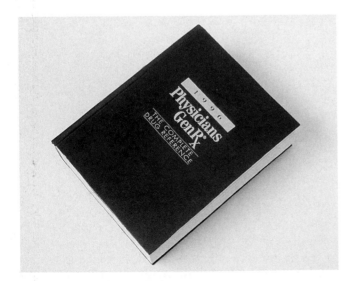

Figure 5-1   *Physicians GenRx: The Complete Drug Reference.*

Pocket mask

Pocket masks are similar to manual bag-valve-mask devices except that the rescuer uses his or her own exhaled air for resuscitation. The pocket mask provides the advantage of avoiding direct contact between the patient and the rescuer. Pocket masks are usually very small and inexpensive so that one can be provided for each mem-

ber of the dental team or placed in each treatment room (Figure 5-3).

Emergency Drug Kit

The emergency drug kit (see Figure 5-2, *A*) is a backup support system designed to provide a variety of drugs in convenient dosage forms for easy administration (Table

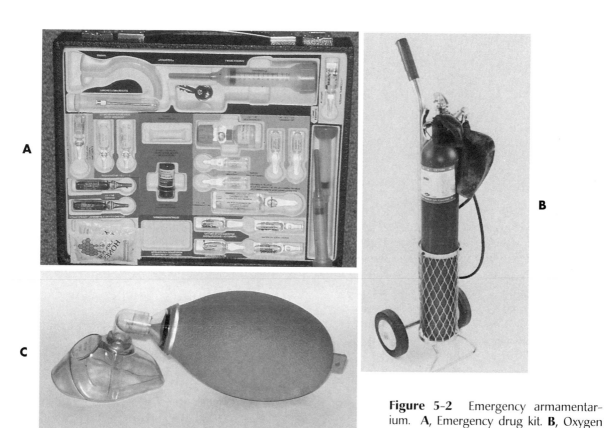

Figure 5-2   Emergency armamentarium.   **A**, Emergency drug kit. **B**, Oxygen unit. **C**, Manual resuscitator (Ambu bag).

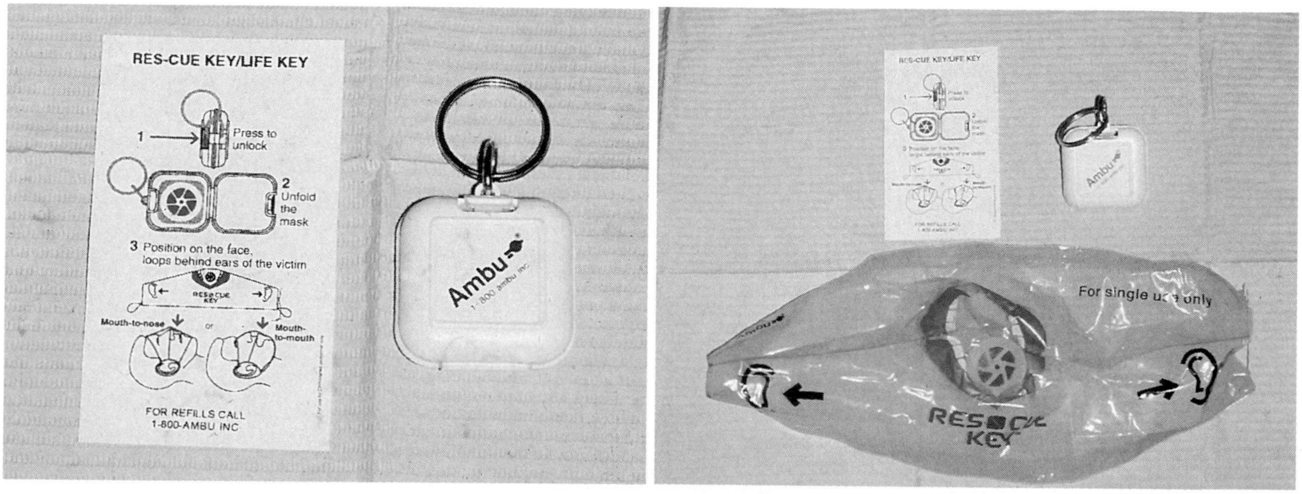

Figure 5-3   Key chain pocket mask.

Table 5-1 Available in the emergency kit

Drug	Types available	Purpose
Epinephrine (Adrenalin)	Injection	Allergic reactions Acute asthma attacks Cardiac arrest
Antihistamine	Injection	Allergy
Vasodilator (nitroglycerin or amyl nitrate)	Spray or tablets	Chest pain (angina) Heart attack
Anticonvulsant	Injection	Prolongation of seizures Hyperventilation
Analgesic (morphine)	Injection	Intense pain or anxiety Heart attack
Antihypoglycemic (dextrose)	Injection	Hypoglycemia
Corticosteroid (hydrocortisone)	Injection	Allergic reactions
Respiratory stimulant ("smelling salts"—aromatic ammonia)	Vapor capsule	Syncope (fainting) Respiratory depression
Antihypoglycemic (sugar)	Beverage, tube frosting, or granulated sugar	Hypoglycemia
Bronchodilator	Inhaler	Asthma

5-1). These kits include syringes and needles needed to administer the drugs and a reference chart to determine proper dosage and route of administration quickly for each drug in the kit. Expiration dates should be checked *at least once each week* by a member of the dental staff. Any drugs that are used from the kit are replaced immediately. It would be a tragedy to discover during an emergency that a badly needed drug was missing from the kit or had passed the expiration date when it could have been used to save a patient's life.

Equipment used in the emergency kit is listed below. The kit must be kept where it is readily accessible to all dental personnel.

Name	Purpose
Oxygen delivery system	Any type of respiratory distress
Suction and suction tips	Aspiration of foreign objects, vomit, blood
Tourniquets	For intravenous (IV) drug administration
Syringes	For injection of drugs
Magill intubation forceps	For removing items blocking the airway
Scalpel or cricothyrotomy needle	To perform a cricothyrotomy for anaphylaxis
Artificial airway	To maintain the victim's airway

Stethoscope and Blood Pressure Cuff

The stethoscope and blood pressure cuff (**sphygmomanometer**) are of value to monitor the patient's blood pressure. Box 5-1 describes the procedure for taking a pa-

tient's blood pressure. A baseline reading should be taken at the patient's first visit and recorded in the medical history. Cuffs of different sizes should be available to fit children and obese patients.

COMMON MEDICAL EMERGENCIES

Many medical emergencies can occur while a patient is in the dental office. Some emergencies are more common than others. It is helpful if the dentist can diagnose the condition causing an emergency. However, it is not necessary that the specific cause of the emergency be determined before treatment is started. It is far more important to diagnose the patient's physical status than to determine the cause of the emergency. For example, if a patient stops breathing, it is more important to begin respiratory support than to determine why breathing has stopped.

All office personnel should be prepared in the event of an emergency. All staff should practice emergency drills. Specific predefined duties can be assigned to each member of the dental team to ensure an efficient response to the emergency. Box 5-2 presents an example of duties that can be assigned to three dental team members.

> ** KEY POINT**
> - The dental office should practice emergency drills on a regular basis. Periodic practice is also necessary for a quick and appropriate response to an emergency.

The telephone number of the emergency medical system should be attached to every telephone in the office.

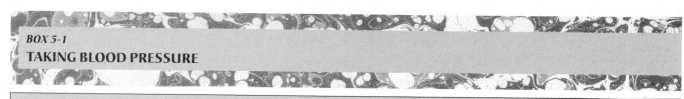

BOX 5-1

TAKING BLOOD PRESSURE

ARMAMENTARIUM

- Blood pressure cuff or sphygmomanometer
- Stethoscope

PROCEDURE	RATIONALE
1. Determine the proper cuff size.	1. The proper cuff size is necessary so that the correct amount of pressure is applied over the artery. The bladder width should be 40% to 50% of the upper arm circumference. Bladder width multiplied by 2.5 defines the ideal arm circumference (e.g., the ideal arm circumference for a bladder width of 15 cm is 15 × 2.5 = 37.5 cm). Cuffs that are too small for a patient's arm produce artificially high blood pressure readings; cuffs that are too large produce artificially low readings.
2. Wash hands with antimicrobial soap.	2. Washing reduces the chances of transmitting infectious microorganisms.
3. Explain the purpose of the procedure.	3. Explanations reassure the patient. Ideally, the patient should not have eaten or smoked 30 minutes before the procedure. The dental assistant must attempt to obtain a blood pressure reading that is representative of the patient's blood pressure under "ordinary" circumstances. The blood pressure should be taken in a quiet area after 5 minutes of rest by the patient. Screen the patient

PROCEDURE	RATIONALE
	for other environmental or biological factors, such as anxiety, distention of the urinary bladder, exertion, pain, changes in climate temperatures, and prescribed drugs or other medications that also may influence blood pressure measurements.
4. Assist the patient to a comfortable sitting position, with arm slightly flexed, forearm supported, and palm turned up.	4. This position facilitates cuff application. Having the arm above heart level would produce a falsely low reading.
5. Expose the upper arm fully.	5. Exposing the upper arm ensures proper cuff application.
6. Palpate the brachial artery. Position the cuff approximately 1 inch above the brachial artery.	6. Proper positioning of the cuff facilitates an accurate reading.
7. Center the arrows marked on the cuff over the brachial artery.	7. Inflating the bladder directly over the brachial artery ensures that proper pressure is applied during inflation.
8. Be sure the cuff is fully deflated. Wrap the cuff evenly and snugly around the upper arm.	8. This ensures that proper pressure will be applied over the artery.
9. Be sure the manometer is positioned at eye level.	9. Eye level placement ensures accurate reading of mercury level.
10. If the patient's normal systolic pressure is not	10. This determines the maximal inflation point

Assessment procedure modified from Potter PA, Perry AG: *Fundamentals of nursing*, ed 3, St Louis, 1993, Mosby, pp 588-589. Description of Korotkoff sounds reproduced and modified with permission from *Recommendations for human blood pressure determination by sphygmomanometers: report of a special task force appointed by the steering committee, American Heart Association*, New York, 1987, The Association, p 4. Copyright American Heart Association.

Continued

BOX 5-1

TAKING BLOOD PRESSURE—*cont'd*

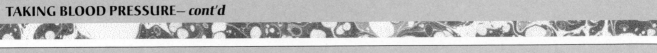

PROCEDURE	RATIONALE
known, palpate the radial artery and inflate the cuff to the point at which radial pulsation disappears. Deflate the cuff and wait 30 seconds.	and prevents auscultatory gap. The 30-second delay prevents venous congestion and falsely high readings.
11. Place the stethoscope earpieces in the ears and be sure sounds are clear, not muffled.	11. Each earpiece should follow the angle of the examiner's ear canal to facilitate hearing.
12. Place the diaphragm (or the bell) of the stethoscope over the brachial artery.	12. Proper stethoscope placement ensures optimal sound reception. The American Heart Association recommends use of the bell for hearing low-pitched Korotkoff sounds clearly.
13. Close the valve of the pressure bulb clockwise until tight.	13. Tightening the valve prevents air leak during inflation.
14. Inflate the cuff to 30 mm Hg above the patient's normal systolic level.	14. Proper cuff inflation ensures accurate pressure measurement.
15. Slowly release the valve, allowing the mercury to fall at a rate of 2 to 3 mm Hg per second.	15. Too rapid or slow a decline in the mercury level may lead to an inaccurate reading.
16. Note the point on the manometer at which the first two consecutive beats are heard.	16. The first Korotkoff sound (heart sound) indicates the systolic pressure. Blood pressure levels should be recorded in even numbers.
17. Continue cuff deflation, noting the point on the manometer at which sound muffles (phase IV) for children or when the sound disappears	17. The American Heart Association recommends recording the fifth Korotkoff sound as the diastolic pressure in adults. In certain patients, such

PROCEDURE	RATIONALE
(phase V) for adults.	as children, the Korotkoff sounds do not disappear and may be heard until the pressure in the cuff falls near to 0 mm Hg. Therefore phase IV, which is a muffled pulse sound heard before the last pulse sound, is a more reliable index for children.
18. Deflate the cuff rapidly. To determine an average blood pressure and to ensure a correct reading, wait 30 seconds and then repeat the procedure for the same arm.	18. Continuous cuff inflation causes arterial occlusion, resulting in numbness and tingling in the patient's arm. The delay prevents venous congestion and falsely high readings and provides an accurate assessment of the patient's blood pressure. The blood pressure reading is repeated on the same arm because there may be as much as 10 mm Hg difference in readings between arms.
19. Remove the cuff from the client's arm. Assist the patient to a comfortable position and cover upper arm.	19. This maintains the patient's comfort.
20. Fold the cuff and store it properly in a cool, dry place.	20. Proper maintenance of supplies contributes to instrument accuracy. Sunlight and heat may compromise rubber tubing.
21. Calculate the average of the two blood pressure readings. Record on the patient's chart the average blood pressure, the date, cuff size, and which arm was used for measurement.	21. Vital signs should be recorded immediately. When phase IV is recorded, phase V (which is when the last sound is heard) is also recorded (e.g., 110/68/52).

DESCRIPTION OF KOROTKOFF SOUNDS

Phase I: First pulse sound—starts faintly and becomes clear tapping sound

Phase II: Second pulse sound—murmur or swishing sound

Phase III: Third pulse sound—sound is crisp and increases in intensity

Phase IV: Fourth pulse sound—muffled sound

Phase V: When the last sound is heard

BOX 5-2

DESIGNATED DUTIES IN EMERGENCY RESPONSE BY DENTAL TEAM

TEAM MEMBER	DUTIES
Team member 1 (usually dentist)	Provide CPR. Stay with the victim. Alert office staff.
Team member 2	Bring emergency kit and oxygen to site of emergency.
Team member 3	Assist with CPR. Monitor vital signs. Prepare emergency drugs for administration. Activate emergency system. Assist as needed. Keep records. Meet rescue team at building entrance.

Modified from Malamed SF: *Medical emergencies in the dental office*, ed 4, St Louis, 1993, Mosby.

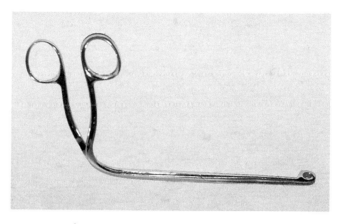

Figure 5-4   Magill intubation forceps.

This service should be called after initial treatment has been started if the dentist needs additional support.

> ➡ **KEY POINT**
> ■ Place emergency telephone numbers on all the telephones in the dental office.

Some common emergency conditions are discussed here because of either their frequency or their life-threatening consequences.

Airway Obstruction

Dental procedures often involve the placement and removal of small objects in the patient's mouth. Therefore these small objects may fall down the patient's throat and be swallowed or **aspirated** into the lungs or become lodged, causing a complete or partial airway obstruction. Measures can be taken to prevent such occurrences. All dental staff should be aware of objects that can fall down the patient's throat. Objects that are still visible are retrieved as follows:

1. *If both assistant and dentist are with patient:*
   a. Do not allow the patient to sit up.
   b. Assistant retrieves **Magill intubation forceps** (Figure 5-4) from emergency kit, or suction is used to retrieve object.
2. *If only one member of dental staff is with patient:*
   a. Do not allow the patient to sit up.

   b. Have patient bend over side of chair with head down.
   c. Encourage patient to cough.

Swallowed objects that do not obstruct the airway

Objects that fall down the patient's throat and that do not obstruct the airway can be either swallowed or aspirated into the lungs. If an object goes down the patient's throat and cannot be seen immediately, place the patient on his or her left side with the head down and initiate the following procedures:

1. Do not allow the patient to sit up.
2. Position the patient on the left side with the head down.
3. Encourage the patient to cough to try to retrieve the object.

If the object cannot be retrieved, dental treatment should be terminated and the patient taken for chest and/or abdominal radiographs to determine the location of the object.

Although it is likely that objects that fall down the patient's throat are swallowed, one cannot assume that this has occurred solely on the patient's statements. Therefore it is essential to follow up with appropriate radiographs.

Partial airway obstruction

Objects that fall down the patient's throat and partially obstruct the airway should be immediately assessed to determine if the patient has good airflow in which a forceful cough can be made. The patient who has good airflow should be allowed to cough in an attempt to dislodge the object without interference from the dental staff. If the patient has poor airflow characterized by a weak cough, a blue face, or an inability to speak, then the emergency must be treated as if it were a complete airway obstruction.

> **↪ KEY POINTS**
> - If the patient has a partial airway obstruction but is able to cough forcefully, do not intervene. Allow the patient to cough in an attempt to dislodge the object.
> - If the patient has a partial airway obstruction and cannot cough forcefully, treat as if it were a complete airway obstruction.

Complete airway obstruction

Signs of complete airway obstruction include an inability to speak, breathe, or cough. Attempts to open the airway must be initiated immediately; otherwise, the patient will lose consciousness and die. The following maneuvers are recommended:

Type of patient	Type of treatment
Infants	Back blows
Adults and children	Manual abdominal thrusts (Heimlich maneuver)
Advanced pregnancy	Chest thrusts
Markedly obese	Chest thrusts
Unconscious	Finger sweep

Abdominal thrusts. If an obstruction of the airway is caused by some foreign material lodged in the patient's airway, an abdominal thrust maneuver is recommended. This maneuver is designed to sharply increase the pressure inside the chest cavity to blow the obstruction out of the patient's trachea (windpipe).

If the patient is already in the dental chair and is unconscious while lying down, the following actions should be taken:

1. Place the patient in the supine position, and remove all articles from the patient's mouth.
2. Sit astride the patient.
3. Form a fist with one hand, and place it on soft tissue between the patient's navel and rib cage. Use the other hand to support the wrist (Figure 5-5).
4. Press the fist into the patient's abdomen with a rapid, upward thrust. Repeat 6 to 10 times.
5. Open the patient's mouth, and use the index finger to sweep the mouth for foreign objects.

If the patient is still conscious, upright, and choking, the following procedure is recommended:

1. Stand behind the patient, and wrap both arms around the patient's waist.
2. Place the thumb of one fist into the soft tissue between the navel and the rib cage. Grasp the fist with the other hand (Figure 5-6). Chest thrusts can be administered to obese or pregnant patients as

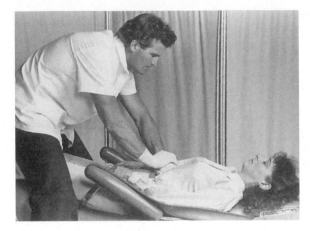

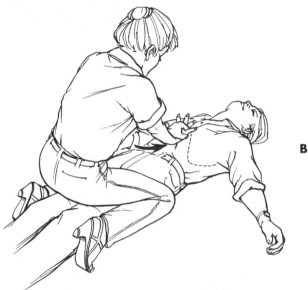

Figure 5-5 **A,** Abdominal thrust performed with patient in dental chair. **B,** Heimlich maneuver administered to unconscious victim (lying down) of foreign-body airway obstruction. (**B** from Chandra NC, Hazinski MF: *Textbook of basic life support for health care providers,* Dallas, 1994, American Red Cross.)

an alternative to the traditional abdominal thrusts (Figure 5-7).

3. Pull the fist quickly into the patient's abdomen with a firm upward movement. Repeat 6 to 10 times.

These rescue techniques are patterned after the recommendations made by Dr. Henry Heimlich in a paper published in 1974 and are often referred to as **Heimlich maneuvers.**

Back blows and chest thrusts are recommended for infants less than 1 year of age. Procedures for delivery of back blows will not be discussed since infants less than 1 year old usually do not receive regular dental treatment.

As with any emergency it is important to assess what type of emergency is occurring. An obstructed airway is

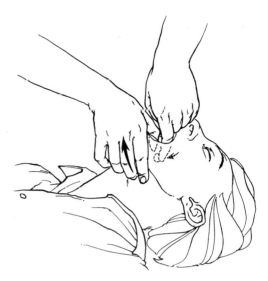

Figure 5-8   Finger-sweep maneuver administered to unconscious victim of foreign-body airway obstruction.

(From Chandra NC, Hazinski MF: *Textbook of basic life support for health care providers*, Dallas, 1994, American Red Cross.)

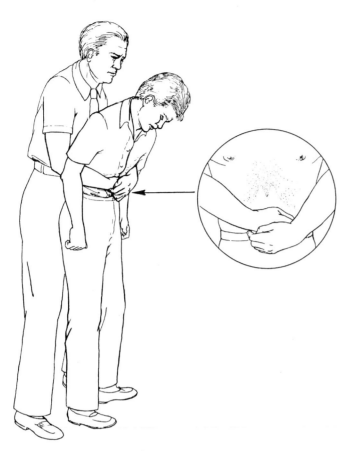

Figure 5-6   Standing abdominal thrust (Heimlich maneuver).

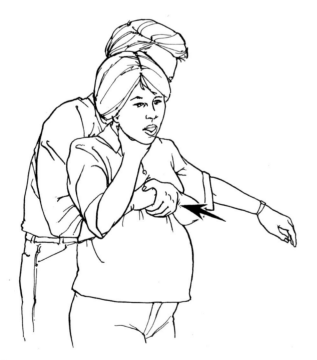

Figure 5-7   Chest thrust administered to conscious victim (standing) of foreign-body airway obstruction.

(From Chandra NC, Hazinski MF: *Textbook of basic life support for health care providers*, Dallas, 1994, American Red Cross.)

more easily assessed if the patient is conscious. If the patient is found unconscious and the cause of the emergency is unknown, breathing and pulse need to be checked immediately. If the patient is not breathing and the rescuer is unable to ventilate the patient, one must assume that the airway is obstructed.

Rescue breathing

If a patient stops breathing, the following steps are recommended:

1. *Evaluate the situation.* Before touching the patient, evaluate the situation for possible danger to yourself, such as live electrical wires.
2. *Determine unconsciousness.* Tap or gently shake the patient and shout, "Are you OK?" in an attempt to wake the patient. If the patient does not awaken, proceed to the following life-support procedures.
3. *Call for help.* Do not leave the patient; instead, call for help from other members of the dental team. The rescuer should summon someone to call the emergency number (usually 911) for an emergency medical system (EMS) rescue unit from the nearest hospital or fire department.
4. *Remove debris from mouth.* Remove any visible foreign debris from the patient's mouth using a "finger sweep" method with the tips of the fingers (Figure 5-8) or an oral evacuator if it is available. Care should be taken not to force foreign debris deeper into the throat.
5. *Use supine positioning.* Place the patient in a **supine** position (Figure 5-9). A woman in the third

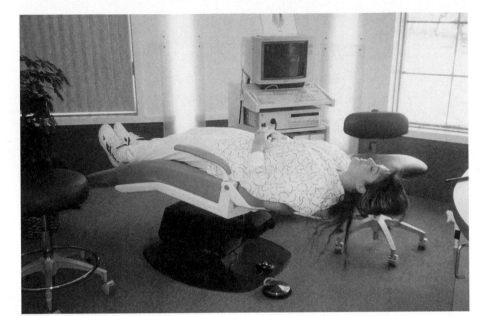

Figure 5-9 Supine position.

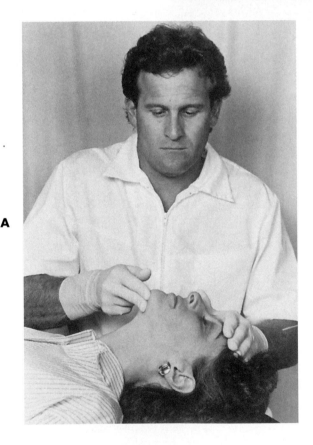

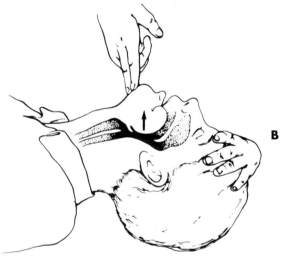

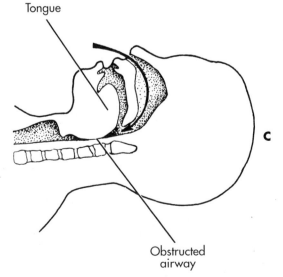

Tongue

Obstructed
airway

Figure 5-10 Head tilt–chin lift maneuver. **A,** Operator's hand positions. **B,** Open airway with head tilt. **C,** Obstructed airway caused by tongue resting against posterior wall of pharynx.

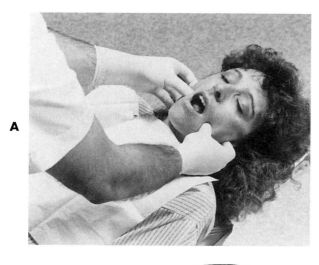

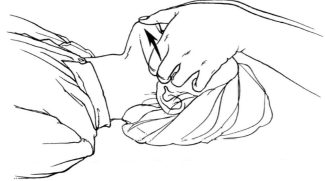

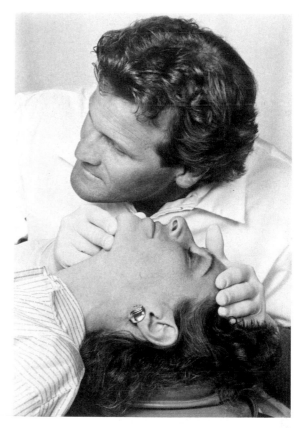

Figure 5-11   **A**, Jaw-thrust method of lifting mandible and tilting head to open airway. **B**, Jaw-thrust maneuver.

(**B** from Chandra NC, Hazinski MF: *Textbook of basic life support for health care providers*, Dallas, 1994, American Red Cross.)

Figure 5-12   Simultaneous observation of chest movement while listening for flow of air through patient's nose or mouth.

trimester of pregnancy should be placed on her side while in the supine position.

6. *Open airway (head tilt–chin lift)*. Tilt the patient's head back by placing one hand on the patient's forehead using firm backward pressure. Lift the chin with the other hand by placing the fingers under the chin and lifting (Figure 5-10, *A* and *B*). This maneuver prevents the tongue from obstructing the airway (Figure 5-10, *C*). If the patient wears complete dentures, they should be removed if they cannot be controlled in their proper position. An alternative maneuver is to simply grasp the patient at the angle of the lower jaw on each side using both hands and lift the mandible upward to tilt the head back and pull the chin forward at the same time (Figure 5-11). In either case the teeth should not be allowed to close completely and the lips should remain parted to allow air to enter through the mouth. The thumb can be used to keep the patient's lips parted if necessary. Since the tongue is attached to the mandible, these maneuvers lift it away from the posterior wall of the

pharynx and open the airway. Success can be determined immediately by placing one ear close to the patient's mouth and nose to listen and feel for airflow. The rescuer can also simultaneously watch for chest or abdominal movement that may indicate that the patient is breathing or attempting to breath (Figure 5-12). This assessment should take only 3 to 5 seconds. If the patient is breathing, keep the airway open until help arrives.

7. *Perform rescue breathing*. If the patient is not breathing, perform rescue breathing by mouth by holding the patient's head in the open airway position and pinching the nostrils closed with the thumb and index finger of the hand used to hold the head in the tilted position. If a ventilation mask is used, place one or two hands to hold the ventilation mask over the patient's mouth and nose.

The rescuer's mouth is placed over the patient's mouth or the ventilation mask is placed over the patient's mouth and nose to form a tight seal (Figure 5-13). The rescuer should blow exhaled air into the patient's mouth two times. The rescuer should allow 1½ to 2 seconds for each breath, and a rise of the patient's chest should be observed to confirm that air is filling the lungs (see Figure 5-12).

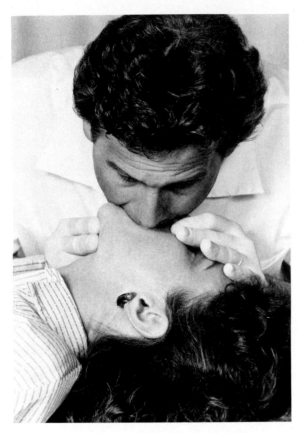

Figure 5-13 Ventilation of patient by sealing nostrils, maintaining head tilt, and blowing air into patient's mouth.

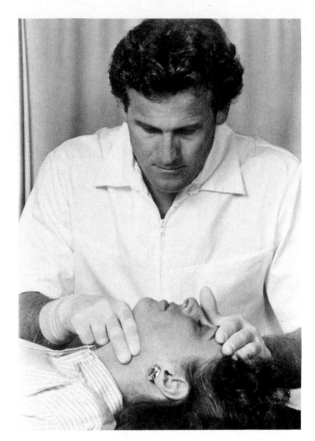

Figure 5-14 Checking for carotid pulse.

Rapid, forceful breaths should be avoided, since the resulting air pressure may open the esophagus and the air will be diverted to the stomach rather than the lungs. A rise in the abdominal area is evidence of such an event.

8. *Check the pulse.* If the airway is unobstructed, the rescuer should hold the patient's head in the tilted position and check the carotid artery on the side of the neck using the first and second fingers of either hand along the side of the patient's neck for evidence of pulse. This procedure must be done within 10 seconds. The artery should be palpated gently to feel for a pulse (Figure 5-14). If the patient has a pulse but is not breathing, perform rescue breathing until help arrives. If the patient has no pulse, initiate chest compressions until the patient recovers or until the rescue team arrives.

Rescue breathing is done at a rate of 12 breaths per minute (one every 5 seconds) while looking for a chest rise and feeling for airflow out of the patient's nose during exhalation. The pulse should be checked periodically to determine whether the heart is still functioning.

Cardiopulmonary Arrest

Cardiopulmonary arrest is a serious emergency that can occur at any time. The stress of dental treatment may increase its possibility during a dental appointment. Technically this condition is a cessation of breathing and heart function. However, the heart may continue to function for a few minutes even though breathing has stopped. Cardiac arrest rarely occurs in the absence of respiratory arrest. If the patient does not receive treatment within 6 minutes, permanent brain damage may occur. Death may occur if the patient does not receive treatment within 4 to 6 minutes. Since time is important in this emergency situation, the operating team must act quickly and efficiently.

Cardiopulmonary resuscitation

External chest compression. If at any time during the rescue procedure a pulse cannot be detected, steps must be taken to support circulation of oxygenated blood to the brain. Rescue breathing is designed to place oxygen in the patient's lungs. External chest compression (ECC) is designed to transport oxygen from the lungs to the brain in the absence of heart function **(cardiac arrest).** The technique for ECC follows:

1. *Patient position.* The patient is kept in the supine position as previously described, and the airway is kept open. Slight elevation of feet into the **Trendelenburg position** (Figure 5-15) may assist circulation.

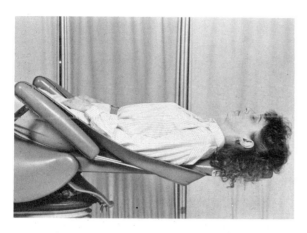

Figure 5-15   Trendelenburg position.

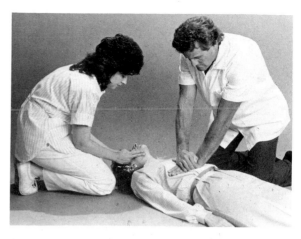

Figure 5-16   Proper positioning of rescue team.

2. *Exposure of the patient's chest.* To accurately determine the correct hand position for chest compressions, the patient's clothing should be removed or lifted away from the chest.

3. *Rescue team position.* Since at least two people are generally present in the office during a dental appointment, a two-person technique of performing **cardiopulmonary resuscitation (CPR)** is described. However, assistants should be familiar with the one-person technique. One person is positioned by the patient's head and maintains the head tilt–chin lift position. This individual does the rescue breathing and monitors the patient for a carotid pulse during each chest compression. The other person assumes a position on the opposite side of the patient next to the patient's chest and does the chest compressions (Figure 5-16).

4. *Hand position.* The "compression" rescuer's hand nearest the patient's legs is used to locate the lower border of the victim's rib cage. Palpating along the rib cage toward the midline, the rescuer can locate the notch formed by the ribs at the patient's sternum (breastbone) in the center of the chest. The middle finger of the rescuer's palpating hand is used to mark a spot just above this notch (Figure 5-17, *A*). The heel of the other hand is placed next to this spot over the lower part of the sternum (Figure 5-17, *A*), and the palpating hand is placed over the back of the first hand. Only the heel of the first hand should contact the patient's chest to avoid damage to the patient's ribs during the compression strokes administered to the sternum (Figure 5-17, *B*).

5. *Compression technique.* Rescuers should kneel and place their shoulders directly over the sternum with

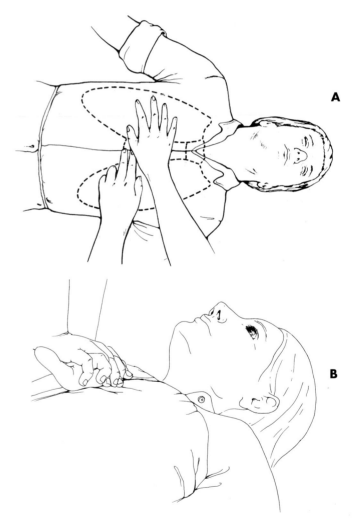

Figure 5-17   Hand positioning for chest compressions. **A,** Location of sternal notch by palpation. **B,** Use of heel of lower hand to compress patient's chest. Upper hand is used to lift fingers of lower hand to prevent rib injuries during compression.

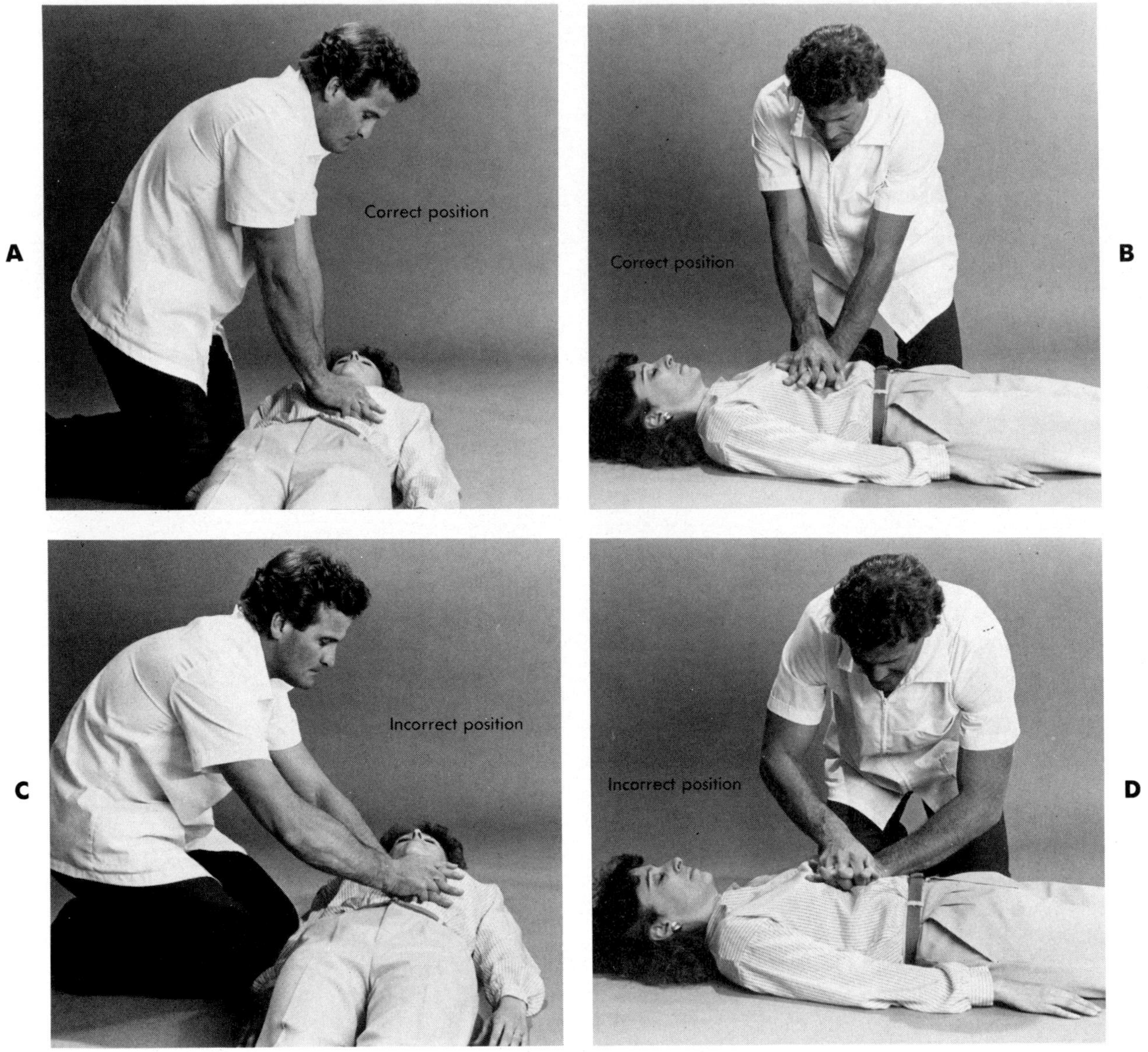

Figure 5-18   Position of rescuer for compression of chest during cardiopulmonary resuscitation (CPR). **A** and **B**, Correct position. **C** and **D**, Incorrect position.

their arms locked in a straight position at the elbows. When downward force is applied to the patient's chest, this position keeps the victim from rolling sideways and reducing the effect of the compression stroke (Figure 5-18).

The rescuer applies the compression stroke to the patient's sternum by rocking forward at the hips to drive the locked arms straight down to compress the sternum by about 1½ to 2 inches. The compression is released by the rescuer rocking backward at the hips while continuing to maintain hand contact with the patient's sternum. Compressions should continue at a rate of 80 to 100 per minute. The other rescuer should palpate for a pulse in the carotid artery to assess the effectiveness of the chest compressions.

At the end of *five* compressions the other rescuer should ventilate the patient through either the patient's mouth or nose as discussed earlier. The compressions should be resumed following the ventilation and continued in a rhythmical manner with a ratio of 5 compressions to 1 breath. Should the rescuers become fatigued, they can change positions following a ventilation. Rescuers need not change sides during a position change. This only adds confusion and delay. The rate of compression can be paced by counting aloud, "one and, two and, three and, four and, five and."

This rescue effort is continued until the patient recovers or until medical personnel with more advanced training arrive. All dental personnel should receive training in cardiopulmonary emergency treatment. This training should include practice sessions using resuscitation manikins. Reading about this rescue technique is no substitute for actual rescue practice.

Angina Pectoris and Myocardial Infarction

Two other serious heart problems are **angina pectoris** and **myocardial infarction,** or heart attack. These conditions result from an inadequate blood supply to the heart muscle through the coronary artery. Often patients are aware of these conditions and carry medication to treat the attacks. Severe chest pains that often spread to the arms and mandible can occur. In the event of an acute anginal episode, initiate the following treatment:

1. Terminate the procedure.
2. Place the patient in a comfortable position, usually sitting upright.
3. Place the patient's dosage (usually 1 to 3 tablets) of nitroglycerin under the tongue.

Symptoms are usually relieved following nitroglycerin administration. Oxygen may be administered to the patient. Nitroglycerin, which is available as a spray or in tablet form, dilates the coronary artery, which increases the flow of blood to the muscle tissue of the heart. A second dose of nitroglycerin should be administered if the angina continues after 5 minutes.

- In patients with a history of angina, medical assistance should be summoned if the pain is not relieved by 3 nitroglycerin tablets or spray doses over a 15-minute period.
- Medical assistance should be summoned at the start of an anginal episode for patients who have had no prior history of angina.

A myocardial infarction should be suspected if the pain is not relieved by nitroglycerin. Patients with a history of a heart attack should not receive dental treatment within 6 months of the heart attack because of the higher incidence of another heart attack within the first 6 months.

↦ KEY POINTS
- Administer nitroglycerin tablets or spray to a patient experiencing angina.
- Delay elective dental treatment for 6 months following a heart attack.

Epilepsy

Epilepsy is a disorder of the central nervous system that results in mild to severe episodes of a convulsive seizure. The medical history should reveal this condition so the operating team can anticipate a seizure during dental treatment. Fear, pain, and even flashing lights can trigger a seizure. Convulsive seizures are transient but can be rather violent while they are occurring. Patients must be protected from harming themselves during the convulsion. Rescuers should never put their fingers or other objects between the patient's teeth during the convulsion stage.

In the event that a seizure occurs, do the following:

1. Terminate the procedure and summon medical assistance.
2. Move all equipment and instruments out of the way to protect the patient.
3. Use limited, not forceful, restraint to minimize excessive movements of the patient's arms and legs. Allow some minor movement of the patient's extremities to prevent injury to the joints.
4. After the seizure activity stops, the dental team should be prepared to provide basic life support for the patient. The patient can lapse into central nervous system depression, which can result in respiratory depression.

Oxygen support or even the head tilt maneuvers described previously may be required. Once the patient recovers, paramedical personnel can evaluate the patient to determine if hospitalization is necessary or if the patient can be discharged from the dental office. If the patient is not hospitalized, it is advisable to have an adult accompany the person home.

Syncope

Syncope (fainting) is probably the most common medical emergency encountered in the dental office. It is usually brought on by fear, anxiety, emotional upset, or pain. Fainting is a result of reduced flow of blood to the brain caused by dilation of blood vessels elsewhere in the body. If the patient is sitting upright, blood tends to pool in the lower portions of the body and the brain is left with a decreased blood supply. The supine position of the patient in the sit-down four-handed dentistry technique helps to prevent fainting, since the patient's head is kept on the same level as the lower part of the body.

The following are some common signs and symptoms of syncope.

Initial changes

1. The patient complains of feeling "funny"; warmth in neck and face is a common symptom. Dizziness, perspiration, and nausea can occur.
2. The facial skin becomes pale (pallor) and clammy.
3. Pulse rate increases markedly (120 beats per minute).
4. Pupils of the eyes become enlarged (dilate).
5. Depth of respiration increases.

Advanced changes

1. Hands and feet become cold.
2. Pulse rate slows markedly (50 beats per minute) and is weak and harder to detect.
3. Pupils of the eyes enlarge markedly.

4. Loss of consciousness occurs; eyes may roll back under lids.
5. Respiration becomes shallow, irregular, and jerky.
6. Muscle convulsions occur in face, hands, and legs.

• • •

Since syncope is a condition that deprives the brain of an adequate blood supply, it must be attended to immediately. The steps in treatment are as follows:

1. Remove all articles from the patient's mouth.
2. Place the patient in a supine position. Women in the third trimester of pregnancy should be placed on their side while in this position. Remove the head support if a contour chair is used.
3. Establish an open airway, and assess breathing and pulse.
4. Administer oxygen.
5. Monitor vital signs.
6. Loosen tight clothing around the neck.
7. Crush an ammonia inhalant from the emergency kit, and hold it under the oxygen mask for a moment to stimulate the patient's breathing.
8. Provide other support measures such as placing a cold towel on the patient's forehead or using a blanket or drape to cover a shivering patient.

This treatment should be continued until the patient recovers completely, with normal respiration, skin color, and awareness of the surroundings. It is advisable to have an adult accompany the patient home.

Often syncope can be anticipated in apprehensive patients. The fear of a dental injection is probably the most common cause of fainting. Use of the hidden syringe transfer, local anesthetic administration in a supine position, and careful injection techniques can help prevent syncope in these patients.

KEY POINTS
- Fainting is the most common medical emergency to occur in the dental office.
- An ammonia inhalant and oxygen can be used to treat a fainting patient.

Hyperventilation

Hyperventilation is essentially an excessive breathing pattern that results in a marked decrease in carbon dioxide levels in the blood. Although unconsciousness rarely occurs, the patient may feel dizzy or have impaired consciousness. The major predisposing factor is anxiety. If a patient's anxiety is managed properly through psychosedative techniques, hyperventilation rarely occurs.

Typically, apprehensive patients begin to breathe more rapidly and deeply in response to their own anxiety. The following signs and symptoms can occur:

1. Pounding of the heart (palpitation)
2. A feeling of a "lump" in the throat
3. A tight feeling in the chest
4. Deep rapid breathing
5. Tingling of the hands, feet, and lips

An apprehensive patient who starts to breathe excessively with a deep, rapid breathing pattern should be treated as follows:

1. Terminate the dental procedure.
2. Place the patient in an upright position.
3. Loosen tight clothing around the neck and remove all articles from the patient's mouth.
4. Reassure the patient, and coach the individual to breathe slowly (4 to 6 breaths per minute). If the patient does not respond, proceed to step 5.
5. Have the patient breathe into a paper bag or paper headrest cover or have the patient cup hands together in front of the mouth and nose until recovery occurs (Figure 5-19). Rebreathing exhaled air, which has a higher level of carbon dioxide, helps to hasten the recovery process.

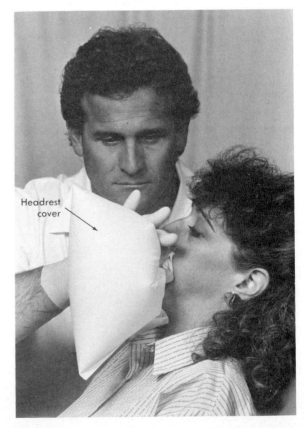

Headrest cover

Figure 5-19 Hyperventilating patient breathing into headrest cover.

Treatment of the patient at future dental appointments should include consideration of treating the patient's anxiety before initiating dental procedures.

> ◆ **KEY POINTS**
> - A hyperventilating patient may use a paper bag or cup the hands over the mouth to alleviate symptoms.
> - Do not use a plastic bag for a hyperventilating patient because the bag can collapse on itself.
> - Do not administer oxygen to a hyperventilating patient. Oxygen may exacerbate the situation.
> - Fainting and hyperventilation are usually caused by fear and anxiety.

Hypoglycemia

Hypoglycemia is a condition frequently associated with patients with diabetes; however, it may also occur in nondiabetic individuals who skip meals. It frequently occurs when there is an abnormally low level of glucose (sugar) in the blood. In patients with diabetes this usually occurs if the amount of insulin administered is excessive for the amount of food eaten or if the diabetic patient fails to eat meals on time. The result is that the patients' blood sugar decreases and they become weak and nervous; vision deteriorates; and the skin becomes pale and clammy. The patient can eventually lose consciousness. If the operating team is aware of the patient's diabetic condition, prevention should be initiated by scheduling the patient's appointments immediately after meals. In the event that a patient becomes hypoglycemic, an oral carbohydrate should be given if the patient is conscious. Every emergency kit should contain a cola beverage, candy bar, lumps of sugar, or tube cake frosting for this purpose. If the patient loses consciousness, basic life support measures should be done to ensure an adequate airway and adequate circulation. A thin strip of decorative cake frosting can be placed in the buccal vestibule of an unconscious or conscious patient. An IV injection of 50% dextrose solution can be administered by a trained dentist. *Do not attempt to administer liquids by mouth to an unconscious patient.*

> ◆ **KEY POINTS**
> - Hypoglycemia is caused by low blood sugar.
> - Hypoglycemia is caused by skipping meals in diabetic and nondiabetic patients.

Anesthetic Toxicity

An overdose of anesthetic solution in the patient's bloodstream causes anesthetic toxicity. This can occur because the anesthetic was inadvertently injected into a patient's blood vessel or because too much anesthetic solution was injected into the patient at one time. The result is that the patient will be stimulated immediately after the injection. Nervousness, talkativeness, and restlessness are early signs of stimulation of the central nervous system with anesthetic solution. The patient may soon begin to convulse. The convulsive episode is often followed by a depression of the central nervous system, which results in respiratory depression and unconsciousness until the anesthetic is detoxified in the system.

Early recognition of the patient's condition is the key to treatment. This is why *a patient must never be left alone after an injection of an anesthetic solution.* Early signs of moderate stimulation should lead the dentist to administer an anticonvulsant intravenously until the patient is calmed. Oxygen should be administered. If severe respiratory depression and unconsciousness occur, emergency measures such as mouth-to-mouth resuscitation or forced oxygen treatment should be carried out until the anesthetic solution clears from the system and the patient recovers.

Asthma

Asthma can be caused by several factors, including allergies, physical exertion, stress, and anxiety. When asthma occurs, the airways in the lungs become narrow, which results in shortness of breath and wheezing. Status asthmaticus is a life-threatening asthmatic condition and occurs when the asthma attack does not respond to the usual drug therapy. Patients with a history of asthma usually carry a bronchodilator aerosol inhaler (Figure 5-20). Patients should be reminded to bring the inhaler to the dental appointment in the event of an asthmatic attack. A patient experiencing an acute asthma attack while receiving dental treatment should be seated upright and use a bronchodilator aerosol inhaler. Dental staff should make all attempts to keep the patient calm because stress and anxiety can make it more difficult to terminate an attack. If the aerosol inhaler is unsuccessful in terminating the attack, the dental assistant may administer an injection of epinephrine (Adrenalin).

Cerebrovascular Accident

A **cerebrovascular accident (CVA)** (stroke) occurs when the brain tissue is destroyed. Strokes often affect only one side of the brain, and if severe they can cause paralysis of one side of the body or death. Strokes can be caused by a lack of oxygen to the brain via a blockage of blood flow to the brain by a blood clot or bleeding to the brain. Patients experiencing a stroke may complain of a headache or difficulty with vision, breathing, or swallowing. The patient

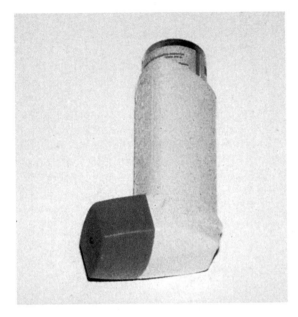

Figure 5-20 Bronchodilator aerosol inhaler.

may be unable to speak or may have slurred speech. A conscious patient experiencing a stroke should be seated upright or semiupright and given oxygen. Medical assistance should be immediately summoned. An unconscious patient is given basic life support until medical assistance arrives. Elective dental treatment should be delayed for 6 months following a stroke because of the higher incidence of another stroke within the first 6 months.

> **⟿ KEY POINT**
> ▪ Patients who have had a stroke should not receive elective dental treatment for 6 months following the stroke.

Allergy

Allergic reactions to drugs and substances in the dental office can range from mild to life threatening. In the dental office the patient can be administered substances that could cause an allergic reaction, such as local anesthetics, antibiotics, narcotics, preservatives, latex gloves, acrylic monomer, and impression materials. Progressive signs and symptoms of an allergic reaction can occur in a few minutes to a day or more. Signs and symptoms of an allergic reaction vary and can range from the formation of a rash, asthma, and swelling of the throat to rapid heart beat and cardiac arrest. Delayed allergic reactions are treated according to the signs and symptoms of the patient. The following medications are used:

Patient reaction	Medication
Asthma	Bronchodilator
Swelling of the throat	Epinephrine and cortico-steroids
Rash	Antihistamine

Acute allergic reactions require quick treatment, which usually consists of administration of epinephrine by injection.

If there is severe swelling of the throat that completely obstructs breathing, a **cricothyrotomy** (surgical opening of the airway) may be performed by a trained dentist or trained medical personnel.

MEDICOLEGAL CONSIDERATIONS

Most lawsuits initiated against dental offices involve undesirable results in treatment; however, an allegedly mishandled medical emergency also poses a risk of the dental staff being sued. Prevention of medical emergencies is the best method to avoid lawsuits. CPR must be provided by the dental staff if needed. Good Samaritan statutes that protect health care providers who perform CPR to the public will not protect a dental staff member who fails to perform CPR for a patient of record. Therefore the dentist and dental staff should be trained in CPR and emergency practice drills should be practiced regularly. After a medical emergency occurs in the dental office, the emergency is documented in the patient's chart. A thorough notation of what occurred may avoid accusations of negligence or wrongdoing later. In the event of a complication, if the dental auxiliary has malpractice insurance, it is best to contact the insurance carrier as soon as possible to discuss potential legal issues. The insurance company may request the auxiliary to complete an incident report form that belongs to the insurance company and cannot be subpoenaed. Avoid notations in the chart that indicate risk management activities such as "malpractice insurance company notified" or "incident report form completed" because they have nothing to do with patient treatment.

BIBLIOGRAPHY

Chandra NC, Hazinski MF: *Textbook of basic life support for health care providers,* Dallas, 1994, American Heart Association.

Chernega JB: *Emergency guide for dental auxiliaries,* ed 2, Albany, NY, 1994, Delmar.

Malamed SF: *Handbook of medical emergencies in the dental office,* ed 4, St Louis, 1993, Mosby.

Miyasaki-Ching CM, Tennenhouse DJ: *Dental risk prevention for dental auxiliaries,* San Rafael, Calif, 1991, Tennenhouse Professional Publications.

QUESTIONS—Chapter 5

1. A patient who has had a heart attack within _____ should not be receiving treatment in a dental office.
   a. 1 month
   b. 3 months
   c. 6 months
   d. 1 year

2. The dental assistant is working alone with a patient, and the temporary crown being placed falls down the patient's throat. Which of the following should the dental assistant do?
   a. Tell the patient to bend over the side of chair and cough.
   b. Get the Magill intubation forceps and retrieve the temporary crown.
   c. Seat the patient upright and tell him to cough.
   d. Go to get the dentist.

3. Respiratory distress frequently may be alleviated by the administration of oxygen. This may be true for all the following *except:*
   a. Hyperventilation
   b. Fainting
   c. Asthma

Questions 4 through 6: A 30-year-old man arrived 10 minutes late for a dental appointment. He was immediately escorted to the treatment room, and the dentist began reviewing the medical history. After 10 minutes the patient complained of nausea, feeling warm, and dizziness.

4. Which of the following could the patient be experiencing?
   a. Fainting
   b. An asthma attack
   c. Epilepsy
   d. *a* and *c*

5. Which of the following might have prevented this medical emergency?
   a. Consulting the patient's physician
   b. Administering oxygen
   c. Placing the patient in the upright position
   d. Reviewing the medical-dental history before treatment

6. How should the dentist manage this emergency?
   a. Call 911.
   b. Leave the room to get help.
   c. Administer oxygen and ammonia immediately.
   d. Place the patient in supine position.

7. Which of the following patients could experience hypoglycemia in the dental office?
   a. A nondiabetic person who does not eat before a dental appointment
   b. A person with diabetes who eats regularly
   c. A person with diabetes who skipped breakfast
   d. *a* and *c*

8. Seating the patient in the _____ position while treating the patient will prevent fainting.
   a. Upright
   b. Supine
   c. Elevated

9. For which of the following medical emergencies would you position the patient on the side?
   a. Aspirated object
   b. Syncope
   c. Asthma
   d. Angina

10. All the following could be administered to a hyperventilating patient *except:*
    a. Paper bag
    b. Plastic bag
    c. Hands cupped over mouth and nose
    d. Paper headrest cover

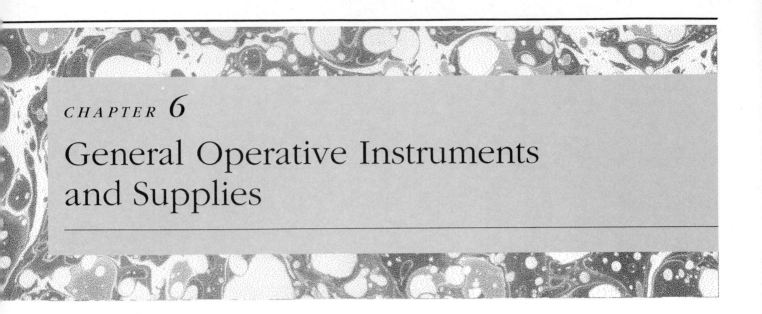

CHAPTER 6

General Operative Instruments and Supplies

KEY TERMS

Autochuck

Burs

Cavity liner

Chuck

Contra-angle attachment

Dental handpiece

Friction-grip bur (short shank)

Illumination

Indirect vision

Latch-type bur

Long-shank bur

Mandrel

Prophy paste

Prophylaxis angle

Retraction

Rheostat

The variety of instruments and supplies used in operative procedures is large and continually growing as new products and techniques are developed. The selection of an armamentarium for a specific procedure is based on a dentist's personal preference, which creates a problem for the beginning dental assistant learning instrumentation. This chapter acquaints the beginning dental assistant with some common instruments and supplies used in operative dentistry. Such a background makes it easier for assistants to adapt to different armamentaria.

Instruments used for specific operative procedures are discussed in later chapters.

DENTAL HANDPIECE

The **dental handpiece** is probably the most frequently used instrument in operative and restorative dentistry. Patients refer to this instrument as the dentist's drill. The handpiece works on a principle similar to a drill. Cutting and polishing instruments are held in the handpiece and spun at various speeds to cut or polish tooth structures or restorations.

> ↠ **KEY POINT**
> - The two types of handpieces used in dentistry are slow-speed and high-speed handpieces.

The slow-speed handpiece can turn a cutting instrument at speeds up to 25,000 rpm, and the high-speed handpiece can operate at 450,000 rpm. Both types are air driven and mandatory in modern dental practice.

Handpieces, whether slow- or high-speed types, are usually activated by a foot control called a **rheostat.** The rheostat works like an automobile accelerator: the more it is depressed, the faster the handpiece will operate. The rheostat frees the dentist's hands to operate the handpiece with greater ease and stability.

Maintenance of handpieces and the attachments is important to ensure proper function and long instrument life. It is important to follow the manufacturer's instructions for cleaning, lubrication, and sterilization.

Slow-Speed Handpiece

The slow-speed handpiece is a multipurpose instrument (Figure 6-1). Slow-speed handpieces are primarily for two purposes: caries removal and fine finishing of the detail of the preparation.

The slow-speed handpiece's relatively slow speed range, coupled with favorable turning power (torque), makes it an ideal instrument for various finishing, polishing, and contouring procedures and for caries removal. These procedures require maximum control by the dentist. When used properly the slow-speed handpiece provides this control.

The basic slow-speed handpiece has a straight-line design with no bends in the working end of the instrument (vs. the high-speed handpiece, which has a slight contra-angle bend). Various long-shafted cutting instruments, such as a **long-shank bur,** can be placed into the nose cone of the slow-speed handpiece (see Figure 6-1, *A*). This is a handy style for polishing, grinding, and adjusting dental restorations both in the oral cavity and at the laboratory bench. The cutting and polishing instruments used in the slow-speed handpiece are designated HP (handpiece) style instruments. An HP designation means that the cutting or polishing instrument has a long, straight shaft that inserts into the handpiece.

> **⟳ KEY POINT**
> - When ordering attachments that are placed into the basic slow-speed handpiece, the dental assistant should order attachments with an HP designation.

Attachments for slow-speed handpiece

Attachments are available for the slow-speed handpiece that expand its use considerably (Table 6-1). Figure 6-1

shows two of the most common attachments: the contra-angle and the prophylaxis angle.

Contra-angle attachment. The **contra-angle attachment** holds a variety of short-shafted burs, grinding stones, and polishing disks for intraoral use. The slight bend in this attachment is the source of its name. This bend, plus the use of short-shafted burs, allows dentists access to all the areas of the mouth.

Two types of contra-angles can be purchased: friction grip (Figure 6-2, *A*) and latch grip (Figure 6-2, *B*).

Friction-grip contra-angles only hold friction-grip burs. Latch-type contra-angles only hold the latch type of burs. A **friction-grip bur** has a smooth shank and is designated FG, whereas a **latch-type bur** has a small groove or "notch" on the end of the bur shank and is given an RA designation.

> **⟳ KEY POINTS**
> - When ordering attachments that are placed into the friction-grip attachment, the dental assistant should specify attachments with an FG designation.
> - When ordering attachments that are placed into the latch attachment, the dental assistant should order attachments with an RA designation.

Burs can be changed in the friction-grip type of contra-angles by pressing a button behind the head of the contra-angle that serves as the **autochuck** (Figure 6-3).

Many FG burs are also available with shorter-than-nor-

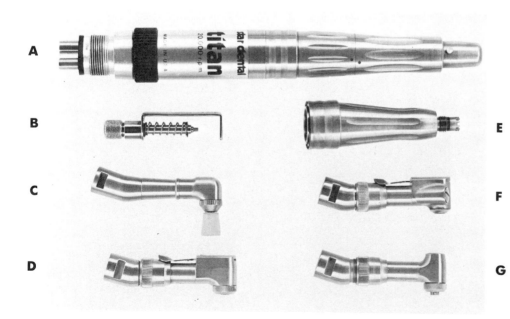

Figure 6-1 Slow-speed handpiece (HP) and accessories. **A,** Handpiece motor with straight HP attachment. **B,** Bur changing tool. **C,** Prophylaxis angle. **D,** Latch-type (RA) contra-angle. **E,** Motor to angle adaptor. **F,** High-torque contra-angle. **G,** Friction-grip (FG) contra-angle.

Table 6-1 Commonly used slow-speed handpiece attachments

Type	Use	Example	Attachment
Long-shafted bur (HP)	Polishing and grinding		None

Prophylaxis angle
  Screw type
  Snap-on type
	Removing plaque and stain during routine prophylaxis		Prophy cup
			Prophy brush

Latch-type contra-angle (FA)	Cutting and polishing		None
Friction-grip contra-angle (RA)	Cutting and polishing		None

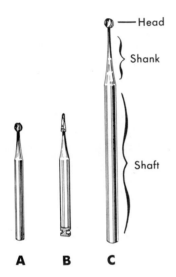

Figure 6-2 Different styles of shafts on rotating cutting instruments. **A,** Friction grip (FG). **B,** Latch (RA). **C,** Handpiece (HP).

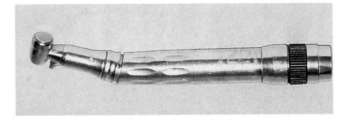

Figure 6-3 Slow-speed handpiece with autochuck feature.

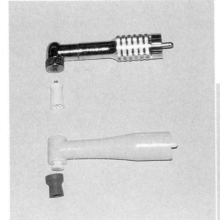

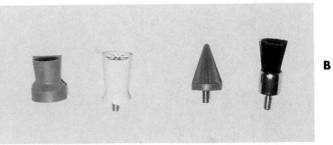

Figure 6-4 **A,** Prophylaxis angles. *Top,* Sterilizable screw type. *Bottom,* Disposable snap-on type. **B,** Various prophylaxis angle attachments.

mal shanks (short shank). These are useful in gaining access to confined areas of the oral cavity.

Prophylaxis angle attachment. The **prophylaxis angle** is a standard attachment for the slow-speed handpiece. It is used to hold polishing cups and brushes needed to remove plaque and stain during the dental prophylaxis procedure. Metal prophylaxis angles can be purchased and used repeatedly. Disposable prophylaxis angles can be purchased for a one-time use, which eliminates the need for cleaning, disinfecting, and sterilization.

Metal and disposable prophylaxis angles are available in two configurations (Figure 6-4). The screw type holds the polishing cup or brush in place by a threaded shaft. The snap-on type has a smooth knob to "snap on" polishing cups or brushes. The assistant must designate which type of prophylaxis angle is in use when ordering replacements for the polishing cups or brushes.

A rubber polishing cup is the most common device used on the prophylaxis angle. It is dipped in a polishing agent often called **prophy paste** and pressed against the surface to be polished. The handpiece is rotated at slow to moderate speeds to achieve a polishing action.

Any part of the slow-speed handpiece that is placed intraorally should be heat sterilized. It is important to follow the manufacturer's recommendations for handpiece sterilization and maintenance.

High-Speed Handpiece

The high-speed handpiece (Figure 6-5) is one of the greatest equipment advancements in recent dental history. This instrument allows the dentist to remove unwanted tooth structure rapidly and accurately.

The fundamental difference between high-speed and slow-speed handpieces is, of course, how fast a cutting instrument can be spun in the handpiece. However, another significant difference should be noted. High-speed handpieces have very little torque. The opposite is true of slow-speed handpieces. Torque is the turning power of the instrument when pressure is applied during the cutting procedure. High-speed handpieces will stop operating if excessive pressure is applied to the cutting instrument during a cavity preparation. Hence a light touch is required so the instrument can function properly.

The high-speed range of the high-speed handpiece per-

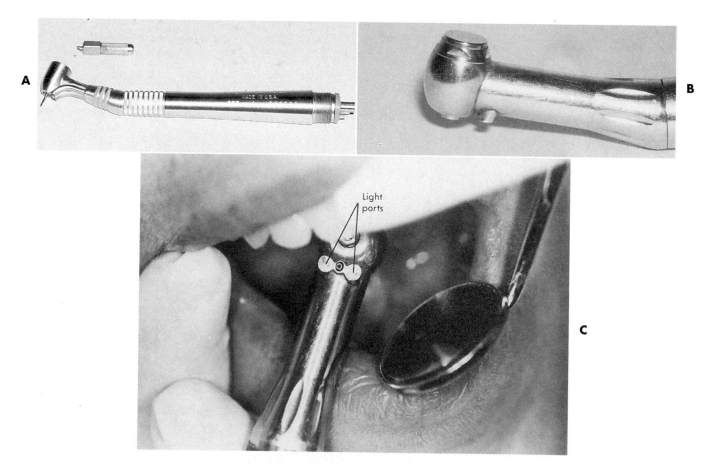

Figure 6-5 High-speed handpieces. **A,** Regular style (nonfiberoptic) with bur changer chuck. **B,** High-speed handpiece with autochuck feature. **C,** Fiberoptic style in use.

mits rapid cutting of tooth structure. Most of the bulk of tooth structure is removed with a high-speed handpiece during cavity preparations. Refinement of the preparation's detail and caries removal are accomplished with both the slow-speed handpiece and hand cutting instruments.

The extremely high speed of this handpiece uses harder, carbon steel burs that do not dull under high-speed use. Carbide burs or diamond stones turning against hard tooth structures at high speed generate a great deal of frictional heat. This heat is significant enough to damage delicate dental pulp. All high-speed handpieces use a water spray to combat frictional heat by constantly spraying the tooth and the cutting instrument with cool water during use. The water also helps to remove debris from the cavity preparation.

Use of water-spray coolant with high-speed handpieces will cause water to accumulate in the oral cavity during cavity preparation. The water spray also obscures the dentist's vision if the dentist is using the mouth mirror for indirect vision. Both of these problems can be solved by a skillful chairside assistant. Careful placement of the oral evacuator tip during cavity preparation removes the excess water coolant. Indirect vision is greatly improved if the dentist positions the mirror as far from the tooth being prepared as possible and the assistant continuously blows water off the mirror surface with air. The need for the use of water coolant with high-speed handpieces has,

in turn, created the need for extremely skillful chairside assistants.

> ### ➼ KEY POINTS
> - The dental assistant uses the oral evacuator or high-velocity evacuator (HVE) to remove water accumulation in the oral cavity from the water spraying out of the high-speed handpiece.
> - When the dentist uses the mirror for indirect vision, the dental assistant sprays the mirror with air to help the dentist see.

The high-speed handpiece uses the friction-grip burs, diamond stones, and polishing devices. Therefore burs ordered for the high-speed handpiece must have the FG (friction-grip) designation. Burs can be changed on older high-speed handpieces with a **chuck.** Newer high-speed handpieces eliminate the need for a chuck and have a pressure-sensitive button behind the head of the handpiece that serves as the autochuck (see Figure 6-5, *B*).

Handpieces are now available with fiberoptic lights that are mounted in the head of the instrument to assist in lighting the cavity preparation (see Figure 6-5, *C*).

It is important to follow the manufacturer's instructions for cleaning, maintenance, and sterilization of the

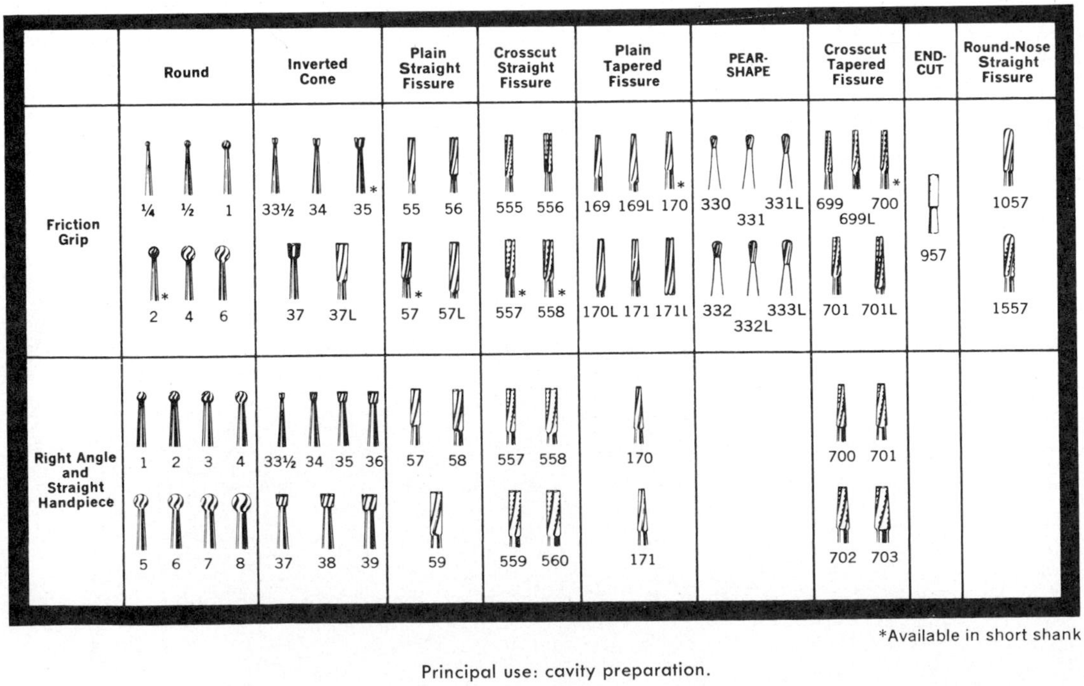

	Round	Inverted Cone	Plain Straight Fissure	Crosscut Straight Fissure	Plain Tapered Fissure	PEAR-SHAPE	Crosscut Tapered Fissure	END-CUT	Round-Nose Straight Fissure
Friction Grip	¼ ½ 1	33½ 34 35	55 56	555 556	169 169L 170	330 331L 331	699 700 699L	957	1057
	2 4 6	37 37L	57 57L	557 558	170L 171 171l	332 333L 332L	701 701L		1557
Right Angle and Straight Handpiece	1 2 3 4	33½ 34 35 36	57 58	557 558	170		700 701		
	5 6 7 8	37 38 39	59	559 560	171		702 703		

*Available in short shank

Principal use: cavity preparation.

Figure 6-6 Common bur styles used for cavity preparation.

(Courtesy Kerr Manufacturing Co, Romulus, Mich.)

handpieces. High-speed handpieces should be sterilized between patients as per recommendations by the Centers for Disease Control and Prevention (CDC).

Burs

Burs are generally made of stainless steel, carbide metal, or diamond chips. Stainless steel burs are used mainly for laboratory purposes and are generally not used inside the mouth. Carbide metal burs and diamond burs are useful for cutting teeth and restorative structures intraorally. Three types of shafts are generally used in dentistry (see Figure 6-2):

1. Friction grip (high- or slow-speed handpiece)
2. Latch type (slow-speed handpiece with contra-angle attachment)
3. Handpiece type (slow-speed handpiece with straight setup)

Friction-grip handpieces can be purchased with a shorter shank, often termed a *mini*.

Burs for slow-speed handpiece

A wide variety of burs can be used in the slow-speed handpiece. These include diamond stones, polishing disks, grindstones, abrasive wheels, and burnishers. Some of these burs are available in all types of shafts (HP, FG, and RA), whereas others are available only in one type or another. Figures 6-6 to 6-10 show a variety of popular rotary instruments available and the common uses of the instruments.

A **mandrel** (see Figure 6-9, *A*) can be used to attach different replacement polishing and grinding devices to the handpiece. Some of the common devices used on these mandrels are polishing disks, rubber abrasive wheels, grinding stones, and separating disks (see Figures 6-9 and 6-10).

Burs for high-speed handpiece

Carbon steel and diamond burs (see Figure 6-8, *A*) are usually used in the high-speed handpiece. Table 6-2 describes

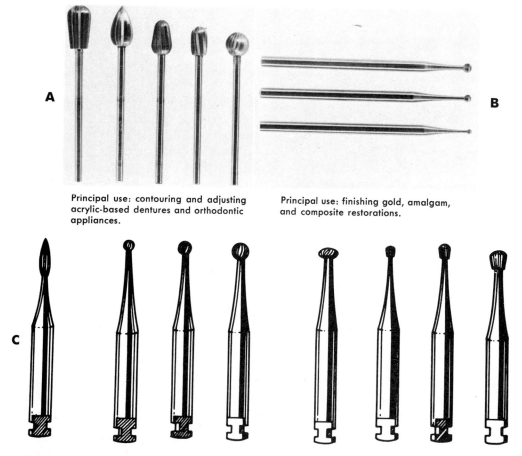

Principal use: contouring and adjusting acrylic-based dentures and orthodontic appliances.

Principal use: finishing gold, amalgam, and composite restorations.

Figure 6-7   Commonly used burs for the slow-speed handpiece. **A,** Acrylic burs. **B,** Straight HP finishing burs. **C,** RA finishing burs.

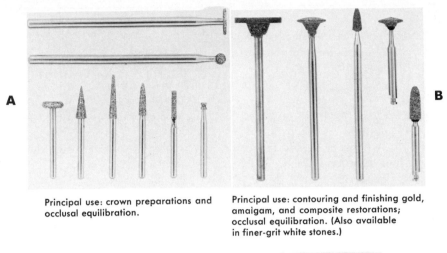

Principal use: crown preparations and occlusal equilibration.

Principal use: contouring and finishing gold, amaigam, and composite restorations; occlusal equilibration. (Also available in finer-grit white stones.)

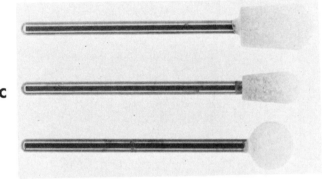

Principal use: contouring and adjusting acrylic-based dentures and orthodontic appliances.

Figure 6-8 Commonly used stones for slow–speed handpiece. **A**, Diamond stones. *Top,* Handpiece style. *Bottom,* FG style. **B**, Green stones. **C**, Acrylic stones.

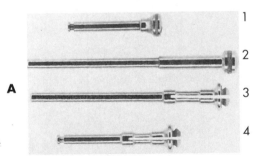

Principal use: attachment of various polishing and cutting wheels and disks to handpiece.

Figure 6-9 Commonly used finishing disks and mandrels. **A**, Mandrels. *1,* RA screw style; *2,* HP screw style; *3,* HP Moore's style; *4,* RA Moore's style. **B**, Assortment of sandpaper disks used with Moore's mandrels.

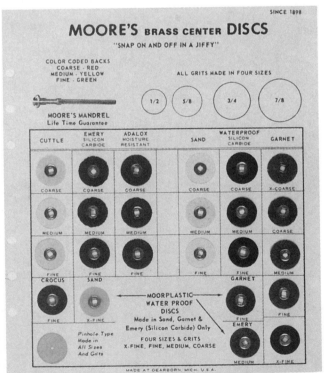

Principal use: finishing and polishing restorations.

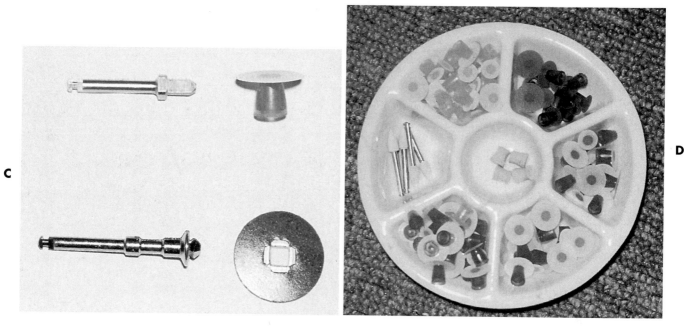

Figure 6-9 cont'd   **C**, Shofu mandrel and abrasive disk *(top)*, Moore's mandrel and abrasive disk *(bottom)*. **D**, Shofu abrasive disks and point.

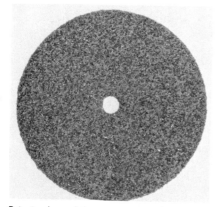

Principal use: laboratory procedures used in finishing gold restorations (used with a screw-type mandrel).

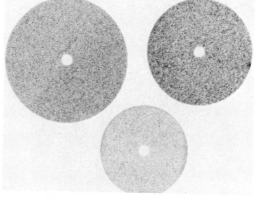

Principal use: crown and inlay preparations; orthodontic slicing (used with a screw-type mandrel).

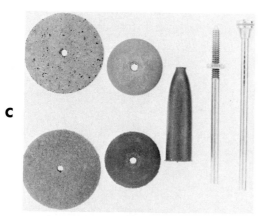

Principal use: finishing metal restorations.

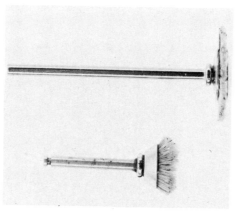

Principal use: polishing teeth and restorations using various polishing pastes.

Figure 6-10   Commonly used finishing and polishing devices. **A**, Carborundum disk. **B**, Lightning disks. **C**, Abrasive impregnated rubber disks and point with mandrels (Craytex). **D**, Bristle brushes.

Table 6-2 Common bur types and uses

Shape	Appearance	Bur no.	Example	Function
Round bur		¼ to 11		Caries removal Opening pulp chamber for root canal
Inverted cone		33½ to 40		Making slight undercuts or retention grooves in cavity preparation Caries removal
Straight fissure, plain cut		55 to 62		Initial opening into tooth for smoothing walls of cavity preparation Axial retention grooves
Straight fissure, crosscut		556 to 563		Same uses as for straight fissure, plain cut Crosscut design enhances cutting ability
Tapered fissure, plain cut		169 to 171		Inlay preparation Opening pulp chamber for root canal
Tapered fissure, crosscut		669 to 703		Same uses as for tapered fissure, plain cut Crosscut design enhances cutting ability
Finishing bur		Round shape: A to D, 200 to 203 Oval shape: 218 to 221 Pear shape: 230 to 232 Flame shape: 242 to 246		Establishing fine detail in amalgam or composite restorations

Figures from Finkbeiner BL, Johnson CS: *Mosby's comprehensive dental assisting: a clinical approach*, St Louis, 1995, Mosby.

the most common carbide bur shapes for the high-speed handpiece.

Bur care

Debris should be removed from burs by placing them in an ultrasonic cleaner. After debris removal the burs should be placed in a heat sterilizer for sterilization. Liquid chemical "cold" sterilization is not ideal for sterilization of burs because the chemicals are corrosive to burs made from carbide steel. Consult the manufacturer's recommendations.

MISCELLANEOUS COMMON OPERATIVE INSTRUMENTS AND SUPPLIES

Many different instruments and supplies are used in operative and restorative dentistry. The instruments presented here are only the fundamental instruments found in most instrument setups for operative procedures. The first two are the most widely used; virtually all instrument setups include a dental mirror and an explorer.

Dental Mirrors

Dental mirrors (Figure 6-11) are used for multiple purposes including indirect vision, illumination, and retraction.

Indirect vision

When the operator can look directly at an area without using a mirror, this is called direct vision. Sometimes the dentist cannot directly see a particular area without straining the back and neck. Dental mirrors are used primarily to allow the dentist to see into the inaccessible areas of the mouth by **indirect vision.**

Illumination

Mirrors can also be used in direct-vision examinations to reflect light into the area being examined or treated. This is called **illumination.**

Retraction

Retraction is done when the dentist or the assistant uses the dental mirror to pull the cheek, tongue, or lips away from the working site for better visibility or to prevent harm to the soft tissues of the mouth. Many problems the dentist and assistant encounter in terms of visibility and access to an area can be solved by use of the retraction function of the dental mirror.

Dental mirrors are available in sizes 2 to 6, with plane or magnifying surfaces. The cone-socket stem is the most popular type used today. This stem screws into a standard-sized handle, which allows the dentist to replace a scratched or damaged mirror without having to replace the still useful handle.

Dental Explorers

Several styles of dental explorers are available (Figure 6-12). All styles have a very fine tip on the working end of the instrument. This fine tip allows the dentist to feel various discrepancies on the surface of the teeth and around

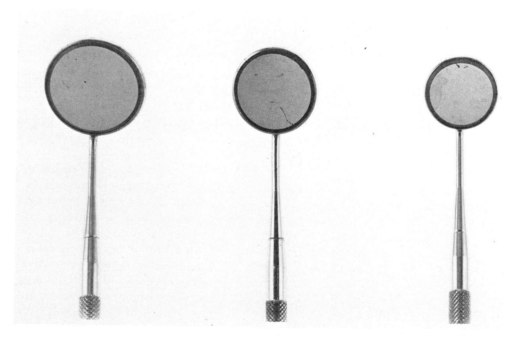

Figure 6-11   Various sizes of mouth mirrors.

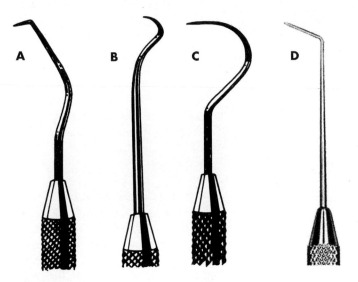

Figure 6-12 Dental explorers. **A**, No. 17. **B**, Cow-horn No. 3. **C**, Shepherd's hook. **D**, No. 11-12 explorer.

(Courtesy Hu-Friedy Manufacturing, Chicago.)

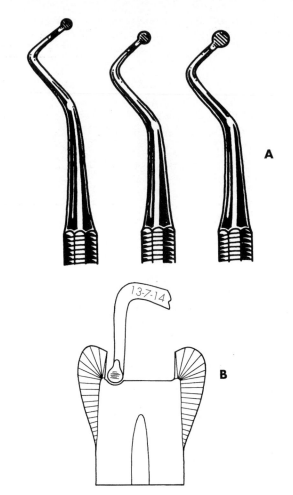

Figure 6-13 **A**, Various sizes of spoon excavators. **B**, Removal of dental caries with spoon excavator.

(Courtesy Sturdevant CM and others: *The art and science of operative dentistry*, ed 3, St Louis, 1995, Mosby.)

dental restorations. Thus the explorer actually becomes an extension of the dentist's hand.

The explorer is a multipurpose instrument. Some of its more common auxiliary uses follow:

1. Explorers are primarily used to detect tooth structure that has been softened by dental caries. The explorer "sticks" to the softened carious area.
2. Excess cement used to seal gold restorations in place can be removed from between the teeth with the explorer.
3. The explorer is useful in carving small areas of amalgam restorations, such as overhangs on the cervical margin, and removing amalgam against a matrix band before the band is removed.
4. Explorers can be used during scaling and root planing to detect calculus on the root surface of the tooth.

Explorers come in many different shapes. One of the most commonly used explorers is shaped like a curly pig's tail. Hence the name *pig-tail* or cow-horn explorer is used (Figure 6-12, *B*).

Another commonly used explorer is shaped like a shepherd's hook. Hence the name *shepherd's hook* explorer is used (Figure 6-12, *C*).

A recently introduced explorer named the 11-12 explorer is used by the dentist or hygienist to detect calculus in deep periodontal pockets (Figure 6-12, *D*).

Spoon Excavator

The spoon excavator is a hand instrument that was originally designed to remove debris and caries from an extensively damaged tooth (Figure 6-13). However, like the explorer, the spoon excavator has been used for other tasks. Following are some common auxiliary uses of this instrument:

1. The spoon excavator is a convenient instrument to use in placement and shaping of cavity liners and cement bases.
2. Like the explorer, the excavator is helpful in placement of gingival retraction cord.
3. Removal of excess cement after cementation of a gold restoration can be accomplished with the spoon excavator.
4. Both temporary and permanent restorations can be removed with the spoon excavator from a prepared tooth in gold and porcelain restorative procedures.
5. The excavator can assist in placing amalgam matrix bands, which are occasionally difficult to seat properly in the cervical area of a preparation.

Chairside assistants should have a gauze sponge ready

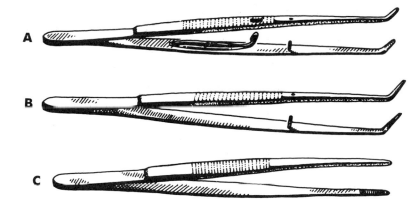

Figure 6-14   Dental pliers (forceps). **A**, Locking-style cotton pliers. **B**, Non-locking-style cotton pliers. **C**, Thumb-style cotton pliers.

to wipe debris from the working end of the excavator when the dentist is using it to debride an area or to place cavity mediations.

Spoon excavators are available in small, medium, and large sizes and are usually double ended.

• • •

There are probably as many uses for the spoon excavator and the explorer as there are dentists. The preceding lists represent only a few of the most common uses of these two popular instruments.

Cotton Pliers (Forceps)

Cotton pliers are standard instruments found on operative and restorative instrument setups (Figure 6-14). They are used to place and retrieve small objects in the oral cavity. Items such as cotton pellets, gingival retraction cord, cotton rolls, articulating paper, matrix bands, and wedges are commonly handled by cotton pliers. The dentist generally uses this instrument when it is more convenient than using fingers to handle these items. Cotton pliers are available in both locking and nonlocking styles.

Straight-beaked forceps (thumb forceps) (see Figure 6-14, *C*) are used to retrieve other instruments, materials, and devices from sterile storage areas to prevent contamination with the fingers.

Burnisher

The burnisher (Figure 6-15) is intended for use in smoothing the surface of dental restorations by rubbing the working end against the restoration surface.

Filling Instruments

Filling instruments are small bladed and are designed to place soft, moldable materials into cavity preparations. These materials include dental cements, composite materials, and acrylic. Filling instruments (Figure 6-16, *A*) are also useful in filling gold and porcelain restorations with cement before seating. Some dentists find the smaller styles convenient for placing gingival retraction cords.

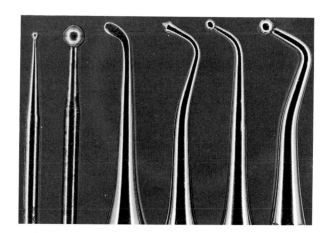

Figure 6-15   Burnishers. *Left to right,* Two ball burnishers (HP style), No. 4 SSW burnisher (hand), anatomic burnisher (hand), two ball burnishers (hand).

A new assortment of composite filling instruments that are used to place and shape composite material during an esthetic bonding procedure is shown in Figure 6-16, *B*. The various blade sizes and angles facilitate convenient access. This procedure is discussed in Chapter 18.

Cement Spatulas

A wide variety of cement spatulas (see Figure 6-16, *A*) is available for mixing dental cements and composite materials. Dental assistants should be familiar with the mixing requirements for the material being prepared. If the material is thin and must be mixed over a wide area, a narrow, flexible spatula should be used for mixing. On the other hand, if the material is thick and heavy textured, a spatula with a thicker blade is more helpful in mixing the material.

Dappen Dish

The dappen dish is a handy item used to dispense various materials during dental procedures (Figure 6-17, *A*). For convenience the dish has a deep well in one end and

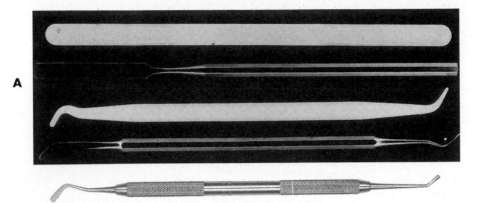

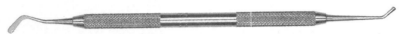

Small universal style features rounded condenser tip and narrow paddle for initial placement and contouring of class 1, 2, and 3 restorations.

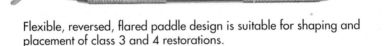

Larger universal style is ideally suited for final placement and contouring of class 1, 2, and 3 restorations.

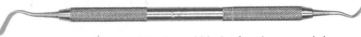

Flexible, reversed, flared paddle design is suitable for shaping and placement of class 3 and 4 restorations.

Flexible, paired, offset, paddle-shaped blades for placing and shaping material on posterior, mesial, and distal surfaces. Reverse angle is also useful for placing and shaping anterior bonded restorations.

Figure 6-16 **A,** Spatulas and filling instruments. *Top to bottom,* Plastic composite spatula, No. 334 SSW cement spatula, composite filling instrument, FP No. 1 filling instrument. **B,** Composite insertion instruments.

(Courtesy Hu-Friedy, Chicago.)

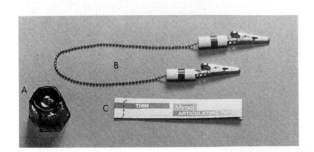

Figure 6-17 *A,* Dappen dish; *B,* napkin holder; *C,* articulating paper.

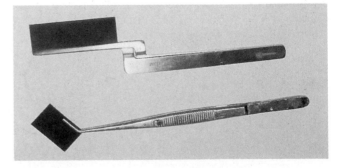

Figure 6-18 Articulating paper held with articulating paper holder *(top)* or cotton forceps *(bottom)*.

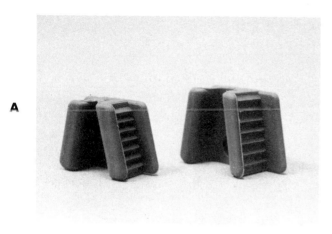
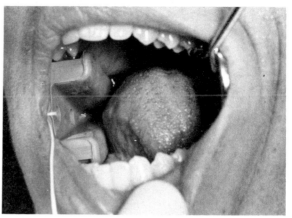

Figure 6-19   **A,** Small and large bite blocks. **B,** Bite block in place with safety floss attached.

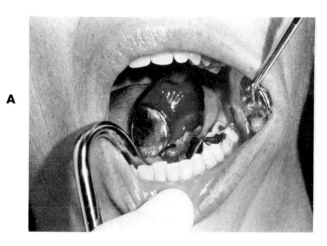
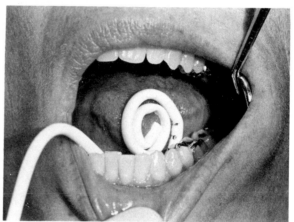

Figure 6-20   Tongue retraction–style saliva ejectors. **A,** Svedopter. **B,** Hygoformic.

a shallow well in the other. Materials often placed in dappen dishes for use during a given procedure are acrylics, alcohol, disclosing solution, various medicaments, amalgam, and tap water.

Napkin Holder

The napkin holder is a standard item available in different styles and used to secure a dental napkin around a patient's neck (Figure 6-17, *B*). Nonmetal types are preferable because they are not as cold on a patient's neck as the metal types.

Articulating Paper

Articulating paper is a fairly heavy-weight paper impregnated with an inklike substance (Figure 6-17, *C*). When the paper is inserted in the patient's mouth and the teeth are closed together, the paper leaves marks indicating where the upper and lower teeth have made contact.

Marks made by articulating paper aid the dentist in establishing a favorable occlusion for patients who have excessive contact on a tooth or restoration. Articulating paper is available in strips or arch shapes, red or blue color,

and thick or thin gauges. It is usually held between cotton forceps or with articulating paper forceps (Figure 6-18).

Bite Blocks

Triangular rubber bite blocks are used to prop open a patient's mouth during a dental procedure (Figure 6-19). A block is placed vertically between the upper and lower teeth on one side of the mouth. To prevent interference with access it is placed on the side of the mouth opposite the area being treated. Various sizes are available to accommodate different patients.

Auxiliaries should be cautioned to tie a length of dental floss through the hole in the block as a safety measure. Some patients experience difficulty swallowing with a block in place while they are in a supine operating position. Thorough oral evacuation procedures can alleviate this problem.

Saliva Ejector

The saliva ejector is connected to a low-velocity vacuum hose to remove saliva from the patient's mouth during a dental procedure (Figure 6-20). Besides their conve-

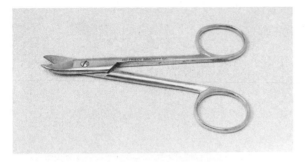

Figure 6-21 Crown and collar scissors.

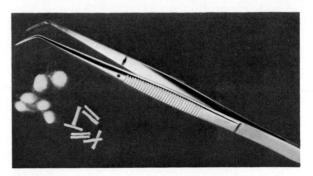

Figure 6-23 Cotton pellets and pledgets, which are handled with cotton pliers.

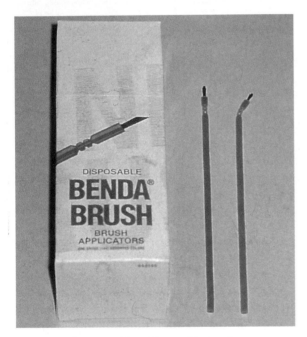

Figure 6-22 Disposable brushes.

nience, disposable saliva ejectors can be adapted to a patient's mouth by being bent into various shapes. The Hygoformic and Svedopter are saliva ejectors that also provide retraction of the tongue.

Crown and Collar Scissors

Crown and collar scissors, sometimes called "crown and bridge" scissors, are short beaked and are used to trim metal matrix bands, temporary crowns, and copper bands (Figure 6-21). Their husky, duck-bill design makes them handy instruments to contour the cervical areas of these devices. The assistant will find crown and collar scissors useful in cutting the various cotton products for use in the oral cavity.

Brushes

Brushes are used to apply various acrylic medicaments and restorative materials to the teeth and existing restora-

tions (Figure 6-22). Sealants, bonding resins, and acrylic can be applied with brushes. Disposable, one-use brushes are convenient, are available in various sizes, and can be bent to adapt to difficult-to-reach areas.

Cotton Pellets

Cotton pellets are one of the most common cotton products used in dentistry (Figure 6-23) and are usually a part of every operative and restorative setup. They are small balls of plain cotton used to clean cavity preparations, apply intraoral medications, and control small areas of hemorrhage. They are available in various sizes and are usually handled in the mouth with cotton pliers.

Mixing Slabs and Pads

Various dental materials are prepared at chairside by dental assistants. These materials include cavity liners, dental cements, surgical dressings, and various impression materials. Some of these materials are mixed on a paper pad, but others must be prepared on a glass mixing slab (Figure 6-24).

Paper pads are convenient because cleanup consists only of disposing of the top sheet of the pad after use. Paper pads are available in various sizes. The amount of material to be prepared determines the size of the pad.

Some materials, such as zinc phosphate cement, are preferably mixed on a cool, dry glass slab. During the mixing procedure these materials produce heat, which must be absorbed by the cool glass slab. Otherwise, the material will set before the dentist can use it.

Cavity Liner Applicators

Cavity liner applicators are handy, tiny-tipped devices for applying a thin layer inside the cavity preparation (Figure 6-25, *A*). This type of material is called a **cavity liner.** Cavity liner applicators are especially useful in the conservative class III, IV, and V cavity preparations.

Some dentists prefer to use a small, hand type of ball burnisher or a spoon excavator for this purpose rather than add another instrument to the preset tray. Some cavity liners are manufactured with a ball burnisher on one end and a small spatula on the opposite end. This type of

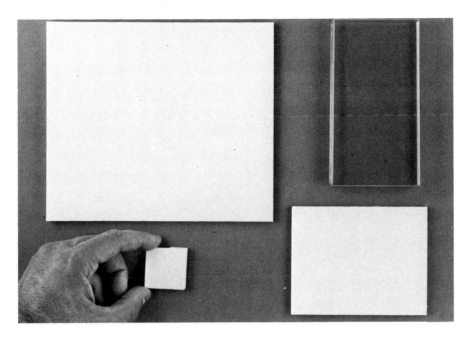

Figure 6-24   Various sizes of paper mixing pads and glass mixing slab.

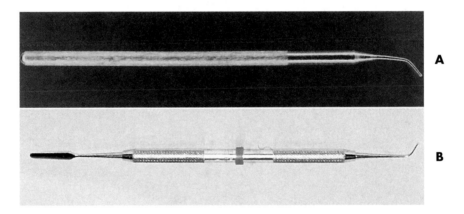

Figure 6-25   **A,** Cavity liner applicator. **B,** Hu-Friedy spatula and cavity liner instrument.

instrument is efficient for mixing and applying dental materials to the tooth (Figure 6-25, *B*).

Isolation Devices

The instruments and devices used for isolation of various teeth are presented in Chapter 8 along with a discussion of their use.

COMMON HAND CUTTING INSTRUMENTS

Hand cutting instruments are operated by hand to remove unwanted tooth structure. The hand cutting instruments were formerly the major means by which a cavity was prepared. Today with the use of both high-speed and conventional-speed handpieces, hand cutting instruments are used primarily to refine the details of the cavity preparation. Figure 6-26 shows the basic parts of these instruments.

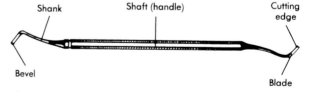

Figure 6-26   Parts of hand cutting instrument.

Within each class of hand cutting instruments further descriptive names are based on the number of angles found in the shank, such as straight, monangle, binangle, and triple angle (Figure 6-27). The shank is defined as the portion of the instrument connecting the blade to the instrument handle or shaft.

Today common reference to instruments by name is a combination of the description of the shank and the class

Table 6-3 Hand cutting instruments

Instrument	Appearance	Example	Function
Hatchet	Cutting edge in same plane as handle Similar to woodsman's tool		To plane cavity walls and cervical floor To sharpen line and point angles in cavity preparation
Chisel	Blade perpendicular to handle		With push motion: Plane enamel margins Trim margins of restorations in anterior areas of mouth
Hoe	Blade perpendicular to handle; bevel opposite that of chisel Resembles garden hoe		With pull motion: Plane cavity walls and floors

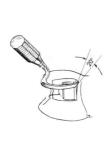

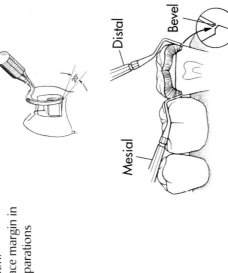

Distal

Bevel

Mesial

Angle former | Similar to chisel but cutting edge at angle

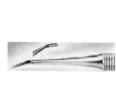

To form sharp internal line and point angles of cavity preparation

Gingival angle former | Similar to hatchet, but working end is curved. Double-ended instruments have one end that curves to right and other end that curves to left. Mesial-style instrument has cutting edge that slopes down and toward instrument handle when in mandibular position. Distal-style instrument has cutting edge that slopes down and away from instrument handle when in mandibular position

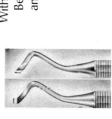

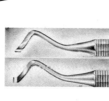

With lateral scraping motion: Bevel cervical cavosurface margin in amalgam and inlay preparations

Figures from Sturdevant CM and others: *The art and science of operative dentistry*, ed 3, St Louis, 1995, Mosby; Carter LM, Yaman P: *Dental instruments*, St Louis, 1991, Mosby.

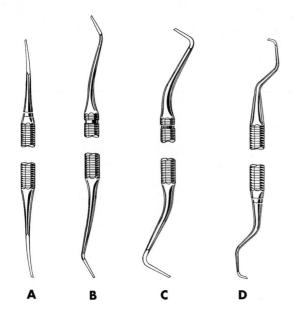

Figure 6-27 Hand cutting instrument shank angles. **A,** Straight: shank containing no angle. **B,** Monangle: shank containing one angle. **C,** Binangle: shank containing two angles. **D,** Triple angle: shank containing three angles.

(Redrawn from Carter LM, Yaman P: *Dental instruments,* St Louis, 1991, Mosby.)

of the instrument. For example, a hatchet with two angles in the shank is called a binangled hatchet; a chisel with one angle in the shank is called a monangled chisel. These references to instruments should be used only among dental personnel out of earshot of the patient. Apprehensive patients may be frightened by the terms *hatchet* and *chisel!* Substitutions such as the instrument number or a special name (e.g., Wedlestaedt) are more acceptable.

Classes of Hand Cutting Instruments

A wide variety of hand cutting instruments is available. For the most part each instrument can be placed in one of five classes:

1. Hatchet
2. Chisel
3. Hoe
4. Margin trimmer
5. Angle former

Each class has basic design features intended to accomplish a specific task. However, with the changes in cavity preparation design and the desire to minimize the number of instruments needed for a given procedure, many of the hand instruments are used for more purposes than their intended one. It is not uncommon to find that the armamentarium of an experienced dentist contains far fewer hand instruments than that of a recent graduate. One way to increase chairside efficiency is to get

maximum use of an instrument during any given procedure. Table 6-3 describes the various hand cutting instruments and their uses.

BIBLIOGRAPHY

Finkebeiner BL, Johnson CS: *Mosby's comprehensive dental assisting: a clinical approach;* St Louis, 1995, Mosby.
Grundy JR, Jones JG: *A colour atlas of clinical operative dentistry: crowns and bridges,* ed 2, London, 1992, Wolfe.
Nield-Gehrig JS, Houseman GA: *Fundamentals of dental hygiene instrumentation,* ed 2, Philadelphia, 1988, Lea & Febiger.
Sturdevant CM and others: *The art and science of operative dentistry,* ed 3, St Louis, 1995, Mosby.

QUESTIONS—Chapter 6

1. The bur shown below is an example of a _____ type.

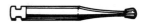

   a. Friction-grip
   b. Latch
   c. Handpiece

2. The bur shown in question 1 is inserted into the _____ attachment for the low-speed handpiece.
   a. Prophylaxis angle
   b. Contra-angle
   c. Straight
   d. Angle former

3. The bur shown below is an example of a(an) _____ that is used to attach sandpaper disks and polishing devices to the handpiece.

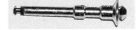

   a. Mandrel
   b. Round bur
   c. Prophylaxis angle
   d. Acrylic bur

4. The high-speed handpiece has _____ torque.
   a. Little
   b. High

5. Which of the following describes the infection control recommendations for high-speed handpieces?
   a. Disinfect between patients.
   b. Flush and disinfect between patients.
   c. Sterilize between patients.
   d. Flush and sterilize between patients.

6. The high-speed handpiece uses _____ burs.
   a. Latch-type
   b. Long-shafted
   c. Mandrel
   d. Friction-grip

7. Which of the following is (are) used to remove soft carious tooth structure?
   a. Spoon
   b. Explorer
   c. Low-speed handpiece and round bur
   d. *a* and *b*
   e. *a* and *c*

8. Explorers are used for all of the following *except:*
   a. To remove excess cement
   b. To remove calculus
   c. To detect caries
   d. To carve amalgam

9. Which of the following is used with a pull motion to plane cavity walls and floors?
   a. Gingival margin trimmer
   b. Angle former
   c. Chisel
   d. Hoe

10. Which of the following is used to bevel the cervical cavo-surface margin in amalgam and inlay preparations?
    a. Gingival margin trimmer
    b. Hatchet
    c. Angle former
    d. Hoe

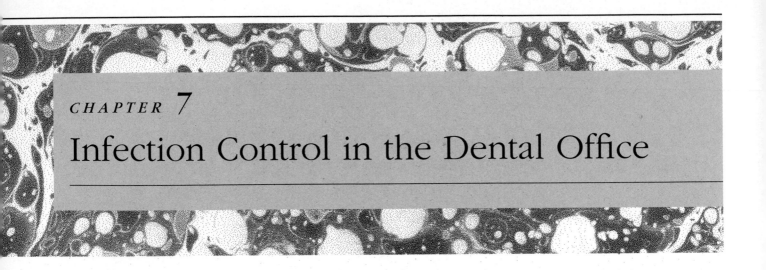

CHAPTER 7

Infection Control in the Dental Office

KEY TERMS
Asepsis
Biological monitor
Chemical monitor
Chemical vapor sterilization
Cleaning
Cross-contamination
Disinfection
Disposable barrier
Dry-heat oven
Ethylene oxide
Infection control
Liquid sterilant
Overgloves
Preset trays
Rapid heat transfer sterilization
Steam autoclave
Sterilization
Ultrasonic cleaner
Unit-dose packaging
Universal precautions

The dental office is a high-risk environment in terms of the spread of disease. It is a facility where patients, staff, delivery people, and material goods come into contact with various microorganisms every workday. This fact should make all dental personnel aware of the need for meticulous infection control measures to protect themselves, their families, their patients, dental laboratory technicians, and the public (Figure 7-1).

A variety of communicable disease poses a threat to the health of patients and members of the dental team. Diseases such as hepatitis B, influenza, tuberculosis, herpes, and acquired immune deficiency syndrome (AIDS) are of ongoing concern (Table 7-1). Renewed concern about the effectiveness of infection control practices occurred in the 1980s when AIDS was first reported and with the emergence of multidrug-resistant tuberculosis.

Although every dental staff member must work to maintain an effective infection control program, the dental assistant is responsible for a major portion of its implementation. This chapter provides information needed to meet this responsibility.

CONCEPT OF INFECTION CONTROL
Microorganisms

Microorganisms are microscopic life-forms such as viruses, bacteria, bacterial spores, and fungi. Some of these microbial forms cause disease and are often referred to as pathogens or pathogenic microorganisms. Some microorganisms are more resistant to destruction than others. The bacterial endospore is a highly resistant microbe, whereas the microorganism that causes AIDS is more easily destroyed. An infection control program is based on targeting the most resistant types of microorganisms.

Universal Precautions

Dental offices must develop stringent infection control programs to destroy the most resistant type of microorganism. Because some infectious diseases exhibit mild to no clinical signs of illness it is not possible to identify all patients carrying an infectious disease. Therefore the dental office must assume that all patients are infectious and practice the same stringent infection control protocol on

Table 7-1 Infectious hazards for both dental personnel and patients in operatory

Infectious organism	Habitat	Transmission	Potential pathology	Vaccine
BACTERIA				
Bordetella pertussis (B)	Nasopharynx	Nasopharyngeal secretions*	Whooping cough	Yes
Cardiobacterium hominis (A)	Nasopharynx	Nasopharyngeal secretions*	Endocarditis	No
Corynebacterium diphtheriae	Nasopharynx	Nasopharyngeal secretions*	Diphtheria	Yes
Enterobacteriaceae (A) *Escherichia coli* *Proteus vulgaris* *Klebsiella pneumoniae*	Mouth, gastrointestinal (GI) tract	Blood, lesion exudate†	Pneumonia, bacteremia, abscesses, wound infections	No
Haemophilus influenzae (C)	Mouth, nasopharynx	Blood, nasopharyngeal secretions*	Pneumonia, meningitis, otitis	Yes
H. parainfluenzae (A)	Mouth, nasopharynx	Blood, nasopharyngeal secretions*	Conjunctivitis, endocarditis	No
H. paraphrophilus (A)	Mouth, nasopharynx	Blood, nasopharyngeal secretions*	Endocarditis	No
Mycobacterium tuberculosis (D)	Pharynx	Pharyngeal secretions*	Tuberculosis	No
Mycoplasma pneumoniae (A)	Pharynx	Pharyngeal secretions*	Primary atypical pneumonia	No
Neisseria meningitidis (C)	Mouth, nasopharynx	Blood, nasopharyngeal secretions*	Cerebrospinal meningitis	Yes
N. gonorrhoeae (D)	Mouth, nasopharynx	Blood, lesion exudate, nasopharyngeal secretions†	Oral lesions, conjunctivitis	No
Pseudomonas aeruginosa (A)	Ubiquitous, sink and drain contaminant	Lesion exudate*	Pneumonia, wound infections	No
Staphylococcus aureus (A) *S. epidermidis* (A)	Mouth, skin, nasopharynx	Lesion exudate*	Suppurative lesions, bacteremia	No
	Mouth, skin, nasopharynx	Lesion exudate*	Endocarditis	No
Streptococcus pyogenes (A)	Nasopharynx	Blood, nasopharyngeal secretions†	Rheumatic and scarlet fever, otitis media, cervical adenitis, mastoiditis, peritonsillar abscesses, meningitis, pneumonia, acute glomerulonephritis	No
S. pneumoniae (A)	Nasopharynx	Blood, nasopharyngeal secretions†	Pneumonia, endocarditis	Yes
S. viridans group (A)	Nasopharynx	Blood, nasopharyngeal secretions†	Endocarditis	No
Treponema pallidum (D) *Actinomycosis* species (sp) *Bacteroides* sp	Blood, oral mucosa	Exudate from oral lesions†	Syphilis	No
Eubacterium sp	Gingival crevice (normal oral flora)	Crevicular exudate†	Abscesses	No
Fusobacterium sp (A) *Peptococcus* sp *Peptostreptococcus* sp *Propionibacterium* sp				No

From American Dental Association Research Institute, Department of Toxicology: *JADA* 117:374, 1988. References: Centers for Disease Control and Prevention: *Reported new U.S. cases for 1987*; Jawetz E, Melnick JL, Adelberg EA: *Review of medical microbiology*, ed 17, Norwalk, Conn, 1987, Appleton and Lange.

A, Nonreportable; *B*, less than 1000; *C*, 1000-9999; *D*, greater than 9999.

NOTE: *Inactivation:* Always use heat sterilization when possible. All of the above organisms can be killed by autoclaving at 121° C, 15 min, 15 psi. Dry-heat sterilization: 170° C, 60 min. Heat-sensitive instruments and surfaces may be disinfected using phenolic or glutaraldehyde-based solutions.
*Infected droplet contact: inhalation, ingestion, direct inoculation.
†Direct inoculation to tissue surface.
‡Inoculation into circulatory system.

Continued

Table 7-1 Infectious hazards for both dental personnel and patients in operatory—cont'd

Infectious organism	Habitat	Transmission	Potential pathology	Vaccine
VIRUSES				
Coxsackie virus (A)	Oropharyngeal mucosa	Ingestion	Hand/foot/mouth disease, vesicular pharyngitis	No
Cytomegalovirus (A)	Salivary gland	Saliva, blood†	Cellular enlargement and degeneration in immuno-compromised individuals	No
Epstein-Barr (A)	Parotid gland	Saliva, blood†	Infectious mononucleosis	No
Hepatitis				
A (D)	Liver, GI tract	Blood (rare), ingestion	Liver inflammation, jaundice	No
B (D)	Liver	Blood, saliva, tears, semen‡	Eventual hepatocellular carcinoma in chronic antigen carriers	Yes
Non-A, non-B (C)	Liver?	Blood‡		No
Delta (A)	Liver	Blood‡	Coinfection with hepatitis B virus (HBV) required	Yes (HBV vac)
Herpes simplex 1 and 2 (A)	Nasopharynx	Lesion exudate, saliva†	Oral lesions, herpetic whitlow, conjunctivitis	No
Human immunodeficiency virus (HIV) (D)	T4 lymphocyte	Blood‡	Acquired immune deficiency syndrome (AIDS)	No
Measles	Nasopharynx	Nasopharyngeal secretions, blood, saliva, vesicle exudate	Generalized vesicular rash	Yes
Rubeola (C)				Yes
Rubella (B)				
Mumps virus (D)	Parotid gland	Saliva, ingestion	Parotitis, meningitis	Yes
Poliovirus (B)	Oropharyngeal mucosa, GI tract	Ingestion	Central nervous system paralysis	Yes
RESPIRATORY VIRUSES (A)				
Influenza A and B	Nasopharynx	Nasopharyngeal secretions*	Flu, common cold	Yes
Parainfluenza				No
Rhinovirus				No
Adenovirus				Yes
Coronavirus				No
Varicella (A)	Skin	Vesicle exudate*	Chickenpox	No
FUNGUS				
Candida albicans (A)	Mouth, skin	Nasopharyngeal secretions*	(Opportunistic) candidiasis, cutaneous infections	No
PROTOZOON				
Pneumocystis carinii (A)	Mouth	Nasopharyngeal secretions*	(Opportunistic) interstitial pneumonia in immuno-compromised individuals	No

BOX 7-1

UNIVERSAL PRECAUTIONS

Each workplace must be safe or free from hazards that could cause harm or death.
Provide personal protective clothing and equipment.

every patient. The term for this type of infection control is **universal precautions.** Universal precautions reduce exposure of patients and the dental staff to infectious disease whether patients are infectious or not. Using universal precautions ensures safety to patients and to the dental staff (Box 7-1). It is not necessary to develop additional measures for patients who report an infectious disease such as AIDS or a hepatitis B carrier state because univer-

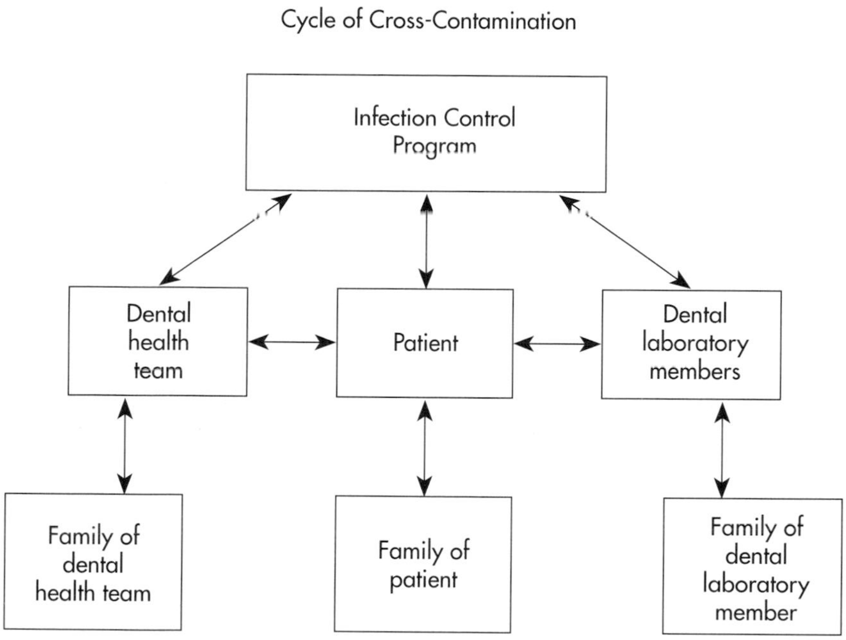

Cycle of Cross-Contamination

Figure 7-1   Cross-contamination cycle.
(From Finkbeiner BL, Johnson CS: *Mosby's comprehensive dental assisting: a clinical approach*, St Louis, 1995, Mosby.)

sal precautions already assume that every patient has these diseases.

> **⇥ KEY POINT**
> ▪ Universal precautions assumes that all patients carry an infectious disease; therefore the same stringent infection control practices are used with every patient.

Routes of Disease Transmission

Microorganisms are everywhere in the environment. They are in the air and on work surfaces, dental and office equipment, skin, hair, instruments, containers, and dental charts. As one might expect, they are also present in saliva and blood. Not all microorganisms thrive in the same surroundings, but several serious infectious viruses, such as hepatitis B, herpes, and AIDS, have been found in body fluids and tissues the dental team comes in contact with during treatment.

Disease can be transmitted in the dental office by the following methods:

1. Direct contact with oral fluids (e.g., blood, saliva, or other secretions)
    a. From patient to dental staff by tiny cuts or cracks in exposed skin while working in the oral cavity
    b. From dental worker to patient by contact with an open wound or sore
    c. Through contact with the eyes by rubbing the eyes with contaminated hands
2. Indirect contact with contaminated items (e.g., instruments, equipment, or environmental surfaces) (Indirect transmission involves an intermediate step. Microorganisms from an infected person are deposited on an object and then infect a second person who comes in contact with the object.)
    a. Cuts from contaminated instruments or needle sticks from contaminated anesthetic needles
    b. Using contaminated instruments and devices from patient to patient
3. Contact with airborne contaminants (e.g., droplets, splatter, or aerosols)
    a. By splatter of blood or saliva to the eye
    b. Through breathing organisms from contaminated air. (Aerosols from the dental handpiece, coughing, and sneezing are common sources of contamination.)

Strategies have been developed to minimize disease transmission by blocking direct, indirect, and airborne routes. Most people are aware of direct route transmission. The indirect and airborne droplet routes of transmission may not be as obvious, since microorganisms are invisible to the naked eye and people may overlook the fact that objects may be contaminated or tiny droplets and aerosols have been released into the air. It is not uncommon for the dental team to return to work in a patient's oral cavity after contact with contaminated objects, such as work surfaces, dental charts, telephones, study models, and dental equipment.

Individuals are usually tolerant of the organisms that normally inhabit their bodies because natural defense mechanisms exist. Organisms foreign to the individual can override these defense mechanisms and are usually the cause of disease. This is the danger of cross-contamination between individuals. However, in some cases an individual's tolerance can be lowered because of stress, fatigue, or body tissue damage to the point where one's own organisms become pathogenic. This change often happens after oral surgical procedures.

INFECTION CONTROL: OVERVIEW

Infection control is a multifaceted effort designed to protect health care workers and patients from cross-contamination in the dental office. It includes the following elements:

1. Reviewing the patient's health status
2. Maintaining an aseptic microorganism-free technique
3. Managing cases sent to the dental laboratory
4. Protecting the operating team
5. Treatment room decontamination
6. Instrument recirculation

Patient's Health Status

The patient's health status should be reviewed at each appointments to determine whether the individual has a condition that precludes dental procedures. For example, a patient with a herpetic oral lesion should not have dental procedures because of the risk of spreading the lesion via dental instruments or gloved hands of the dental staff to other areas of the patient's mouth or possibly eye.

If the patient reports a history of an infectious disease it is not necessary to take additional infection control measures such as wearing two pairs of gloves or repeated sterilization of the instruments. This is not the purpose of the medical history. Remember that a patient may have an infectious disease and may not be aware of it or may not report it because of the stigma associated with it.

Aseptic Technique

The operating team should avoid **cross-contamination** of their gloves, instruments, devices, and materials during treatment to prevent the spread of an infectious disease from one person or inanimate object to another. Common examples of cross-contamination with contaminated gloves follow:

- Handling dental charts
- Touching your face, mask, or protective eyeglasses
- Retrieving instruments or supplies from drawers

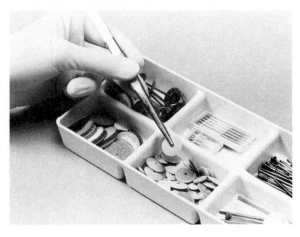

Figure 7-2 Preventing contamination of dental supplies by using sterile forceps to retrieve needed items.

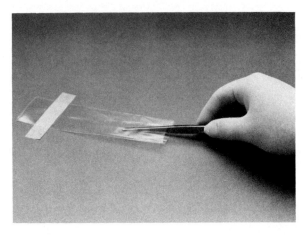

Figure 7-3 Use of protective sleeve to maintain cleanliness of retrieval forceps.

Inexpensive plastic food handlers' gloves, often called **overgloves,** can be used to retrieve objects or instruments, to write in the chart, or to dispense materials from bulk containers.

Instruments, burs, diamond stones, cotton products, and other small items can be retrieved using overgloves or sterile forceps to prevent contamination of adjacent items in the container (Figure 7-2). Likewise, only clean forceps should be used to dip cotton pellets into bottles of liquid such as cavity varnish. Such forceps must be kept in a clean area on the dental assistant's cart. A small storage sleeve can be made from a 5 × 2-inch plastic autoclave bag (Nyclave) (Figure 7-3). The bag can be creased in the middle to hold it open and taped to the work surface for storage of the forceps. Individually wrapped cotton swabs and gauze squares prevent contamination during retrieval (Figure 7-4).

Whenever possible, a rubber dam and high-volume evacuation should be used to minimize the escape of mi-

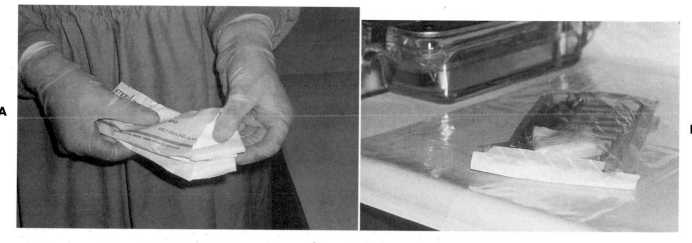

Figure 7-4 **A,** Unit-dose package of disposables. **B,** Packaging of gauze with instrument pack.

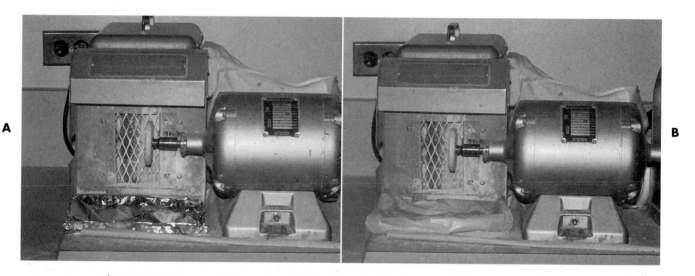

Figure 7-5 Covered lathe pan. **A,** Pan covered with aluminum foil. **B,** Pan covered with plastic.

croorganisms from the patient's mouth via droplets or aerosols. Using a rubber dam and high-volume evacuator can reduce aerosols and splatter by over 90%.

Laboratory Case Management

All laboratory items such as impression trays, models, appliances, and dentures should be decontaminated before and after laboratory processing to protect the laboratory technician and the patient. Table 7-2 summarizes the recommended disinfection methods for impressions and prostheses and appliances.

Impressions

After the impression is removed from the mouth, it is rinsed with running tap water to remove blood and saliva and shaken to remove excess water.

After rinsing, impressions are disinfected by immersion

in an appropriate disinfectant (see Table 7-2). After immersion disinfection the impression is rinsed again before pouring with plaster or stone.

Prostheses and appliances

Partials, dentures, retainers, and other appliances should be cleaned and disinfected before and after sending to the dental laboratory. After removal from the mouth, clean the prosthesis or appliance with a brush and antimicrobial handwash. Immerse the prosthesis or appliance in an appropriate disinfectant. Removable prostheses can be immersed in iodophor or chlorine compounds. Fixed metal or porcelain prostheses can be immersed in glutaraldehydes or heat sterilized. The prosthesis or appliance should only be placed in the disinfectant for the recommended tuberculocidal inactivation and then removed from the disinfectant to avoid corrosion or other

Table 7-2 Guide for selection of disinfectant solutions

Items	Glutaraldehydes[a]	Iodophors[b]	Chlorine compounds[c]	Complex phenolics[a]
IMPRESSIONS[d]				
Alginate	−	+	+	−
Polysulfide	+	+	+	+
Silicone	+	+	+	+
Polyether	+[e]	+[e]	+	+[e]
ZOE impression paste	+	+	−	?
Reversible hydrocolloid	−	+	+	?
Compound	−	+	+	
PROSTHESES AND APPLIANCES[f,g]				
Fixed (metal/porcelain)	+	?	+[h]	?
Removable (acrylic/porcelain)	−	+	+	−
Removable (metal/acrylic)	−	+[h]	+[h]	−
Appliances (all metal)	+	?	?	?

Modified from Merchant: *Compend Contin Educ Dent* 14:382-391, 1993.

+, Recommended method; −, not recommended; ?, data not available or inconclusive.

[a]Prepared according to manufacturer's instructions for disinfection.

[b]1:213 dilution.

[c]1:10 dilution of commercial bleach or prepared according to manufacturer's instructions for disinfection.

[d]Impressions and prostheses should be rinsed under running tap water and then immersed for the time recommended for tuberculosis disinfection with the selected product. Thorough rinsing of impressions and prostheses under running tap water after disinfection is necessary to remove any residual disinfectant.

[e]Use with caution. Consult manufacturer's recommendations.

[f]Also may be ethylene oxide sterilized.

[g]Prostheses or appliances that have been worn by patients must be cleaned thoroughly before disinfection.

[h]Use minimal exposure time (10 minutes) to avoid damage to metal.

adverse effects. After immersion disinfection the prosthesis or appliance is rinsed again and dried. Removable prostheses are placed in diluted mouthwash for storage if necessary. Sodium hypochlorite or other chlorine compounds are not recommended for a prosthesis fabricated with metal because the solution is corrosive to the metal. Laboratory pans should be cleaned and disinfected after each use.

Polishing

Many dental offices have a dental lathe for polishing and grinding. Polishing agents such as pumice should be distributed in **unit-dose packaging** to limit cross-contamination. Dry polishing agents such as pumice can be moistened with a disinfecting agent to reduce exposure to pathogenic microorganisms. Lathe attachments such as rag wheels and stones should be sterilized between uses or disposable attachments thrown away after each case. The pan below the lathe that collects the used polishing agent should be lined with aluminum foil (Figure 7-5, *A*) or plastic (Figure 7-5, *B*), and the liner containing the polishing agent should be discarded after each use.

Laboratory burs are cleaned and sterilized after each use. Laboratory handpieces are cleaned and disinfected after each use. Gloves, masks, protective eyewear, and a spray bottle of disinfectant should be made available in the dental laboratory area.

Sending items to the private dental laboratory

If contaminated items are to be shipped or transported to a private dental laboratory, the contaminated items must be placed in a closed, leakproof, red color-coded container. A biohazard label is placed on containers that are not color coded red.

Protection of the Operating Team
Immunization

As shown in Table 7-1, dental personnel are vulnerable to a wide variety of diseases. Immunization against such diseases is an important line of defense. Of particular concern is the hepatitis B infection. Hepatitis is a serious disease that can be prevented by vaccination. Dental auxiliaries should consult a physician to review their status of immunity to rubella, hepatitis B, influenza, measles, polio, tetanus, and diphtheria and should update vaccinations when needed.

Personal barrier techniques

Physical barriers between patients and operating teams are another line of defense against contagious disease.

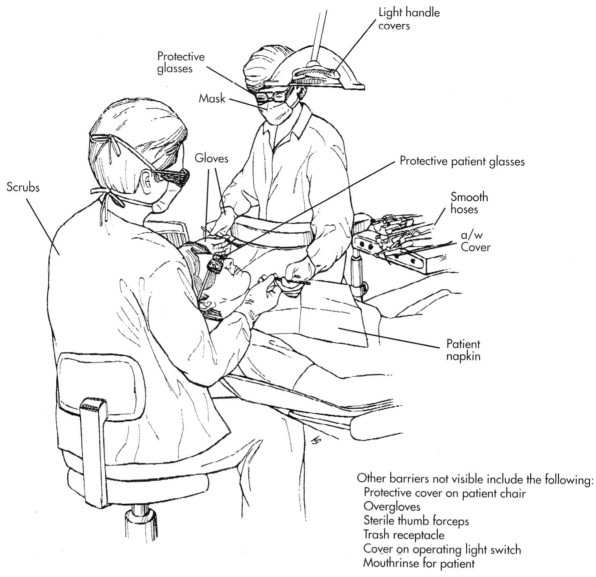

Figure 7-6 Dental assistant and dentist using standard barrier techniques, including protective eyewear, face mask, gloves, and clinic attire.

(From Finkbeiner BL, Johnson CS: *Mosby's comprehensive dental assisting: a clinical approach*, St Louis, 1995, Mosby.)

Such barriers that protect the individual are called personal protective equipment (Figure 7-6). Personal protective equipment consists of protective eyewear, face masks, protective clothing, and gloves.

Protective eyewear

Protective eyewear is worn whenever there is risk of splatter from the patient's oral cavity during treatment. Use of the dental handpiece, the air-water syringe, and the ultrasonic scaler may cause splatter and spray. The eye can be infected by splatter. Protective eyewear prevents such infections by providing a barrier and reminds staff members not to rub their eyes. Protective eyewear includes normal eyeglasses with additional side protection, safety goggles, and face shields.

Safety goggles and face shields offer both top and side shielding and are preferable to normal eyeglasses with additional side protection. Contaminated eyewear should be washed with soap and water, rinsed, and disinfected or sterilized.

Protective eyewear is also worn when there is danger of damage to the eyes by propelled objects during grinding or polishing in laboratory or other procedures. Patients should also be offered protective eyewear to prevent accidental splatter or damage to the eyes by dental procedures.

Face masks

Face masks, like protective eyewear, provide a barrier against splatter of infectious organisms to susceptible mucous membranes. In addition, masks provide a filter against aspiration of microorganisms that are sprayed in the air by aerosol from the dental handpiece, the ultrasonic scaler, or the air-water syringe.

Masks should be changed between patients to prevent cross-contamination. During longer procedures masks are changed hourly to maintain filtration quality because moisture from breathing causes deterioration of quality.

Protective clothing

Protective clothing is worn during treatment of dental patients so organisms are not carried to or from the dental office on street clothes. Likewise, dental assistants should avoid wearing clinic attire outside the office. Protective clothing is changed at least once each day for routine dental procedures. Clothing is changed during the day if visibly soiled.

The U.S. Occupational Safety and Health Administration (OSHA) blood-borne pathogens standard mandates that the employer is responsible for the laundering of protective clothing. The employee should not be taking contaminated clothing or linens home to launder.

> ➡ **KEY POINTS**
> - Wear protective clothing only at the dental office.
> - If you go to lunch or out of the office, change out of your protective clothing.
> - Before leaving the office at the end of the day, change out of your protective clothing.

Gloves

Gloves are an essential part of an infection control program. They protect the dentist and the dental auxiliary from organisms that can enter through small cuts, scratches, hangnails, and sores on the hands. Gloves also protect the patient from pathogenic microorganisms that could be present on the ungloved hands of the dental care worker. Gloves are worn when there is exposure or potential for exposure to blood, oral fluids, or contaminated objects or surfaces. Common types of gloves and their uses are described in Box 7-2.

Nonsterile latex rubber examination gloves are used during routine dental procedures. Examination gloves are worn for all intraoral procedures and changed after every patient. If a glove becomes torn during a procedure, the glove is removed, hands are washed, and new gloves are put on. Jewelry such as a ring is removed when wearing gloves because of the potential to puncture the glove and also because of the potential to develop fungal infections under the ring. Vinyl gloves, nonpowdered gloves, and hypoallergenic gloves are available for dental personnel

---

BOX 7-2

COMMON TYPES OF GLOVES AND THEIR USES

TYPE	USE
Nonsterile latex rubber or vinyl examination gloves	Routine dental treatment
Plastic overgloves	Prevention of cross-contamination
Sterile surgical gloves	Surgical procedures
Heavy-duty neoprene utility gloves	Instrument decontamination
Autoclavable polynitrile gloves	

---

who develop an allergic reaction to latex gloves or the glove powder. Gloves are rinsed in cool water to remove excess powder from the glove. Do not wash latex gloves in soap and water, which could cause minute breaks in the gloves.

Sterile surgical gloves are available for treatment procedures that require surgical **asepsis.**

Plastic overgloves are worn over treatment gloves when there is potential for cross-contamination. Plastic overgloves can be worn over treatment gloves when writing in the dental chart, reaching into drawers for instruments, or dispensing dental materials from bulk containers.

Heavy-duty gloves are used for decontamination of the treatment room and dental instruments and equipment. Neoprene or autoclavable polynitrile gloves are both suitable.

> ➡ **KEY POINTS**
> - Wear a new pair of gloves for each patient.
> - Do not wash gloves with soap and water because it causes small breaks in the gloves; instead rinse with cool water.
> - Remove torn or punctured gloves, and replace with a new pair after washing hands thoroughly.

Handwashing

Hands should be washed with an antimicrobial soap containing chlorhexidine gluconate, para-chlorometaxylenol (PCMX), or iodophors (Figure 7-7). Antimicrobial soaps can make the skin of the hands very dry and cause cracking. The Centers for Disease Control and Prevention (CDC) recommendations state that a nonantimicrobial liquid soap is sufficient to wash hands between patients and antimicrobial soap can be reserved for critical times dur-

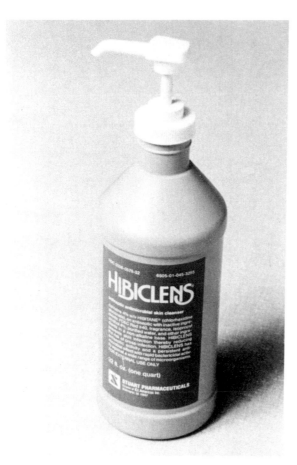

Figure 7-7   Antimicrobial hand soap.

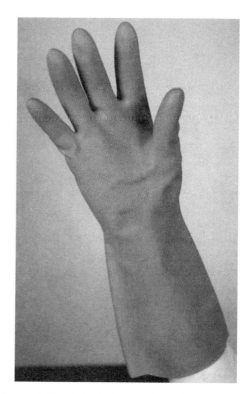

Figure 7-8   Polynitrile autoclavable gloves
(Courtesy Health Sonics Corporation, Pleasanton, Calif.)

ing the day, such as beginning and end of day or before and after surgical procedures.

Hands should be washed at the following times:
- At the beginning of the day (surgical scrub)
- Between each patient (at least 15 seconds)
- Before and after wearing gloves at the end of the day

When washing hands, use cool water and dry hands with disposable paper towels. Sinks, faucets, and soap dispensers that are foot controlled avoid the risk of cross-contamination.

Treatment Room Decontamination Procedures
Cleaning

Cleaning is the process of removing debris and some organisms from instruments, devices, and work surfaces. Debris such as blood, plaque, residual cement, impression material, and salivary mucus harbors microorganisms. Debris interferes with disinfection and sterilization procedures and must be removed before such procedures.

The surface of large dental equipment and countertops can be cleaned with 4×4–inch gauze sponges and a disinfectant. Several sponges are recommended to prevent smearing debris instead of removing it. Gloves, a mask, protective eyewear, and protective clothing are worn dur-

ing all cleaning and disinfection procedures. Heavy, household-style neoprene gloves or polynitrile gloves are worn during treatment room decontamination and instrument cleaning (Figure 7-8).

The central oral evacuation system often becomes highly contaminated. Debris from the patient's oral cavity is drawn into tubing that extends from the dental unit. This system must be cleaned thoroughly each day by flushing with commercially available cleaners designed for this purpose. The evacuator holding device and the tubing must be flushed between patients.

The high-speed handpiece tubing and air-water syringe should also be flushed for 3 minutes at the beginning of the day and at least 20 to 30 seconds between patients.

Disinfection

Disinfection is the chemical destruction of most forms of microorganisms. A disinfectant does not kill all microorganisms regardless of the amount of time they are exposed to the chemical. Table 7-3 lists approved disinfectants.

The surface of countertops and large dental equipment should be cleaned and disinfected with a suitable disinfectant applied with a spray bottle or aerosol can. Disinfection is a two-step process—a cleaning step and a disinfecting step. For the cleaning step the item is sprayed and wiped with the disinfectant. The item is then sprayed

Table 7-3 Office sterilization asepsis procedures (OSAP): representative agents for surface cleaning and disinfection

Chemical classification	Products Name	EPA reg. no.	TB directions Dilution	Time	Temperature	Test*	Hydrophilic virucide**	Cleaning ability
CHLORINES								
Sodium hypochlorite	Bleach (5.25%)	–	1:100	10 min	20° C	–	Yes	Good
	Dispatch (0.55%)	56392-7	none	2 min	20°–25° C	–	Yes	Good
Chlorine dioxide	Exspor	45631-03	4:1:1	3 min	20° C	AOAC	Yes	Good
IODOPHORS	Iodofive	1677-22	1:213	5 min	20° C	AOAC	Yes (10 min)	Good
	Biocide, Bi-Arrest	4959-16	1:213	10 min	20° C	AOAC	Yes	Good
	Surf-A-Cide	4959-16	1:213	10 min	20° C	AOAC	Yes	Good
	Asepti-IDC	303-63	1:256	10 min	–	AOAC	Yes	Good
	Wescodyne	52-150	1:213	25 min	25° C	Quant	Yes	Good

PHENOLIC COMBINATIONS†
Water-based pump spray

Phenyl	Amyl	Chloro	Name	EPA reg. no.	Dilution	Time	Temperature	Test*	Hydrophilic virucide**	Cleaning ability
9.0%	–	1%	Omni II, ProPhene	46851-1	1:32	10 min	20° C	AOAC	Yes	Good
			Vital Defense-D	46851-1	1:32	10 min	20° C	AOAC	Yes	Good
0.28%	–	0.03%	ProSpray	46851-5	None	10 min	20° C	AOAC	Yes	Good
12.0%	4.0%	10.0%	Top-Cide	11725-7	1:256	10 min	20° C	AOAC	Yes	Good
2.94%	1.49%	4.56%	Asepti-phene 128	303-223	1:128	10 min	20° C	AOAC	Yes	Good

The following products in this group do not demonstrate a hydrophilic virus kill:

Phenyl	Amyl	Chloro	Name	EPA reg. no.	Dilution	Time	Temperature	Test*	Hydrophilic virucide**	Cleaning ability
2.23%	13.12%	7.24%	Lysol IC Disinfectant Cleaner	675-46	1:128	10 min	20° C	AOAC	No	Good
10.5%	13.12%	5.0%	Lysol IC Disinfectant	675-43	1:200	10 min	20° C	AOAC	No	Good

Alcohol-based pump spray

Phenyl	Amyl	Ethanol	Name	EPA reg. no.	Dilution	Time	Temperature	Test*	Hydrophilic virucide**	Cleaning ability
0.216%	0.054%	66%	Coe Spray-The Pump	334-417	None	10 min	20° C	AOAC	Yes	Fair
0.216%	0.054%	66%	Novospray	334-417	None	10 min	20° C	AOAC	Yes	Fair

Alcohol-based aerosol

Phenyl	Amyl	Ethanol	Name	EPA reg. no.	Dilution	Time	Temperature	Test*	Hydrophilic virucide**	Cleaning ability
0.1%	–	79%	Lysol IC Disinfectant	777-53	None	10 min	20°	AOAC	Yes	Poor
0.12%	–	66.6%	Citrace	56392-2	None	10 min	20°–25° C	AOAC	Yes	Poor
0.176%	0.045%	49.95%	Asepti-Steryl	706-69	None	10 min	25° C	AOAC	Yes	Poor

The following products in this group do not demonstrate a hydrophilic virus kill:

Phenyl	Amyl	Ethanol	Name	EPA reg. no.	Dilution	Time	Temperature	Test*	Hydrophilic virucide**	Cleaning ability
0.176%	0.044%	52.79%	Medicide/ADC Disinfectant Deodorant	334-214	None	10 min	–	AOAC	No	Poor

Copyright March 1995, OSAP Research Foundation. All rights reserved.
NOTE: Chlorines and iodophors must be diluted daily (when dilution required) to be tuberculocidal. 20° C = 68° F. Other products are to be used as disinfectants on pre-cleaned surfaces. Listing does not imply endorsement, recommendation, or warranty. Purchasers are legally required to consult the package insert for changes in formulation and recommended product uses. Check compatibility of material before use on dental equipment. Updated tables are available from the OSAP Research Foundation 800-298-OSAP (6727); FAX: 410-798-6797.
*Tests for TB label claim: AOAC = Association of Official Analytical Chemists; Quant = Quantitative.
**Hydrophilic viruses include various strains of polio, coxsackie, rhinovirus, and rotavirus.
†Phenyl = ortho phenylphenol; amyl = tertiary amylphenol; chloro = benzyl chlorophenyl.

again with the disinfectant, which is allowed to remain on the surface for the recommended disinfection time as specified by the manufacturer. Spraying the chemical helps place it in inaccessible areas such as instrument holders and evacuator tips. Caution must be exercised to avoid spraying hot operating light bulbs and electrical switches. Iodophor disinfectants, chlorine dioxide disinfectants, synthetic phenols, and household bleach (1:5 to 1:100) are the chemicals currently recommended for surface disinfection (Table 7-4). Unacceptable solutions for disinfection include isopropyl or rubbing alcohol and quaternary ammonium compounds. Although 2% glutaraldehyde solutions are preferred for sterilant instrument baths, they are not recommended for surface disin-

fection because of their corrosiveness, their odor, and the potential toxicity if a significant volume evaporates into surrounding air.

•❖ KEY POINT
- **The following is a summary of the correct technique for surface disinfection:**
  1. **Spray surface with disinfectant.**
  2. **Wipe surface with gauze or paper towel.**
  3. **Spray surface again with disinfectant.**
  4. **Allow disinfectant to remain on surface for recommended tuberculocidal action.**

Table 7-4 Characteristics of surface disinfectants

Advantages	Disadvantages
IODOPHORS	
EPA-registered surface disinfectant	Not a sterilant
Broad spectrum: bactericidal, tuberculocidal, and virucidal against hydrophilic and lipophilic viruses	Unstable at high temperatures
	Dilution and contact time critical
Biocidal activity within 5-10 min	Daily preparation necessary
Effective in dilute solution	Discoloration of some surfaces
Few reactions	Rust inhibitor necessary
Surfactant carrier that maintains surface moistness	Inactivated by hard water (1:200)
Residual biocidal action	
HYPOCHLORITES	
EPA-registered surface disinfectant	Chemically unstable solution
Rapid antimicrobial action	Necessary to prepare diluted solutions fresh daily
Broad spectrum: bactericidal, tuberculocidal, and virucidal (also sporicidal under certain conditions)	Diminished activity by organic matter
	Unpleasant, persistent odor in high concentrations
Effective in dilute solution	Irritating to skin and eyes
Economical	Corrosive to metals
	Damaging to clothing
	Degrading to plastics and rubber
CHLORINE DIOXIDE	
EPA-registered surface disinfectant	Discarded daily
Instrument or environmental surface germicide	24-hr sterilant use life
Rapid acting: 3 min for disinfection; 6 hr for sterilization	Inability to readily penetrate organic debris
	Protective eyewear and gloves required
	Closed containers
	Adequate ventilation necessary for surface disinfection
	Corrosive to aluminum containers
	Not sporicidal
	Daily fresh preparation necessary for most diluted solutions
SYNTHETIC PHENOLS	Able to degrade certain plastics and etch glass with prolonged exposure
EPA-registered surface disinfectant	
Broad antimicrobial spectrum	Difficult to rinse off certain materials
Tuberculocidal	Film accumulation
Useful on metal, glass, rubber, and plastic	Skin and eye irritation
Residual biocidal action	

From Cottone JA and others: *Practical infection control in dentistry*, ed 2, Media, Pa, 1996, Lea & Febiger.

BOX 7-3
INSTRUMENT PROCESSING

PROCEDURE	RATIONALE
1. If contaminated instruments can not be cleaned immediately, place them in holding (presoaking) solution.	1. To prevent drying of biological debris (blood and saliva) on instruments.
2. Put on heavy-duty utility gloves and safety glasses.	2. To reduce risk of accidental injury while decontaminating instruments.
3. Place instruments in basket for ultrasonic cleaner, and rinse with cool running water.	3. To remove gross debris. Cold water is best to remove blood.
4. Place instrument basket into ultrasonic cleaner and activate for 6-10 minutes (cassette systems may require longer cleaning time; check with manufacturer for details), or hand scrub instruments individually with long-handled brush. Rinse instruments with cool running water.	4. To remove biological debris on instruments. This alternative is only recommended if ultrasonic cleaner is not available; it is a less desirable option because risk of injury increases as handling of instruments increases.
5. Dry instruments thoroughly for sterilization in chemical vapor or dry-heat sterilizer. Remove excess water for sterilization in steam autoclave.	5. It is necessary to dry instruments thoroughly when using a chemical vapor or dry-heat oven because it will inhibit sterilization.

6. Package instruments in appropriate wrap.
a. Steam autoclave
  (1) Paper
  (2) Plastic
  (3) Surgical muslin
b. Dry heat
  (1) Paper
  (2) Muslin
  (3) Aluminum foil
c. Chemical vapor
  (1) Perforated metal trays
  (2) Paper
  (3) Paper or plastic bag
	6. Steam must be allowed to penetrate packaging material for steam autoclave sterilization. Packaging material should not insulate instruments from heat and also must not be destroyed by temperature. Chemical vapor must be able to penetrate packaging for chemical-vapor sterilization.

PROCEDURE	RATIONALE
7. Place autoclave tape or other process indicator on instrument package before placing in sterilizer.	7. Although process indicators such as autoclave tape do not indicate sterilization, they are useful to indicate that instruments have been exposed to sterilizing conditions.
8. Once each week, insert appropriate biological indicator into heat sterilizer and process with normal load of instruments. a. Steam autoclave—*Bacillus stearothermophilus* strips or vials b. Dry heat—*Bacillus subtilis* strips c. Chemical vapor—*Bacillus stearothermophilus* strips	8. Biological monitoring is recommended weekly by CDC.

9. Sterilize instruments for appropriate time.
a. Steam autoclave
  (1) 15-20 minutes
  (2) 121° C (250° F)
  (3) 15 psi
b. Dry heat
  (1) 2 hours, 160° C (320° F), *or*
  (2) 1 hour, 170° C (340° F)
c. Rapid heat transfer
  (1) Wrapped instruments—12 minutes, 190° C (375° F)
  (2) Unwrapped instruments—6 minutes, 190° C (375° F)
d. Chemical vapor
  (1) 20-40 minutes
  (2) 131° C (270° F)
  (3) 20 psi	

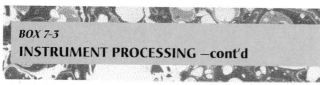

BOX 7-3
INSTRUMENT PROCESSING —cont'd

PROCEDURE	RATIONALE
10. After appropriate sterilization cycle, allow instruments to cool and dry if necessary; then remove from sterilizer.	10. Too rapid cooling of warm instruments may produce condensation inside instrument pack. Wet instrument packing such as absorbent paper material may tear easily or may draw microorganisms into packet if placed on contaminated surface.
11. Store sterile instrument package in dry, covered area away from heat or moisture for no more than 30 days.	11. Sterility is compromised when absorbent packages become wet or moist. Heat may make packaging material brittle.

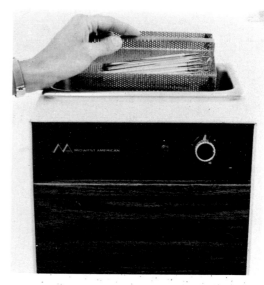

Figure 7-9   Ultrasonic cleaner.

Table 7-5   Summary of methods for decontamination in the dental office

Item category	Item definition	Is item used in the mouth?	Potential risk of disease transmission*	Method of decontamination
Critical	Touches bone or penetrates soft tissue	Yes	Very high to high	Sterilization
Semicritical	Touches mucous membranes but will not touch bone or penetrate soft tissue	Yes	Moderate	Sterilization or high-level disinfection†
Noncritical‡	Has contact with intact skin	No	Low to none	Intermediate to low-level disinfection or simple cleaning§

From Cottone JA and others: *Practical infection control in dentistry,* ed 2, Media, Pa, 1996, Lea & Febiger.
*Depends on nature and amount of contamination and how item or surface is used.
†Depends on whether instruments are damaged by heat.
‡Includes environmental surfaces, which carry an even lower risk of disease transmission than medical instruments.
§Depends on whether items are contaminated visibly by blood.

Instrument Recirculation
Sorting instruments and devices for processing

Although infection can occur through any of the routes mentioned previously, open wounds expose the individual to the greatest risk of infection. This is why effective infection control programs involve sorting instruments and devices for sterilization and disinfection according to how they are used (see Box 7-3 for the appropriate procedure). This sorting is done using a classification system based on the potential risk of disease transmission (Table 7-5).

Although heat is the best method of sterilization, it may destroy some devices, and therefore alternative methods must be used. The sorting scheme just discussed may assist the infection control assistant in processing instruments and preparing the treatment room.

Cleaning

Whenever possible an **ultrasonic cleaner** (Figure 7-9) should be used to clean instruments. Ultrasonic cleaners replace the need to hand scrub instruments. Hand scrubbing instruments increases the risk of injury from the instruments. The ultrasonic cleaner contains a special cleaning solution and vibrates at a high frequency, which shakes debris loose from items placed in it. It is best to use an ultrasonic solution recommended by the manufacturer rather than using a plain disinfectant or any other solution not indicated for the ultrasonic cleaner. Never use a glutaraldehyde solution in the ultrasonic cleaner. Glutaraldehyde solutions can give off noxious vapors from the heat and vibrations created by the ultrasonic cleaner.

Hand scrubbing instruments with a long-handled brush is a less desirable but alternative method. The long-handled brush protects the assistant from the sharp tips of instruments. Heavy, household-style neoprene or polynitrile gloves should be worn during instrument cleaning, and instruments should be scrubbed one at a time to minimize the risk of accidental injury (Figure 7-10).

Sterilization

Sterilization is the process of destroying all living microorganisms, including viruses and bacterial spores. True sterilization can be achieved with sterilant solutions or by various means of heat sterilization. Most dental offices achieve sterilization by several forms of heat with or without chemicals. A less desirable method of sterilization is the use of liquid sterilant solutions. **Ethylene oxide** is a room temperature gas that can also be used for sterilization; however, because it emits a poisonous gas, is costly, and takes 10 to 16 hours per cycle, its use is limited to hospitals, dental schools, and large clinics. Table 7-6 summarizes the major methods of sterilization.

Heat sterilization. Heat sterilization is the most practical method to sterilize dental instruments. All microorganisms die in extreme heat. When temperature exceeds their tolerance level, sterilization occurs. Autoclaving (moist heat), dry heat, and chemical vapor are the three most common methods of heat sterilization used in most dental offices.

STEAM AUTOCLAVE. A **steam autoclave,** or moist-heat sterilizer, is an effective and efficient method of sterilization.

Depending on autoclave size, large quantities of instruments can be sterilized quickly. Figure 7-11 depicts a combination autoclave and dry-heat sterilizer.

The autoclave is a steam chamber where the instruments are placed. During the sterilization cycle, water flows into the chamber and is heated to the boiling point to create steam. Since the chamber is sealed, pressure increases to approximately 15 pounds per square inch (psi). This increase in pressure raises steam temperature to approximately 250° F (121° C). When instruments are exposed to steam, sterilization occurs. Usually this requires about 15 to 20 minutes for resistant bacterial spores and viruses. Porous materials such as cotton goods and surgical sponges may require 30 minutes for steam to penetrate them and render them sterile. It is unfortunate that steam has a corrosive effect on metal instruments. Instruments rust and lose sharp edges when repeatedly exposed to steam. Table 7-6 describes characteristics of autoclave sterilization.

A general guideline for autoclaving is to sterilize a light, well-spaced load of instruments for 15 to 20 minutes at 250° F (121° C) and 15 psi. The size of the load, the type of instruments or materials processed, and the method of placement may alter the time required for sterilization.

The steam must penetrate the entire load to achieve sterilization. Therefore it is important to avoid overloading the steam chamber and wrapping instruments too tightly, which reduces the penetration of steam around the instruments being processed.

After the cycle the pressure is released from the steam chamber through a vent, and the door can be opened to allow the instruments to dry.

Manufacturer's instructions should be followed closely when autoclaves are used.

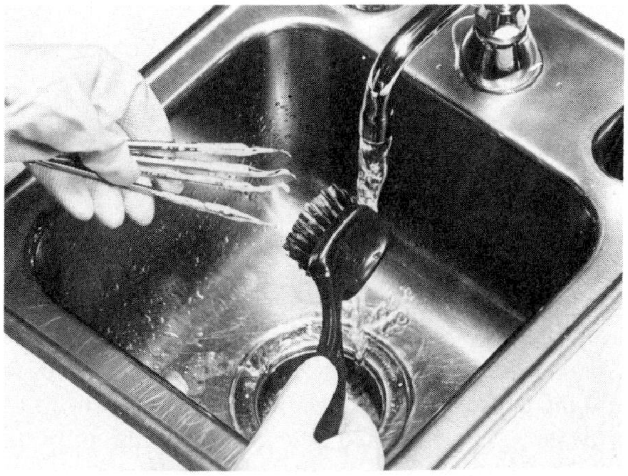

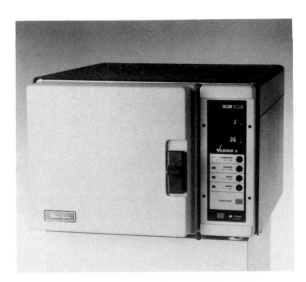

Figure 7-10 Use of household gloves and long-handled brush to clean dental instruments.

Figure 7-11 Steam/dry-heat sterilizer.
(Courtesy Pelton Crane, Charlotte, NC.)

Table 7-6 Major methods of sterilization

Method	Temperature	Pressure	Cycle time	Advantages	Disadvantages	Spore test
Steam autoclave	121° C (250° F)	15 psi	15–20 min	Rapid turnaround Low cost per cycle No toxic or hazardous chemicals	Corrodes carbon steel instruments or burs (stainless steel ok)	*Bacillus stearothermophilus*
Dry-heat oven (rapid dry heat)	160° C (320° F) 170° C (340° F) 190° C (375° F)	None used	2 hr 1 hr 6 min unwrapped; 12 min wrapped	Does not corrode instruments No toxic or hazardous chemicals	Long cycle time May char paper packaging material	*Bacillus subtilis*
Unsaturated chemical vapor	131° C (270° F)	20 psi	20–40 min	Lowest cost per cycle Faster cycle time Does not corrode carbon steel instruments or burs	Uses toxic or hazardous chemicals Requires fume ventilation in area used	*Bacillus stearothermophilus*
Ethylene oxide	Room temperature	None used	10–16 hr	Can sterilize almost anything because does not use heat	Slow cycle time Poisonous gas Needs special ventilation Expensive—limited to hospitals and dental schools	None available
Chemical sterilization (glutaraldehyde)	Room temperature	None used	10 hr	Can use for dental items that may melt with heat sterilizers	No way to test for effectiveness Often misused Harmful chemical if mishandled	None available

DRY-HEAT STERILIZATION. Dry heat sterilization is a popular method of sterilization that is essentially a process of "baking" instruments in a special **dry-heat oven** at 320° F (160° C) for 2 hours or 340° F (170° C) for 1 hour (see Figure 7-12). Because no moisture is used in the process, instruments do not corrode. Table 7-6 describes characteristics of dry-heat sterilization.

The choice of which heat method to use for sterilization may be based on either personal preference or the type of item being sterilized. For example, some items made of paper, cloth, or plastic or some metal impression trays with solder joints may be destroyed at the extreme temperatures used in the dry-heat method. On the other hand, instruments such as endodontic files and reamers are so vulnerable to corrosion they should be sterilized by dry heat to preserve their usefulness.

Instruments processed by dry-heat methods must be cleaned and dried before being placed in the dry-heat oven. Covered metal preset trays can be processed in the dry-heat oven and stored without handling the contents.

A **rapid heat transfer sterilization** method has recently been introduced (Figure 7-12) that works in a manner similar to a convection oven. Instruments can be sterilized at 375° F (190° C) for 12 minutes for wrapped items and 6 minutes for unwrapped items.

CHEMICAL VAPOR STERILIZATION. Another method of sterilization is a combination of heat and chemical vapor. This sterilizer (Figure 7-13) is used with a special solution containing alcohol, acetone, ketone, formaldehyde, and some distilled water (9.25%). Because the water content is below 15%, corrosion and dulling of instruments do not occur. Table 7-6 describes various characteristics of **chemical vapor sterilization.**

Instruments must be scrubbed thoroughly or cleaned in an ultrasonic cleaner, rinsed with cold water, and towel dried before placement in the sterilizer. Failure to prepare instruments properly can result in incomplete sterilization, damage to instruments, or both.

Clean items being sterilized are packaged loosely in the usual containers such as autoclave bags or towel wraps and placed in the sterilizer. The sterilization cycle is run according to the manufacturer's instructions (usually about 20 to 40 minutes at 131° C [270° F] with 20 psi of pressure).

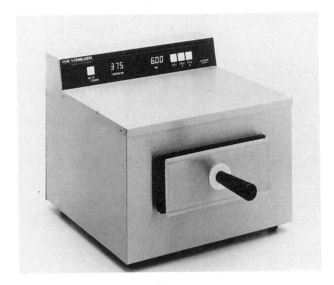

Figure 7-12   Rapid heat transfer sterilizer.

(Courtesy Bowmar Technologies, Fort Wayne, Ind.)

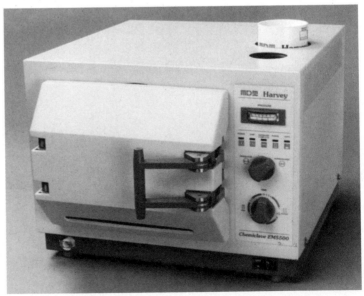

Figure 7-13   Chemical vapor sterilizer.

(Courtesy MDT Corporation, Gardena, Calif.)

Table 7-7   Glutaraldehydes for instrument sterilization (EPA-registered sterilant reuse for 28–30 days)

| Chemical classification | Product | EPA reg. no. | High-level tuberculocidal disinfection | | | Sterilization | |
			Temperature	Time	Test*	Temperature	Time
ALKALINE							
3.4%	Cidex Plus	7078–14	25° C	20 min	Quant	20°–25° C	10 hr
	Maxicide Plus 30	7078–14	25° C	20 min	Quant	20°–25° C	10 hr
3.2%	CoeCide XL Plus	46781–4	25° C	90 min	Quant	20°–25° C	10 hr
	Metricide Plus 30	46781–4	25° C	90 min	Quant	20°–25° C	10 hr
2.5%	Cidex 7	7078–4	25° C	90 min	Quant	20°–25° C	10 hr
2.0%	Asepti-Steryl 28	62329–1	25° C	25 min	AOAC	20° C	10 hr
	Glutall 28	62329–1	25° C	25 min	AOAC		10 hr
	Baxter/Omnicide	46851–2	20° C	45 min	AOAC	20° C	10 hr
	Omnicide	46851–2	20° C	45 min	AOAC	20° C	10 hr
	ProCide	46851–2	20° C	45 min	AOAC	20° C	10 hr
	Vital Defense-S	46851–2	20° C	45 min	AOAC	20° C	10 hr
	CoeCide XL	46781–2	25° C	90 min	AOAC	20°–25° C	10 hr
	Maxicide	46781–2	25° C	90 min	AOAC	20°–25° C	10 hr
	Metricide	46781–2	25° C	90 min	AOAC	20°–25° C	10 hr
	Protec-top	46781–2	25° C	90 min	AOAC	20°–25° C	10 hr
2% ACIDIC	Banicide	15136–1	20° C	30 min	Quant	21° C	10 hr
	Sterall	15136–1	20° C	30 min	Quant	21° C	10 hr
	Wavicide 01	15136–1	20° C	30 min	Quant	21° C	10 hr

Copyright March 1995, OSAP Research Foundation. All rights reserved.
20° C = 68° F; 25° C = 77° F.

NOTE: All products are to be used full strength, undiluted on precleaned instruments. All products meet former ADA acceptance criteria. Other products are available. Listing does not imply endorsement, recommendation, or warranty. Purchasers are legally required to consult the package insert for changes in formulation and recommended product uses. Updated tables are available from the OSAP Research Foundation 800-298-OSAP (6727); FAX: 410-798-6797.

*Tests for TB label claim: Quant = quantitative; AOAC = Association of Official Analytical Chemists. Products withdrawn from U.S. market: 1992: CoeSteril, ColdSpor (55195-2), Glutarex (7182-4); 1991: all sporicidin brand products (8383).

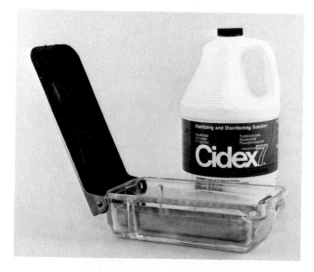

Figure 7-14   Sterilant bath.

A well-ventilated sterilization area is recommended to reduce odor produced by the sterilization solution.

An advantage of this type of system is not only that corrosion and dulling of instruments are eliminated, but also that the sterilized items are dry at the end of the cycle because of the low water content of the sterilization solution. Any items that can be sterilized in an autoclave can usually be safely sterilized in the chemical vapor sterilizer.

Liquid sterilants. Liquid sterilants are chemicals that destroy all microorganisms if they are exposed long enough. Table 7-7 lists approved sterilants. **Liquid sterilant** solutions are used only when heat sterilization would destroy the instruments or devices. Use of this method of sterilization is time consuming, and its effectiveness is difficult to monitor. Successful sterilization depends on the concentration and freshness of the solution and the time of exposure. For maximum effectiveness the manufacturer's directions should be followed precisely. The procedure is outlined in Box 7-4. Instruments and devices must be cleaned before immersion in a sterilant solution (Figure 7-14).

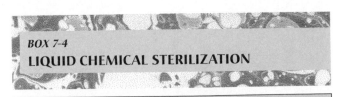

BOX 7-4
LIQUID CHEMICAL STERILIZATION

PROCEDURE	RATIONALE
1. Clean and dry instruments as indicated in Box 7-3, steps 1-4.	1. Organic debris, such as blood and saliva, inhibits the sterilization process.
2. Dry instruments thoroughly.	2. Placing wet instruments into chemical solution will dilute solution and compromise sterilization.
3. Remove undisturbed items after appropriate time as recommended by manufacturer's instructions. Sterilization in liquid chemical solutions requires 10 hours.	3. If additional instruments are later added to solution, removal time must be readjusted.
4. Rinse items thoroughly with water.	4. Glutaraldehydes can be irritating to mucous membranes if residual amounts are left on instruments.
5. Dry instruments and place in clean packaging.	5. Placing instruments in clean packaging will help to maintain sterility.

Monitoring of sterilization. Several devices have been developed to assist dental personnel in monitoring heat and ethylene oxide sterilization (Figure 7-15). At present it is not possible to monitor sterilization for liquid sterilants, which is one of the reasons why that method is less desirable than heat sterilization.

Chemical monitoring. Chemically treated tape or other monitors on heat sterilization wraps change color when exposed to certain sterilization conditions. Although the color change identifies instrument packs that have been exposed to heat, it does not guarantee that the instruments inside the pack have been sterilized. A **chemical monitor** should be used on each sterilization wrap. Chemical monitors are most useful in dental offices with more than one dental auxiliary who is responsible for instrument cleaning and sterilization. Contaminated instrument packs are often stored in the heat sterilizer until the unit is closed and the sterilization cycle has been started. An assistant can quickly check to see if the instruments in the heat sterilizer are contaminated and need to be sterilized or the instruments have been sterilized and the heat sterilizer should be emptied.

Biological indicators. Commercially prepared bacterial spores, often called spore tests, are used as a **biological monitor** and are the most accurate method of determining whether sterilization has occurred in a heat sterilizer. Spores are available either in glass ampules or on spore strips enclosed in glassine envelopes. Weekly spore tests are recommended by the CDC. These tests are conducted by placing the test device in the center of an instrument pack during a normal sterilization cycle. Test spores are

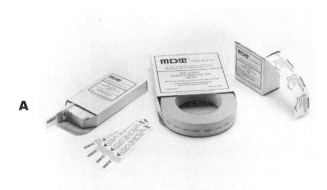

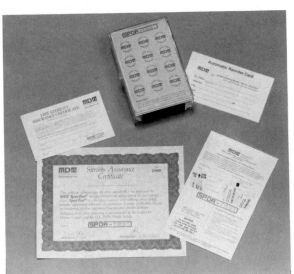

Figure 7-15 Sterilization indicators. **A,** Autoclave tape and heat test strips. **B,** Complete Spor-Test program.
(Courtesy MDT Corp, Gardena, Calif.)

either sent to the laboratory or incubated at the office to determine whether they were destroyed during the cycle.

> ## ☞ KEY POINTS
> - Autoclaves and chemiclaves should use *Bacillus stearothermophilus* spore tests.
> - Dry-heat ovens should use *Bacillus subtilis* sport tests.

Packaging dental instruments

The best way to maintain sterile instruments is to sterilize them in some sort of container. The instruments can remain in the container until they are used. Paper and steam-permeable plastic bags, cloth towel wraps, plastic instrument cassettes, and covered metal trays are commonly used (Figure 7-16). No impermeable containers should be used in the autoclave or the vapor sterilizer.

Towel wraps of two layers are useful for surgical instrument setups. An entire setup of heavy surgical instruments can be placed in a towel wrap secured with autoclave tape. The towel wrap also serves as a sterile surface during treatment.

Metal or plastic cassettes (Figure 7-17) that can serve as an instrument tray are rapidly becoming popular. Cassettes reduce the amount of instrument handling because the cassettes can close and lock the instruments into place. The closed cassette can be placed directly into the ultrasonic cleaner and heat sterilizer. Before placement into the sterilized the cassette can be wrapped and taped closed. The wrap allows the instrument cassette to be sterilized but prevents contamination after removal from the sterilizer. Like towel wraps, autoclave paper can be used on a dental assistant's cart to provide a sterile work surface. One disadvantage of cassette systems is the cost. Some offices will need to purchase larger heat sterilizers or ultrasonic cleaners to accommodate cassettes, which are bulkier than most instrument packages.

Covered metal preset trays have instrument racks similar to cassettes. No autoclave paper is needed to wrap the tray. When the tray is processed and cooled, it can be stored until needed.

INFECTION CONTROL MEASURES RELATED TO PATIENT TREATMENT

Equipment Barriers

Frequently touched equipment that is either too large to fit into a heat sterilizer or cannot be disconnected from the operatory area should be wrapped with a **disposable barrier** (Figure 7-18) such as aluminum foil, plastic, or impervious paper.

Plastic food wrap can also be used to cover dental chair switches and x-ray tube heads (Figure 7-19). Large clear plastic bags can be used as an alternative to cover the head of the dental chair and the switches.

Disposable barriers should be carefully removed and discarded after each patient. A new barrier should be placed before each patient.

> ## ☞ KEY POINT
> - Place disposable barriers on items or equipment that is touched frequently.

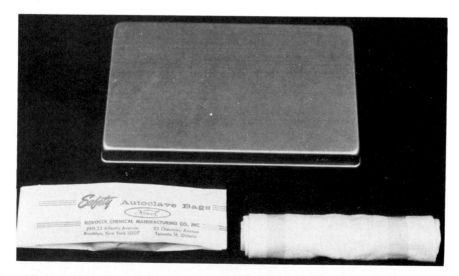

Figure 7-16 Methods of packaging instruments for sterilization. *Top,* Covered metal tray. *Bottom left,* Paper autoclave bag. *Bottom right,* Towel wrap.

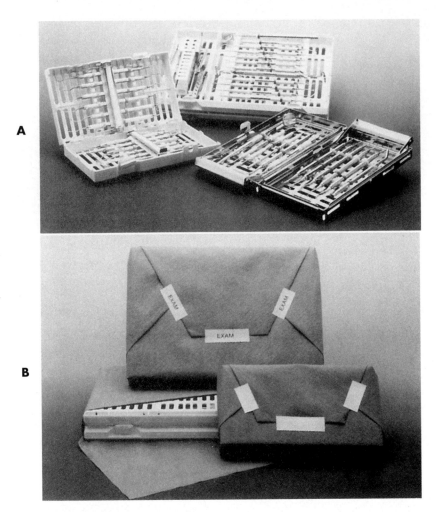

Figure 7-17   Cassette instrument sterilizing system. **A,** Unwrapped. **B,** Wrapped in autoclave paper and labeled for storage.

(Courtesy Hu-Friedy, Chicago.)

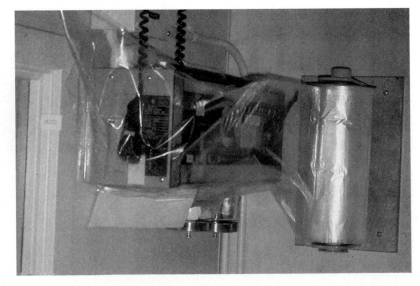

Figure 7-18   Disposable equipment barrier for x-ray control unit.

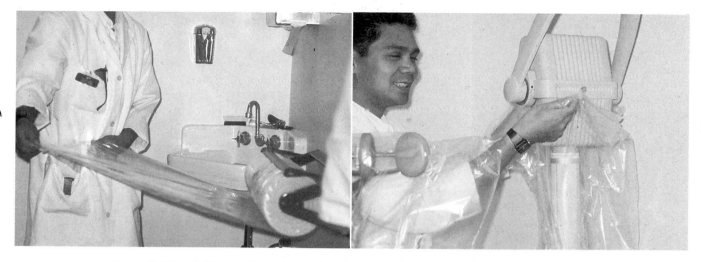

Figure 7-19   **A**, Disposable equipment barriers for large equipment. **B**, Wrapping x-ray head with large plastic bag.

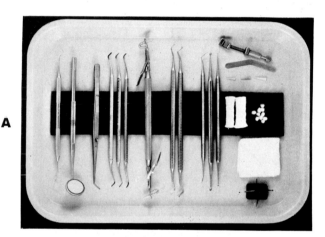

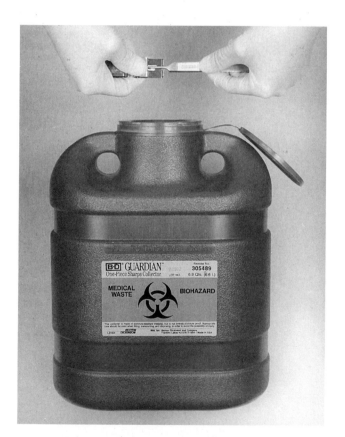

Figure 7-20   Sharps container.

(Courtesy Becton-Dickinson, Franklin Lakes, N.J.)

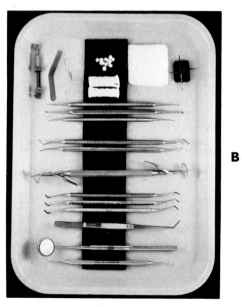

Figure 7-21   **A**, Preset tray in horizontal orientation with instruments arranged from left to right in sequence in which they are used. **B**, Preset tray in vertical orientation with instruments arranged from bottom to top in sequence in which they are used.

Sharps

A color-coded red, leakproof, closable, and secured sharps container (Figure 7-20) should be located as close as possible to the work area. If the sharps container is not color coded red, it must be labeled with a biohazard label. A sharps container is located ideally in the dental operatory for immediate disposable of sharps. Another less desirable alternative is to have the sharps container located in the sterilization area. Sharps containers should be discarded in compliance with local, state, or federal regulations. Broken glass, orthodontic wires, anesthetic cartridges visibly contaminated with blood, and anesthetic and suture needles should routinely be placed in a sharps container.

Handpiece Asepsis

High-speed handpieces are heat sterilized after each patient. Attachments to the low-speed handpieces that are placed intraorally are also sterilized, including the reusable prophy angle and contra-angles. Before sterilization the handpiece is flushed, cleaned, and/or lubricated according to the manufacturer's recommendations.

Radiology Procedures

Because radiographic procedures require the placement of film intraorally, careful aseptic technique must be practiced. Plastic barriers can be placed on the x-ray unit, control panel, and exposure button (see Figures 7-19 and 7-20). The barriers should be changed for each patient. Surfaces that are not covered and are contaminated should be disinfected. Reusable film placement holders should be sterilized.

Dental films should be developed with minimal contamination of the darkroom equipment and film developing unit (Box 7-5).

Dental film can be purchased already enclosed in a plastic pouch. After the film is exposed the outer contaminated plastic pouch can be carefully removed and the dental film developed.

Daylight Loader

Daylight loaders attached to dental film processors can pose a difficult problem in maintaining aseptic techniques. It is not possible to disinfect the cloth arm cuffs that prevent light from entering the area where the film is unwrapped and placed in the film developer. Therefore contaminated gloves or dental film should not be passed through the arm cuffs. Plastic dental film packets can be disinfected by soaking for 10 minutes with an iodophor disinfectant or sodium hypochlorite (household bleach) in a 1:10 dilution. As an alternative, contaminated film packets can be placed into the daylight loader through the top lid, which avoids passing contaminated material through the cloth arm cuffs.

OCCUPATIONAL SAFETY AND HEALTH ADMINISTRATION AND DENTISTRY

OSHA is concerned about the safety and health of employees in the work setting. OSHA rules and regulations protect employees in general industry as well as in health care fields. OSHA has rules and regulations concerning general safety standards and hazardous chemicals in the workplace (Hazard Communication Standard). OSHA has also enacted rules and regulations to protect workers from contracting diseases by blood and body fluids (Bloodborne Pathogens Standard).

OSHA's Bloodborne Pathogens Standard

OSHA's Bloodborne Pathogens Standard became effective in 1992 to protect workers from contracting diseases transmitted by blood and other body fluids. Box 7-6 summarizes this standard.

OSHA's Safety and Health Requirements for the Dental Office

OSHA also mandates that dentists provide a safe general working environment for their employees, which in-

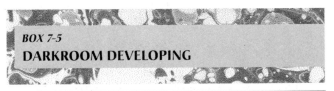

BOX 7-5
DARKROOM DEVELOPING

PROCEDURE	RATIONALE
1. Exposed dental film should be transported to darkroom in disposable container such as paper or plastic cup.	1. To avoid cross-contamination.
2. Enter darkroom wearing overgloves over contaminated latex gloves, or remove contaminated gloves to prevent cross-contamination of darkroom door handle.	2. To avoid cross-contamination of door handle
3. On paper towel or patient napkin, open film packets and drop films onto paper towel or napkin without touching films.	3. To avoid contamination of film inside film packet
4. Discard contaminated film packets and container, remove gloves, wash hands, and place film into developer.	4. To avoid cross-contamination of developer

cludes fire, building, and equipment safety. Box 7-7 summarizes the most important points of OSHA's General Safety Standards.

OSHA's Hazard Communication Standard

OSHA's Hazard Communication Standard was developed to protect employees from hazardous chemicals in the workplace. All employees should be aware of any hazardous chemicals in the workplace and be trained in the handling of these chemicals. Box 7-8 summarizes important points concerning OSHA's Hazard Communication Standard.

PRESET TRAY SYSTEM

An important part of instrument processing is the maintenance of a preset tray system. A **preset tray** is a well-organized group of instruments and supplies needed for a dental procedure. They are stored on a labeled tray for use when that procedure is performed (Figure 7-21). Ad-

vantages and disadvantages of using a preset tray system follow.

Advantages

- Reduced downtime
- Improved procedural flow
- Easier instrument cleaning and processing

Disadvantage

- Increased initial cost

The advantages of using a preset tray outweigh the disadvantage of the initial cost. Preset trays reduce downtime because less time is used to prepare the operatory for the next patient. A preset tray helps promote the orderly flow of treatment procedures. Preset trays are also easier to clean and process as a group and can be maintained in a sterile state until they are used at chairside.

Instruments on preset trays should be arranged in the same sequence that has been established by the dental team for each procedure. The most frequently used items,

---

BOX 7-6

1992 OVERVIEW OF REQUIRED FEDERAL OSHA STANDARDS

- Employers must identify and train workers who are *reasonably anticipated* to be at risk of exposure; reduce or eliminate exposure; and offer medical care and counseling.
- Employers must have written exposure control plans that will identify workers with occupational exposure to blood and other infectious materials and will identify the means to protect and train those workers.
- Employers must have a plan that includes a protocol for barrier techniques; sterilization; disinfection; hepatitis B vaccination; handling of office accidents, including postexposure to infectious materials; and plans to protect and train employers, with annual reviews and updates of the plan that are readily available to employees.
- Puncture-resistant containers must be used, hands must be washed as gloves are changed, and proper personal protective equipment is required to be worn.
- To launder protective clothing at home is prohibited.
- Recapping of sharps must be accomplished with a one-handed technique or by using a mechanical recapping device.
- Employees are required to wear gowns and gloves when there is risk of exposure of skin to blood, body fluids, or saliva.

- General work clothes are not considered protection against exposure to blood, body fluids, or saliva.
- Employees must wear masks, eyewear, or a face shield during exposure to splashes, spray, spatter, droplets of blood, body tissue, or saliva.
- Solid eyewear must have sideshields.
- Employers must provide personal protective equipment to be worn by all employees, including gowns, gloves, masks, and eyewear, at no expense to employees.
- Sharps containers must be labeled and easily accessible to the area of sharps use.
- Hepatitis B vaccinations must be offered to employees at no cost after training is completed but within 10 days of placement in a position that involves occupational exposure. If a worker declines the hepatitis B vaccination, access is still required if the employee has a change of mind.
- Employers must provide a training program during working hours to all employees in occupational exposure positions by June 4, 1992 and annually in subsequent years.
- Training records must be kept for 3 years following the training sessions.
- The standard requires that the following be handled as infectious waste by placement in special, labeled containers: pathological waste; sharps; blood and body fluids; items that release blood, body fluid, or saliva when compressed; items caked with dried blood, body fluid, or saliva if they can release these materials during handling.

From Finkbeiner BL, Johnson CS: *Mosby's comprehensive dental assisting: a clinical approach*, St Louis, 1995, Mosby.

BOX 7-7

OSHA'S GENERAL SAFETY STANDARDS

- Workplaces with 11 or more employees should have a written emergency action plan and also train employees in the event of a fire, tornado, hurricane, earthquake, or other natural disaster.
- A fire prevention plan must be developed, and all employees should be trained concerning workplace fire hazards and how to prevent fires.
- All fire suppression and detection equipment must be working and properly maintained.
- A first aid kit should be available and at least one person trained in first aid.
- Eyewash facilities should be located within 25 feet or 10 seconds of employees.
- Eyewash stations should flow for 15 minutes and be labeled.
- Doors and exits must be kept open during office hours and kept free of obstructions.
- All exits must be clearly marked with a readily visible sign.
- Documentation of building hazards to the owner of the building must be maintained.
- Electrical outlets and appliances must be grounded and properly maintained.
- Circuit breakers and main power switches must be marked clearly for on-off positions and also labeled according to what each switch controls.
- All equipment and machinery should be inspected for proper working condition and safety.
- Employees should use stepladders instead of other equipment to reach items, and stepladders should:

Be maintained in good condition
Be placed on the floor and not on other equipment to reach a higher level
Have nonslip safety feet
Be free of grease or oil
Be labeled *"Caution:* Do Not Use Around Electrical Equipment"
Not be used in front of a door that could open (ladder could be knocked down)
- Gas cylinders should be labeled and secured from tipping. The valves on the containers should be covered with a valve protector and closed when moved or when empty. Cylinders should not be placed near heat sources and should be kept in a secure area to prevent tampering or unauthorized use.
- Air compressors should:
Have pressure relief valves and gauges
Have air filters in the air intake
Have a drain pipe and valve at the lowest point for oil removal
Be drained of oil and water periodically
Be bled of pressure and turned off for repair work
- In addition, employees should be informed that compressed air should not be used for cleaning purposes and should never be directed toward another person except in the case of dental procedures.
- Trash cans should never be overfilled and should also be checked for dried blood or liquid inside the trash can after removing the trash bag.

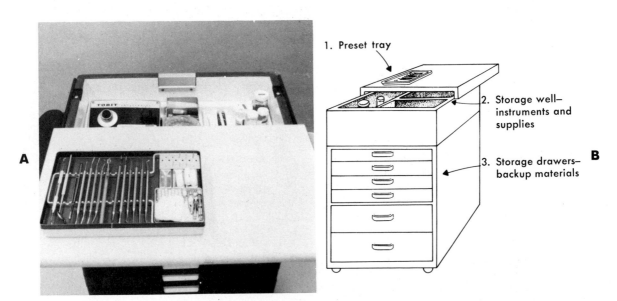

Figure 7-22 **A,** Preset tray in working position on assistant's mobile cabinet. **B,** Instruments and materials arranged according to their priority in mobile cart.

BOX 7-8

OSHA'S HAZARD COMMUNICATION STANDARD

The employer must ensure that the following are achieved.
- A list or inventory of all hazardous chemicals that are found in the dental office must be maintained. All hazardous chemicals must be labeled with specific information. If hazardous chemicals are transferred to a secondary container, that container must be labeled unless the chemical is for immediate use.
- A material safety data sheet (MSDS) that contains relevant information concerning the chemical (e.g., fire and explosion information, health hazards, carcinogenicity, precautions for safe handling, and emergency and first-aid procedures) must be kept for each hazardous chemical in the workplace, and the employee must be trained as to the whereabouts of the MSDS forms and how to read them.
- Employees must be trained about hazardous chemicals in the workplace at the time of initial assignment and when a new hazardous chemical is introduced in the workplace. Training sessions must be documented and maintained.
- A written hazard communication program must be developed, implemented, and maintained by the dentist/employer. This document must describe how employees are trained, labeling of hazardous chemicals, and MSDS information.

such as the mirror, explorer, and cotton pliers, should be placed nearest the patient (Figure 7-21, *B*). After an instrument is used, it should be returned to the same location on the tray in case it is needed again. Maintenance of a neat, orderly tray permits the chairside assistant to retrieve instruments quickly as they are needed, without the delay involved in searching though all the instruments for the desired one. Chairside assistants who become familiar with an orderly arrangement of instruments on a tray can substantially reduce the scanning time required to find any instrument in the setup. New employees can learn to work with an operator more quickly if a specific treatment sequence is followed and the instruments are arranged on the tray to match that sequence.

Preset trays are usually assembled according to procedures performed frequently during the normal workday. For an average dental office preset trays might include the following:
- Crown and bridge preparation
- Crown and bridge cementation
- Amalgam
- Composite

- Endodontic procedures
- Examination or emergency
- Oral prophylaxis

Each tray can be color coded to identify the procedure for which it is used. An identification code is selected for convenient labeling of trays according to their intended use. Color coding is a popular labeling method.

General Considerations

Preset trays should be kept as simple as possible and stocked only with items usually needed in a given procedure. Preset trays are usually assembled in the sterilization area with disposable items readily available to place on the tray. Items that are generally placed on preset trays include the following.
- Hand instruments
- Burs
- Cotton products
- Interproximal wedges
- Matrix bands
- Evacuator tips
- Articulating paper

Items that are impractical to place on a preset tray or are only used occasionally are kept in the assistant's mobile cabinet or in the operatory (Figure 7-22), such as the following:
- Restorative materials
- Cements
- Cavity liners
- Impression material
- Anesthetic cartridges

The final choice of which items to include on a given tray must be made by the dentist according to individual technique.

Tray Maps

A key requirement of any system is coordination among personnel who use it. To ensure uniformity in the preparation of preset trays, it is helpful to develop guides for sterilization personnel to use when setting up instrument trays. The tray map or an enlarged photograph of the tray setup is such a guide (Figure 7-23). Tray maps are particularly helpful for new employees or employees who are assigned to sterilization only occasionally.

V Arrangement

Still another method of organizing instruments on trays is to place color-coding identification tape carefully on the handles of the instruments so that they form a distinct V pattern (Figure 7-24, *A*). The assistant can tell at a glance if the instruments are properly arranged on the tray. Figure 7-24, *B*, is the same instrument setup but placed out of sequence on the tray.

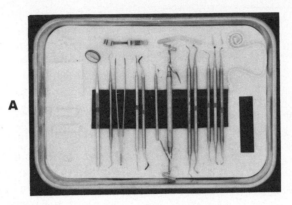

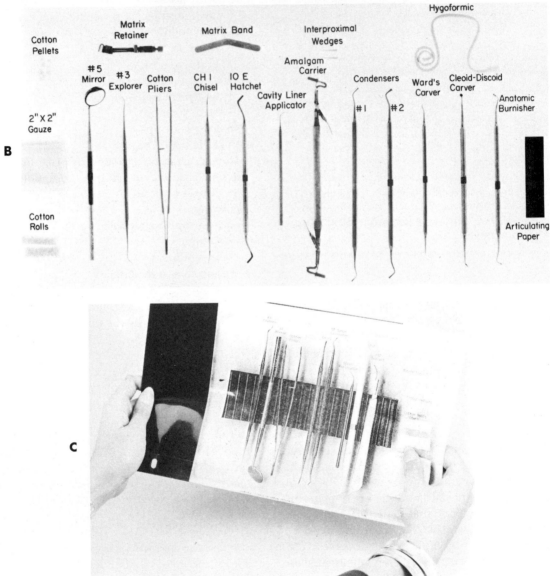

Figure 7-23 **A,** Sample preset tray for amalgam procedure. **B,** Tray map for amalgam preset tray. **C,** Photocopy of tray setup in protective cover.

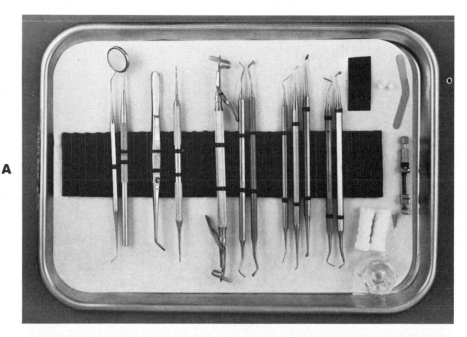

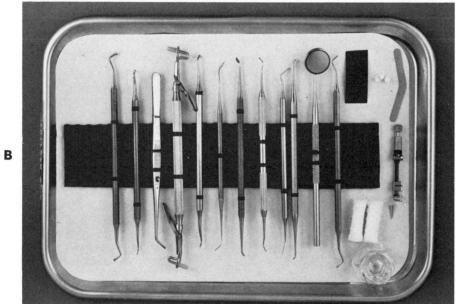

Figure 7-24   **A,** V pattern indicates instruments are in proper order. **B,** Same preset tray but instruments are out of order.

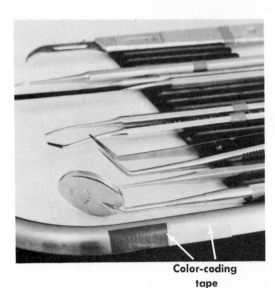

Figure 7-25   Stainless steel open-style tray with color-coding tape on edge.

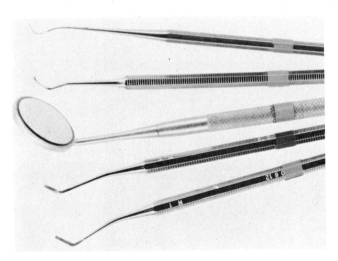

Figure 7-26   Color-coded instruments with colored identification tape on handles.

Color-Coding Systems
Color-coding preset trays

Color coding is one of the most convenient ways to identify the intended use of any preset tray (Figure 7-25). Colors can be arbitrarily assigned to the various procedures. For example, blue might be assigned to amalgam restorations, yellow to cast-gold restorations, and pink to composite restorations.

Color-coding instruments

Colored identification tape or rubber rings can be placed on the handles of instruments to match the color code on the tray (Figure 7-26). Although this may be helpful

for quickly locating the tray on which a stray instrument may belong, it is not absolutely necessary if the contents of each preset tray are processed together and tray maps are used. Color-coding instruments with identification tape or rubber rings requires continuous maintenance, since tape or rubber rings become discolored or sometimes separate from instruments after repeated sterilization. Choosing whether to code individual instruments is left to the operatory team.

BIBLIOGRAPHY

ADA Council on Dental Therapeutics: Infection control recommendations for the dental office and the dental laboratory, *JADA* (Suppl):1-8, 1992.

Centers for Disease Control and Prevention: Recommended infection control practices for dentistry, *MMWR* 42:1-12, 1993.

Cottone JA and others: *Practical infection control in dentistry,* ed 2, Media, Pa, 1994, Lea & Febiger.

Department of Labor, Occupational Safety and Health Administration: 29 CFR Part 1910. 1030: Occupational exposure to bloodborne pathogens: final rule, *Federal Register* 56(235):64004-64182, 1991.

Finkbeiner BL, Johnson CS: *Mosby's comprehensive dental assisting,* St Louis, 1995, Mosby.

QUESTIONS—Chapter 7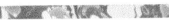

1. The *Bacillus subtilis* spore test is used for which of the following sterilization methods:
   a. Dry heat
   b. Steam autoclave
   c. Chemical vapor
   d. Liquid chemical sterilant

2. Which of the following are requirements for steam autoclaving?
   a. 1 hour, 340° F
   b. 20 minutes, 270° F, 20 psi
   c. 15-20 minutes, 250° F, 15 psi
   d. 2 hours, 320° F

3. Which of the following is the term used to describe the fact that dental staff must follow stringent infection control procedures for every patient whether or not the patient reports or exhibits an infectious disease?
   a. Universal precautions
   b. Cross-contamination
   c. Disinfection
   d. Sterilization

4. The destruction of all forms of life including bacterial endospores is described by which of the following terms:
   a. Universal precautions
   b. Cross-contamination
   c. Disinfection
   d. Sterilization

5. Which of the following methods of sterilization can cause corrosion of instruments?
   a. Steam autoclave
   b. Dry-heat oven
   c. Chemical vapor

6. Which of the following types of disinfectant can cause corrosion of metals and damage clothing?
   a. Iodophors
   b. Chlorines
   c. Quaternary ammonium compounds
   d. Synthetic phenols
   e. Alcohol

7. All of the following are not acceptable for surface disinfection *except:*
   a. Quaternary ammonium compounds
   b. Alcohol
   c. Household bleach
   d. 2% Glutaraldehyde

8. Which of the following solutions can be used in the ultrasonic cleaner?
   a. Iodophor
   b. Household bleach
   c. A solution recommended by the manufacturer
   d. 2% Glutaraldehyde

9. Which of the following describes the recommended disinfection technique?
   a. Spray, wipe
   b. Spray, wipe, spray
   c. Spray, wipe, spray, wipe immediately
   d. Spray, let air dry

10. All of the following are recommendations for handling
sharps *except:*
   a. Dispose of in a puncture-proof container.
   b. Recap using a one-handed technique.
   c. Recap immediately after use.
   d. Bend the needle before throwing it away.

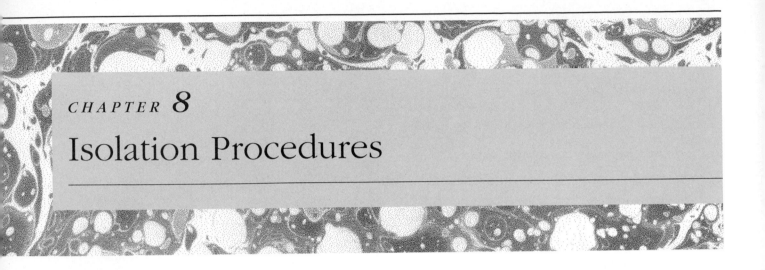

CHAPTER 8

Isolation Procedures

KEY TERMS

Dental compound
Inverting/everting
Ligature
Rubber dam
Rubber dam clamps
Rubber dam forceps
Rubber dam lubricant
Rubber dam napkins
Rubber dam punch
Rubber dam stamp
Rubber dam (Young) frame

Isolation of an operating field is the process of retracting soft tissue to gain access and visibility. Since the oral cavity is a wet environment, an important function of isolation procedures is controlling salivary contamination of the operative field. Virtually all restorative materials require a clean, dry environment at the time of insertion into a prepared cavity. Hence effective isolation is integral to all restorative procedures. Isolation of the operating field also provides protection to the patient and the dental staff. The patient can be protected from harm to the soft tissue or aspirating small objects and aerosols. Certain techniques, such as using the rubber dam, can minimize exposure of the dental staff to aerosols and droplets.

Many devices and methods are available to isolate an operating field. This discussion is limited to cotton roll isolation and rubber dam isolation.

COTTON ROLL ISOLATION

The still-popular cotton roll method is one of the oldest isolation methods. It is a simple and rapid way to isolate the operative field. However, it is by no means the most reliable isolation method. The cotton roll method does not prevent the patient from inadvertently contaminating the operative field while swallowing or with a "curious tongue." This method does not prevent debris from the operative procedure from dropping into the throat or under the tongue. Various sizes of cotton rolls are available. Some are wrapped in cotton thread to prevent them from sticking to the mucosa when removed. Dry cotton rolls should be moistened with a water syringe before removal. This prevents the cotton roll from pulling off the delicate epithelial covering of the mucosa.

Isolation of Maxillary Arch

A typical cotton roll isolation in the maxillary arch is accomplished by placing an appropriate-sized cotton roll in the mucobuccal or mucolabial area of the region being treated (Figure 8-1, *A* and *B*).

Isolation of Mandibular Arch

A little more gadgetry is required to isolate the mandibular arch because of the tongue and the pooling of saliva in the floor of the mouth. A comfortable method of isolating the mandibular posterior area is to place a cotton roll on the buccal aspect of the arch and an additional cotton roll between the teeth and the tongue.

An aspirating tongue retractor can be placed on the lingual aspect (Figure 8-1, *C* and *D*) to help keep the working area dry. These retractors are available in two styles (Figure 8-2). The disposable types are preferable because they can adjust to fit the patient and can be thrown away after use. They are connected to the saliva-ejector hose.

A triangular absorbent paper disk (Dri-Angle) is an auxiliary device that helps isolate posterior areas (Figure 8-3). The disk aids retraction of buccal mucosa. The disk is thin, and when it is used in conjunction with cotton roll isolation it provides excellent visibility.

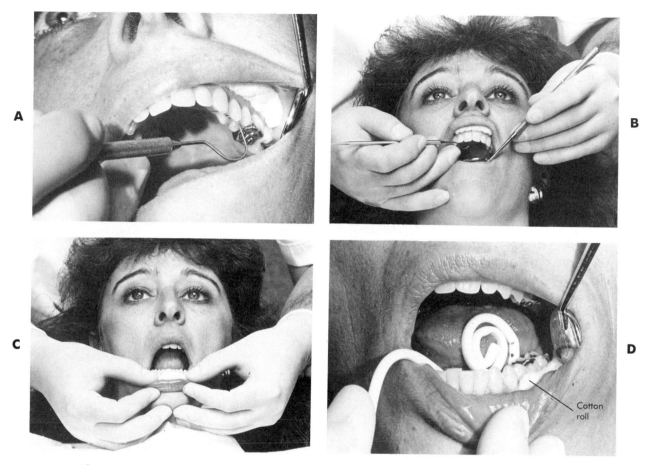

Figure 8-1   Cotton roll isolation. **A,** Maxillary posterior area. **B,** Maxillary anterior area. **C,** Mandibular anterior area. **D,** Mandibular posterior area along with hygoformic saliva ejector.

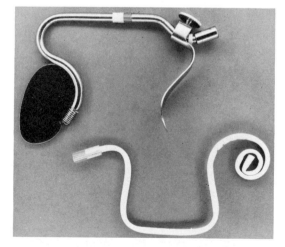

Figure 8-2   Aspirating tongue retractors. *Top,* Svedopter. *Bottom,* Hygoformic.

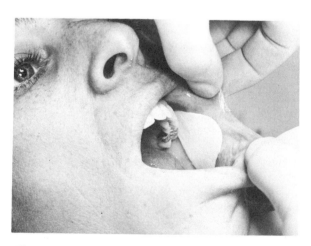

Figure 8-3   Absorbent paper triangle (Dri-angle)

One disadvantage of the cotton roll isolation is that cotton rolls must be replaced after they are wetted by the handpiece water coolant or saliva during the cavity preparation phase. The new dry cotton rolls ensure a dry field during the insertion of restorative material.

RUBBER DAM ISOLATION

The rubber dam isolation method is much more complicated but provides better isolation quality as well as a barrier between the patient's oral tissues and the operating team. This arrangement is often cited as one of the barrier devices that protect the operating team from saliva splatter associated with restorative procedures. A rubber dam used in conjunction with an oral evacuator can reduce aerosols and droplet spray by over 90%. Rubber dams also prevent patients from inadvertently swallowing or aspirating materials and debris during treatment. There is no doubt that the rubber dam is the best isolation method in dentistry. It requires a little more time to apply than the cotton roll method, but the time saved during the restorative procedure makes up for the additional effort required in the application.

Armamentarium

The rubber dam procedure requires a separate tray setup for convenience (Figure 8-4).

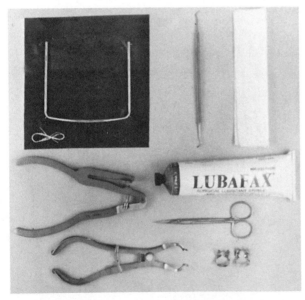

Heavy rubber dam (prestamped)
Young frame
Dental floss
Spoon excavator
Gauze napkin (or rubber dam napkin)
Rubber dam punch
Water-soluble lubricant
Rubber dam forceps
Scissors
Clamps

Figure 8-4 Rubber dam armamentarium.

Rubber dam clamps

Rubber dam clamps are used to anchor the rubber dam to the teeth (Figure 8-5). Various clamps are available to meet the particular needs of any restorative procedure. The points of the clamp (Figure 8-6, *A*) engage the cervical portion of the tooth to hold it in place.

Rubber dam clamps come in various sizes and are available either *winged* (Figure 8-6, *B*) or *wingless* (Figure 8-6, *C*). It is a personal preference whether the dentist uses winged or wingless clamps. Winged clamps allow the dentist or assistant to place the rubber dam and the clamp onto the clamp tooth simultaneously. Wingless clamps are

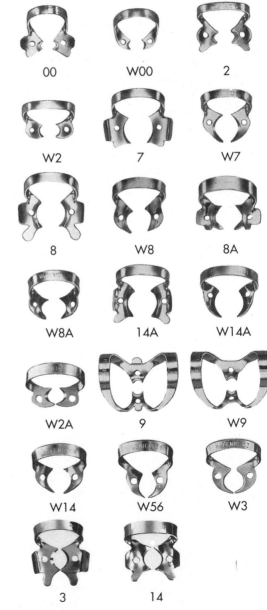

Figure 8-5 Rubber dam clamp assortment.
(Courtesy The Hygienic Corp, Akron, Ohio.)

placed onto the clamp tooth before slipping the rubber dam over the teeth. Wingless clamps have a letter *W* preceding the clamp number. Double-bowed clamps (Figure 8-6, *D*) are used for anterior teeth and assist with retraction of the gingiva for class V restorations.

Rubber dam punch

The **rubber dam punch** is used to punch holes in the dam so that it can be placed over the teeth. The punch has an adjustment wheel on it so that proper-sized holes can be made (Figure 8-7). There are five to six punch holes, each slightly larger than the next on the rubber dam cutting table. Figure 8-8 demonstrates guidelines for a five-hole punch.

Rubber dam stamp

The **rubber dam stamp** (Figure 8-9) is helpful in positioning holes properly on the dam. Although the arrangement of hole markers on the stamp does not fit every case, they are valuable as a guide. The rubber dam can be stamped before the procedure.

In situations involving malposed or missing teeth in the area to be isolated, the positions of the holes must be altered to accommodate changes. For example, if a tooth is located more buccally than normal, the hole that will be punched for it must be punched in a more buccal position. Holes are not punched in areas where teeth are missing.

> **⚬◦ KEY POINT**
> ▪ Using a rubber dam and an oral evacuator reduces exposure to aerosols and splatter by over 90%.

It is helpful to attach the dam to the frame while it is being punched. This makes it easier to visualize the desired position of the holes.

Rubber dam forceps

Rubber dam forceps are used to spread the beaks of a rubber dam clamp when the clamp is placed on and removed from the anchor tooth (Figure 8-10). The tips of the forceps are inserted into the two holes located on the beaks of the clamp. The clamp beaks are spread open with the forceps and locked in this position with a locking device on the forceps. After the clamp is placed over the anchor tooth, the locking mechanism is released and the clamp closes around the cervical area of the tooth.

Rubber dam

Rubber dam material is available in light or heavy weights, in light or dark colors, and in either sheet or roll form. Most dentists prefer 5- or 6-inch square, dark-col-

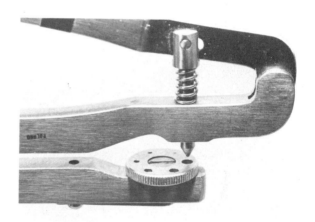

Figure 8-7 Rubber dam punch, showing various sizes of holes that can be punched in dam.

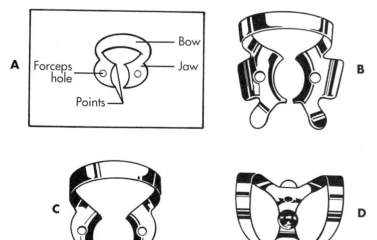

Figure 8-6 Rubber dam clamps. **A,** Bow of clamp is placed distally. **B,** Winged clamp. **C,** Wingless clamp. **D,** Anterior double-bowed clamp.

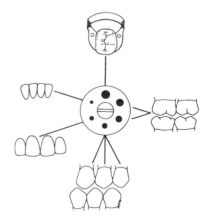

Figure 8-8 Cutting table on rubber dam punch illustrating use of hole size.

(From Sturdevant CM and others: *The art and science of operative dentistry,* ed 3, St Louis, 1995, Mosby.)

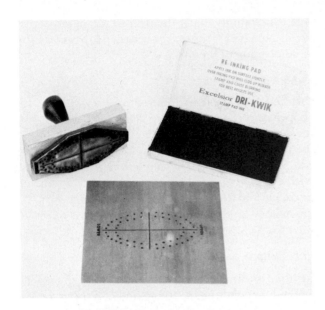

Figure 8-9   Rubber dam stamp.

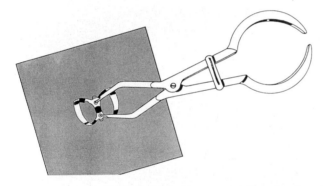

Figure 8-10   Rubber dam forceps spreading beaks of rubber dam clamp.

(From Miller D: *Dental dam procedures,* ed 8, Akron, Ohio, 1990, The Hygienic Corp.)

ored sheet forms. Heavy-weight dam material is preferred because it resists tearing and provides better soft tissue retraction. The dark color is a better background, since it contrasts with white teeth. Precut sheets are convenient to handle. The sheets can be stamped with the rubber dam stamp (see Figure 8-9) at the convenience of the assistant before they are needed.

Rubber dam napkins

Rubber dam napkins are disposable cotton preformed sheets that are placed under the rubber dam. These napkins provide patient comfort during the procedure.

Rubber dam frame

The **rubber dam (Young) frame** is used to support the dam on a patient's face. It maintains isolation by holding the dam out of the way.

Dental floss ligature

A dental floss **ligature** is tied to the rubber dam clamp as a safety feature in the event that the clamp falls down the patient's throat. The dental floss is also used to slip the septal portion of the rubber dam down between the teeth.

Rubber dam lubricant

Lubricating the rubber dam with a water-based **rubber dam lubricant** helps to slip the septal portion of the rubber dam down between the teeth.

Dental compound (optional)

If necessary, **dental compound** (a waxlike material) is softened and used to anchor the rubber dam clamp.

Rubber Dam Procedure

The detailed explanation of the rubber dam procedure that follows is intended to give assistants a thorough understanding of the technique so greater assistance can be offered to increase the efficiency of the rubber dam technique. In addition, many dentists are using dental assistants to apply the dam by themselves as a part of patient preparation.

Rubber dam application

The following is a step-by-step procedure used for rubber dam application. It is by no means the only method that can be used, but it is one of the most common techniques. Isolation of the mandibular left quadrant with a winged rubber dam clamp will be used as an example (Figure 8-11).

   1. Attach rubber dam to the frame. Attach the prestamped rubber dam to the rubber dam frame (Young frame) by stretching the material over the metal pegs along the sides and bottom of the frame. The dam is oriented so that the top of the frame is the open end that will rest under the patient's nose. The curved lower portion of the frame rests over the patient's chin, with the frame curving toward the patient's face (Figure 8-11, *A*). The rubber dam has a dull side and a shiny side. The dull side is placed up to help to prevent glare.

   2. Use the rubber dam punch to punch the holes for the teeth to be isolated. Punch holes in the dam in the area being isolated using the rubber dam punch at the hole marks made by the stamp. *The largest hole is generally used for the clamp tooth, the next largest for molars, a medium-sized hole for premolars, canines, and upper incisors and the smaller holes for lower incisors (Figure 8-11, B).*

   3. Attach the floss ligature to the rubber dam clamp. Tie a 12-inch strand of dental floss around the bow of a wing-style clamp before testing the fit on the patient's tooth. This is a safety precaution in the event the clamp

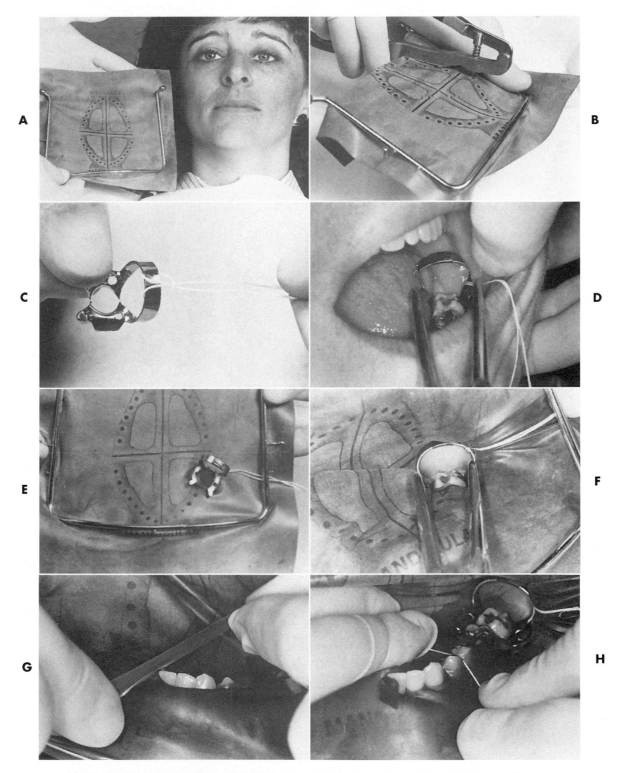

Figure 8-11   Application of rubber dam. **A,** Proper orientation of dam on frame. **B,** Use of rubber dam punch. **C,** Placing safety floss on clamp. **D,** Testing clamp for fit. **E,** Placement of clamp in dam. **F,** Placement of clamp on anchor tooth. **G,** Placement of anterior ligature. **H,** Pulling dam between teeth using dental floss.

Continued

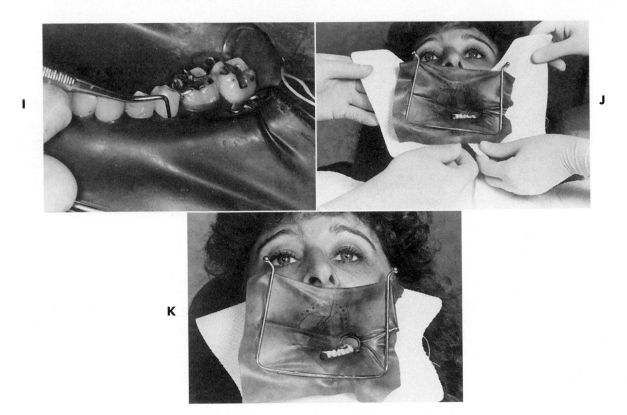

Figure 8-11, cont'd   **I,** Tucking (everting) dam around teeth. **J,** Placing gauze napkin. **K,** Rubber dam assembly in place.

becomes dislodged and is either swallowed or aspirated by the patient (Figure 8-11, *C*).

4. Try the rubber dam clamp on the tooth. Using rubber dam forceps, place the clamp on the selected anchor tooth. Usually the second molar is used as the anchor tooth if an entire quadrant is isolated. A proper fit is achieved when the beaks contact the anchor tooth at four points around the cervical area and the clamp does not rock when finger pressure is applied (Figure 8-11, *D*).

5. Place the rubber dam clamp in the rubber dam. Once the proper clamp is selected and tested for fit, it is removed from the patient's mouth and placed in the most posterior hole in the punched rubber dam. The clamp should be oriented so that the bow is on top for lower teeth and on bottom for upper teeth. The wings on the clamp serve as holding points to secure the clamp in the dam (Figure 8-11, *E*).

6. Lubricate the punched holes. The dam is lubricated lightly with a water-soluble lubricant such as shaving cream or soap slurry around the punched holes. Only the tissue surface of the rubber dam is lubricated. This lubrication aids in passing the rubber dam between the teeth during application. Do not use oil-based lubricants such as petroleum jelly (Vaseline) or cocoa butter because they can degrade the latex of the rubber dam.

7. Floss the teeth to remove debris. Floss the interproximal areas of the teeth being isolated. This removes debris from between teeth, which may interfere with the passage of rubber dam material past the contact areas.

8. Place the clamp on the rubber dam forceps. Place the tips of the forceps in the holes located on the beaks of the clamp. Spread the clamp beaks, and lock the forceps open.

9. Place the clamp on the anchor tooth. Place the open clamp on the anchor tooth. *The lingual beak is seated first followed by the buccal beak.* Slowly close the clamp on the tooth by releasing the lock on the forceps (Figure 8-11, *F*). (Optional: stabilize clamp with dental compound.)

10. Anchor the rubber dam on the most anterior tooth to be isolated. Center the most anterior hole over the lateral incisor, and pass the dam through the interproximal areas mesial and distal to the incisor. This can be done by pulling the border of the rubber between the teeth with dental floss. Once the rubber is between the teeth it can be held in place by stretching a 1- x 1/4-inch strip of rubber dam material and pulling it through the mesial contact of the lateral incisor (Figure 8-11, *G*). This serves as a ligature.

11. Isolate the remaining teeth. Now center the remaining holes over the corresponding teeth between the first molar and lateral incisor, and pass the rubber between the holes through interproximal contacts, using dental floss. This is more easily accomplished if one member of the operating team stretches the dam over the teeth while the other passes the floss between the teeth to pull the rubber dam through the contacts (Figure 8-11, *H*).

12. Invert the edges of the rubber dam around the teeth. Once the dam is over the teeth, form a seal around each tooth to prevent salivary leakage by tucking the dam toward the gingiva around each tooth. This step is called **inverting/everting** the rubber dam. It is accomplished with a blunt instrument such as a spoon excavator, beaver-tail burnisher, fishtail burnisher or plastic instrument to invert the dam while the assistant dries the dam with an air syringe (Figure 8-11, *I*). The dam is lifted off the wings of the clamp to allow a seal to form around the anchor tooth.

13. Place the rubber dam napkin on the patient's face. Apply the gauze napkin for patient comfort (Figure 8-11, *J*).

14. Adjust the dam. Wrinkles can be eliminated by reorienting the rubber dam on the frame as needed. The upper border of the dam should not cover the patient's nasal passages. If necessary, cut away or fold the upper portion of the dam to open the airway (Figure 8-11, *K*).

15. Heat the end of a stick of dental compound, and place in water to cool slightly. Pinch off a small piece of dental compound. Form a 1/2-inch cone and place it on the bow of the clamp and on the occlusal/incisal surface of the clamped tooth.

Problem solving

In any application of a rubber dam some common problems may be encountered during the application and use of the dam. Some of these problems are listed with suggested solutions.

Problem: clamp slipping off anchor tooth
1. Try a different style of clamp or grind the beaks of the clamp in use to improve the fit.
2. Allow a little slack in the dam by loosening it on the Young frame to lessen tension on the clamp.
3. Stabilize the clamp by drying the anchor tooth and adding dental compound around the tooth to hold the clamp in place.

Problem: difficulty in pulling dam through contact areas
1. Separate the teeth slightly by forcing a plastic instrument toward the contact area (Figure 8-12).
2. Sometimes it is necessary to polish rough margins of old restorations before dam application to allow the rubber to slip between the teeth.
3. In extremely difficult situations the preparations can be roughed-in without the dam. Then the dam is applied after the contacts are opened.

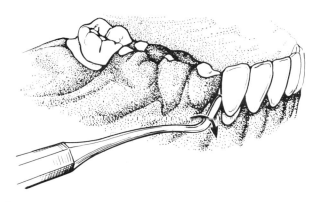

Figure 8-12   Separating teeth with plastic filling instrument.

Problem: difficulty in tucking or inverting dam around teeth
1. Pull the rubber dam away from the teeth so that the hole around the tooth is enlarged. Using the air-water syringe, dry the undersurface of the dam and the cervical area of the tooth. Relax the dam, and proceed with the tucking process.
2. Some patients who salivate excessively may require an unfolded 2- x 2-inch gauze sponge placed in the mucobuccal fold under the dam to keep the teeth dry until the eversion procedure is complete.

Problem: wrinkling or creasing of dam
1. Punch the holes closer together.
2. Reorient the dam on the frame.

Problem: spaces between dam and teeth
1. The holes have been punched too close together. Remove the dam and apply a new dam with holes farther apart.

Problem: rotary instruments catching interproximal rubber
1. Place a wooden wedge between the teeth to force the dam cervically. The bur may cut into the wedge during the preparation of class II cavities, but it will not tangle in the dam.

Problem: saliva accumulation in patient's mouth
1. Since the patient's saliva is free of contamination when the dam is in place, instruct the patient to swallow in a normal manner.
2. If the patient is still reluctant to swallow, slip a saliva ejector underneath the dam or cut a hole in the lingual area of the dam and insert a saliva ejector through the dam.

Removal of rubber dam

After the restorations have been placed, the dam must be removed to check the patient's occlusion, or biting relationship, on the new restorations. The removal sequence is as follows:

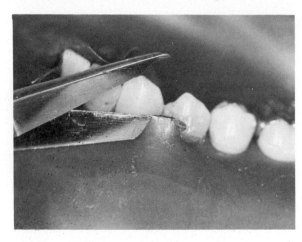

Figure 8-13 Cutting interproximal rubber dam material before removal.

1. Pull the dam in a buccal direction so that the interproximal rubber can be cut with the scissors (Figure 8-13). This prevents fracture of newly placed restorations such as temporary dressings and amalgam.
2. Remove the anterior rubber dam retention strip (ligature) mesial to the lateral incisor.
3. Remove the rubber dam clamp with rubber dam forceps.
4. Remove the entire rubber dam and napkin assembly. Check the interproximal areas to make sure no rubber has been torn and trapped between the teeth. Also, inspect the rubber dam itself for pieces of rubber that may be missing between the holes.
5. Rinse and evacuate the mouth.

> ➦ **KEY POINT**
> ▪ When cutting the septal portion of the rubber dam, protect the gingiva by placing a gloved finger between the dam and the gingiva.

BIBLIOGRAPHY

Finkbeiner BL, Johnson CS: *Mosby's comprehensive dental assisting: a clinical approach,* St Louis, 1995, Mosby.

Miller D: *Dental dam procedures,* ed 8, Akron, Ohio, 1990, The Hygienic Corp.

Sturdevant CM and others: *The art and science of operative dentistry,* ed 3, St Louis, 1995, Mosby.

QUESTIONS—Chapter 8

1. Which of the following describes the purpose of inverting the rubber dam?
   a. To anchor the rubber dam to the tooth
   b. To prevent accidental aspiration of the clamp
   c. To support the rubber dam on the patient's face
   d. To prevent salivary leakage

2. Which of the following instruments can be used to invert the rubber dam?
   a. Spoon excavator
   b. Probe
   c. Fishtail burnisher
   d. *a* and *b*
   e. *a* and *c*

3. Which of the following is used to help slip the rubber dam between the interproximal areas?
   a. Dental floss
   b. Burnisher
   c. Lubricant
   d. *a* and *c*
   e. *a* and *b*

4. Which of the following appropriately describes cotton roll isolation for tooth #19?
   a. Cotton roll in mucobuccal fold
   b. Theta Dri-angle on buccal mucosa
   c. Cotton roll in mucobuccal fold and Theta Dri-Angle in lingual area
   d. Cotton roll in mucobuccal fold and between teeth and tongue in lingual area

5. Which of the following describes the correct placement of the rubber dam clamp?
   a. Lingual to buccal
   b. Buccal to lingual
   c. Lingual and buccal together

6. Which of the following describes the correct removal of the rubber dam?
   a. Pull dam off in one piece.
   b. Cut the interproximal rubber on the lingual aspect.
   c. Cut the interproximal rubber on the buccal aspect.
   d. Cut the interproximal rubber on the buccal and lingual aspects.

7. It is the clamp _____ that engages the cervical portion of the tooth.
   a. Bow
   b. Wing
   c. Beak

8. Which of the following would be an appropriate lubricant for the rubber dam?
   a. An oil-based lubricant
   b. Petroleum jelly (Vaseline)
   c. Cocoa butter
   d. A water-based lubricant

9. The rubber dam clamp can be stabilized using which of the following:
   a. Dental floss
   b. Dental compound
   c. A small piece of rubber dam
   d. A cotton roll

10. The largest hole in the rubber dam punch is generally used for which of the following teeth:
    a. Cuspids
    b. Premolars
    c. Molars
    d. Clamp tooth

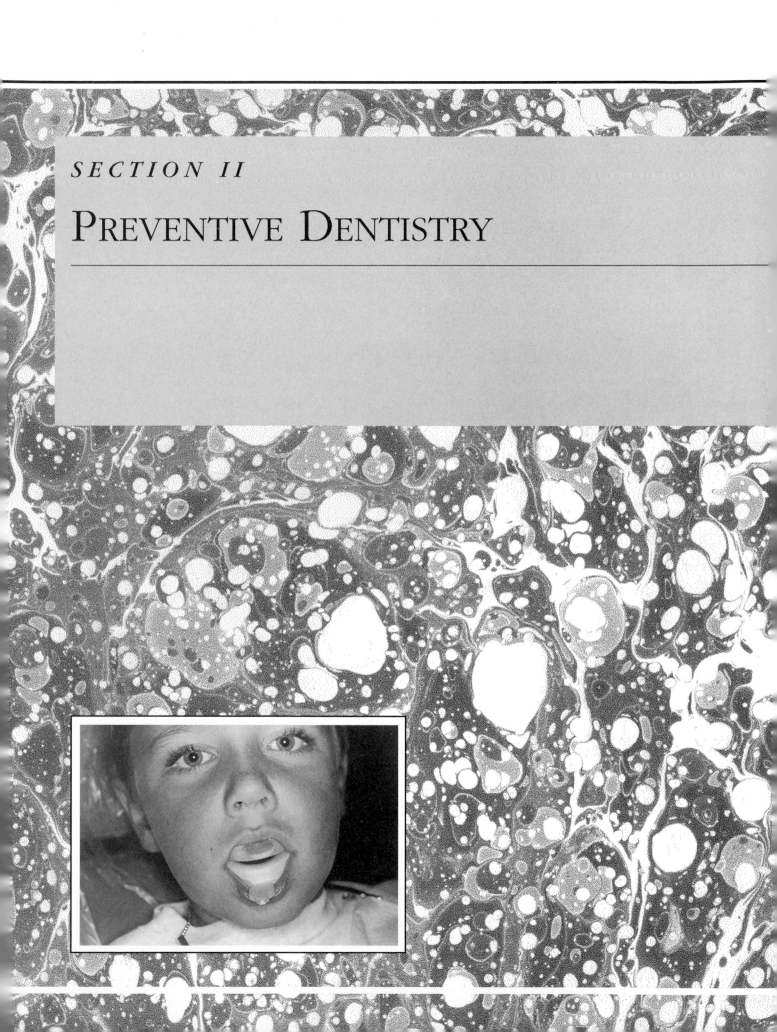

SECTION II

PREVENTIVE DENTISTRY

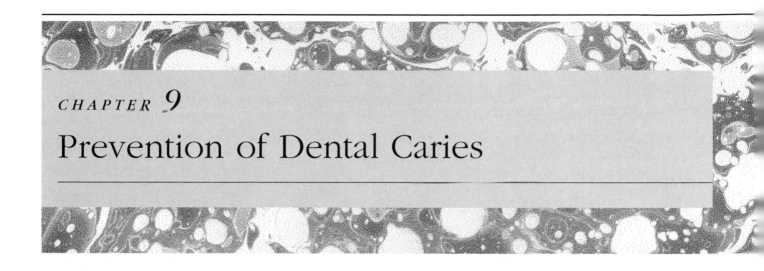

CHAPTER 9

Prevention of Dental Caries

KEY TERMS

Caries
Demineralization
Enamel pits and fissures
Fluoride
Fluorosis
Mottling
Pellicle
Periodontal disease
Pit and fissure sealants
Plaque
Subgingival plaque
Supragingival plaque
Topical fluoride

It was recognized long ago that the best treatment for any disease is to prevent it from occurring. The alternative to disease control is treatment after the disease occurs. This alternative is less desirable because of the destructive nature of dental disease. The two most common dental diseases, dental caries and periodontal disease, result in loss of normal tissue. In both disease categories the damaged tissue can never be regained. At best, dentists can only halt the progress of the disease before more damage occurs. The damaged tissue is gone forever. It seems reasonable to approach dental health by protecting the hard and soft tissues one is given in the first place. This is the basis of preventive dentistry.

The dental assistant is a key person in the incorporation of dental disease prevention programs. Increasing numbers of dental practices are establishing formal prevention programs for their patients. The dental assistant is

frequently placed in charge of this function. Therefore it is essential that the fundamentals of prevention be clearly understood before the assistant assumes these responsibilities.

DENTAL PLAQUE

Discussion of the prevention of dental disease first involves identifying one of the main causes of dental decay and periodontal disease, namely, **plaque**—a soft, adherent collection of salivary products and bacterial colonies on the teeth. It accumulates in varying degrees on the surface of the teeth continuously throughout the life span of most people. A patient's only hope in eliminating this disease-producing material is to continually remove it by toothbrushing and dental flossing.

Plaque re-forms rapidly after a thorough cleaning of the teeth. The first phase of plaque development is the deposition of adherent products from the saliva. These products are primarily composed of protein components, which form a thin, noncellular, adherent layer on the teeth, called the **pellicle.** Once the pellicle has been formed on the clean tooth surface, bacteria that inhabit the oral cavity attach themselves to the pellicle. After attachment the bacteria multiply to form large masses of bacterial colonies. This begins rapidly after a thorough cleaning of the teeth and continues until the plaque is fully matured by the end of 3 weeks.

Mature plaque consists primarily of bacteria of various types. Each type of organism functions in a different way. Some bacteria produce harmful chemical substances, and others produce substances that are needed by neighboring bacteria to survive. Still other organisms produce adherent substances that are interspersed with the bacteria and hold the plaque intact on the surface. Additional minor components of plaque include salivary mucin, dead epithelial cells, and food debris. Mature plaque is in reality a microscopic community of different bacteria and other substances that function to produce dental disease.

➡ KEY POINTS
- Plaque is a combination of bacteria, bacterial by-products, and salivary components.
- The pellicle is a thin, noncellular material that forms on the tooth and lies underneath the plaque.
- Plaque is able to adhere to the teeth by a sticky polysaccharide produced by the bacteria, primarily *Streptococcus mutans*.

Research has revealed that plaque located above the gingiva (**supragingival plaque**) consists of a different combination of bacteria than does plaque below the free gingival margin (**subgingival plaque**) (Figure 9-1). In patients who experience dental **caries** (decay), the bacteria found in supragingival plaque are capable of producing acids that can erode the surface of the tooth. On the other hand, subgingival plaque does not produce acids but rather other chemical compounds that penetrate the soft gingival tissue and cause it to become inflamed. Therefore current thinking regarding the disease-producing potential of dental plaque is that supragingival plaque, because of its acidic nature, is responsible for the pro-

duction of dental caries. Subgingival plaque, because of its capacity to produce substances that are toxic to soft tissue, is responsible for **periodontal disease** (gum disease). Plaque is extremely adherent and cannot be washed away by simply rinsing the mouth. More vigorous methods such as toothbrushing and dental flossing are required to remove it. These are discussed in detail in Chapter 10.

➡ KEY POINTS
- Supragingival plaque is formed above the gumline.
- Subgingival plaque is formed below the gumline.
- Bacteria in plaque causes periodontal disease and dental caries.

Dental Plaque and Dental Caries

Streptococcus mutans is one of the first organisms to attach to the pellicle and multiply. The streptococci are capable of producing both polysaccharides and acids from carbohydrates that are consumed by the patient. This is important because the polysaccharides help attach the streptococci to the pellicle. The acid they produce is capable of demineralizing the enamel layer of the tooth. This **demineralization** is the first stage of dental caries. Demineralization can appear as a white to brown lesion. Fortunately, research has found that demineralization is a reversible process. Therefore if the patient makes an improvement in his or her oral hygiene by thorough brushing and flossing, the demineralized areas may remineralize and actually become a more caries-resistant area. However, once the caries process has progressed beyond demineralization, the process is no longer reversible.

Other organisms in dental plaque produce various substances that help the bacterial mass attach to the pellicle. The fact that acid-producing bacteria are attached to the tooth surface contributes to a greater effectiveness of acid demineralization of tooth enamel. Because of its thickness and density the plaque prevents acid produced within it from being diluted by saliva or neutralized by chemicals contained in the saliva. Therefore the acid remains rather concentrated adjacent to the tooth surface and can break down the enamel more quickly.

Once the caries process is initiated, another organism, *Lactobacillus*, can be retained in the decayed area (carious lesion). Since the lesion is acidic, these organisms thrive, and like those of *Streptococcus mutans*, they convert sugar to acid, which in turn attacks tooth structure. It is also believed that *Lactobacillus* organisms can become

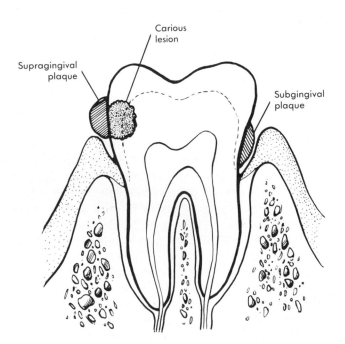

Figure 9-1 Common sites for accumulation of dental plaque.

Carious lesion

Supragingival plaque

Subgingival plaque

lodged in the retentive pits and fissures in the tooth surfaces, where they multiply and the acid they produce attacks tooth structure.

Dental Plaque and Periodontal Disease

The irritating effect of subgingival plaque on soft gingiva that surrounds the teeth is rather profound. If the plaque is allowed to remain in contact with this delicate tissue for prolonged periods of time, the gingiva becomes inflamed. The potential for serious damage to all the supporting structures around the teeth exists when the gingiva is inflamed for sustained periods. Thus the initiation of two of the most common periodontal diseases, gingivitis and periodontitis, is caused by plaque. The present strategy for the prevention of these periodontal diseases is continuous removal of plaque from the surfaces of the teeth through various oral hygiene methods such as toothbrushing and flossing between the teeth. Again, plaque cannot be removed from the teeth by vigorous rinsing; it must be mechanically removed by a toothbrush, floss, or other oral hygiene aid.

> **◆ KEY POINT**
> - **Plaque cannot be removed by vigorous rinsing alone.**

A discussion of periodontal disease and its treatment is presented in Chapter 21.

Dental Plaque and Mouth Odors

Dental plaque, beside being a factor in dental disease, is also a major contributor to breath odors. In fact, most mouth odors stem from the accumulation of dental plaque. The plaque mass has an unpleasant odor. If it is allowed to accumulate on the teeth and tongue, it will create an unpleasant mouth odor. This fact can be easily demonstrated by brushing the teeth without the use of dentifrice and then smelling the bristles of the brush. The unpleasant odor is readily detectable.

DIETARY CONTROL OF DENTAL CARIES

Although research is ongoing into the cause of dental caries a basic understanding of the disease can be explained by the following formulas:

Carbohydrates + Bacteria → Acids (dental plaque)

Acids + Susceptible tooth structure → Decay

In essence the first formula states that some bacteria living in the oral cavity can convert carbohydrates to organic acids. When these acids are produced in close contact with the tooth, as in a plaque mass or in pit and fissure areas, they are capable of demineralizing tooth

enamel. In other words they cause tooth decay. Without intervention, the progress of dental caries continues through the enamel and into the dentin layer, and the tooth is progressively destroyed.

From a caries prevention standpoint, plaque control programs and periodic dental prophylaxis are both directed toward eliminating the plaque mass so that acids cannot be produced in significant quantities in contact with the tooth surface.

Because bacteria can be harbored in the many pits and fissures found in normal tooth anatomy and because plaque control may not be 100% effective, further attention must be paid to controlling tooth decay by other means. These include controlling the diet of the patient and protecting the teeth through the use of fluoride and sealant materials.

One of the most effective ways to control dental caries is to regulate the dietary habits of the patient. Diet influences caries prevention in two ways:

1. *Tooth development and maturation.* Proper dietary intake of vitamins A, C, and D, calcium, phosphorus, and fluoride during tooth formation and maturation influences the resistance of tooth structure to future caries.
2. *Local effects of food on caries susceptibility.* Carbohydrates can be converted by certain bacteria into acids that demineralize the tooth structure. This local effect often overrides the resistance that the teeth acquire during their formation.

The local effect of food on the tooth surface is instrumental in initiating tooth decay, whereas the progress of decay in the tooth structure is greatly influenced by resistance the tooth acquired during its formation.

Dietary control of dental caries is primarily directed toward controlling the local effect that food has on caries production, since it tends to override the resistance of the tooth to decay to some extent. A reasonable approach to any dietary regimen requires that the basic nutritional needs of the patient be met while caries control is being accomplished. Therefore it is extremely important that the patient's present diet is analyzed for food value and carbohydrate intake.

Dietary changes should consider the fact that each time the patient ingests a carbohydrate type of food the oral bacteria produce a 20-minute acid attack on the teeth. A soda sipped over a long length of time will prolong an acid attack vs. drinking the soda all at once or having it with a meal in which the patient will experience an acid attack with the meal anyway. It is also important for patients with high caries rates to eliminate hidden sugars, such as nondairy creamer, pretzels, and chewing gum.

Although dietary control of dental caries is used less today than in the past, it should not be overlooked as an effective preventive measure. The impact of fluoride and pit and fissure sealants on caries prevention is the major reason for the decrease in dietary strategies to reduce dental decay. However, a prevention-oriented dental practice should be prepared to employ diet control techniques with patients who have a high caries rate.

FLUORIDE

Probably no single public health measure has been as effective in reducing dental caries as the use of fluoride. **Fluoride** compounds such as sodium fluoride, stannous fluoride, and acidulated phosphate fluoride react with tooth enamel to make it more resistant to demineralization by bacterial acid. In other words, fluorides make teeth less vulnerable to decay.

Fluorides are natural minerals found in certain foods or beverages, such as broccoli, tea, water, and fish. Fluorides are incorporated into the crystal structure of tooth enamel. The existence of fluoride in the crystal structure makes the enamel less soluble in bacterial acids. Further, recent studies have revealed that the presence of fluoride in the enamel layer of a tooth may actually inhibit acid-producing bacteria in dental plaque. A tooth whose enamel contains no fluoride will be far more vulnerable to caries than a fluoridated tooth, such as a recently erupted tooth. A tooth can have fluoride incorporated in the enamel crystal structure in three ways: by ingestion, by topical application of dentifrice or mouthrinse, or by both ingestion and topical application.

Ingestion in Fluoridated Drinking Water

The history of fluoride is long and interesting. The first indication that some substance (later found to be fluoride) could inhibit or eliminate dental caries was discovered in 1916 in Colorado. Residents of certain areas of Colorado had a curious stain in their enamel, but at the same time their teeth were resistant to dental caries. This aroused the curiosity of researchers to determine what caused this phenomenon. After much research it was discovered that all these patients with stained teeth and resistance to dental caries drank well water most of their lifetime. Continued research demonstrated that if persons consumed fluoride during the years of tooth development and for a few years after eruption, their teeth would be more resistant to dental caries.

During the course of experiments to determine the favorable effect of fluoride on tooth enamel it was also discovered that excessive ingestion of fluoride could result in staining (**fluorosis**) and pitting of the teeth (**mottling**) (Figure 9-2). The Colorado residents were found to have consumed excessive concentrations of fluorides in their water supply. Through experimentation it was discovered that a concentration of 1 part fluoride in 1 million parts of water (1 ppm) was the most favorable concentration. This 1 ppm concentration makes the teeth resistant to caries without causing staining and pitting.

> ↬ **KEY POINTS**
> - A concentration of fluoride at 1 ppm is the most favorable concentration for caries inhibition without causing any damage to the teeth.
> - Concentrations over 1 ppm have been found to cause dental fluorosis and mottling of the enamel.

Many communities now provide their residents with the 1 ppm fluoride concentration in the water supply so that they can benefit from this caries prevention phenomenon. In rural areas where well water is consumed or in cities without fluoridated water supplies, children should be given dietary supplements of fluoride during the tooth-developing years (birth to 21 years of age). The water supply should be tested for its present level of fluoride and the dietary supplement prescribed to adjust the concentration up to the equivalent of 1 ppm (Table 9-1).

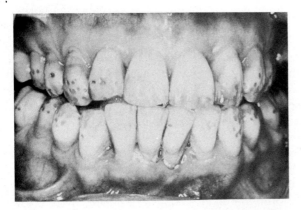

Figure 9-2 Consumption of excessive concentrations of fluoride can result in both fluorosis (dark-stained areas) and mottling of enamel (pitted areas).

Table 9-1 Dosage schedule for fluoride supplements*

Age of child (yr)	Water fluoride concentration (ppm)		
	<0.3	0.3-0.7	>0.7
Birth to 3	0.25 drops	0†	0†
3-5	0.50 drops or tablet	0.25	0
5-16	1.00 tablet	0.50	0

*Recommendations from the American Dental Association, Chicago. In milligrams of fluoride per day; 2.2 mg sodium fluoride provides 1 mg fluoride ions.
†Infants receiving their total diet from breast-feeding need a 0.25 mg supplement.

This testing service is provided by most state laboratories. If well water contains a natural fluoride concentration of 1 ppm, supplemental fluoride should be avoided to prevent staining (fluorosis) and possible mottling.

Repeated studies on the effectiveness of ingested fluorides have indicated that there is approximately a 50% to 65% reduction in caries in patients who have consumed 1 ppm fluoride during the tooth-developing years. The reason for such a high reduction in caries is that the fluoride is incorporated throughout the entire layer of enamel. This renders the entire enamel layer more resistant to demineralization by bacterial acids.

➥ KEY POINT
- Fluoridated drinking water produces the highest reduction of dental caries vs. home or office topical application of fluoride and is highly cost-effective.

Topical Application

After the discovery of the effectiveness of ingested fluoride on inhibiting dental caries, other ways of using fluoride in caries prevention were explored. It was discovered that patients who did not benefit from ingested fluoride could receive some caries-inhibiting effect by painting a clean tooth with a high concentration of fluoride. A caries reduction of approximately 40% to 50% can be achieved with this topical application method.

Topically applied fluoride penetrates only the outermost portion of the enamel layer, and hence it is less effective than ingested fluoride. Newly erupted teeth allow better incorporation of fluoride in the crystal structure than do more mature teeth. Topical fluoride must be applied to a clean tooth on a semiannual or an annual basis to achieve maximum effect.

Some of the agents that are used today are 2% sodium fluoride, 10% stannous fluoride, and 1.23% acidulated phosphofluoride gels and foams. The gels and foams are probably the most widely used today because of their convenience and pleasant taste. These preparations are available in 1-minute and 4-minute formulas.

The gel or foam technique of fluoride treatment follows:

1. Give the patient prefluoride treatment instructions such as the following:
   a. The fluoride is a gel/foam that helps to prevent dental decay.
   b. Do not eat, drink, or rinse for 30 minutes after the fluoride treatment to get the maximum benefit from the treatment.
   c. Try not to swallow the fluoride.

2. The gel or foam is placed in polyvinyl trays that will cover the teeth. The trays should be filled approximately one third full. If the gel is used, the sides of the trays should be squeezed to distribute the gel.
3. The teeth are isolated with cotton rolls on the buccal surfaces of both arches and on either side of the tongue.
4. The teeth are dried with the air-water syringe.
5. The gel- or foam-filled trays are placed over the dry teeth. Maxillary and mandibular arches can be done at the same time. It is advisable to pump the trays up and down on insertion to force the gel/foam into the less accessible areas in and around the teeth. One manufacturer provides trays with padded liners and instructs the patient to bite up and down on the trays after insertion to accomplish this task (Figure 9-3).
6. Place two cotton rolls between the upper and lower arches. Instruct the patient to bite down gently on the cotton rolls. Bend the saliva ejector into a U shape, and place inside the patient's mouth. Give the patient a paper towel for any excess saliva that may leak out.
7. After the waiting period (usually 1 to 4 minutes) is complete, the trays are removed, and the mouth is evacuated but not rinsed.
8. The patient can expectorate the excess gel but is cautioned not to eat, drink, or rinse for 30 minutes after the fluoride application.

Topical Fluorides Applied at Home

In addition to periodic fluoride treatments done in dental offices, supplemental applications of **topical fluoride** may benefit patients with a high caries rate. Daily use of dentifrice that contains fluoride has proved effective in the prevention of dental caries. A list of fluoridated den-

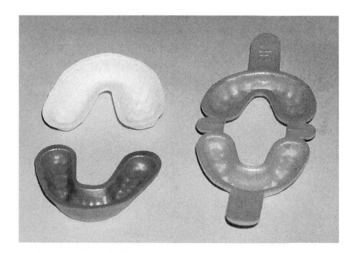

Figure 9-3 Polyvinyl trays for topical application of fluoride gel.

tifrices can be obtained by calling the American Dental Association, Council on Dental Therapeutics, and requesting an "Accepted Products" list.

Patients with severe caries susceptibility also benefit from daily rinses with over-the-counter mouthwashes containing either 0.05% sodium fluoride or 0.1% stannous fluoride. A list of fluoridated daily rinses can be obtained by calling the American Dental Association, Council on Dental Therapeutics, and requesting an "Accepted Products" list. A weekly rinse is also available. Fluoride rinses should not be given to children under 6 years old because of the risk of accidentally swallowing the rinse. Children over 6 years old should be carefully monitored to prevent accidental ingestion.

Use of additional forms of fluoride-containing agents seems to benefit caries-susceptible patients. However, such use should be monitored by a dentist.

Combined Ingestion and Topical Application

There is some debate as to whether patients who have ingested fluoride throughout their lifetime benefit from topical fluoride applications. It is important to remember that fluoride is a natural mineral that can also be found in certain foods and beverages, such as tea. Newly erupted teeth are more susceptible to decay than teeth that have been erupted for some time because as we grow older the outer layer of the enamel becomes fluoride rich and caries resistant. However, some research indicates that some additional benefit can be derived from this practice. The benefit is minimal but probably worthwhile.

Fluoride Supplements

Studies have shown that fluoride supplements given from birth through the teenage years can equal or exceed the caries reduction rate for water fluoridation. However, supplements must be given continuously and conscientiously during this period of life. The dosage of fluoride supplements is determined based on the patient's age and also the amount of fluoride the patient is exposed to in the drinking water. See Table 9-1 for a dosage schedule recommended by the American Dental Association. Children should be instructed to chew the tablet and swish the slurry before swallowing to get an added topical benefit from the fluoride.

ENAMEL PIT AND FISSURE SEALANTS

The enamel layer of the tooth does not provide a perfect covering for all teeth. Particularly in posterior teeth, the occlusal surfaces contain several voids in the enamel called **enamel pits and fissures** (Figure 9-4). These pits and fissures vary in extent from one tooth to another. Some teeth do not contain any.

Teeth that contain rather deep pits and fissures have been shown to be more vulnerable to dental caries in these voids. Oral bacteria and their nutrients can easily enter the fissures and initiate decay. It is nearly impossible to clean these voids adequately by toothbrushing or conventional prophylaxis procedures. Hence the bacteria are harbored in the pits and fissures and can create the acid environment that initiates dental caries. Dental caries studies have demonstrated that approximately 44% of all carious lesions in young patients occur in occlusal surfaces with deep pits and fissures.

Although fluorides have significantly reduced overall decay experienced by individuals, they do so primarily by reducing caries on smooth surfaces. Close analysis of studies of caries reduction with the various fluoride methods demonstrates clearly that tooth surfaces with pits and fissures do benefit from the fluoride protection but not as greatly as smooth tooth surfaces. Therefore **pit and fissure sealants**, along with fluoride, make up an important dentistry measure used in the prevention of dental decay.

Research on pit and fissure sealants so far seems to indicate as much as a 17% to 54% reduction in occlusal caries when sealants are used.

Materials

Sealants are made of a material similar to composite materials used for esthetic anterior restorations. Sealants are basically "runny" composites. They can be clear or opaque in color and should feel smooth and glasslike on the tooth (Figure 9-5).

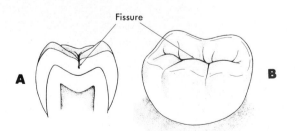

Figure 9-4 Enamel pits and fissures. **A,** Longitudinal section. **B,** Buccal view.

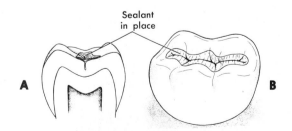

Figure 9-5 Pit and fissure sealant in place. **A,** Longitudinal section. **B,** Buccal view.

Two commercially available products use two different methods of hardening the sealant after it is applied:

1. Chemical cure: this product has chemicals within the product that when mixed together automatically harden it.
2. Light cure: this product uses intense visible light to activate the chemical within the product to form a hard, glasslike seal (Figure 9-6).

The sealant is bonded to the enamel to form an adequate seal. The tooth is conditioned by cleaning it with a pumice polishing paste followed by an etching procedure. Etching is accomplished by applying a 35% to 50% solution of phosphoric acid to the enamel, which forms pores in the enamel surface. After a thorough rinsing, the sealant is placed, penetrating these pores and bonds to the enamel when it hardens.

Technique of Application

The armamentarium for application of pit and fissure sealants is shown in Figure 9-7. The technique for application is described in Box 9-1.

The patient should be checked at 6-month intervals to evaluate the sealant. If there is evidence of loss or damage to the seal, the sealant is replaced by the procedure just described.

Indications and Contraindications

Not all posterior teeth are candidates for the sealing procedure. The selection of teeth should be based on the following considerations:

1. *Patient's oral hygiene.* Pit and fissure sealants should be considered as only one part of a total prevention scheme. It would be futile to protect the pit and fissure areas of teeth if other tooth surfaces and oral tissues are neglected.
2. *Patient's caries activity.* Sealants would be helpful in patients with high caries rates and deep occlusal fissures. However, it again would be futile without other preventive measures such as fluorides, diet control, and proper oral hygiene.
3. *Caries susceptibility of individual occlusal surfaces.* Only deep enamel pits and fissures need treat-

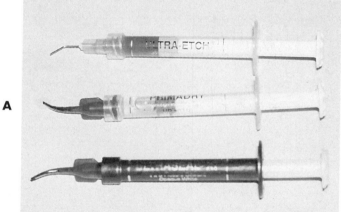
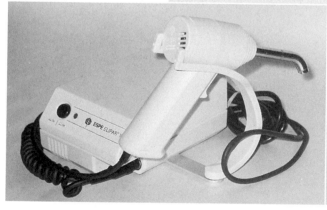
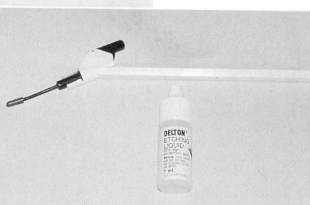

Figure 9-6   Pit and fissure sealing agents. **A,** Sealant base material in syringes. *Top:* Etchant; *middle:* priming and drying agent; *bottom:* sealant material. **B,** Curing light used to set sealant material. **C,** Unit-dose, light-cured sealant material.

(**A** and **B** courtesy L.D. Caulk Dental Manufacturing, Milford, Del. **C** courtesy Lee Pharmaceuticals, South El Monte, Calif.)

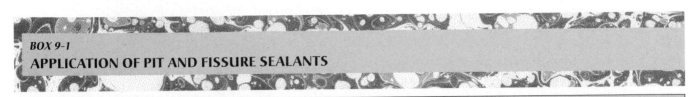

BOX 9-1

APPLICATION OF PIT AND FISSURE SEALANTS

PROCEDURE	RATIONALE
1. Isolate teeth. Small children may need to have sealants applied by separate quadrants. Full arches can usually be sealed in older children.	1. Teeth must be kept dry to ensure proper adhesion of sealant.
2. Polish teeth with rubber cup and flour of pumice moistened with water. Avoid prophylaxis paste containing oils, fluoride, or glycerin. Dry teeth.	2. Polishing teeth removes plaque and debris from tooth surface. Oils, fluoride, or glycerin prevents material from making proper seal.
3. Apply liquid etching agent with cotton pliers and cotton pellets. Gently move cotton over enamel surface, which will be covered by sealant. Manufacturers' instructions vary on time interval for etching, which can range from 60 to 90 seconds. *Note:* A recently introduced alternative method dispenses acid etch in a syringe. Syringe is used to apply acid etch directly to tooth.	3. Vigorous rubbing will defeat purpose of etching by collapsing microscopic pores being formed by etching agent.
4. Rinse teeth for 30 seconds with aerated spray and then dry teeth. Etched surfaces should appear frosty white. If saliva contaminates area to be sealed, tooth must be reetched for 10 seconds.	4. Teeth must be rinsed thoroughly to remove etchant and must not be contaminated with saliva.

PROCEDURE	RATIONALE
5. Sealant is prepared and applied to thickness that just clears occlusion. Dentist may use explorer or small brush to gently spread sealant on occlusal surface.	5. Only thin layer of sealant material is needed to seal teeth effectively. Too much sealant placed on tooth will require occlusal adjustment.
6. Sealant is allowed to harden if it is self-curing type, or it is hardened using appropriate light source.	6. Manufacturer's instructions should be consulted concerning setting time for self-curing types of sealants. Light-cured sealants usually require a 40-second cure.
7. Dentist checks sealant with explorer to see if sealant is properly hardened.	7. To check if sealant has cured properly.
8. Articulating paper is used to check occlusion. Round bur and slow-speed handpiece are used to adjust high spots.	8. Sealant should not interfere with patient's occlusion.
9. Patient is instructed to return to office if it is found that sealant interferes with patient's occlusion after patient has left office.	9. Sealants that interfere with occlusion can cause trauma to tooth and periodontium.
10. Patient is instructed to avoid chewing ice or hard candy.	10. Sealant will break from pressure.

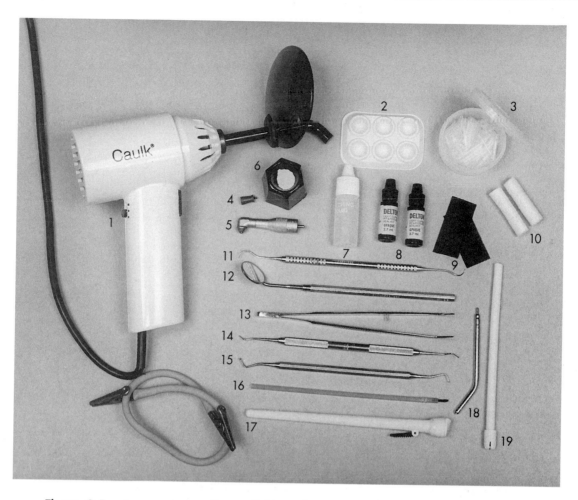

Figure 9-7 Armamentarium for application of pit and fissure sealants. *1,* Light-curing device. *2,* Welled-solution devices. *3,* Tubes for pit and fissure application. *4,* Prophylaxis cup. *5,* Prophylaxis angle. *6,* Dappen dish, with nonfluoridated paste. *7,* Acid etch solution. *8,* Sealant. *9,* Articulating paper. *10,* Cotton rolls. *11,* Explorer. *12,* Mirror. *13,* Cotton pliers. *14,* Spoon excavator. *15,* Ball burnisher. *16,* Brush. *17,* Sealant applicating device. *18,* Air-water tip. *19,* Saliva ejector.

ment. Occlusal surfaces with shallow grooves do not harbor caries-producing bacteria and are far more resistant to decay.

4. *Caries history of the individual tooth.* There is little reason to seal a tooth that has been in the mouth 4 years or more without developing occlusal decay. Chances are minimal that it will develop occlusal decay if it has not already done so by this time.

Newly erupted posterior teeth should be sealed routinely if they have deep pits and fissures because of their known vulnerability to occlusal decay.

Role of Dental Assistant

The role of the dental assistant in applying pit and fissure sealants depends greatly on the laws governing dental practice in each state. Most states now allow auxiliaries to assist the dentist in this procedure. An extra pair of hands is needed during the prophylaxis and isolation phases. This procedure is ideal for consideration as an expanded duty for dental auxiliaries.

BIBLIOGRAPHY

Council on Dental Therapeutics: *Accepted dental therapeutics,* ed 40, Chicago, 1995, American Dental Association.

Darby ML, Walsh MM: *Dental hygiene theory and practice,* Philadelphia, 1995, WB Saunders.

Englander HR and others: Incremental rates of dental caries after repeated topical sodium fluoride applications in children with lifelong consumption of fluoridated water, *JADA* 82:354, 1971.

Erlich AE: *Nutrition and dental health,* ed 2, Albany, NY, 1994, Delmar Publishers.

Horowitz HS, Creighton WE, McClendon BJ: The effect on human dental caries of weekly oral rinsing with a sodium fluoride mouthwash: a final report, *Arch Oral Biol* 16:609, 1971.

Horowitz HS, Heifetz SB: Evaluation of topical applications of stannous fluoride to teeth of children born and reared in a fluoridated community: final report, *J Dent Child* 36:65, 1969.

Horowitz HS, Heifetz SB: The current status of topically applied fluorides in preventive dentistry. In Newbrun E, editor: *Fluorides and dental caries,* Springfield, Ill, 1975, Charles C Thomas.

Horowitz HS, Heifetz SB, Poulsen S: Retention and effectiveness of a single application of an adhesive sealant in preventing occlusal caries: final report after five years of a study in Kalispell, Montana, *JADA* 95:1133, 1977.

Loesche WJ: The bacteriology of dental decay and periodontal disease, *Clin Prev Dent* 2:18, 1980.

Newbrun E: Sugar and dental caries, *Clin Prev Dent* 4:11, 1982.

Newbrun E: *Fluorides and dental caries,* ed 3, Springfield, 1986, Charles C Thomas.

Newbrun, E: *Cariology,* Chicago, 1989, Quintessence Publishing.

Nizel AE, Papas AS: *Nutrition in clinical dentistry,* ed 3, Philadelphia, 1989, WB Saunders.

Wilkins EM: *Clinical practice of the dental hygienist,* ed 7, Baltimore, 1994, Williams & Wilkins.

QUESTIONS–Chapter 9

1. The ideal concentration of fluoride in the drinking water for the prevention of dental caries is:
   a. 0.5 ppm
   b. 1 ppm
   c. 1.5 ppm
   d. 2 ppm

2. When applying the acid etch to prepare the tooth for a pit and fissure sealant, the tooth must be rinsed for a minimum of _____ seconds.
   a. 10
   b. 15-20
   c. 30
   d. 60

3. The tooth became contaminated with saliva after it had been acid etched, rinsed, and dried. What should be done next?
   a. Apply the sealant.
   b. Dry the tooth, and then apply the sealant.
   c. Reetch the tooth.
   d. Rinse and dry the tooth again.

4. When placing a pit and fissure sealant the tooth should look _____ when dried after acid etching.
   a. Brown
   b. Blue
   c. Frosty white
   d. Normal

5. Which of the following is the best caries-inhibiting preventive measure?
   a. Daily over-the-counter fluoride rinse
   b. In-office fluoride treatment
   c. Fluoridated drinking water

6. Permanent discoloration of the enamel that is caused by too much ingested fluoride is called:
   a. Fluorosis
   b. Demineralization
   c. Dental caries
   d. Erosion

7. A thin, noncellular layer that is produced from products in the saliva and is attached directly onto the tooth is called:
   a. Plaque
   b. Supragingival plaque
   c. Subgingival plaque
   d. The pellicle

8. The dissolution of minerals from the enamel by acid-producing bacteria is called:
   a. Fluorosis
   b. Demineralization
   c. Mottling
   d. Remineralization

9. The bacterium that has been associated with dental decay is:
   a. *Actinobacillus actinomycetemcomitans*
   b. *Bacteroides gingivalis*
   c. *Streptococcus mutans*
   d. Spirochetes

10. Following a fluoride treatment, the patient must be instructed to do which of the following:
    1. Do not eat for 30 minutes.
    2. Do not rinse for 30 minutes.
    3. Do not drink for 30 minutes.
    4. Do not smoke for 30 minutes.
       a. *1* and *3*
       b. *2* and *4*
       c. *1, 2,* and *3*
       d. *4* only

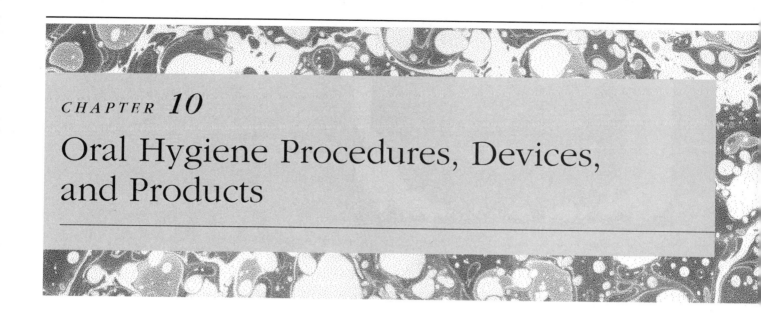

CHAPTER *10*

Oral Hygiene Procedures, Devices, and Products

KEY TERMS

Air-powder abrasive polisher
Bass method of toothbrushing
Bridge threader
Calculus
Curette scaler
Dental floss
Dentifrice
Disclosing solution
Electric toothbrush
Explorer
Floss holder
Gingival stimulators
Gracey curette
Interdental brushes
Mouthrinse
Oral irrigator
Plaque
Polishing
Prophylaxis
Root planing
Rotary scrub method of toothbrushing
Scaling
Sickle scaler
Universal curette

DENTAL PROPHYLAXIS

The term **prophylaxis** means the prevention of disease. A dental prophylaxis is a procedure to prevent dental disease. The objective of the procedure is to identify and eliminate undesirable substances from the surfaces of the teeth. These substances include plaque, stain, calculus, and food debris. Patients refer to this procedure as a "cleaning of the teeth." It is indeed a teeth cleaning that has as its primary purpose the prevention of periodontal disease and dental caries.

The need for this valuable service varies with the individual. To a great extent the frequency of needing a prophylaxis is determined by the effectiveness of a patient's personal oral hygiene efforts. Most patients need this service twice each year. However, some patients require it only on a yearly basis, and still others should have a prophylaxis every 2 to 4 months.

A dental prophylaxis is usually reserved for patients who seek regular periodontal maintenance. Some patients need more than just a regular cleaning and may require quadrant root planing (smoothing of the root surfaces of the teeth) with local anesthesia.

Armamentarium for Routine Prophylaxis

A suggested setup for performing a routine prophylaxis is shown in Figure 10-1.

A **sickle scaler** is a hand instrument with two cutting edges and a pointed toe (Figure 10-2). Sickle scalers are used primarily to scale under the interproximal contact mainly in the anterior region of the mouth.

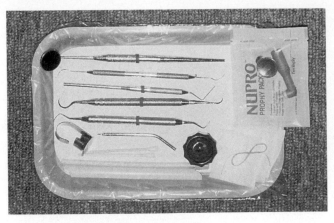

Mirror
Explorer
Peridontal probe
Sickle scaler
Universal 3/4 curette
Prophy paste ring holder
Air/water syringe tip
Cotton swabs
Dappen dish/disclosing
    solution

Saliva ejector
HVE tip
Disposable prophy angle
Prophy paste
Gauze sponges
Dental floss

Figure 10-1   Prophylaxis armamentarium: preset tray (optional fluoride setup not shown).

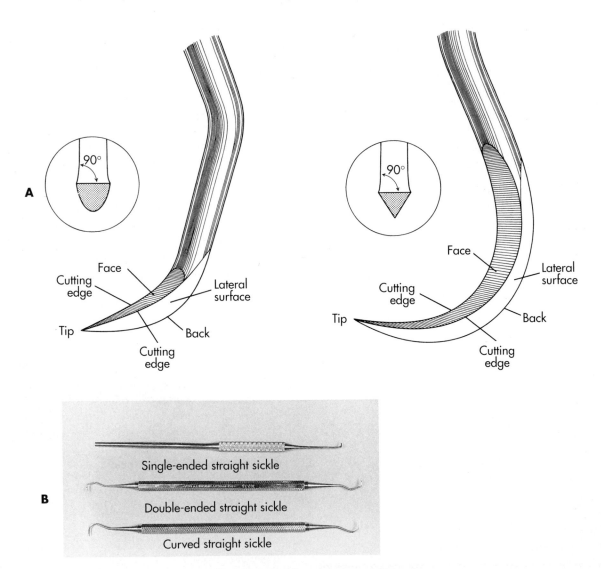

Figure 10-2   A, Sickle scalers. **B,** Three common sickle scalers.

(**A** from Genco R, Goldman HM, Cohen DW: *Contemporary periodontics,* St Louis, 1990, Mosby.)

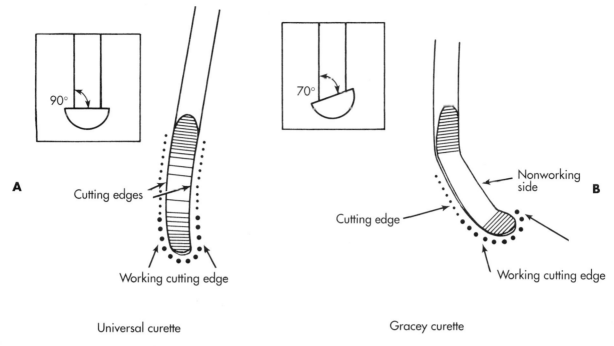

Figure 10-3 Curette scalers. **A**, Universal curette. **B**, Gracey curette.

> **KEY POINT**
> ▪ Sickle scalers are generally not used for root planing because the pointed toe can gouge the root surface.

Curettes are used for scaling and root planing. A **curette scaler** has two cutting edges and a rounded toe (Figure 10-3). Two types of curettes may be used by the dentist or dental hygienist:

1. A **universal curette** can be used in all areas of the mouth and is often used for routine prophylaxis because this one instrument can be used to clean the entire mouth (see Figure 10-3, *A*).
2. A **Gracey curette** is site specific. Each Gracey curette can be used to scale certain surfaces of the tooth (see Figure 10-3, *B*). For example, the 11/12 Gracey curette is used to scale the mesial surfaces of the posterior teeth. Gracey curettes are often used for quadrant root planing appointments, and the dentist may use a Gracey curette during a routine prophylaxis to scale an area that is difficult to access. Figure 10-4 shows a variety of Gracey curettes. A typical tray setup for quadrant root planing may contain the Gracey 5/6, 7/8, 11/12, and 13/14 curettes (Figure 10-5).

Local anesthesia is usually administered to the patient for comfort.

> **KEY POINTS**
> ▪ A universal curette can be used in all areas of the mouth.
> ▪ A Gracey curette is site specific.

Technique

Generally the methods used to perform a prophylaxis contain the following phases.

1. *Assessment phase*
   a. *Disclosing phase*. The patient's lips are coated with lubricant to prevent staining. Disclosing solution is painted on the patient's teeth with a cotton swab. After the solution is rinsed off with the air-water syringe and oral evacuator or saliva ejector, the areas of plaque accumulation appear stained (Figure 10-6). This is an opportune time to demonstrate the results to the patient with a hand mirror and a mouth mirror.

      With the hand mirror, the patient is given oral hygiene instruction. The patient can see the disclosed plaque being removed with the toothbrush. This patient education effort clearly demonstrates that the toothbrush will do the job if it is used properly.

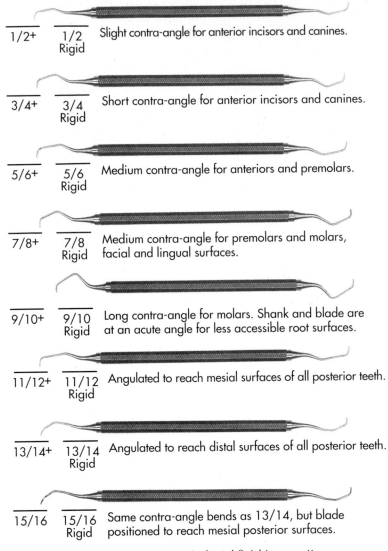

1/2+ 1/2 Rigid Slight contra-angle for anterior incisors and canines.

3/4+ 3/4 Rigid Short contra-angle for anterior incisors and canines.

5/6+ 5/6 Rigid Medium contra-angle for anteriors and premolars.

7/8+ 7/8 Rigid Medium contra-angle for premolars and molars, facial and lingual surfaces.

9/10+ 9/10 Rigid Long contra-angle for molars. Shank and blade are at an acute angle for less accessible root surfaces.

11/12+ 11/12 Rigid Angulated to reach mesial surfaces of all posterior teeth.

13/14+ 13/14 Rigid Angulated to reach distal surfaces of all posterior teeth.

15/16 15/16 Rigid Same contra-angle bends as 13/14, but blade positioned to reach mesial posterior surfaces.

Figure 10-4 Gracey periodontal finishing curettes.

(Courtesy Hu-Friedy, Chicago.)

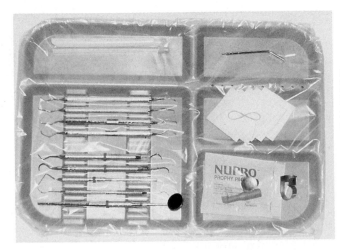

Mirror	HVE tip
Explorer	Saliva ejector
Probe	Air/water syringe tip
Sickle scaler	Gauze
Universal curette scaler	Dental floss
7/8 Gracey curette	Prophy paste
5/6 Gracey curette	Prophy angle
11/12 Gracey curette	Prophy paste ring holder
13/14 Gracey curette	Additional items: Local anesthetic setup

Figure 10-5 Quadrant root planing armamentarium.

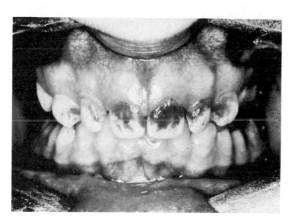

Figure 10-6 Disclosed dental plaque on maxillary anterior teeth.

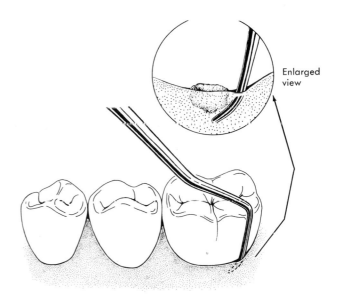

Figure 10-7 Curette scaler placed in gingival crevice to remove existing calculus.

2. *Treatment phase*

a. *Scaling phase.* **Scaling** is the process of scraping plaque (soft) and **calculus** (hard) adherent substances off the surface of the teeth. There are many designs of scalers for scaling and root planing. These instruments are introduced into the gingival crevices and interproximal areas to remove irritating debris (Figure 10-7). Visibility and access are important during this phase. Efficient use of the oral evacuator and retraction of the lips and cheeks are of great assistance to the operator.

As debris is removed from the teeth, the dental assistant should quickly remove it from the scaler with either the oral evacuator or 2- × 2-inch gauze sponges. Accumulations of blood and saliva must be constantly removed during the scaling phase.

The **explorer** is a valuable instrument for checking the presence of calculus in subgingival areas.

During the scaling phase the patient may need root planing in certain areas. **Root planing** is the smoothing of the root surfaces of the tooth. Root planing can be accomplished with the same instruments used to scale the teeth. Patients who need root planing for many teeth are usually scheduled for quadrant root planing appointments and are given local anesthesia.

As with toothbrushing techniques, a pattern should be established for scaling and polishing. This is helpful to the assistant in anticipating the operator's needs.

b. *Polishing phase.* After all areas of the mouth have been scaled, the teeth may be polished using either the slow-speed handpiece with a rubber cup or the newer air-powder abrasive technique. Polishing is done selectively because enamel is worn by abrasives used to remove stain from tooth surfaces.

Polishing is primarily a "super toothbrushing" of the teeth. The action of polishing removes residual plaque and stain and leaves a smooth surface on the enamel.

Constant oral evacuation by the assistant is usually needed during this phase to prevent spattering of polishing paste and saliva. Patients tend to salivate more during polishing procedures. This calls for an increase in evacuation of the lowest posterior regions of the mouth. A good oral rinse with the syringe and evacuator is helpful at this point before flossing.

c. *Flossing phase.* Dental flossing is the best way to ensure that plaque is removed from between the teeth. Neither rubber cup nor scalers can completely clean the tight contact areas between the teeth. A thorough cleaning should include the flossing phase.

Once again, with patients using a hand mirror to observe their own mouths, a flossing demonstration can be given by either the prevention assistant or the hygienist.

Following the demonstration it is advisable to have the patient floss various areas of the mouth while the assistant holds the mirror. This offers the assistant an opportunity to evaluate the patient's technique and to correct any mistakes.

d. *Fluoride treatment.* Once the prophylaxis is complete, an optional fluoride treatment can be performed using one of the methods discussed in Chapter 9.

Dental Prophylaxis Devices
Ultrasonic scaler

The ultrasonic scaler (Cavitron) is useful for removing debris from tooth surfaces (Figure 10-8). Like the ultrasonic cleaner discussed in Chapter 7, the ultrasonic scaler vibrates rapidly and removes adherent substances such as calculus and stain from tooth surfaces. Many dentists prefer to use hand-operated scalers after ultrasonic scaler use to refine the scaling process.

A significant amount of coolant water is used with ultrasonic scalers. Dental assistants should drape patients to protect their clothing and should provide patients with protective eyewear to prevent aerosol from getting in their eyes. The operating team should use standard barrier techniques to protect themselves from aerosol produced by the scaler.

Intraorally, accumulation of water must be controlled by the dental assistant through the use of oral evacuation devices.

The dental assistant often sets up the ultrasonic scaler. Figure 10-9 demonstrates this procedure.

Two types of ultrasonic scaler tips are available for the ultrasonic scaler (Figure 10-10):

1. Universal tips can be used in all areas of the mouth.
2. Slimline tips are thinner than universal tips and are available in the universal style or in a right and left pair. Slimline tips may be useful for reaching tooth surfaces under tight gingiva.

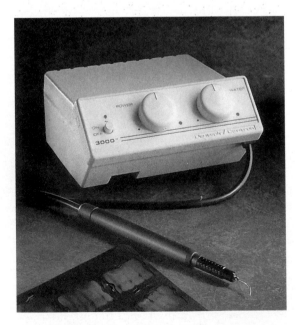

Figure 10-8   Ultrasonic scaler.

(Courtesy Dentsply International, Milford, Del.)

Sonic scaler

The sonic scaler (Figure 10-11) works on the same concept as an ultrasonic scaler but is less powerful. The sonic scaler is an air-driven handpiece that fits directly into the handpiece lines of the dental unit. There is no bulky unit attached to the sonic scaler as with the ultrasonic scaler, which offers the advantage of increased mobility.

Air-powder abrasive polisher

The **air-powder abrasive polisher** (Prophy-Jet) (Figure 10-12, *A*) is the polishing device that removes stain and plaque in less time than do handpieces and rubber cups. It is also generally more effective in removing stain from pit and fissure areas. The device uses air pressure to force water that contains fine particles of sodium bicarbonate against tooth surfaces and in effect "sandblasts" the stain away. As with the ultrasonic scaler, some precautions are recommended. The same draping and barrier techniques should be used. The aerosol produced by this device tends to leave abrasive sodium bicarbonate dust throughout the treatment room and creates a need for maintenance. Patients should remove contact lenses before air-powder abrasive polishing and wash eyeglasses after polishing to prevent scratching the lenses with residual dust. Since the patient may swallow some sodium bicarbonate during the procedure, this polisher should not be used for patients on a restricted sodium diet. The fine aerosol mist may preclude use of this polishing technique on patients with severe respiratory illness. Use of an effective oral evacuation technique can help control fluids produced by this polishing device.

Because of the abrasive nature of this polishing technique, soft root surfaces, composite restorations, and the gingiva should have minimal exposure to direct spray from the instrument nozzle.

Air-powder abrasive polishers are available as either separate polishing units or in combination with an ultrasonic scaler (Figure 10-12, *B*).

Oral irrigator

An **oral irrigator** (Figure 10-13, *A*) is a device designed to pump water or special irrigating solutions into the oral cavity to flush debris from inaccessible areas around teeth. Although more discussion on the home use of these devices is presented later in this chapter, mention of irrigation in conjunction with dental prophylaxis is warranted here.

Interest has emerged recently regarding use of antimicrobial agents to flush the periodontal pocket. Antimicrobials such as chlorhexidine, tetracycline, and stannous fluoride are currently being used. Following the dental prophylaxis procedure, periodontal pockets can be flushed with an antimicrobial solution using a fine tip on the irrigator (Figure 10-13, *B*). Use of special mouth-

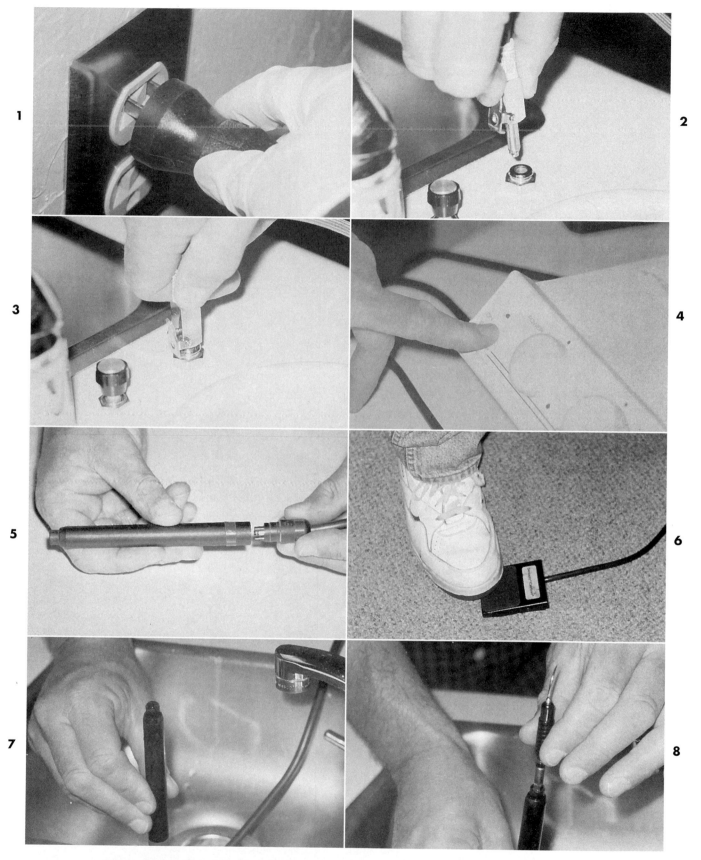

Figure 10-9 Steps in setting up ultrasonic scaler. *1,* Insert electrical plug into outlet. *2,* Insert water connector of ultrasonic unit into dental unit water supply. *3,* Lock water connector. *4,* Turn on ultrasonic unit. *5,* Attach autoclavable/sterile handpiece to ultrasonic unit. *6,* Step on foot pedal to activate. *7,* Hold handpiece upright until filled with water. *8,* Plunge sterile ultrasonic insert into handpiece.

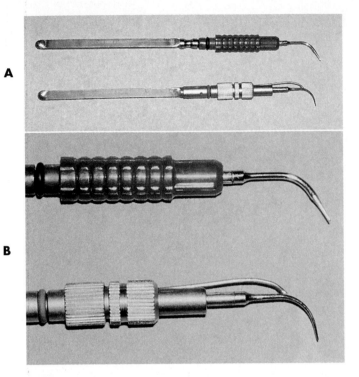

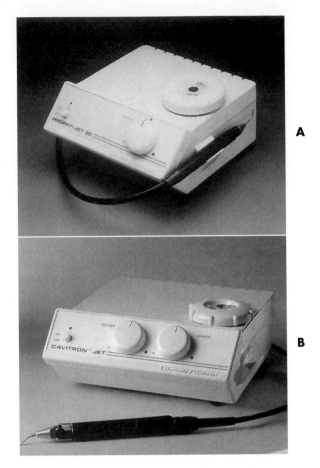

Figure 10-10 Ultrasonic tips. **A**, Universal tip (top); slimline tip (bottom). **B**, Closeup view of universal and slimline tips.

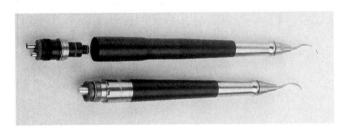

Figure 10-12 **A**, Air-powder abrasive polisher. **B**, Ultrasonic scaler and air polishing system.

(Courtesy Dentsply International, Milford, Del.)

Figure 10-11 Sonic scaler.

(Courtesy Star Dental, Lancaster, Pa.)

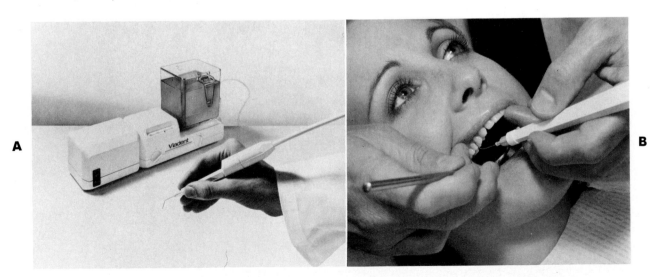

Figure 10-13 **A**, Professional model oral irrigator with gingival sulcus cannula attached. **B**, Cannula in working position.

(Courtesy Viadent Inc, Fort Collins, Colo.)

washes as an adjunct to traditional periodontal therapy is an interesting frontier of dental care.

Dental Assistant's Role

As mentioned in the description of the prophylaxis procedure, the assistant is of great value in retraction and oral evacuation. The necessary instrument exchanges are accomplished through standard exchange techniques (see Chapter 15).

Both the disclosing phase and the flossing phase can and should be done by the assistant. If a topical fluoride treatment is desired after the flossing phase, the assistant can accomplish this task also if state dental law allows assistants to provide this service.

TOOTHBRUSHING TECHNIQUES

Dental assistants are frequently called on to provide oral hygiene instructions for patients. Therefore the "prevention assistant" should be well informed regarding common techniques that can be used by patients to clean their teeth on a daily basis.

During the instructional phase of the plaque-control program, a specific technique of brushing the teeth should be taught for the individual patient's needs. There are only two guidelines to toothbrushing: the method should remove plaque from teeth and should not harm the patient's tissues. Beyond that, several methods can be used. Select the method that works best for the patient you are teaching.

Probably the best starting point is to have patients demonstrate the method they are currently using. Evaluate the effectiveness of the method by using a disclosing agent. Key areas that are often missed are the cervical areas and interproximal regions. This is especially true on the lingual surfaces of all teeth and the most posterior teeth. Never make a final judgment of the effectiveness of any toothbrushing technique by looking only at the anterior teeth. These areas are easiest to reach and therefore are usually better cared for than less accessible areas of the mouth.

An intelligent approach to proper oral hygiene instruction is to recognize that often patients already possess the ability to adequately care for their teeth. It is not unusual to discover that many patients already meet the two guidelines previously mentioned. They thoroughly remove plaque from their teeth without harming their tissues. These patients need no further instruction. They should be encouraged to continue with their own method for ongoing success.

A second group of patients may accomplish plaque removal fairly well but may be skipping a few areas. Teaching efforts should be directed toward telling them how well they are doing generally and where they can perfect their technique. Emphasis should be on the positive side by encouraging patients to continue their successful technique with a few helpful improvements.

Another group of patients who make a valiant effort at oral hygiene are the overzealous brushers. These patients do an excellent job of plaque removal but in doing so damage their own tissues. Help from the dentist in making this judgment is essential, since some of the early signs of tissue damage are often too subtle for recognition by dental assistants. Some obvious signs of tissue damage are soft tissue laceration, gingival recession, and tooth abrasion. Since this technique does not meet the two criteria of toothbrushing, a more favorable method should be taught to prevent further tissue damage while continuing successful plaque removal. Study models are helpful because they record the present condition of the tissues for future reference and also because a judgment can be made in the future as to whether tissue damage has been halted with the new brushing techniques.

Still another group of patients are those who do not meet either brushing guideline adequately. This group should be taught safe, effective brushing techniques. It is unfortunate that many people are in this category. Most patients in plaque-control programs start in this category.

The key to all effective oral hygiene instruction is to recognize the plaque status of each patient and then proceed according to individual needs. Proper recording of the plaque status of each patient should be done as a part of the individual's permanent dental record for future reference. This is essential for the evaluation of patients on future recall visits.

Several techniques can be employed to brush the teeth. The key to success is to choose a specific technique to meet the patient's needs. Generally speaking, most dentists agree that a brush with soft nylon bristles should be used to accomplish adequate plaque removal without tissue damage. After toothbrush selection, the brushing technique should be taught. Popular techniques taught currently are directed primarily toward ensuring adequate cleaning of the cervical and interproximal areas of the teeth. These are the areas most commonly missed by the patient. The following methods achieve this goal if they are properly done. Remember that variations of the basic techniques must be employed to meet the special needs of individual patients resulting from differences in dexterity, arch form, and tooth position; missing teeth; and restorative devices.

Bass Method

The **Bass method of toothbrushing** has gained great popularity in recent years because it is effective in cleaning the cervical and much of the interproximal areas of the teeth (Figure 10-14, A). Any portion of the interproximal area not cleaned by this technique is cleaned with dental floss and other interproximal aids.

1. Place bristles at a 45-degree angle to the long axis of the tooth (Figure 10-14, B).
2. The brush is then shimmied in a gentle but firm vibratory motion. This action forces the bristle tips

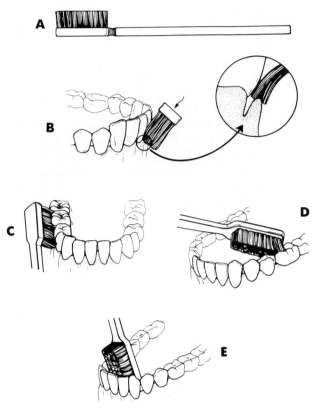

Figure 10-14 Bass toothbrushing technique. **A,** Favorably designed toothbrush. **B,** Proper placement of bristles against buccal and lingual aspects of teeth so that bristles slip into gingival crevice. **C,** Proper buccal position of brush. **D,** Proper lingual position of brush. **E,** Proper lingual position for upper and lower anterior areas.

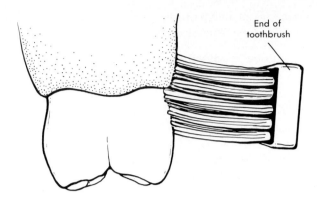

Figure 10-15 Brush placement for rotary scrub toothbrushing technique.

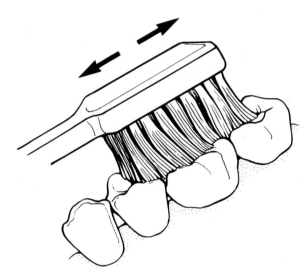

Figure 10-16 Brush placement and action for cleaning occlusal surfaces.

into the gingival sulcus to remove the adherent plaque. Figure 10-14, *C* to *E*, shows proper brush placement. The brush head should be vibrated 6 to 10 times before moving on in overlapping strokes to the adjacent area.

3. The toothbrush is in a horizontal position for the buccal and lingual aspects of posterior teeth (see Figure 10-14, *C* and *D*). The brush should be placed in a vertical position for the anterior teeth (see Figure 10-14, *E*).

If the patient has difficulty moving the brush in tiny circles, a modified Bass technique can be used. This method simply calls for moving the bristles back and forth across the tooth surface using extremely short strokes.

◆● KEY POINT
  ▪ The Bass method is sometimes called sulcular brushing.

Rotary Scrub Method

The **rotary scrub method of toothbrushing** is a composite of several other toothbrushing techniques (Figure 10-15). The basic idea is to use a soft nylon brush as previously described.

1. Place the bristle at a right angle to the facial and lingual surfaces (see Figure 10-15).
2. Scrub the tooth surface using small, gentle circular strokes.
3. Apply gentle pressure. Care must be taken to avoid strong horizontal scrubbing motions, which can cause tooth abrasion and gingival trauma.

This is an easy technique to learn. Therefore it is an excellent choice to teach young children with primary teeth. See Figure 10-8 for brush placement.

General Toothbrushing Considerations

The brushing methods just described are not foolproof. Their effectiveness depends primarily on the skill of the

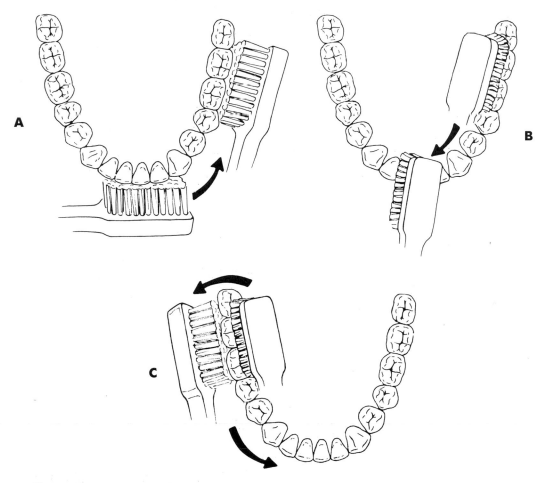

Figure 10-17   Suggested toothbrushing pattern for upper and lower dental arches. **A,** Start on facial aspect and proceed posteriorly. **B,** Brush occlusal surfaces on left side; then brush lingual surfaces as brush is advanced around arch. **C,** Brush occlusal surfaces on right side; then brush facial surfaces as brush is advanced anteriorly to starting point.

patient. Although the techniques differ, they have the following steps in common:

1. *Brushing the occlusal surfaces.* Any technique requires that the biting surfaces be cleaned, as well as the facial and lingual surfaces. This can be done by placing the bristle tips on the occlusal surfaces (Figure 10-16) and scrubbing with forceful horizontal strokes. The action drives the bristle tips into the pit and fissure areas.

2. *Overlapping brush strokes.* Regardless of what technique is used or what area is being brushed, it is wise to brush an area approximately the length of the brush head at a time. When this area is cleaned, move the brush ahead to the next area by two thirds the length of the brush head. This produces an overlapping of the cleaning effect. Overlapping helps to prevent areas from being skipped.

3. *Number of brush strokes.* Most techniques call for 6 to 10 strokes on each area before moving on to the next. It is a good idea to have patients mentally count the strokes during the early learning phase for any technique.

4. *Brushing pattern.* One of the most important fundamentals of toothbrushing and flossing is to develop a pattern of cleaning the mouth that is repeated every time. This is essential so that no areas are skipped because the patient forgets that an area has not been brushed. The order in which areas are cleaned is not critical, but the repetition of whatever pattern is selected is essential for a successful result.

Figure 10-17 suggests a pattern of brushing that begins on the facial surfaces of lower anterior teeth and proceeds posteriorly. When the last molar is reached, the occlusal surfaces are brushed. The position of the brush is then changed as shown, and the lingual surfaces are brushed around the entire arch. After the last molar on the opposite side is reached, the occlusal surfaces are brushed. The brush position is changed again, and the facial surfaces are brushed as the brush is moved anteriorly back to the starting point. The same sequence is followed in the upper arch. Repeating this pattern each time the teeth are brushed will help to avoid skipping areas where the brush is repositioned or entire segments of the mouth, which often happens when haphazard patterns are used. After the teeth are brushed, the upper surface of the tongue should be brushed to remove debris that accumulates on its rough surface.

5. *Rinsing.* The patient should always rinse with mouthwash or warm water after brushing and flossing to remove loose debris.

6. *Time of day for oral hygiene.* The practicalities of everyday life often interfere with ideal timing of when to brush. It is unrealistic to expect patients to carry out oral hygiene procedures during the busiest times of the day. A more effective approach is to suggest a thorough morning cleaning before beginning daily activities. Oral rinsing can easily be accomplished throughout the day to remove loose food debris after a meal. Patients should be told to brush before retiring at night. A close look at the patient's daily schedule can serve as a guide as to when the individual can brush and floss.

7. *Type of toothpaste.* There are many types and brands of **dentifrice** (toothpaste) available. Although a dentifrice is not necessary for plaque removal, it offers a pleasing taste and a mild abrasiveness that facilitates plaque removal. Many patients will ask the dental assistant about which toothpaste is best to use. If the patient has good oral hygiene habits, just about any toothpaste will be fine. Patients who accumulate supragingival calculus, especially on the lingual surfaces of the lower anterior teeth, can use a "tartar control" toothpaste. A patient who is experiencing decalcification or caries should use a fluoridated toothpaste. Baking soda is the least abrasive agent and can be used if a patient has abrasion and/or gingival recession. Patients with dentinal sensitivity can use an over-the-counter or office-prescribed dentifrice that can decrease the sensitivity.

Problem Solving

Patients encounter difficulties with virtually every toothbrushing technique. The following are some common problems that are encountered and their solutions.

Problem: Skipping the last maxillary molar on the facial aspect. The problem is usually caused by the coronoid process of the mandible moving forward when the jaws are open. Simply place the brush in the approximate area. Then close the jaws nearly together. The coronoid process moves out of the way so that the brush can be properly positioned for adequate cleaning.

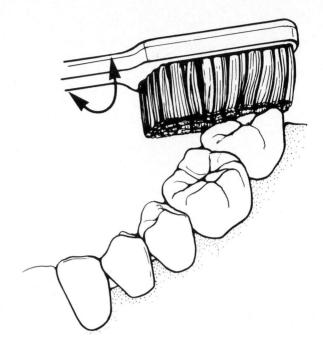

Figure 10-18 Cleaning distal surfaces of last molars. Brush is swept back and forth in buccolingual direction.

Problem: Skipping the distal surfaces of last molars. The tufts at the tip of the toothbrush should be "dangled" onto the distal surface by raising the handle of the brush relative to the biting surfaces (Figure 10-18). Use a buccolingual sweeping motion to clean the distal surface.

Problem: Inadequate space on the facial surfaces for brush placement and proper movement. Usually the lingual surfaces present little problem insofar as gaining access to cleaning is concerned. Occasionally patients complain that they do not have enough space to maneuver their brush on the facial aspects of the teeth. Closing the jaws together partially or completely after placing the brush in the buccal area gives greater access to the facial surfaces. This maneuver gives greater slack to the cheek and allows more movement. In cases where the lip interferes (usually the lower lip), the patient can be instructed to hold down the lip with one hand while manipulating the brush with the other.

Problem: Gaining access to the lingual surfaces in patients with narrow arches. Brushing the lingual surfaces is usually accomplished with the top two thirds of the brush head. In patients with narrow arches, a standard brush does not allow access on the lingual aspect of anterior teeth. This problem can be solved by using a small child's brush or using a standard-size brush in a vertical position and using a vibratory scrubbing motion.

Problem: Missing the gingival portion of the teeth in various areas. The patient should feel the bristles of the brush contact the gingiva while brushing the entire arch, except while brushing the occlusal surfaces. This will

BOX 10-1
FLOSSING TECHNIQUE

PROCEDURE	RATIONALE
1. Dispense adequate length of floss. Approximately 24 inches of floss is required.	1. It is recommended to use clean piece of floss between each interproximal contact.
2. Wrap strand of floss around first joint of middle finger of each hand (see Figure 10-19, *A*), with approximately 4 inches of floss extending between your hands.	2. This method allows positive grip on floss.
3. A 4-inch portion of floss can then be guided between teeth in each quadrant of mouth by using index fingers of each hand, thumbs, or combination of finger and thumb (see Figure 10-19, *B*). These fingers then become guides to force floss through contact area. Choice of which combination of guiding fingers to use is left to patient, based on convenience.	3. Passing floss through contact area should be done with great care so that floss does not snap through contact area and injure interdental papillae, which is painful and discouraging to patients.
4. Place guiding fingers on each side of teeth to be flossed. Fingers should be as close to teeth as possible.	4. Floss is pulled back and forth in buccolingual seesaw direction as floss is forced toward gingiva (see Figure 10-19, *C*).

PROCEDURE	RATIONALE
	Seesaw motion helps to slide dental floss through contact.
5. Once floss is through contact area, it is pulled against proximal surfaces being cleaned. It is most important that floss be "wrapped around" tooth surface. (see Figure 10-19, *D*).	5. Floss must be "wrapped around" tooth surface to ensure effective cleaning of entire proximal area.
6. When floss is properly positioned, it should be moved up and down to shave away plaque. Wrapping and cleaning movements are repeated for both proximal surfaces that border interproximal space. Only move floss up and down once floss is through interproximal contact.	6. Seesaw motions can wear notch in root surface of tooth.
7. Floss can be removed by gently pulling it in occlusofacial direction with back-and-forth motion. If tight contact makes this difficult, simply unwind floss from one hand and pull free end in facial direction to remove it from interproximal area.	7. Pulling floss out from side will avoid shredding it.

help ensure that the gingival or cervical areas of the teeth are cleaned, which is critical for the prevention of periodontal disease (see Figure 10-13, *B* through *D*). Caution should be exercised so that gentle brush movement is used to prevent damage to the soft tissue. In addition, the brush should not be placed too far down on the gingiva, so that damage to the unattached gingiva can be prevented (see Figure 10-14 for correct toothbrush placement).

DENTAL FLOSSING TECHNIQUES

The two vulnerable areas on tooth surfaces where plaque accumulation can cause irritation of the gingiva are the cervical region and the proximal surfaces. The cervical areas on the facial and lingual aspects of the tooth are cleaned effectively with one of the toothbrushing methods just described. However, brushing does not clean the proximal surfaces adequately. The most effective way to clean the proximal surfaces is through the use of a durable string called **dental floss**.

Dental floss is placed between the teeth in the interproximal areas and then rubbed against the two proximal surfaces on each side of the space. The floss acts as a scraping device to "shave" the plaque off the tooth surfaces. Since most periodontal disease begins in the interproximal area as a result of plaque accumulation, flossing is an extremely important preventive measure. The key to learning proper flossing technique is to maintain control of the floss (Box 10-1 and Figure 10-19).

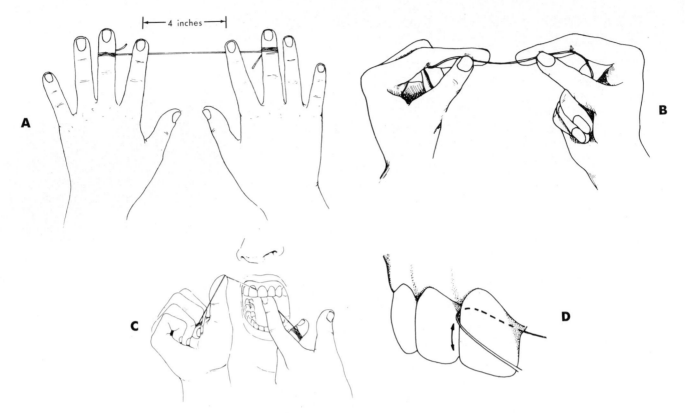

Figure 10-19   Method of dental flossing. **A,** Wrap floss around middle finger of each hand, leaving approximately 4 inches of floss between index fingers. **B,** Use index fingers, thumbs, or a finger and a thumb to guide floss between teeth. **C,** Keep guide fingers (thumbs) as close to teeth as possible to prevent snapping floss through contact area. **D,** Once floss is below contact area, wrap it around proximal surface of each adjacent tooth and move it in an occlusal (incisal)–cervical direction to scrape surface clean.

Flossing at least once each day is recommended. Patients can do this while watching television or during other relaxation periods.

If patients have difficulty using the hands to floss, a floss-holding device can be used instead. (See discussion of oral hygiene devices and products.)

Patients with fixed bridges find bridge-cleaning aids helpful in threading floss under these appliances.

ORAL HYGIENE DEVICES AND PRODUCTS

Since the basis for oral health is the patient's ability to maintain adequate oral hygiene, some guidance should be offered on the selection and use of various oral hygiene aids. Patients can make a more intelligent approach to maintaining a high level of oral hygiene if they understand the purpose and use of these aids.

The selection of an oral hygiene regimen depends greatly on the individual patient's needs. Much has been written about various hygiene aids. The effectiveness of most devices can be debated because there is wide variability in patients' use of these devices. Generally speak-

ing, most dentists agree that any device is acceptable as an oral hygiene aid if it aids in plaque control and does so without harming the patient.

Toothbrushes

Many types and styles of toothbrushes are on the market today. An appropriate toothbrush is made of end-rounded nylon filaments.

Floss

Floss is thinner than dental tape (Figure 10-20) and usually passes more easily through the contact area between teeth. The wax coating on dental floss helps make passing floss through the contact area easier. In addition, waxing helps prevent fraying of floss.

Polytetrafluoroethylene floss (e.g., Glide) has been recently introduced into the market (see Figure 10-20). This type of floss is made of a Gore-Tex type of material. It slips easily between tight contacts and resists fraying.

Tufted floss (e.g., Super Floss) is also available. A strand of tufted floss has three parts (Figure 10-20, *B*). One end is rather stiff and acts as a floss threader. The other end is a

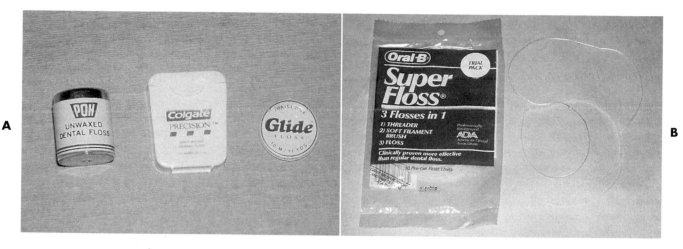

Figure 10-20   Dental floss. **A,** Unwaxed floss, waxed floss, and Glide floss. **B,** Tufted floss.

length of regular floss. The middle section is made of a thicker nylon mesh. Tufted floss is most useful under fixed bridges, implants, and open contacts.

Studies have shown that there is no difference in plaque removal for waxed vs. unwaxed floss. Rather, effective removal of interproximal plaque depends on the patient's dedication to routine flossing rather than on the specific product used. If a patient has rough areas or tight contacts that cause unwaxed floss to fray or break, then waxed floss should be recommended to prevent frustration that could discourage the patient from flossing.

Disclosing Agents

Any preventive regimen must educate patients as to the presence of dental plaque on their teeth. Since **plaque** is usually a translucent or white material, it is difficult to see on a tooth surface. **Disclosing solution** and tablets are principally vegetable dyes that are absorbed by plaque when they are applied to the teeth. These dyes are usually red or blue and give the patient an excellent color display of the accumulated plaque on the teeth (see Figure 10-6). Disclosing solutions that stain early and late plaque are also available to give the patient an idea about the formation of plaque on the teeth. A plaque-free tooth will not stain. The patient can use these disclosing dyes as a guide for brushing and flossing by brushing and flossing until the color is gone from the teeth.

Disclosing dyes are available in disclosing solutions visible under normal light, disclosing solutions visible under ultraviolet light, and disclosing tablets visible under normal light. Disclosing solutions are generally more effective than tablets because they penetrate plaque better than a dissolved disclosing tablet. Disclosing solutions are usually limited to use in the dental office because they are more difficult for the patient to apply and they can be messy. Disclosing tablets, on the other hand, are conve-

nient for home use. Patients simply chew and dissolve a tablet in their mouths. They then swish the dissolved tablet around the teeth and expectorate the excess.

The principal complaint of patients about disclosing solution and tablets that are visible under normal light is that they also stain the tongue, lips, and gingiva. A patient who goes out in public after using these disclosing agents can find the stain embarrassing. A good recommendation is to advise a patient to use these agents before bedtime. The stain is usually gone by morning.

A solution to this problem is a disclosing solution that is applied to teeth and absorbed by plaque but is not visible under normal light. The dye is visible only when it is exposed to ultraviolet light. Thus any inadvertent staining of the soft tissue is not visible under normal lighting conditions. However, because these disclosing solutions are visible only under ultraviolet light, the less accessible posterior areas of the mouth are sometimes overlooked.

Mouth Mirrors

For patients to accurately assess their effectiveness in oral hygiene procedures, they must be able to inspect their teeth thoroughly. This inspection is accomplished by using disclosing agents and a mouth mirror. Inexpensive plastic mouth mirrors can be obtained through various companies. Some mirrors have flashlights built into the handle to make it easier for the patient to see into the posterior region of the mouth.

Bridge Threaders

Patients with fixed bridges and splints in the mouth should be encouraged to clean around and under these restorations. Plaque accumulates on these restorations as it does on natural teeth.

Floss must be threaded under the bridge with a floss threader or **bridge threader** (Figure 10-21) because of

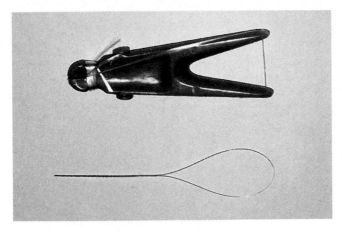

Figure 10-21 Floss holder *(top)* and floss threader *(bottom)*.

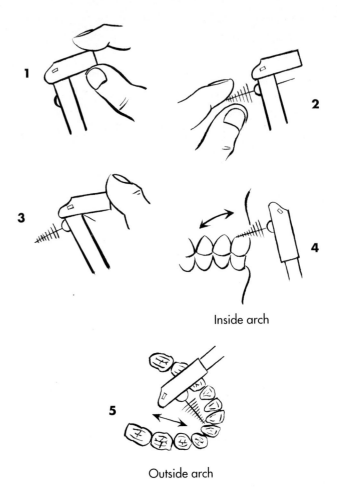

Inside arch

Outside arch

Figure 10-23 Steps in use of interdental brush. *1,* Flip up locking clip. *2,* Insert wire end of brush through hole opposite clip. *3,* Press clip back down against handle, locking brush into position. *4,* Insert brush between teeth. Move back and forth several times at horizontal angulation with slightly vertical tilt, using minimum pressure. *5,* Again insert brush between teeth and tongue and move back and forth several times. Brush at horizontal angulation.

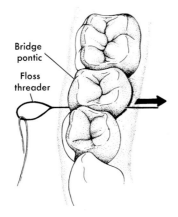

Figure 10-22 Floss threader in use. Flexible plastic loop is used to guide floss under fixed bridges and splinted contacts.

the soldered contacts present in a bridge. After the floss is threaded under the bridge, the gingival surface of the restoration can be cleaned with the floss. Figure 10-22 demonstrates the use of a floss threader.

Interdental Brushes

Straight or conical-shaped **interdental brushes** can be inserted into a plastic or metal reusable handle. Interdental brushes are effective when used in a back and forth motion to clean between the teeth when the interdental papillae do not completely fill the interdental space (Figure 10-23). Interdental brushes can also be used around implant abutments and fixed dental appliances.

Floss Holders

A complaint frequently voiced by patients is the difficulty of getting both hands in the mouth to introduce floss between the teeth. Other patients find placing their fingers in their mouths objectionable for various reasons, which discourages them from flossing routinely. Several manu-

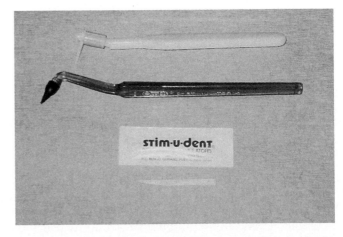

Figure 10-24 Gingival stimulators. *Top:* Perio-aid; *middle:* rubber tip; *bottom:* wooden tip.

perio-aid® 2°& 3° patient instructions

...use as recommended by your dentist

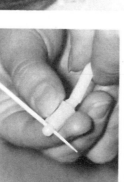
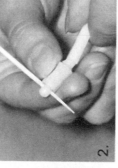
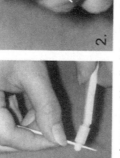
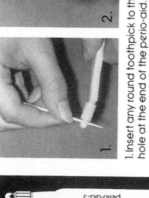
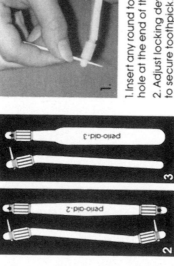
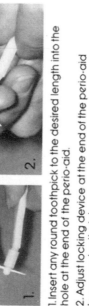
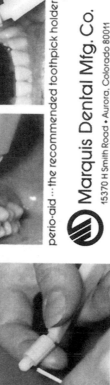
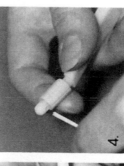
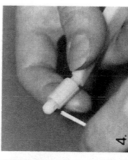
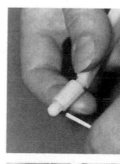
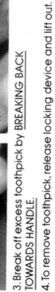

1. Insert any round toothpick to the desired length into the hole at the end of the perio-aid.
2. Adjust locking device at the end of the perio-aid to secure toothpick.

3. Break off excess toothpick by BREAKING BACK TOWARDS HANDLE.
4. To remove toothpick, release locking device and lift out.

perio-aid...the recommended toothpick holder

Marquis Dental Mfg. Co.
15370 H Smith Road • Aurora, Colorado 80011

If you are interested in having your local drug store or pharmacy carry the perio-aid, have them contact us.

® Registered Trademark in The U.S. And Canada
• U.S. Patent No. 3,892,040 Canadian Patent No. 1,020,380

Figure 10-25 Use of gingival stimulator.

facturers have attempted to circumvent these problems by designing a **floss holder** (see Figure 10-21) to guide the floss between the teeth.

Care should be exercised when these devices are used so that the floss does not lacerate the interdental papillae.

Gingival Stimulators

Several devices are available for patient use to encourage an increase in circulation of blood to the gingiva. These devices are referred to as **gingival stimulators**. They are in the form of rubber tips, soft wooden sticks, and toothpicks (Figure 10-24) in plastic holders. Circulation of blood to the soft tissue is encouraged by massage of the gingiva with these devices. They are not in widespread use, but the dentist should select these devices in specific cases. Figure 10-25 demonstrates the use of Perio-aid.

Oral Irrigators

As discussed previously, oral irrigation devices (Figure 10-26) are useful in flushing debris from teeth and delivering therapeutic agents to inaccessible spaces between teeth and in the gingival sulcus. Home versions of these products offer patients the opportunity to supplement daily oral hygiene procedures with irrigations prescribed by the dentist. The most frequently used irrigating agents prescribed are sanguinarine, chlorhexidine gluconate, commercial mouthwashes, and plain warm water. For safety reasons home models of oral irrigators have blunter tips on the working end than do professional models.

Oral irrigators may also be helpful to patients who wear orthodontic appliances or fixed bridgework, which may be difficult to clean.

➡ KEY POINT
- Oral irrigators are effective only in removing loose adherent debris and food from the teeth and have not been proven effective in the removal of dental plaque.

Mouthrinses

Like dentifrices, **mouthrinses** have changed. A variety of products available to the public offers different benefits. Fluoride mouthrinses offer caries-reduction benefits, whereas some commercial mouthwashes do nothing but temporarily refresh the mouth. Mouthwashes that contain either sanguinarine, phenolic compounds (Listerine), or chlorhexidine gluconate prove beneficial in controlling mouth odors and minimizing plaque accumulation when used in conjunction with traditional brushing and flossing techniques.

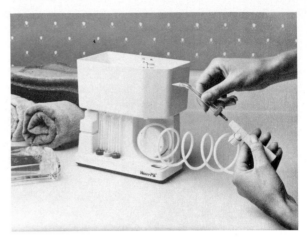

Figure 10-26   Home-style oral irrigator with sulcus tip that replaces cannula used in dental office.

(Courtesy Teledyne Water Pik, Fort Collins, Colo.)

Although many mouthrinses are available, currently only two products have been shown to prevent gingivitis. Listerine is an over-the-counter product, and chlorhexidine gluconate is a rinse that must be prescribed by the dentist.

BIBLIOGRAPHY

Boyd RL and others: Effect on periodontal status of rotary electric toothbrushes versus manual toothbrushes during periodontal maintenance. II. Microbiological results, *J Periodontol* 60:396, 1989.

Carranza FA: *Glickman's clinical periodontology*, Philadelphia, 1990, WB Saunders, pp 684-711.

Ciancio SG, editor: Oral irrigation—a current perspective, *Biol Thera Dentistry* 3:33, 1988.

Ciancio SG: Effect of a chemotherapeutic agent delivered by an oral irrigation device on plaque, gingivitis, and subgingival microflora, *J Periodontol* 60:310, 1989.

Darby ML, Walsh MM: *Dental hygiene theory and practice*, Philadelphia, 1995, WB Saunders.

Flemming TF and others: Chlorhexidine and irrigation in gingivitis. I. Six months of clinical observations, *J Periodontol* 61:112, 1990.

Gibson JA, Wade AB: Plaque removal by the Bass and Roll brushing techniques, *J Periodontol* 48:456, 1989.

Kleber CJ, Putt MS: Evaluation of a floss-holding device compared to hand-held floss for interproximal plaque, gingivitis, and patient acceptance, *J Clin Prev Dentistry* 10:6, 1988.

Ong G: The effectiveness of three types of dental floss for interdental plaque removal, *J Clin Periodontol* 17:463, 1990.

Spindel L, Person P: Floss design and effectiveness of interproximal plaque removal, *J Clin Prev Dentistry* 9:3, 1987.

Stevens AW: A comparison of the effectiveness of variable diameter vs. unwaxed dental floss, *J Periodontol* 51:666, 1980.

Wilkins EM: *Clinical practice of the dental hygienist*, ed 7, Philadelphia, 1994, Lea & Febiger.

QUESTIONS—Chapter 10

1. An instrument used to remove plaque and calculus that has two cutting edges and a rounded toe is called a (an) _____.
   1. Sickle scaler
   2. Universal curette
   3. Explorer
   4. Gracey curette
   a. *1* and *3*
   b. *2* and *4*
   c. *1, 2,* and *3*
   d. *4* only

2. A device that vibrates rapidly and uses water coolant to remove calculus and stain from the tooth surface is called a (an) _____.
   1. Ultrasonic scaler
   2. Universal curette
   3. Sonic scaler
   4. Air-powder abrasive polisher
   a. *1* and *3*
   b. *2* and *4*
   c. *1, 2,* and *3*
   d. *4* only

3. A toothbrushing technique that places the toothbrush at a 45-degree angle to the long axis of the tooth and uses a vibratory motion is called the _____.
   a. Rotary scrub method
   b. Bass method

4. Which of the following types of toothbrush bristles should you recommend to your patients?
   a. Natural bristles
   b. Boar bristles
   c. Hard nylon bristles
   d. Soft nylon bristles

5. Which of the following is the most appropriate method of placing the dental floss through the interproximal contact?
   a. Snap the floss through the contact.
   b. Push the floss up and down through the contact.
   c. Seesaw the floss through the contact.
   d. Thread the floss under the contact.

6. Patients should floss at least _____.
   a. Once each day
   b. Three times each week
   c. Once each week

7. The interproximal areas of fixed bridges can be cleaned by the patient with which of the following:
   1. Bridge threader
   2. Oral irrigator
   3. Tufted floss
   4. Floss holder
   a. *1* and *3*
   b. *2* and *4*
   c. *1, 2,* and *3*
   d. *4* only

8. A patient with a high caries rate should use which of the following types of toothpaste?
   a. Baking soda
   b. Tartar control
   c. Hydrogen peroxide
   d. Fluoridated

9. Which of the following could be suggested for a patient who is having difficulty using dental floss?
   a. Floss threader
   b. Floss holder
   c. Oral irrigator
   d. Mouthwash

10. Which of the following types of dental floss could be recommended to a patient who complains of floss shredding in tight interproximal contacts?
    1. Unwaxed floss
    2. Waxed floss
    3. Tufted floss
    4. Polytetrafluoroethylene floss
    a. *1* and *3*
    b. *2* and *4*
    c. *1, 2,* and *3*
    d. *4* only

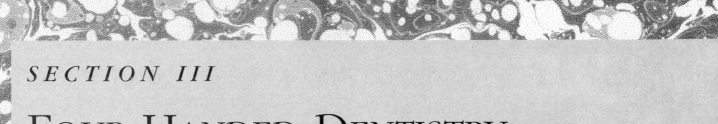

SECTION III

FOUR-HANDED DENTISTRY

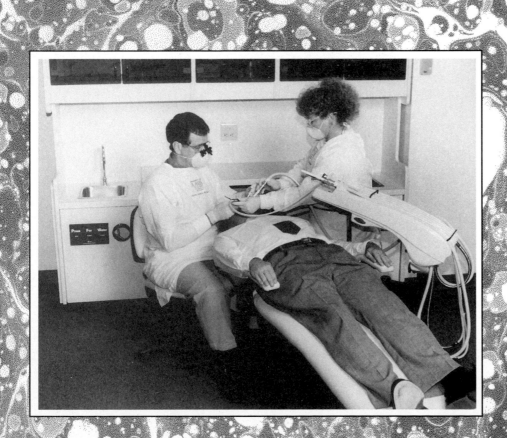

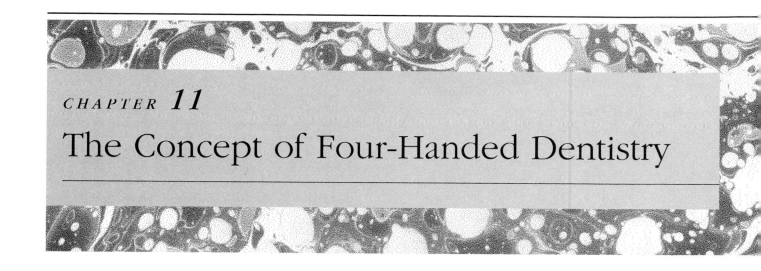

CHAPTER 11

The Concept of Four-Handed Dentistry

KEY TERMS

Class I movements
Class II movements
Class III movements
Class IV movements
Class V movements
Four-handed dentistry
Motion economy
Standardization
Time management
Work simplification

Since the early 1940s, considerable interest in the mode of dental practice has developed. The interest has centered on two basic issues that confront the practicing dentist every day: minimizing stress and fatigue for the dentist during the process of delivering dental services to patients and increasing the productivity of a dental practice while maintaining a high standard of quality in the services delivered.

The nature of dentistry creates a high potential for stress and fatigue for the practicing dentist. To provide quality dental services for patients the dentist must maintain a high level of concentration throughout the workday. In addition, the achievement of clinical excellence is predicated on the dentist's ability to meet the wide variety of dental needs of individual patients and perform delicate manual skills within fine tolerances while working with limited access and visibility in the oral cavity. These clinical demands are superimposed on demands to meet a busy patient schedule and to manage the practice itself.

Trying to meet the combination of clinical and management demands can result in severe stress and fatigue. The four-handed dentistry concept derives its name from the fact that the hands of both the dentist and dental assistant are used to provide patient care. This method of practice is more efficient and reduces stress and fatigue for the dentist over an entire practice life span.

> ➤ KEY POINT
> - The dentist and the dental assistant provide the four hands for four-handed dentistry.

A second reason for practicing four-handed dentistry is to provide the dentist with a means of becoming more productive through increased efficiency in the dental practice. Increased productivity is important to dentists because of economic implications and because of ever-increasing demands by the public for dental services. In effect, four-handed dentistry is part of good practice management.

PRINCIPLES OF FOUR-HANDED DENTISTRY

The term **four-handed dentistry** has evolved during the past 30 years to the point at which it now represents an entire concept of delivering dental services. Modern dentistry should be based on the concept of four-handed dentistry, which has the following four basic principles:
1. Operating in a seated position
2. Employing the skills of trained dental auxiliaries
3. Organizing every component of the practice
4. Simplifying all tasks as much as possible

Sit-Down Dentistry

Working in the proper seated position reduces stress and fatigue for the dentist and the assistant (Figure 11-1). Balanced posture for both the dentist and the assistant is described in detail in Chapter 13.

Auxiliary Utilization

To practice dentistry efficiently, the modern dentist must make maximum use of the skills of dental auxiliaries. The days when a dentist could operate a busy practice alone have long since passed. Solo operating is an inefficient use of a practitioner's valuable time. Today dentists must delegate duties to auxiliaries to increase the efficiency and productivity of a dental practice.

Practice Organization

The process of organization is never-ending. As a practice grows and changes or when initial plans fall short of expectations, reorganization of certain aspects of the practice is warranted. Once major elements are organized, the operating team can begin to reorganize dental treatment rooms and methods of delivering dental services. This level of organization is critical to the success of four-handed dentistry. The following key areas require organization:

1. Dental treatment room contents and arrangement
2. Complete preplanning of treatment to provide efficient delivery of dental services
3. Planning work patterns to standardize as many procedures as possible; this enables the operating team to work in a predictable sequence
4. Placement of instruments and materials on preset trays in a convenient arrangement that is consistent with the sequence of the standardized work pattern

Work Simplification

Just as the term implies, **work simplification** is the process of finding an easier way to do any task. Work simplification is learning to work smarter, not harder. In major industries, work simplification studies have been used for years to make workers more comfortable, more productive, and safer during the workday. The principles used in industry can be adapted in varying degrees to the practice of dentistry. Dentistry is hard, tension-producing work, and every effort should be made to make it more comfortable for the operator, the auxiliaries, and the patient. As a result of work simplification studies, four basic processes that the dental team can follow to make dentistry easier have been established:
- Rearrangement
- Elimination
- Combination
- Simplification

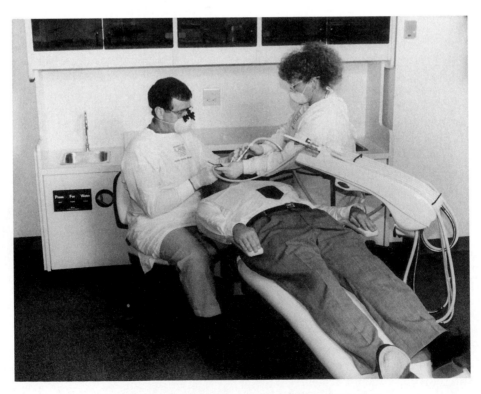

Figure 11-1 Properly positioned operating team.

Rearrangement

Equipment, instruments, and materials essential to operating procedures should be positioned in a favorable relationship to the operating team. Favorable positioning of these items helps to minimize movements of the operating team (Figure 11-2). For example, an amalgamator located out of easy reach of the dental assistant causes unnecessary movement and delay in every amalgam procedure done in the operatory.

The rearrangement of treatment plans and patient scheduling can add to the convenience of many treatment regimens. A patient who needs multiple restorations in all areas of the mouth can be scheduled for quadrant dentistry. This scheduling minimizes the need for repeated injections of local anesthesia or repeated placement of the rubber dam. Longer dental appointments also help to minimize the number of times the operatory room is set up and broken down.

As dental materials and products improve and change, the dental assistant plays a key role in the arrangement of instruments and materials on preset trays and in the storage cabinetry. Maintenance of a favorable arrangement of these items is clearly the responsibility of the dental assistant.

❖ KEY POINT
- Rearrangement of items, materials, and equipment is an ongoing task often delegated to the dental assistant.

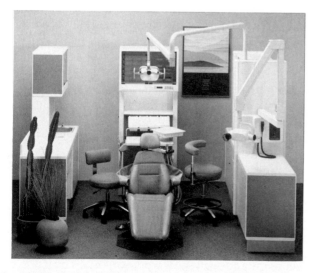

Figure 11-2   Favorable operatory design, conducive to practice of four-handed dentistry.
(Courtesy Adec Inc, Newburg, Ore.)

Elimination

The practicing dentist begins the process of work simplification by engaging in task analysis. Every procedure, system, movement, and piece of equipment should be analyzed to assess its value and necessity in daily office activities. A great deal of time and effort can be saved by eliminating unnecessary movements, procedural steps, instruments, and equipment.

Dentists tend to make many more movements than necessary to accomplish tasks. Excessive reaching for instruments and supplies and to make operating-light adjustments can be eliminated by having a chairside assistant deliver instruments to the operator and adjust the light. As mentioned previously, arranging equipment in favorable locations around the operating area can reduce unnecessary movements for operating team members.

Often steps in a procedure can be eliminated so that valuable chair time can be used more productively. The following are some examples of such eliminations:

1. Unnecessary bur changes in a procedure can be eliminated by using more than one handpiece with the burs placed ahead of time. An exchange of handpieces between the dentist and assistant is much quicker than a bur change when only one handpiece is used.
2. Unnecessary instrument exchanges can be eliminated by using an instrument to the maximum before returning it to the dental assistant. Frequent instrument switching is a rather common, time-consuming habit among dentists.
3. Supplies and materials that may save steps in a procedure should be used whenever possible. For example, the use of preformed aluminum shell crowns can eliminate, or at least minimize, the contouring of crowns during a procedure. Using premeasured materials, such as alginate and amalgam capsules, and disposable items can eliminate unnecessary steps.

When reviewing the contents of an instrument setup, a dentist often discovers that some of the equipment is not used routinely and consequently could be eliminated. Thus the number of instruments purchased and processed can be reduced. Plan for the usual, not the unusual or occasional, need for certain instruments.

Common areas in which the process of elimination can save time and cost are the equipment, supplies, and devices stored in the operatory. Many items that are seldom used or, in some cases, not used at all can be eliminated from the operatory. These items simply add to clutter and tend to bog down entire operations.

Combination

Using one step or instrument to serve multiple functions has real value in work simplification. Even greater reductions in the number of instruments required for a given procedure are made when the operator becomes proficient at using instruments for more than one purpose or double-ended instruments. Amalgam condensers are handy for placing cement bases and driving interproximal wedges into place, as well as for condensing amalgam. To have all sizes of round burs available on a tray setup is not really necessary since one size suffices in most restorative situations.

Simplification

The simplification aspect of the entire work simplification process is the actual determination how a job should be done. Simplification is listed last because it takes place after the rearranging, eliminating, and combining activities have been completed. The basic idea of simplification is to minimize the number of variables in every aspect of the practice. It is a streamlining process geared to promote predictable routines in the work pattern.

Plan for the usual, not the unusual. The majority of procedures and activities in a dental office can be standardized. **Standardization** involves the following:

1. Analyzing a procedure to determine the steps necessary to accomplish the task and then arranging steps in a smooth sequence that minimizes movements, verbal communication, and delays
2. Determining what instruments and materials are used in the procedure (The selected instruments are then assembled on a preset tray in the order they are to be used, from left to right.)

Instruments such as the mirror, explorer, and cotton pliers are used at various stages of a procedure and placed in the first three positions on the left side of the tray (Figure 11-3). This standardization process simplifies a procedure by making the operator predictable. The dental assistant can easily follow a standardized sequence, thus minimizing delays, verbal communication, and misunderstanding. The standardized procedure is smoother than a haphazard approach to accomplishing a task.

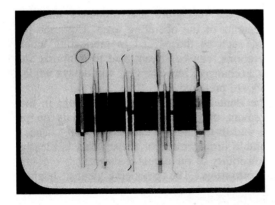

Figure 11-3 Simple but well–organized preset tray.

(Modified from Chasteen JE: *DAU manual of four-handed dentistry*, Ann Arbor, Mich, 1977, University of Michigan School of Dentistry.)

> **➥ KEY POINT**
> ■ Plan for the usual, not the unusual.

Ultimately, this effort creates a more consistent flow from the start to the completion of a procedure and usually results in greater productivity. Further, a new chairside assistant can adapt more readily to a dentist's techniques if they are standardized.

In offices with multiple operatories it is highly recommended that each operatory be standardized by identical equipment and identical arrangement. This permits the same predictable work pattern to be followed in each operatory without change. Special equipment that may not be used routinely can be moved from one operatory to another as needed (e.g., electrosurgery units, nitrous oxide machines, and salt sterilizers). If these items are used routinely, each operatory should be outfitted with them. All operatories should be the operating team's "favorite." This not only makes the work pattern easier to maintain but also simplifies the scheduling of patients by permitting their placement in any operatory regardless of the service rendered.

MOTION ECONOMY

The practice of dentistry cannot be discussed without repeated references to conservation of motion. Movements consume time and can produce fatigue. This does not imply that all movement is undesirable; movements that are productive, purposeful, and not harmful to the health of the operating team are entirely acceptable. However, movements that place the dentist or assistant in a contorted posture for substantial amounts of time are unnecessary and harmful over a long period. Dentists and assistants who can exercise daily should be encouraged to do so.

As a result of research on the subject of time and motion in dentistry, a classification of common movements used during dental procedures was developed as follows:
- **Class I movements**: movements of only the fingers
- **Class II movements**: movements of the fingers and wrist
- **Class III movements**: movements of fingers, wrist, and elbow
- **Class IV movements**: movements of the entire arm from the shoulder
- **Class V movements**: movements of the entire arm and twisting of the trunk

This classification is helpful in the discussion of motion economy and analysis of work patterns. The basic idea of **motion economy** is to design an office facility and work patterns that minimize the number of class IV and V movements required for any procedure. These movements are the most fatiguing and time consuming. They require the operator to look away from the brightly illuminated operative field and then to refocus, resulting in eye strain and subsequent headache. A dentist can substantially reduce the number of class IV and V movements through the effective use of a chairside assistant.

> ↠ **KEY POINT**
> ▪ Class IV and V movements should be avoided because the movements repeated during the day will cause fatigue.

In most instances Class I, II, and III movements are preferable for both the operator and assistant because they involve less muscular activity, save time, and allow the eyes to remain fixed on the operative field.

> ↠ **KEY POINT**
> ▪ Use class I, II, and III movements as much as possible during the workday.

Implementation of the work simplification and motion economy concepts should not be interpreted as an attempt to convert the operating team into statuelike figures at chairside. On the contrary, it is an attempt to guide the team into a comfortable, relaxed method of working that is free of wasted movements.

ELEMENTS OF FOUR-HANDED DENTISTRY

The performance of four-handed dentistry requires certain basic elements to be effective (Table 11-1). These el-

ements are a mixture of mechanical, technical, and attitudinal factors that must be combined if the concept is to succeed, and they are listed as follows:

1. Positive team attitude
2. Favorable work environment
3. Proper positioning of the patient and operating team
4. Simplified instrumentation
5. Standardized operating procedures
6. Use of preset trays
7. Efficient instrument delivery
8. Effective oral evacuation and debridement
9. Proper time management

Positive Team Attitude

Both the dentist and the dental assistant must make a commitment to work as a team. Working in a team configuration requires skills that must be acquired by both team members. Teamwork skills take time to develop. Each member of the team must be willing to communicate openly with one another and to help other members daily. Dental personnel who do not make this commitment often find themselves in frustrating circumstances that can lead to failure.

Favorable Work Environment

Various equipment and treatment room configurations work well in the four-handed dentistry concept. Regardless of which configuration is selected, the end result should be that both the dentist and the assistant can gain access and visibility during any procedure while maintaining comfort throughout the workday. Chapter 12 offers specific guidelines that have proved helpful in this regard.

Proper Positioning of Patient and Operating Team

Studies have been done to identify the most favorable positions to use while working in the different segments of the oral cavity. Guidelines are presented in Chapter 13.

Table 11-1 Concept of four-handed dentistry

Sit-down dentistry	Auxiliary utilization	Organization	Work simplification
Proper equipment Proper positioning of patient and operating team	Delegation of as many duties as possible Instrument transfer Oral evacuation and debridement Retraction Preparation of dental materials Preparation of operatory and patients	Time management Treatment planning Design of facilities Business procedures Staff recruitment and assignments Recall Inventory control Establishment of work pattern Preset tray system	Rearrangement Elimination Combination Simplification

Simplified Instrumentation

Dentists develop their own methods of accomplishing a given task. They may select a battery of instruments that differs from other dentists, but the same result is achieved. One goal is to reduce the number of instruments to only those needed for the procedure at hand. Using instruments and materials to the maximum and using them for several functions usually result in fewer instruments being included on a preset tray. This practice is consistent with work simplification principles discussed earlier in this chapter.

Standardized Operating Procedures

Most procedures performed in general practice are rather straightforward and can be done with minimal variation. As mentioned previously, common procedures can be standardized to the extent that the dental team can perform them predictably and efficiently. A little planning and arranging are required, but the effort is certainly worthwhile for both the dentist and the assistant.

Use of Preset Trays

The convenience of placing the most common items needed for a dental procedure on a preset tray during instrument processing is significant. Specific details of how preset trays are prepared and used during a procedure are presented in Chapter 7.

Efficient Instrument Delivery

The transport of instruments and other items to and from the patient's oral cavity constitutes a great deal of movement by the dentist who works alone. One of the most effective ways of reducing the amount of movement by the dentist during a procedure is to develop an efficient instrument transfer method in which the chairside assistant transports needed items to the hands of the dentist near the patient's oral cavity. Guidelines for effective instrument transfer are presented in Chapter 15.

Effective Oral Evacuation and Debridement

Control of fluids and debris during a dental procedure is mandatory for favorable visibility and for patient comfort and safety. Details on rinsing and evacuating the patient's mouth are presented in Chapter 14.

Proper Time Management

Time is the most valuable commodity in a dental practice. Proper **time management** allows the dentist to provide the best care for the most people. Any effort to eliminate the waste of the operator's time is worthwhile. Disorganized treatment areas, poor appointment scheduling, lack of standardized procedures, and interruptions of the dentist are common examples of poor time management that should be eliminated.

BIBLIOGRAPHY

Chasteen JE: *DAU manual of four-handed dentistry*, ed 2, Ann Arbor, Mich, 1982, University of Michigan, School of Dentistry.

Finkbeiner BL, Johnson CS: *Mosby's comprehensive dental assisting: a clinical approach*, ed, St Louis, 1995, Mosby.

Golden SS: Engineering comfort into dentistry, *Mechanical Engineering* 86:38, 1964.

Green EJ, Brown ME: Body mechanics applied to the practice of dentistry, *J Am Dent Assoc* 67:679, 1963.

Green ES, Lynam LA: Work simplification: an application to dentistry, *J Am Dent Assoc* 57:242, 1958.

Hoffman DA: Time and motion study in dentistry, *Bull Greater Milwaukee Dent Assoc* 23:101, 1957.

Klein H: Civilian dentistry in war-time, *J Am Dent Assoc* 31:648, 1944.

Pollack R: Ergonomics: efficiency without strain, *Dental Team*, Sept-Oct 1993.

Robinson GE and others: *Four-handed dentistry manual*, ed 2, Birmingham, Ala, 1971, University of Alabama School of Dentistry.

Schmid W, Stevenson SB: Dynamic instrument placement and operator's and assistant's stool placement, *Dent Clin North Am* 15:145, 1971.

Sharma DS, Kuster CG: Basic principles of four-handed sit-down dentistry and effective utilization of a chairside dental assistant, *J Wisc State Dent Soc* 50 (6):252-254, 1974.

Torres HO and others: *Modern dental assisting*, ed 5, Philadelphia, 1995, Saunders.

Waterman GE: Effective use of dental assistants, *Public Health Rep* 67:390, 1952.

QUESTIONS—Chapter 11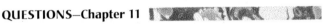

1. It is good to use four-handed dentistry because _____ _____.
   a. It increases productivity
   b. It increases efficiency
   c. It frees the dental assistant to do other tasks
   d. *a* and *b*

2. With multiple operatories it is best to have each operatory _____.
   a. Standardized
   b. Different

3. Movement of the fingers, wrist, and elbow is considered a _____ movement.
   a. Class I
   b. Class II
   c. Class III
   d. Class IV
   e. Class V

4. Class _____ movements should be avoided.
   a. I and II
   b. II and III
   c. III and IV
   d. IV and V

5. Unnecessary bur changes could be eliminated by _____.
   a. Using two assistants
   b. Using two handpieces
   c. Using one bur
   d. *a* and *b*
   e. *b* and *c*

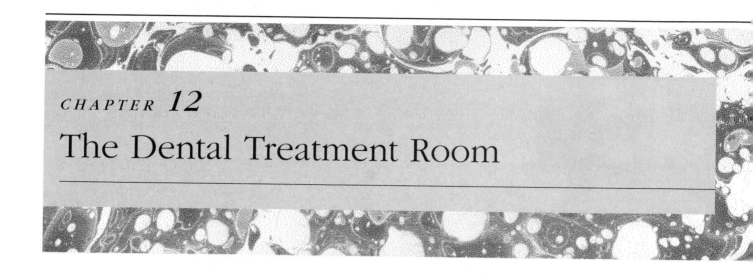

CHAPTER 12

The Dental Treatment Room

KEY TERMS

Air-water syringe
Articulating headrest
Assistant's stool
Dental chair
Dental operatory
Dental unit
Fixed consoles
Mobile carts/cabinets
Operating light
Operating stools
Oral evacuator
Programmed-setting feature
Radiographic view box
Rear delivery system
Saliva ejector
Side delivery unit
Transthorax delivery style

The dental treatment room, or **dental operatory**, is the primary work environment for dentists and their assistants. Its size, layout, and contents should be designed and organized to provide comfort and convenience for the operatory team. In other words, work environments should be adapted to workers instead of having the workers adapt to environments.

Once the functional aspects of a treatment room have been included in the design, an attractive decor should be added to create a pleasant ambience to the room. Such factors as lighting, color, textures, window treatments, sound systems, and floor coverings must be considered when decorating treatment areas. Room decor has a sig-

nificant psychological effect on both patients and operating teams.

ROOM DESIGN

New innovations in office design have prompted dentists to create treatment areas instead of conventional rooms. Today dental offices may have an open design (Figure 12-1). This design concept eliminates walls between the treatment stations and creates a feeling of openness that many dentists prefer. However, some dentists object to the lack of privacy associated with this design.

A compromise between the open design and the conventional treatment room is the semiopen design, which uses higher barriers between treatment stations. These barriers may be partial walls or dental cabinetry (Figure 12-2).

Figure 12-3, *A*, shows an example of a conventional design 9 × 11–foot room that functions quite well. Two doors at the rear of the room create a favorable traffic pattern for the operating team. Two sinks add convenience by providing two washing stations and auxiliary counter space. Figure 12-3, *B*, shows an example of how a conventional design works in a dental office.

Regardless of which design exists in a dental office, the contents of the treatment area should be kept as simple as possible. Only those items that are used routinely should be kept in this prime work space. A cluttered environment should be prevented.

Treatment areas should be kept spotlessly clean. Constant assessment of the room is necessary to ensure a desirable appearance. It is a good idea to sit in the dental chair occasionally to see what patients see during treatment. That dusty operating light or the cobweb on the ceiling becomes quite obvious from this position. Maintenance of treatment areas is a responsibility of the dental assistant throughout the workday.

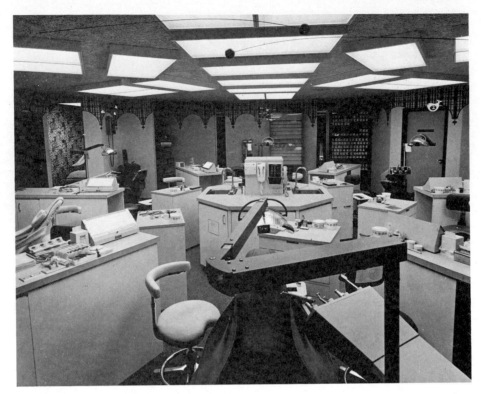

Figure 12-1   Open clinic design.
(From Wolff RM: *Dent Surv* 49:44, Jan 1973. Courtesy Roy M. Wolff, DDS, Creve Coeur, Mo.)

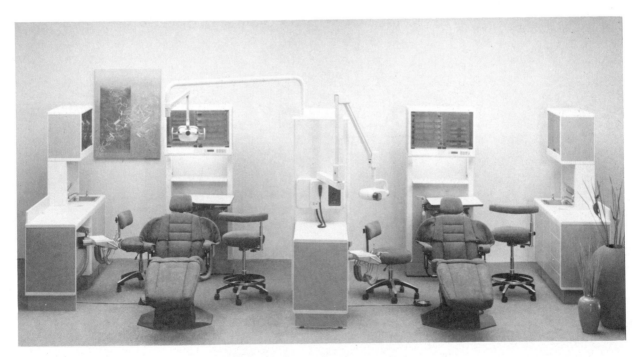

Figure 12-2   Semiopen design.
(Courtesy Adec, Inc, Newburg, Ore.)

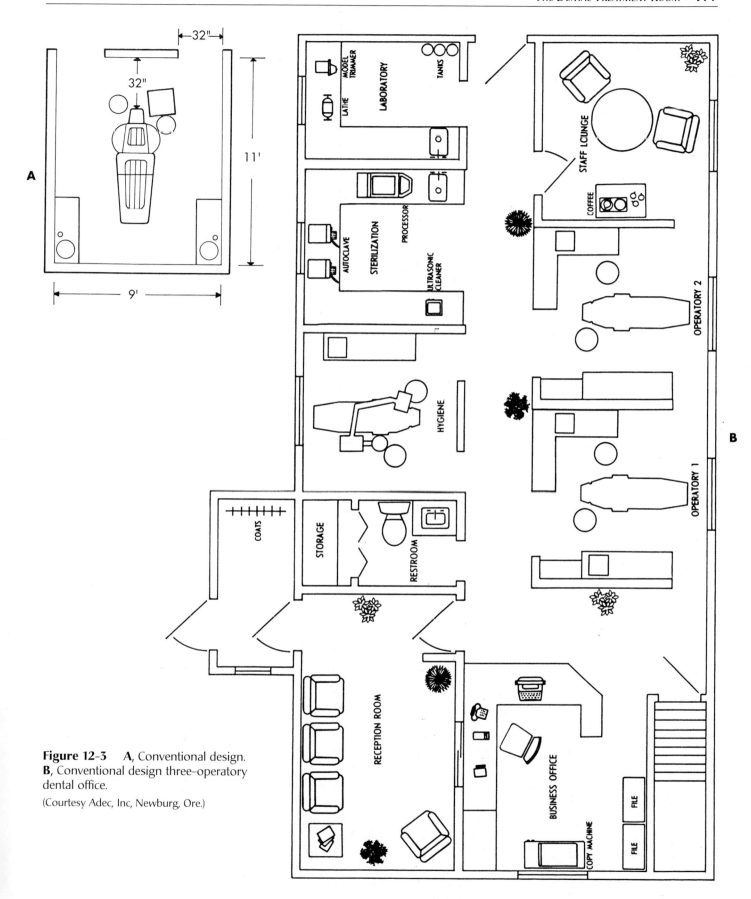

Figure 12-3   **A**, Conventional design.
B, Conventional design three-operatory
dental office.

(Courtesy Adec, Inc, Newburg, Ore.)

3 operatories, 1152 sq. ft.

Patients With Disabilities

The dentist is legally bound to provide a barrier-free environment for patients with disabilities; whether the patient is in a wheelchair, uses crutches, or uses a walker, the dental office must be constructed for free and easy accessibility to all areas. Doorways must be at least 32 inches wide to accommodate a patient in a wheelchair. The dental chair should be able to be lowered to 19 inches from the floor to provide for transfer of the patient from the wheelchair to the chair.

➤ KEY POINTS
- The dental office must accommodate patients with disabilities.
- Doorways must be at least 32 inches wide to accommodate a wheelchair.

BASIC OPERATING EQUIPMENT

To suggest there is only one equipment setup suitable for four-handed dentistry is just as hazardous as suggesting there is only one automobile design for all drivers. However, certain fundamental design features are essential to allow an operating team to work comfortably and have favorable access to a patient's oral cavity. Many brands of equipment meet these basic requirements. The following is a discussion of basic treatment room equipment required in a general practice.

A basic equipment setup used in a modern dental office generally includes the following items:
- Dental chair
- Dental unit
- Operating stools
- Storage cabinets
- Air-water syringe
- Oral evacuator
- Operating light
- X-ray machine
- Sinks
- Radiographic view box
- Communication system
- Preset trays

Common optional items include the following:
- Nitrous oxide machine
- Ultrasonic scaler
- Composite light (fiberoptic)
- Vitalometer
- Computer video system

Dental Chair

The **dental chair** is the center of activity for all treatment procedures. Its design is critical to successful four-handed dentistry.

The most important features of the dental chair are those that allow access to the patient's oral cavity while the operating team is seated in a comfortable position. Of lesser significance are features that provide patient comfort, since the patient is seated in the chair for only a short time. Fortunately a chair such as the one shown in Figure 12-4 provides both excellent operator access and patient comfort.

Analysis of a desirable dental chair reveals the following features:

1. The dental chair should allow the patient to be placed in a supine position (see Figure 12-4, *B*).
2. The back of the chair should be thin and narrow in the headrest area (see Figure 12-4, A). This allows the dentist and the assistant to position themselves as

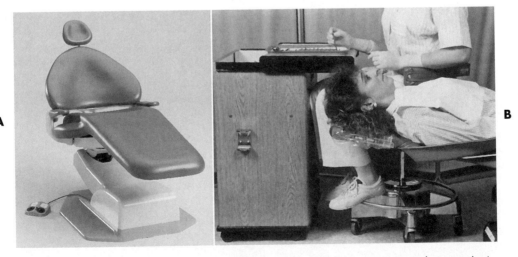

Figure 12-4 Favorable dental chair provides complete patient support and convenient access to adjustment controls.

(Courtesy Adec, Inc., Newburg, Ore.)

close to patients as possible without leaning and reaching to gain access. The ability to see into the oral cavity is determined by how close the operating team can get to the patient. Therefore the thin, narrow back design is essential, since it permits the operating team to get closer to the patient.

3. Once the patient is supine, the chair base must allow the patient to be lowered so that the person's head is actually located in the lap of the dentist. Therefore the base of the chair should allow the chair to be lowered to a position 14 to 16 inches above the floor.

4. The patient should be as comfortable as possible without the dentist's sacrificing access and visibility. The chair shown in Figure 12-4 supports patients very well in a supine position.

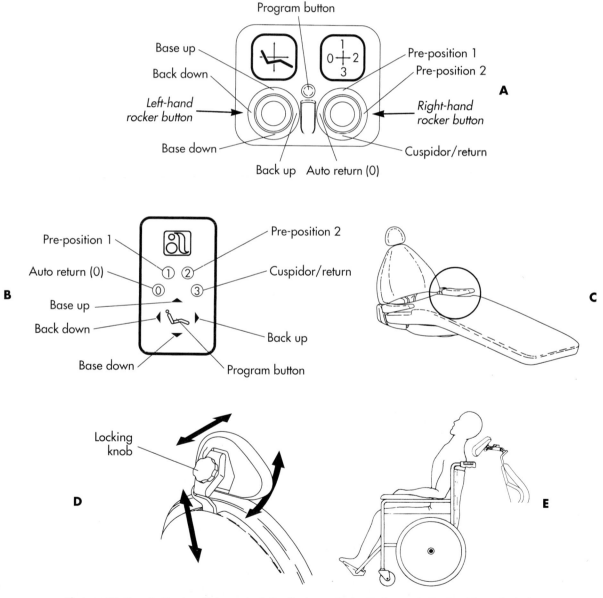

Figure 12-5 **A,** Foot switch control. **B,** Chair controls. **C,** Armrest. **D,** Double articulating headrest. **E,** Headrest position for wheelchair usage.

(Courtesy Adec, Inc, Newburg, Ore.)

5. The controls should be located so that both the assistant and the dentist can reach them conveniently. A good arrangement is to have a foot switch control that changes the position of the chair (Figure 12-5, *A*). An alternative option is to have the controls located along the side of the headrest area for easy access (Figure 12-5, *B*).

6. The armrests should slide backward (Figure 12-5, *C*) or lift upward to allow easier seating of the patient and also to allow a patient in a wheelchair to transfer to the dental chair.

7. The headrest should ideally be removable for children or shorter patients (Figure 12-6). An **articulating headrest** allows the patient's head to be placed at various angles during treatment (Figure 12-5, *E*). An articulating headrest also allows treatment of patients who cannot be transferred to the dental chair for one reason or another (Figure 12-5, *D*).

⊷ KEY POINTS
- Foot controls for the dental chair minimize cross contamination.
- Hand controls along the side of the headrest must be covered with plastic or other disposable barriers to prevent cross contamination.

An optional item available in newer dental chairs is a **programmed-setting feature** that allows the chair to be automatically placed in preselected positions with one touch of an activation switch. This adds to the convenience of seating and dismissing a patient.

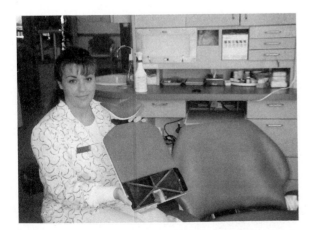

Figure 12-6 Removable headrest.

Another feature that is rather popular is a traverse function that moves the seat of the chair forward toward the foot board while the back of the chair is being reclined. This maintains the head of the chair at a uniform distance from any cabinetry or dental unit located behind the chair.

The dental chair can be kept clean with special upholstery cleaners or mild soap solutions. The crevices in the seat portion of the chair should be kept free of waste amalgam particles that may be dropped during an amalgam restorative procedure. To prevent cross contamination between patients, a clear plastic bag should be placed over the head of the chair to cover the switches.

Dental Unit

The **dental unit** is the control center for dental handpieces. Its primary function is to control the flow of air and water to these instruments and provide a holder to position them within reach of the operating team. Dental units vary in design and instrument configuration. Some units contain not only the dental handpieces but also such items as the oral evacuator, air-water syringe, saliva ejector, ultrasonic scaler, and fiberoptic composite light probe.

Since the dental assistant may encounter a variety of dental units in general practice, a review of the basic design concepts is worthwhile. Three common concepts are in use today, grouped according to the location of the unit relative to the patient in the dental chair. The following is a description of the three concepts:

1. Figure 12-7, *A*, is an example of a **rear delivery system**. Instruments are delivered to the dentist from a unit located behind the patient.

2. Figure 12-7, *B*, is a **side delivery unit** that is placed on the dentist's side of the chair. Side delivery units are mounted on either bracket arms or mobile carts.

3. Figure 12-8 is an example of an over-the-patient style, or **transthorax delivery style**, which is located over the patient's chest between the dentist and the assistant.

Each concept has advantages and disadvantages, but all three function well in the four-handed dentistry concept if they are used properly in a favorable treatment room.

Dental units that do not house an air-water syringe, a saliva ejector, or an oral evacuator must be used with a mobile cart that does contain these devices (Figure 12-9). The basic dental unit should contain at least the following:

- Two high-speed handpieces
- One slow-speed handpiece
- An air-water syringe

Some operating teams find two air-water syringes helpful. One is located on the unit, and the other is mounted on the assistant's mobile cabinet.

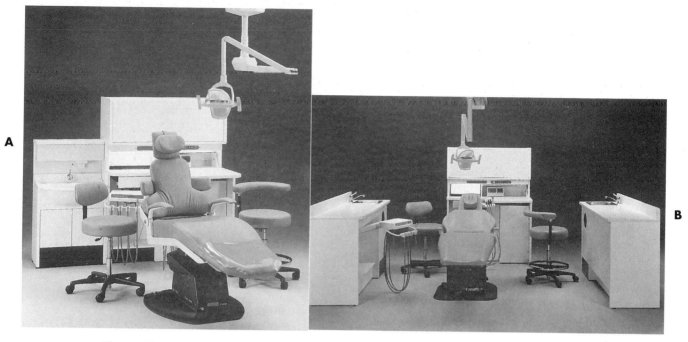

Figure 12-7 Common dental unit designs. **A,** Rear delivery system. **B,** Side delivery system.
(Courtesy Adec, Inc, Newburg, Ore.)

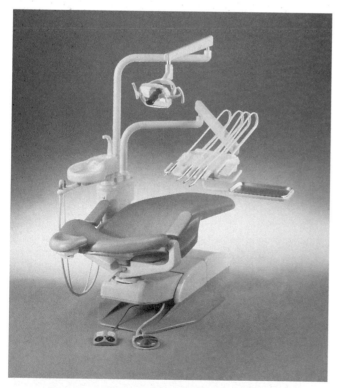

Figure 12-8 Transthorax delivery system.
(Courtesy Adec, Inc, Newburg, Ore.)

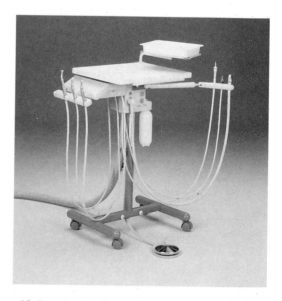

Figure 12-9 Assistant's mobile cart, available with or without dental handpieces.
(Courtesy Adec, Inc, Newburg, Ore.)

Handpieces are controlled by two switches. The switch on the unit programs which handpiece is used (Figure 12-10). The second switch is located on the foot control, often called a rheostat (Figure 12-11), which the dentist uses to activate the handpiece and to make the bur spin at various speeds. If fiberoptic handpieces are used, the light in the handpiece can be activated by the foot control. Some fiberoptic handpieces light when they are touched by the dentist.

Maintenance of the dental unit involves routine cleaning and periodic inspection of pressure gauges to ensure all instruments are working according to manufacturers' specifications.

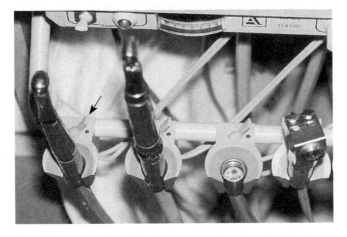

Figure 12-10 Handpiece control on wall-mounted dental unit.

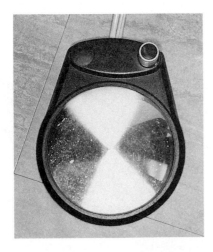

Figure 12-11 Accelerator-style foot control.
(From Chasteen JE: *DAU manual of four-handed dentistry*, Ann Arbor, Mich, 1977, University of Michigan School of Dentistry.)

> **KEY POINT**
> ▪ The switch that controls which handpiece is used is also used by the assistant as a safety feature to change burs on a handpiece when the dentist is using another handpiece from the dental unit.

At the beginning of every workday, water should be run through the handpiece hoses and air-water syringe into a receptacle for at least 3 minutes to clear the unit of any stagnant water. Some manufacturers provide a water reservoir, which can be filled with sterile water to flush the dental unit. Such systems can be used to flush the system with disinfectants before the reservoir is filled with sterile water.

Operating Stools

Operating stools should be selected with as much care as is taken to select lounge chairs for a cozy living room. Comfort is the key factor in stool selection. Remember that nearly a full workday is spent sitting on operating stools.

The operator's stool should have the following features to ensure comfort and convenience (Figure 12-12):

1. The seat should be padded adequately to support the operator. The seat can be flat surfaced or contoured (saddle type).
2. A broad base with at least five casters on the stool is recommended to prevent tipping and allow mobility.
3. The seat should be adjustable from 14 to 21 inches. A lever located beneath the seat is used to activate

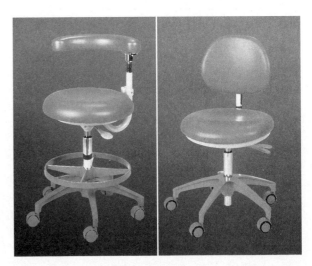

Figure 12-12 *Left,* Assistant's stool; *right,* operator's stool.
(Courtesy Adec, Inc, Newburg, Ore.)

a hydraulic system for raising or lowering stool height.

4. The back support must be adjustable both vertically and horizontally to adapt to individual operators.

An **assistant's stool** must be designed a little differently from the operator's stool because of the position of the assistant at chairside. The following features are important when selecting an assistant's stool (see Figure 12-12):

1. The base of the stool should be broad to prevent tipping. A stool with five casters is recommended. An adjustable foot ring is desirable to allow for the adaptation of the stool to fit the lower leg length of the assistant.

2. The seat should be adjustable to a height of approximately 27 inches. This can be accomplished using the same hydraulic lever system found on operator stools.

3. The seat should be padded sufficiently for comfort.

4. A body support is recommended for the assistant's stool. This allows support for the upper portion of the trunk when the assistant leans forward. The body support must be adjustable horizontally and vertically.

The ability of the operating team to see into the oral cavity was mentioned during the discussion of dental chair design. Likewise, stool design and proper positioning contribute greatly to visibility. The design features listed permit the mobility, height adjustment, and body support necessary to achieve comfortable visual access to the oral cavity. Comfort and visibility are two critical goals that must be achieved if four-handed dentistry is to succeed. Obviously equipment design is only part of gaining comfort and visual access to the oral cavity. Proper positioning of the patient and the operating team is discussed in detail in Chapter 13.

Storage Cabinets

Organizing auxiliary instruments and materials in appropriate cabinetry in the operatory results in chairside efficiency. Only commonly used items should be stored in the operatory. The main supply inventory should be kept in other storage areas in the office.

Dental cabinets can be divided into two categories—**fixed consoles** attached to the wall (Figure 12-13) and **mobile carts/cabinets** that can be moved around the operatory on casters. It is common to use a combination of both types to provide convenient storage.

Generally speaking, items kept in the fixed cabinetry are those used to prepare the operatory for treatment. Items such as preset trays and disposable paper goods are kept here.

The mobile cabinet is reserved for auxiliary items needed during the treatment procedure (Figure 12-14, *A*). These cabinets have a sliding top that can be pulled over the assistant's lap to create a convenient work surface. The preset tray is placed on this surface for maximum access during procedures. There is a deep well under the top. Since the cabinet can be moved anywhere, it is the most accessible storage space in the operatory. Therefore only the most frequently used auxiliary items should be kept here. These items include such articles as gauze sponges, cotton rolls, extra anesthetic cartridges, various bases and cavity liners, amalgamator, amalgam materials, and mixing pads. The operating team should analyze its procedures to determine what items should be kept in this prime storage space. Access can be gained to all areas

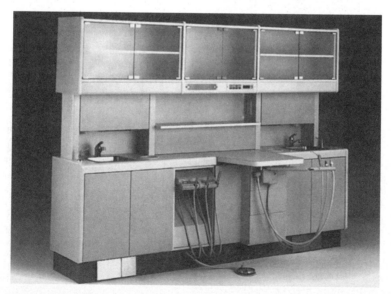

Figure 12-13 Dual treatment console with dentist's and assistant's wash stations.
(Courtesy Adec, Inc, Newburg, Ore.)

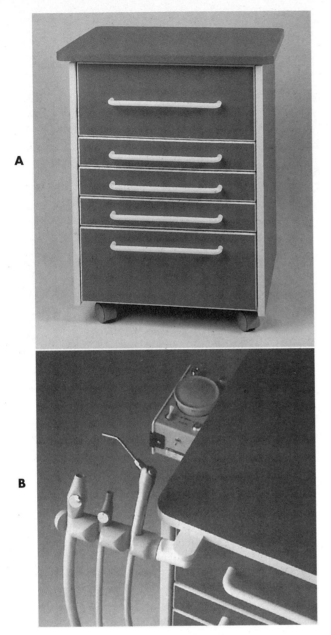

Figure 12-14 **A**, Assistant's mobile cabinet. **B**, Oral evacuator, saliva ejector, and air-water syringe optional attachment to mobile cart.

(Courtesy Adec, Inc, Newburg, Ore.)

of the well by simply sliding the top back and forth as needed.

The mobile cabinet can be fitted with an oral evacuator, a saliva ejector, and an air-water syringe; however, this limits the mobility of the cabinet because it will not be removable from the operatory (Figure 12-14, *B*).

Cabinet drawers should contain auxiliary instruments that can be used if an instrument from the preset tray is dropped during a procedure. Since these drawers are less convenient to reach, frequently used items should not be placed here. A good guide to cabinet organization is to

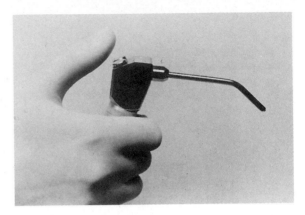

Figure 12-15 Pistol type of air-water syringe.

place the more frequently needed items in the uppermost drawers and the less frequently needed items in the lower drawers. "Frequently needed items" refers to auxiliary items only. The primary instruments commonly used in any procedure are placed on a preset instrument tray.

Air-Water Syringe

The **air-water syringe** (Figure 12-15) can deliver a stream of air into the mouth to dry a preparation or a stream of water into the mouth for rinsing; or a combination of air and water spray can be created by activating the air and water buttons at the same time. The water spray produced can be used to rinse the oral cavity vigorously.

The pistol style of syringe offers convenience in handling that cannot be matched by other designs. It is easy to transfer between operator and assistant, and it is comfortable to use. Activation buttons are located on top of the syringe. The thumb is used to activate the syringe.

The syringe tip should be removable for sterilization and should have a slight bend in it to assist in gaining access intraorally. In addition, the tip should be capable of swiveling 360 degrees to orient the tip to any area of the mouth. The proper use of the syringe and the method of transfer between the dentist and the assistant are discussed in Chapter 15.

Oral Evacuator and Saliva Ejector

The **oral evacuator** (Figure 12-16) and **saliva ejector** constitute a suction instrument used to remove fluids and debris from the patient's mouth. Modern evacuation systems have virtually eliminated the need for the time-honored cuspidor. Oral evacuation is the responsibility of the chairside assistant. The technique of using this important instrument is discussed in detail in Chapter 14.

↪ KEY POINT
- The air-water syringe tip should be sterilized after each patient.

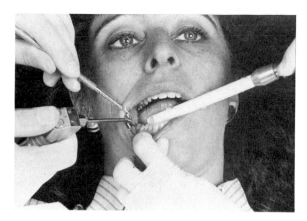

Figure 12-16   Oral evacuator in use.

Operating Light

The **operating light** (Figure 12-17) is an important factor in visibility. A ceiling-mounted type is preferred. Favorable light design dissipates heat away from patients. Since the positioning of the light is primarily the assistant's responsibility, the light should have handles on both sides for use by the dentist and the assistant.

Maintenance of the light is limited to cleaning the heat shield and occasional bulb changes. The light switch and handles can be disinfected between patients. As an alternative, the light handles can be covered with aluminum foil, plastic wrap, or plastic bags after each patient.

X-Ray Machine

X-ray machines are essential in a dental office. The valuable diagnostic information they provide is critical to dental treatment. Dental offices may have an x-ray machine in every treatment area or limit x-ray service to one room.

The dental assistant should receive adequate training in the use of radiographic equipment. Many courses and texts deal with this important aspect of dental assisting.

X-ray machines require little maintenance beyond disinfecting between patients. Plastic food wrap or bags can be wrapped around the machine head and control unit to prevent cross-contamination.

Sinks

Two key points should be emphasized regarding sinks in the dental operatory. There should be two sinks in the operatory—one for the dentist and one for the assistant (see Figure 12-13). This eliminates wasted time spent waiting for a turn to wash. Each sink should be located to provide convenient access to the operating team. In addition, the water controls on the sink should be operated by a knee or a foot control (Figure 12-18). This prevents recontamination of the hands after washing by avoiding controls that require use of the hands to turn off the water. A good compromise is to use a hand control like the one shown in

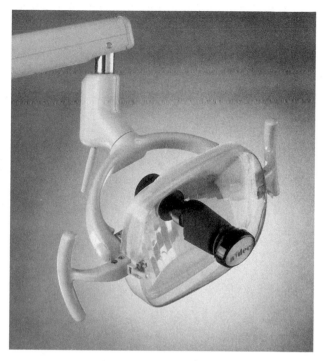

Figure 12-17   Operating light.
(Courtesy Adec, Inc, Newburg, Ore.)

Figure 12-19, which can be turned off using only the wrist. A few other considerations regarding sinks are as follows:

1. Small, stainless steel sinks are good because they require little space and are relatively easy to keep clean.
2. The dentist's sink can be either at stand-up or sit-down height, depending on personal preference. The assistant's sink is usually at stand-up height.
3. Each sink cabinet should contain a disposal hole without a cover to permit easy discarding of towels.
4. Soap and paper towel dispensers should be located conveniently at each sink.

The team should wash their hands in the presence of the patient just before starting an examination or a treatment. This reassures the patient of the team's concern for cleanliness. If dentists wash in another room, when they enter the operatory, a patient is not sure whether their hands have been washed or not. Hands should be rewashed whenever they touch an unclean object, such as the telephone, hair or face, or the chair. Sinks should be cleaned, and disposal receptacles should be emptied several times each day to maintain a tidy appearance and prevent unpleasant room odors.

↝ KEY POINT
- A no-hands type of paper towel dispenser is desirable to prevent cross contamination of the towel dispenser.

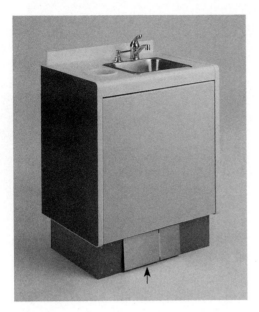

Figure 12-18 Free-standing wash station with foot control *(arrow).*

(Courtesy Adec, Inc, Newburg, Ore.)

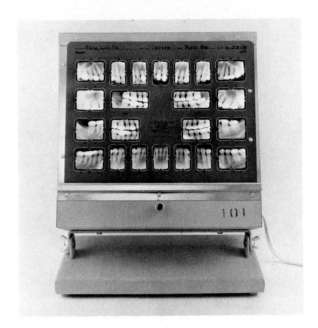

Figure 12-20 Radiographic view box.

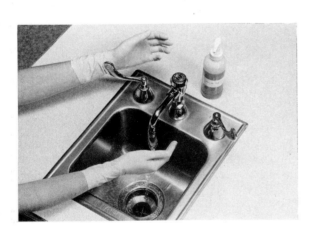

Figure 12-19 Faucet control that can be turned off with wrist.

Radiographic View Box

Dental radiographs can be more accurately interpreted by the dentist if they are viewed with a diffused light source. A **radiographic view box** (Figure 12-20) is such a light source.

View boxes are available in different shapes that fit different sizes of radiographic mounts. The surface glass of the view box should be kept free of any spots or smudges that could be mistaken for dental disease when a radiograph is placed over it.

Communication System

Communication within the dental office is required for coordination of activities among the staff members. It is helpful to have some type of communication system located in each treatment room. This allows the dental team to communicate with other areas in the office.

Color-coded light signals and intercom systems are commonly used. The system shown in Figure 12-21, *A*, is an example of a combination light signal and intercom system. Figure 12-21, *B*, depicts a no-button type of light signal. Each color-coded light is used to designate a specific message, such as "the next patient has arrived" or "the hygienist is ready for the dentist to examine a patient." The appropriate color is illuminated to convey the necessary message. The light is turned off when the message is acknowledged.

BIBLIOGRAPHY

Combs R: Openness provides privacy, efficiency. In *Dental economics,* 1992, Pennwell.

Finkbeiner BL, Johnson CS: *Mosby's comprehensive dental assisting: a clinical approach,* St Louis, 1995, Mosby.

Torres HO and others: *Modern dental assisting,* ed 5, Philadelphia, 1995, WB Saunders.

QUESTIONS—Chapter 12

1. When the instruments are delivered to the dentist from behind the patient, this is called a _____.
   a. Side delivery system
   b. Rear delivery system
   c. Transthorax delivery system

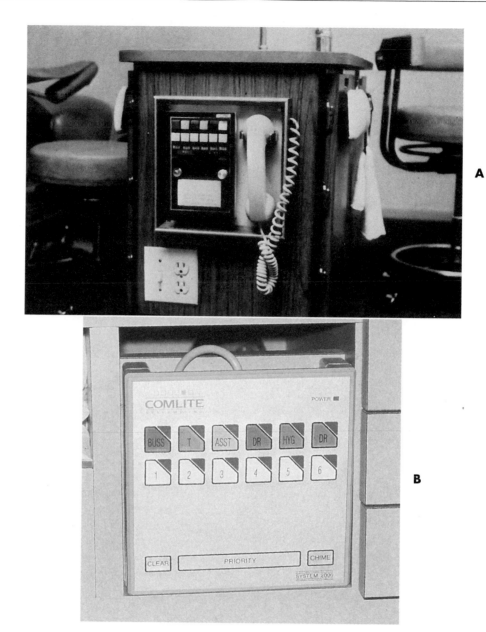

Figure 12-21 **A,** Combination light signal and intercom system located in treatment area. **B,** No-button type of light signal.

2. A movable cart that is used by the assistant to hold the pre-set tray and adjunctive items is called a(n) _____.
   a. Wall mount system
   b. Mobile cabinet
   c. Articulating headrest

3. Doorways must be at least _____ inches wide to accommodate a disabled person.
   a. 20
   b. 30
   c. 32
   d. 40

4. All of the following characteristics describe an operator's stool *except* _____.
   a. Broad base
   b. Adjustable seat
   c. Adjustable back support
   d. Adjustable foot ring

5. The best type of sink to use is one that is _____.
   a. Foot controlled
   b. Hand controlled
   c. Knee controlled
   d. *a* and *c*

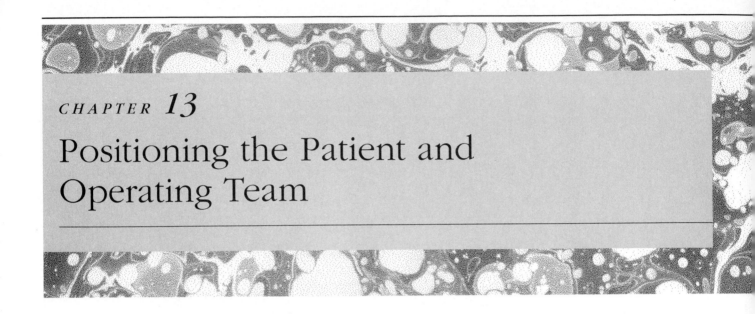

CHAPTER 13

Positioning the Patient and Operating Team

KEY TERMS
Assistant's zone
Delivery corridor
Operator's zone
Semisupine position
Static zone
Supine position
Transfer zone
Work circle
Zones of activity

A great deal of research has been done to determine the most favorable working position for the operating team and patient. The results of these studies have shown the seated position is generally best for both dentists and chairside assistants. Although there is no perfect operator-patient-assistant position, the sit-down approach fulfills the demands of most clinical problems.

However, comfortable, stress-free four-handed dentistry requires more than simply sitting down to operate. The manner in which dentists and chairside assistants sit relative to their patients is the most significant factor in achieving comfort for the operating team. As with many other aspects of dentistry, it is not just a matter of doing, but rather how well it is done, for success to be achieved. This chapter suggests how an operating team should be positioned relative to each other and the patient.

THE WORK CIRCLE

The focal point of activity in the treatment room is the patient's oral cavity. By placing the operating team and instrumentation close to the patient's head the following objectives can be achieved:
1. Favorable access to the operative field
2. Good visibility
3. Reduction of class IV and V movements
4. Comfort for the operating team
5. Comfort and safety for the patient

Arranging the treatment room so that the operating team can work around the patient's head within an imaginary circle with a 20-inch radius is helpful. This is referred to as the **work circle** (Figure 13-1).

Delivery Corridor

The arrow from the instrument tray to the patient's mouth in Figure 13-1 identifies the primary route of instruments and materials to and from the oral cavity during a treatment procedure. By keeping the end of this **delivery corridor** within 18 inches, excessive movements can be eliminated when transporting items to and from the operative field.

Zones of Activity

The work circle can be divided into **zones of activity** that are used to describe the working positions of both the equipment and operating team.

Four major zones of activity are visualized around a patient in a supine position. If one visualizes the patient's

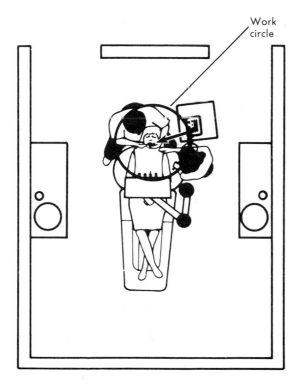

Work circle

Figure 13-1 Work circle.

face located in the center of the face of a clock, these zones may be designated as follows (Figure 13-2):

- Operator's zone (7 to 12 o'clock position)
- Static zone (12 to 2 o'clock position)
- Assistant's zone (2 to 4 o'clock position)
- Transfer zone (4 to 7 o'clock position)

With this standard reference, the location of the operating team and equipment relative to the patient's face can be stated as positions on the clock. For example, the operator in Figure 13-2, *A*, is in the 11 o'clock position, and the assistant is in the 3 o'clock position.

Operator's zone

The **operator's zone** is the part of the work circle where the dentist is positioned to gain access to various segments of the patient's oral cavity. Patients enter and leave the dental chair through this zone.

Transfer zone

The **transfer zone** is the area where instruments and materials are transported to and from the oral cavity. It is also an excellent area for the location of the dental unit so that it is within easy reach of either the assistant or the dentist.

Assistant's zone

The **assistant's zone** is rather small because the dental assistant remains in the 3 o'clock position throughout a

procedure regardless of the operator's position. It is critical to have a work surface extend into this zone over the assistant's lap for convenience and reduction of excessive motion.

Static zone

The **static zone** is a nontraffic area where equipment, such as a nitrous oxide machine or a mobile cabinet, can be placed with the top extending into the assistant's zone. Rear delivery dental units are also placed in this zone.

> **→ KEY POINTS**
> - The operator's zone is 7 to 12 o'clock.
> - The static zone is 12 to 2 o'clock.
> - The assistant's zone is 2 to 4 o'clock.
> - The transfer zone is 4 to 7 o'clock.

POSITIONING THE OPERATOR

It is important to adapt the work environment to the operator, instead of having the operator adapt to a fixed environment. This concept requires the dentist to assume a favorable seated position and then arrange the patient, assistant, and equipment in relationship to that position.

The process of preparing for any chairside procedures should begin with the seating of the dentist in a position of balanced posture, which is described by the following characteristics:

1. Stool height should be adjusted so that the tops of the operator's thighs are parallel to the floor or sloping slightly downward (Figure 13-3).
2. The entire surface of the seat of the stool should be used to support the operator's weight.
3. A backrest to support the operator's back without interfering with movement of the arms is recommended.
4. The patient should be positioned so that the operator's forearms are parallel with the floor or sloped slightly upward when the hands are in operating position. The operative field should be located in the dentist's midline to maximize visibility.
5. The elbows should be close to the body.
6. The operator's back and neck should be straight, with the top of the shoulders parallel to the floor.
7. A distance of 14 to 18 inches between the operator's nose and the patient's oral cavity should be maintained so that the operator does not encroach on the patient's breathing space (see Figure 13-3). The distance is dictated somewhat by the focal distance of different dentists. Several optical devices that magnify the operative field are available (Figure 13-4).

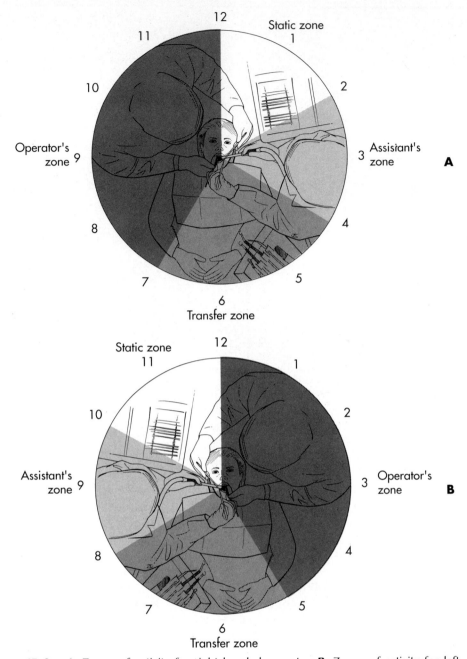

Figure 13-2 **A,** Zones of activity for right-handed operator. **B,** Zones of activity for left-handed operator.

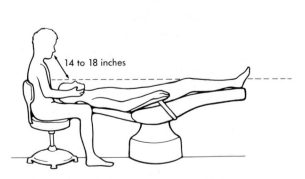

Figure 13-3 Operator–patient relationship with operator in balanced posture and patient in supine position.

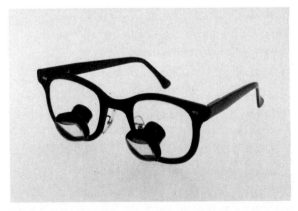

Figure 13-4 Surgical telescopes used to magnify operative field. (Courtesy Designs for Vision Inc, Rokonkoma, NY.)

The essence of balanced posture is having the dentist positioned so that favorable body mechanics are at work, permitting comfort for the operator and minimizing fatigue.

This description of balanced posture is not intended to imply that operators must sit in a statuelike manner but rather to establish a set of guidelines that is helpful in achieving comfort while the operator works at chairside.

POSITIONING THE PATIENT

One of the most important steps in adapting the work environment to the dentist is proper positioning of the patient relative to the balanced posture of the dentist. The patient is positioned so that the oral cavity is centered over the operator's lap at the height of the operator's el-

bow (Figure 13-5). Remember that the forearms of the dentist should be parallel to the floor or sloping slightly upward when the hands are in working position in a patient's oral cavity. A thin back on the dental chair permits most operators to fit their legs underneath the chair while working in the 10 to 12 o'clock positions (Figure 13-6). However, a dentist with short, large thighs and a short upper body may have to place the chair back between the thighs to position the patient properly (Figure 13-7).

A lounge-style chair has proved a favorable design for sit-down four-handed dentistry. Its low base and thin, narrow chair back allow the operator to be positioned close to the patient's oral cavity not only in the vertical relationship just discussed but also in the horizontal relationship of the dentist to the patient. Access and visibility often involve fractions of inches. This fact should not be

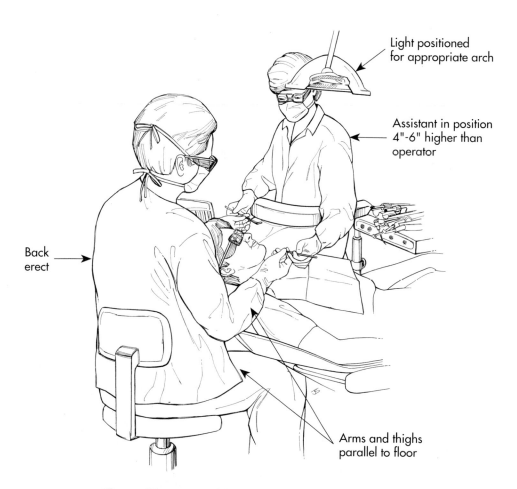

Light positioned for appropriate arch

Assistant in position 4"-6" higher than operator

Back erect

Arms and thighs parallel to floor

Figure 13-5   Favorable working position for operating team.

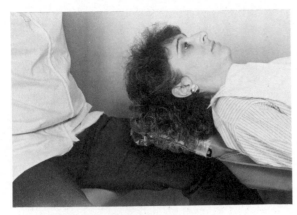

Figure 13-6 Thin back of dental chair resting on top of operator's left thigh.

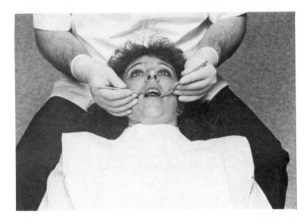

Figure 13-7 Chair back positioned between operator's legs.

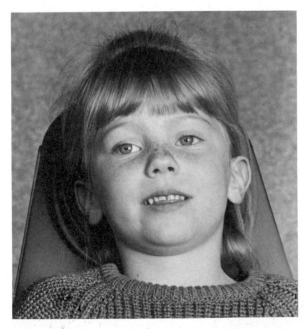

Figure 13-8 Pediatric patient's head placed in working position.

overlooked when purchasing the appropriate equipment for four-handed dentistry. The narrow chair back not only adds to the convenience of the dentist but also affords the chairside assistant similar access and visibility.

To benefit from the thin, narrow design of the chair back, the patient's head must be placed at the upper end of the chair and slightly to the operator's side. This is referred to as the working position for the patient (Figure 13-8). Patients are placed in the working position regardless of their height. In other words, short adults and children must be positioned in the chair from the head down. If they are always placed so that the buttocks are resting on the seat of the chair, the head of a short patient is located in a wider portion of the chair back, tending to limit the access of the operating team to the oral cavity.

The force of gravity prevents patients in a supine position from sliding down in the chair. Very small children (3 to 4 years of age) can simply bend their knees (Figure 13-9).

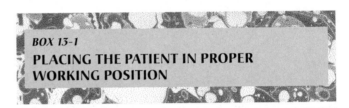

BOX 13-1

PLACING THE PATIENT IN PROPER WORKING POSITION

PROCEDURE	RATIONALE
1. Adjust chair back so it is at approximately 60 degrees to vertical.	1. This is comfortable seated position for patient.
2. Raise chair height.	2. Allows patient to be easily seated.
3. Raise arm of chair.	3. Removes barrier that could make seating difficult for elderly or disabled patients.
4. Once patient is seated, raise chair approximately 10 inches.	4. Allows room for dentist to slide under chair back.
5. Lower back of chair in increments, pausing at each increment until patient is in desired position. a. In maxillary position, patient is supine. b. In mandibular position, patient is semiupright.	5. Pausing at each increment allows patient to adjust to change in position.
6. Lower chair onto operator's lap.	6. Allows dentist to work comfortably in patient's oral cavity.

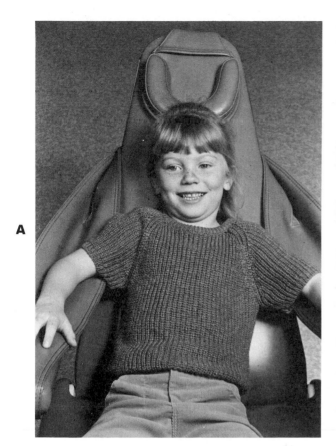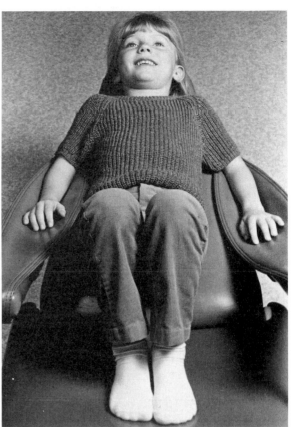

Figure 13-9 Small child in adult-sized chair. **A**, Seated too low with head out of working position of chair. **B**, Head in working position with knees bent as shown or cross-legged.

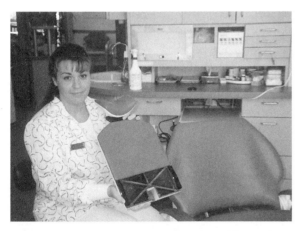

Figure 13-10 Dental chair with removable headrest.

Alternative types of dental chairs are designed so that the headrest is removable for short adults or children (Figure 13-10).

Actually a dental chair does not function as a chair per se in the practice of four-handed dentistry. For the most part it becomes a kind of operating table when the dentist places the patient in the proper position (Box 13-1).

Placing a patient in the proper working position is far more acceptable if the patient is not "thrown" into this position. With the chair back at 60 degrees before the patient enters the chair and a momentary pause halfway to supine position, the patient can adjust to the change. Some chairs with programmed positions place patients in a supine position too quickly, and they may object. Similar responses often occur when patients are rapidly returned to an upright position at the conclusion of treatment.

In the **supine position** a patient's legs and head should be at the same level (Figure 13-11). The patient should lie flat in the chair with little bending at the waist. This duplicates the position most people assume while sleeping for several hours without impairment of circulation. A patient whose legs are higher than the head is not supine, and such placement for long periods is not recommended.

Once the patient is placed properly in the working position, the chair base is lowered to place the head of the patient in the lap of the dentist. This height should be low enough that the operator's forearms are reasonably

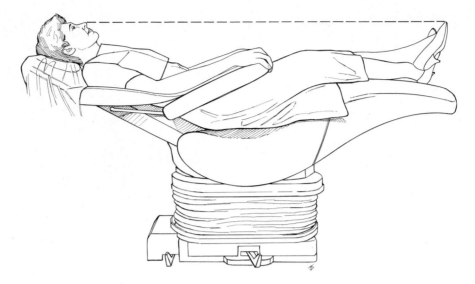

Figure 13-11 Plane of patient's head approximately parallel with floor.

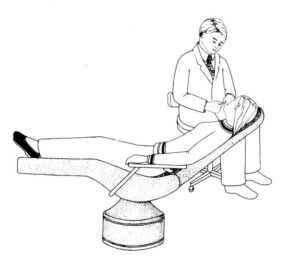

Figure 13-12 Operator–patient relationship while dentist is working on mandibular arch.

parallel or sloping slightly upward with the floor when the hands are in working position. Final adjustments for visibility and access to all quadrants of the mouth can be achieved by having the patient turn the head toward or away from the operator as needed. The patient's head can also be tilted backward or forward as needed to assist in improving visibility and access.

The supine position is considered a universal position for working in the maxillary quadrants (see Figure 13-11). The **semisupine position,** or semiupright position, is used for the mandibular quadrants. The operator is placed in the 7 or 9 o'clock position (Figure 13-12). Access is fur-

ther improved when the patient's head is turned slightly toward the operator and the chin is lowered.

> ### ➡ KEY POINTS
> - **For treatment on the maxillary quadrants, the patient is placed in the supine position.**
> - **For treatment on the mandibular quadrants, the patient is placed in the semisupine position.**

At this point it should be emphasized that once the patient is properly placed in either the supine position or some modification of it, assessment of proper patient positioning is accomplished by analyzing the operator and not the patient. The dentist should mentally go through the following positional checklist:

1. Thighs somewhat parallel to floor
2. Forearms somewhat parallel to floor
3. Elbows close to side
4. Neck and back straight
5. Distance of 14 to 18 inches between the operator's nose and patient's face
6. Operative field in dentist's midline

Adjustments in the position of the patient should be made until these relations are established. The chairside assistant can help the dentist by observing these relationships. The assistant who sees marked deviation from these guidelines can politely communicate this to the dentist by asking, "Are you comfortable?" This is a signal that perhaps a reassessment of position is needed.

POSITIONING THE DENTAL ASSISTANT

The dental assistant must be able to see and have favorable access to the oral cavity. The assistant needs to retract tissues, evacuate fluids, keep the mirror free from water drops, debride the operative site, and view the progress of any procedure to anticipate the operator's needs. Although it is not absolutely necessary that the assistant see every detail the operator can see, the assistant must at least be able to see the tooth or area being treated. The following are recommended considerations

for positioning the right-handed dental assistant for all quadrants of the mouth:

1. The assistant should be in the 3 o'clock position for working in all quadrants (Figure 13-13).
2. The assistant's stool should be placed so that the edge that is toward the top of the patient's head is in line with the patient's oral cavity (Figure 13-14).
3. The stool should be as close to the dental chair as possible.
4. To enhance visibility, the height of the stool should be elevated so that the top of the assistant's head is 4 to 6 inches higher than that of the dentist while they are working in most areas of the mouth (Figure 13-15). However, on occasion, improved vision can be achieved by lowering the stool so that the assistant's head height is the same as the operator's.
5. The assistant's back should be rather erect, with the body-support arm adjusted to support the upper body just under the rib cage.
6. The assistant's legs should be directed toward the head end of the chair with the sides of the thighs parallel with the chair back. The feet should rest on the foot support at the base of the stool.
7. When the assistant's stool is properly positioned, the mobile cabinet top can be placed over the lap of the assistant, thus putting instruments and materials within comfortable reach (Figure 13-16).

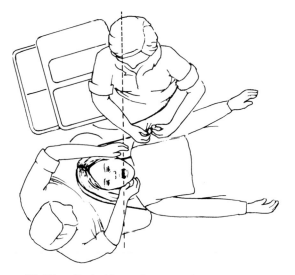

Figure 13-13   Chairside assistant maintains same position while working in all areas of mouth.

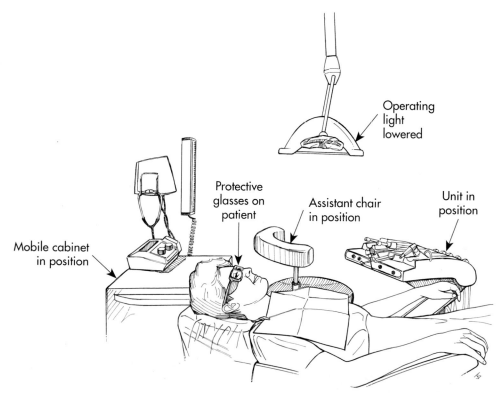

Figure 13-14   Chairside assistant's stool properly positioned relative to patient's oral cavity.

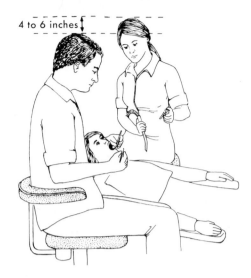

Figure 13-15 Proper vertical relationship between dentist and assistant to enhance assistant's visibility.

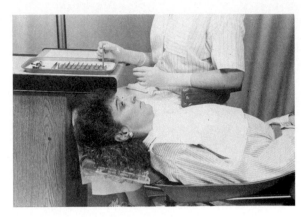

Figure 13-16 Properly positioned assistant's stool puts tray within comfortable reach.

> **KEY POINT**
> ■ The assistant's head is 4 to 6 inches higher than that of the dentist to allow the assistant better access to the oral cavity.

LIGHTING THE OPERATIVE FIELD

Operating lights should deliver at least 1200 footcandles to the operative field at a distance of 3 feet from the patient's face. Most modern operating lights have this capacity.

In general, the operating light should be directed over the patient's oral cavity when working on the mandibular arch (Figure 13-17). When working on the maxillary arch, the operating light should be placed over the patient's chest and the light directed toward the oral cavity (Figure 13-18).

When both the dentist and assistant are properly positioned, they should not block the path of the operating light into the oral cavity. Leaning forward over the patient by either the operator or the assistant is not only uncom-

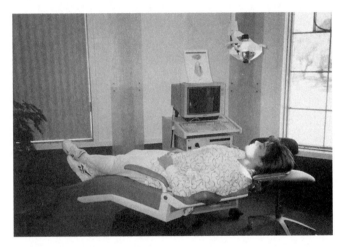

Figure 13-17 Operating light placed directly over patient's oral cavity for treatment on mandibular arch.

> **KEY POINTS**
> ■ The operating light should be placed directly over the patient's oral cavity for treatment of mandibular areas.
> ■ The operating light should be placed over the patient's chest and pointed toward the oral cavity during work on maxillary areas.

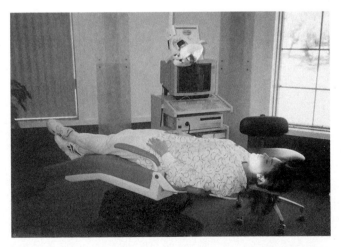

Figure 13-18 Operating light placed over patient's chest for treatment on maxillary arch.

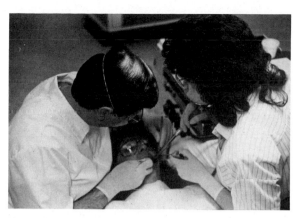

Figure 13-19   Operating team leaning too far forward and blocking light. Note light on top of operator's head.

fortable; it also tends to obstruct light and impair visibility (Figure 13-19).

DISMISSING THE DENTAL PATIENT

After the dental procedure has been completed, all isolation materials are removed, and a complete mouthrinse is done to remove debris and freshen the patient's mouth. The patient's face is wiped clean of any debris.

All operating equipment is moved out of the way of the patient, and the dental chair is slowly returned to a rather upright position. The right arm of the chair should be raised, but the patient is encouraged to remain seated for a moment until the circulatory system has had sufficient time to readjust to the upright position of the body. During that time the patient's napkin can be removed. Individuals often appreciate the use of a hand mirror to inspect their appearance before departing the operatory.

BIBLIOGRAPHY

Darby ML, Walsh MM: *Dental hygiene theory and practice,* Philadelphia, 1995, WB Saunders.

Finkbeiner BL, Johnson CS: *Mosby's comprehensive dental assisting: a clinical approach,* St Louis, 1995, Mosby.

Golden SS: Engineering comfort into dentistry, *Mechanical Engineering* 86:38, Aug 1964.

Green EJ, Brown ME: Body mechanics applied to the practice of dentistry, *J Am Dent Assoc* 67:679, 1963.

QUESTIONS–Chapter 13

1. The transfer zone is the _____ position for a right-handed operator.
   a. 7 to 12 o'clock
   b. 12 to 2 o'clock
   c. 2 to 4 o'clock
   d. 4 to 7 o'clock

2. The assistant's zone is the _____ position for a right-handed operator.
   a. 7 to 12 o'clock
   b. 12 to 2 o'clock
   c. 2 to 4 o'clock
   d. 4 to 7 o'clock

3. The static zone is the _____ position for a right-handed operator.
   a. 7 to 12 o'clock
   b. 12 to 2 o'clock
   c. 2 to 4 o'clock
   d. 4 to 7 o'clock

4. A distance of _____ inches between the operator's nose and the patient's oral cavity should be maintained during the delivery of dental treatment.
   a. 4 to 6
   b. 6 to 10
   c. 14 to 18
   d. 16 to 20

5. The patient should be placed in the _____ position for dental treatment on the mandibular arch.
   a. Upright
   b. Supine
   c. Semisupine
   d. Subsupine

6. The patient should be placed in the _____ position for dental treatment in the maxillary arch.
   a. Upright
   b. Supine
   c. Semisupine
   d. Subsupine

7. The height of the dental assistant's stool should be elevated so that the top of the assistant's head is _____ inches higher than that of the dentist during the delivery of dental treatment.
   a. 2 to 4
   b. 4 to 6
   c. 6 to 8
   d. 14 to 16

8. The operating light should be positioned _____ when working on the mandibular arch.
   a. over the patient's chest
   b. directly overhead

9. The assistant should place the patient in the supine position _____.
   a. Quickly
   b. With pauses in between
   c. Slower than normal

10. The assistant's legs should be directed toward the _____ of the dental chair.
   a. Head end
   b. Foot end
   c. Armrest

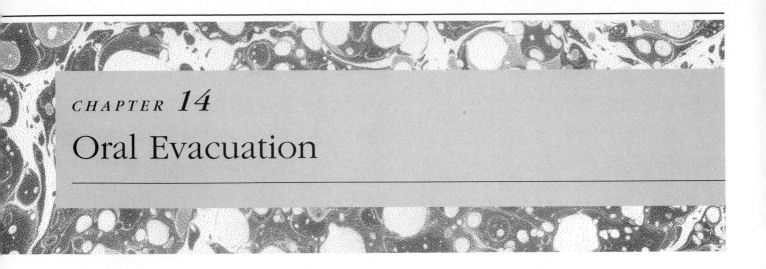

CHAPTER 14

Oral Evacuation

Bevels
Evacuation
Oral evacuator tips
Retraction
Solids trap

It is interesting to note how the various elements that make up the concept of four-handed dentistry relate to each other. Comfort and access to the patient's oral cavity are essentially achieved by placing the patient in a supine position while the operating team sits as close to the patient's head as possible. However, it would be nearly impossible to treat a patient in the supine position successfully without some way to control the accumulation of saliva, blood, water, and debris in the posterior region of the mouth. Therefore the oral **evacuation** system is used to remove fluids and debris from the oral cavity while a patient remains in the supine position throughout a dental procedure.

Oral evacuators are high-velocity vacuum systems that create enough suction to remove fluids and debris from the mouth. They work on a principle similar to that of household vacuum cleaners. High volumes of air are moved into a vacuum hose at rather low negative pressure. A vacuum cleaner is capable of picking up debris when the opening of the hose is placed near, but not actually touching, the debris. Likewise, the oral evacuator can pull fluids into the evacuation hose without making contact with a pool of fluid. This phenomenon is possible because of the movement of massive volumes of room air at normal pressure into the vacuum system, which has a low negative pressure.

Evacuation systems consist of a main vacuum pump, vacuum lines to each operatory, and an evacuation hose that the assistant manipulates to remove oral debris. The vacuum pump is usually placed in the basement or utility room of the office near a sewer line. The vacuum lines draw debris from each operatory to the pump, where it is exhausted into the sewer (Figure 14-1). Evacuation hoses are connected to the vacuum lines via a solids trap connector that catches most solids in the operatory (Figure 14-2).

Most modern dental units have a **solids trap** attached to the unit assembly itself. This makes it convenient to retrieve a solid object such as an inlay that may be inadvertently picked up by the oral evacuator. The solids trap should be cleaned daily, or disposable solid traps should be replaced regularly (Figure 14-3).

The evacuator hose in the operatory is a flexible hose that does not collapse when it is manipulated. It has a

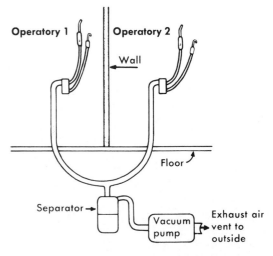

Figure 14-1   Semiwet oral evacuation system.

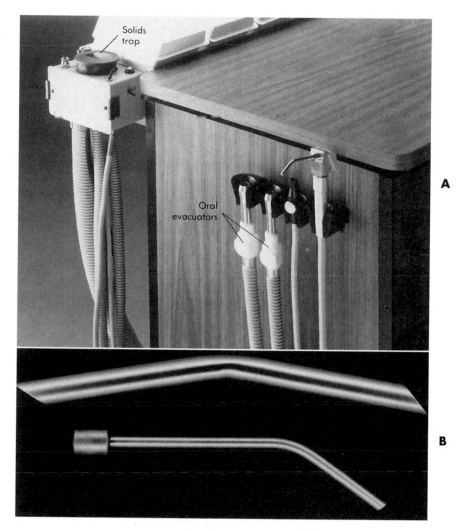

Figure 14-2   A, Assistant's mobile cabinet with solids trap and oral evacuators attached. **B,** Evacuator tips. *Top,* Universal style (stainless steel); *bottom,* surgical cannula style.

control on the operating end of the hose, which has an on-off valve to control airflow into the hose while the pump is running. An electrical control switch should be conveniently located on or near the dental unit so that the vacuum pump can be turned on or off with ease.

There are two types of evacuation:

1. A high-velocity oral evacuator is used for most dental procedures when four-handed dentistry is being used. An oral evacuator tip (disposable or sterilizable) is inserted into this control for use in the oral cavity.

2. A saliva ejector (Figure 14-4) does not have as strong a suction as the oral evacuator. Hence the tubing to the saliva ejector is smaller in diameter. The saliva ejector is used as an adjunct to the high-velocity oral evacuator.

The evacuator tip or saliva ejector tip is changed for each patient. If the tip is disposable, it is thrown away. If the tip is sterilizable, it is cleaned and sterilized before use on the next patient.

▪◇ **KEY POINTS**
- The evacuator tip and saliva ejector are replaced after each patient.
- When cleaning the vacuum lines do not use solutions that are not indicated for use in the oral evacuator; for example, iodophor solutions have a foaming action that can burn out the evacuation system.

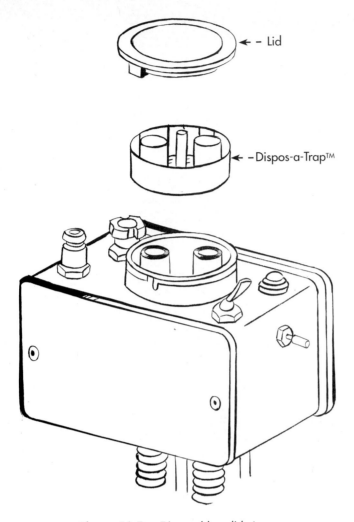

Figure 14-3   Disposable solids trap.

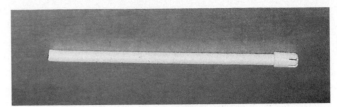

Figure 14-4   Saliva ejector.

Maintenance of evacuation systems generally includes daily cleaning of the solids trap or replacement of the disposable traps and flushing the vacuum hose and lines with a special cleaner. This routine procedure maintains cleanliness, prevents odors, and keeps the system from clogging with debris.

The oral evacuator control should be disinfected after each use along with other parts of the dental units.

ORAL EVACUATOR TIPS

Several styles of **oral evacuator tips** are available (see Figure 14-2, *B*). Some are made of plastic, and others are stainless steel. Some tips are disposable, and others are sterilizable. Every dental assistant soon establishes a preference for a certain style of evacuator tip, but regardless of personal preferences, the following key features must be considered in the initial purchase of evacuator tips.

Diameter of the Opening

Universal tips (see Figure 14-2, *B*) are used for operative and other restorative procedures.

Surgical tips (see Figure 14-2, *B*) are often used when suction is required in a small area. Such is the case during surgical or endodontic procedures. The effectiveness is reduced considerably for generalized evacuation purposes, but these tips are excellent for concentrated evacuation in and around surgical sites.

Metal vs. Plastic Tips

Metal evacuator tips are durable and can be sterilized in an autoclave. However, patients sometimes complain about the coldness of the metal on their faces when air is constantly rushing through the tip, cooling the metal. Plastic tips eliminate this minor problem; however, some of them cannot be put in the autoclave. Consult the manufacturer's recommendations for the disposal or sterilization of the evacuator tips.

Plastic evacuator tips are recommended during electrosurgery because they do not conduct electricity. This is a safety precaution to prevent burning patients should the electrosurgery probe come in contact with the evacuator tip. Plastic evacuator tips are also recommended during laser procedures because there is danger of reflecting the laser beam toward undesirable areas.

Straight vs. Bent Styles

Depending on the dexterity of the individual assistant, the suction tips bent in the center are usually more convenient to use. The bend is an aid to the assistant to properly place the tip and avoid blocking the operating light (Figure 14-5).

Design of the Tip Opening

Many unique and even bizarre designs for suction tip openings have been created to assist in retraction and prevent tissue grabbing while the evacuator is in use. Again, personal preference plays an important role here. A standard tip design with opposite **bevels** on each end (Figure 14-6) works well in the hands of most people. Proper tip placement, not the paraphernalia on the end of the tip, is the greatest factor in oral evacuation.

ORAL EVACUATION TECHNIQUE

The natural salivation of a patient during dental procedures plus the use of a constant water coolant sprayed into the patient's mouth from ultraspeed handpieces have created a profound need for effective oral evacuation. In addition, rinsing techniques using an air-water syringe with the patient remaining in the supine position require an oral evacuator. Both patients and dentists truly appreciate assistants who master an effective oral evacuation technique. Efficient evacuation prevents the patient from "drowning" in oral fluids and maintains a clear, visible operating field for the dentist.

The principal responsibility for oral evacuation falls on the chairside assistant. The following discussion of technique serves as a guide to effective evacuation during most dental procedures. Slight modifications are needed in individual cases.

Holding the Oral Evacuator

The thumb-to-nose grasp, or palm-thumb grasp (Figure 14-7, *A*), and the modified pen grasp (Figure 14-7, *B*) are two popular methods to hold the oral evacuator.

Both methods give the assistant control of the evacuator tip. This is essential for patient safety. A secondary

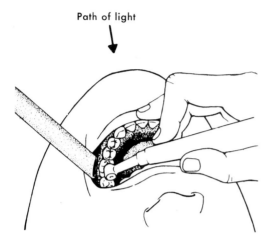

Path of light

Figure 14-5 Proper placement of evacuator tip so that path of light is not blocked.

> ◆ **KEY POINT**
> - The evacuator tip should be held with a thumb-to-nose grasp (palm-thumb grasp) or a modified pen grasp with the right hand.

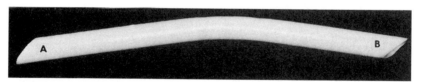

Figure 14-6 Universal-style evacuator tip. End *A* is generally used in posterior areas and end *B* in anterior areas.

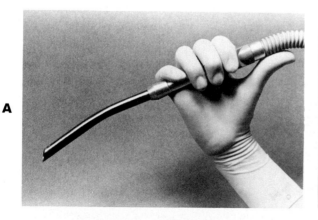
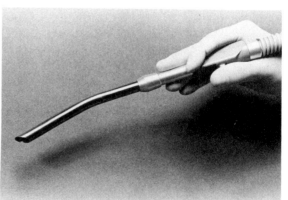

Figure 14-7 Common methods of holding oral evacuator. **A,** Thumb-to-nose grasp. **B,** Modified pen grasp.

function of the evacuator tip is to retract the soft tissues. This retraction requires a firm grip on the evacuator. Most assistants switch back and forth between the two grasps depending on the resistance of the tissues to **retraction** and the area being treated. The thumb-to-nose method is best used when more leverage is needed for retraction.

> ➠ **KEY POINT**
> ▪ The evacuator tip also retracts the soft tissue.

The assistant holds the evacuator in the right hand when assisting a right-handed dentist and in the left hand when assisting a left-handed dentist. The discussion here applies to a right-handed dentist.

The universal, or standard, evacuator tip is commonly used for most dental procedures. It has two functional ends (see Figure 14-6). An important relationship to remember is which end of the beveled evacuator tip should be used in a given area of the oral cavity. Figure 14-6 demonstrates that bevels are in opposite directions on the ends of the tip. Generally, one end (*A*) is used in all posterior segments, and the other end (*B*) is used in all anterior regions. A model is used in Figure 14-8 to demonstrate proper evacuator tip placement while assisting a right-handed operator.

When a dental handpiece is used with water coolant, the assistant must remove the water continuously to

> ➠ **KEY POINT**
> ▪ With the universal-style evacuator tip (see Figure 14-6), end *A* is used in the posterior segments and end *B* is used in the anterior segments.

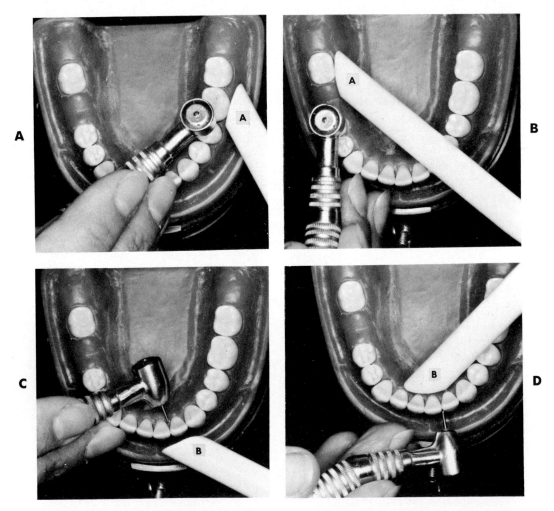

Figure 14-8 Proper placement of universal-style evacuator tip. **A,** For posterior areas on assistant's side of patient's mouth. **B,** For posterior areas on dentist's side of patient's mouth. **C,** For anterior areas when dentist is using lingual approach. **D,** For anterior areas when dentist is using either labial or incisal approach. (End *A* is used in posterior areas; end *B* is used in anterior areas.)

BOX 14-1

USE OF UNIVERSAL EVACUATOR TIP

PROCEDURE	RATIONALE	PROCEDURE	RATIONALE
1. Select appropriate end (A or B) for use in segment being treated.	1. End A is for posterior areas, and end B is for anterior areas.	6. d. For posterior teeth, place upper edge of tip slightly beyond occlusal surface (Figure 14-9).	6. a. Evacuator tip should be thought of as a scoop to catch water spray from handpiece after it strikes tooth being prepared. Suction tip is held on labial surface for lingual preparations to keep tip from interfering with dentist's vision. Tip also helps to retract lip. Suction tip is held on lingual surface for labial preparations to keep tip from interfering with dentist's vision; tip also helps to retract tongue for mandibular preparations.
2. Hold evacuator in either thumb-to-nose or modified pen grasp.	2. Depending on area, dental assistant chooses one that is most comfortable.	b. For anterior teeth: (1) If dentist is preparing tooth from lingual approach, hold beveled suction tip (end B) parallel with labial surface of tooth being prepared. Tip is held slightly beyond incisal edge (Figure 14-8, C).	
3. Place suction tip near working area.	3. It is best to place tip into mouth first to retract soft tissue and also because it is awkward to place bulky evacuator tip in mouth after dentist has placed handpiece and mirror or has already started delivery of treatment to area.	(2) If dentist is preparing a tooth from either labial or incisal approach, hold tip parallel with lingual surface. Again, place tip slightly beyond incisal edge (Figure 14-8, D).	
4. Place tip as close as possible to tooth being treated (usually slightly distal when occlusal approach is used).	4. In this position evacuator draws water coolant into opening immediately after it cools tooth being prepared.		
5. Position bevel of suction tip so that it is parallel to buccal or lingual surface of tooth being prepared.	5. This increases efficiency of evacuator. Tip is placed on buccal aspect of posterior teeth being prepared on assistant's side of patient's mouth and on lingual aspect of posterior teeth being prepared on dentist's side of patient's mouth (Figure 14-8, A and B).		

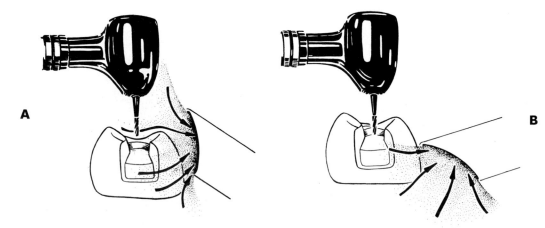

Figure 14-9 Vertical orientation of evacuator tip relative to buccal (or lingual) surfaces for maximum efficiency. **A,** Opening of evacuator tip is placed slightly beyond occlusal surface for maximum efficiency. **B,** Placing opening too far cervically reduces efficiency.

maintain a clear field of operation for the dentist. See Box 14-1 for the six basic steps to follow in positioning the evacuator tip.

Evacuator Tip Placement

Figure 14-10 demonstrates placement of the universal evacuator tip in various areas of the oral cavity for various approaches with the dental handpiece. Note the relationships among the handpiece, the tooth being prepared, the mouth mirror when used, and the evacuator tip.

One problem that is encountered by dentists using a mouth mirror for indirect vision is the collection of water drops on the surface of the mirror. Water drops obscure vision, but this problem can be eliminated by holding the mirror as far from the tooth being prepared as possible. The assistant should use the left hand to operate an air-water syringe and maintain a constant stream of air on the mirror to prevent water drops from collecting on the surface while the right hand operates the oral evacuator (Figure 14-10, *C*).

The mandibular lingual surfaces are difficult to treat. It is often helpful to have the assistant retract the tongue and evacuate intermittently as fluid accumulates in this area. Further, use of a conventional-speed handpiece with-

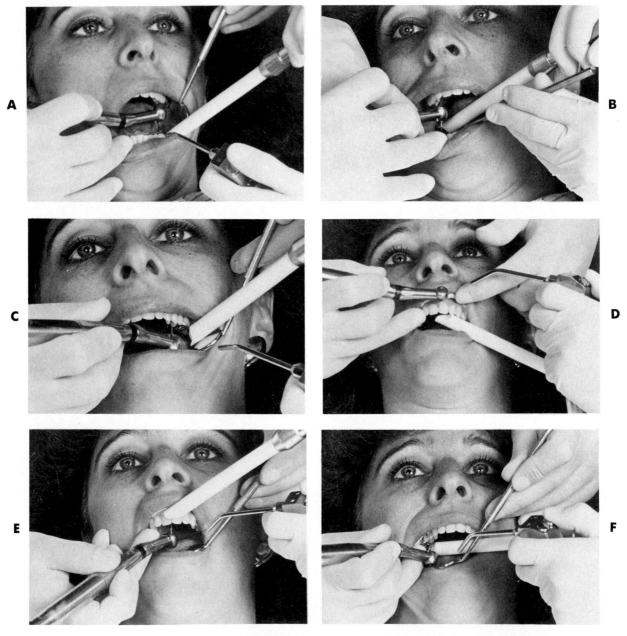

Figure 14-10 Guide to proper evacuator tip placement. **A,** Lower left posterior segment. **B,** Lower right posterior segment. **C,** Upper left posterior segment. **D,** Upper anterior segment (labial approach). **E,** Upper anterior segment (lingual approach). **F,** Upper right posterior segment.

KEY POINT
- The assistant holds the air-water syringe with the left hand and blows air on the dentist's mirror to clear the water that accumulates from the handpiece water spray.

out water coolant is recommended for cavity refinement. Evacuator tip placement for the mandibular anterior area is similar to that shown in Figure 14-10, *E*, for the maxillary anterior area.

This technique has proved effective. In summary, it should provide the following results:

1. Removal of both fluids and debris from the oral cavity
2. Retraction of soft tissues for better access and visibility
3. Placement of the evacuator tip in such a way as not to interfere with access and visibility for the operator
4. Control of the suction tip by the assistant's right hand with the left hand free to retract, operate the air-water syringe, or transfer instruments to the operator
5. Comfort for the patient during dental procedures

ORAL RINSING TECHNIQUE

Oral rinsing maintains a clear operating field for the dentist and frees the patient's mouth of debris before dismissal. The two basic types of rinsing procedures in dentistry are limited-area rinsing and complete-mouth rinsing.

Limited-Area Rinsing

As the name implies, limited-area rinsing is limited to a small area of the mouth being treated. It is used to maintain a clear operating field for the dentist as treatment progresses. The debris that accumulates in a tooth as a preparation proceeds can be removed quickly and conveniently, without significant delay in the procedure. This rinsing should be done automatically when the operator pauses during cavity preparation to inspect the detail of the cavity.

The limited-area rinse is accomplished by having the assistant operate the air-water syringe with the left hand and the oral evacuator with the right hand while the dentist may retract the cheeks or lips as needed to give the assistant access (Figure 14-11). If the assistant can keep the syringe in the left hand during the preparation phase, limited-area rinsing and drying can be done rapidly every time the dentist pauses for cavity inspection. Fluids that accumulate in the posterior region of the patient's mouth should be removed after each rinse.

Complete-Mouth Rinsing

The complete-mouth rinsing technique is designed to eliminate the need for patients to rinse and expectorate into a cuspidor. It is used whenever it is desirable to freshen the patient's entire mouth. Prolonged restorative procedures,

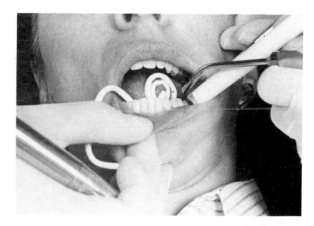

Figure 14-11 Limited-area rinse.

periodontal treatment, and routine dental prophylaxis often require this rinsing technique. Before the patient is dismissed after any dental procedure, it is a good idea to rinse the mouth completely, allowing the patient to leave the office with a comfortable, fresh feeling in the mouth. The method by which this can be accomplished is a matter of choice, but one of the most convenient is as follows:

1. The dentist operates the air-water syringe with the right hand and retracts the lips and cheeks with the mouth mirror held in the left hand.
2. The assistant retracts the lips and cheeks with the left hand and operates the oral evacuator with the right hand.
3. The combination of air and water produces a vigorous spray to dislodge debris.
4. Starting at the maxillary midline, the operator rinses the mouth by quadrants, finishing one side completely before proceeding to the other side (Figure 14-12).
5. The pattern of rinsing should force the water to loosen and push debris posteriorly. The water collects in the posterior region, since this is the lowest part of the mouth. The assistant can easily evacuate the accumulation, and the dentist can assist in the evacuation by gently blowing the accumulation of water into the evacuator tip with air from the air-water syringe.
6. The last action of the assistant with the evacuator tip should be to remove all the accumulated water in the posterior region until the evacuator just picks up the mucosa. This must be done quickly and gently. It ensures removal of all the water and leaves the patient dry and comfortable.
7. Immediately after removal of the water, it is helpful for the assistant to suggest that the patient swallow by saying, for example, "Your mouth is clean, you can swallow if you like." This reassures patients their mouths are clean and it is safe to swallow. Hence, they are less likely to look for a place to expectorate.
8. Patients who still feel the need to rinse at the end of treatment can simply use a cup of water and one of the sinks in the operatory before they leave.

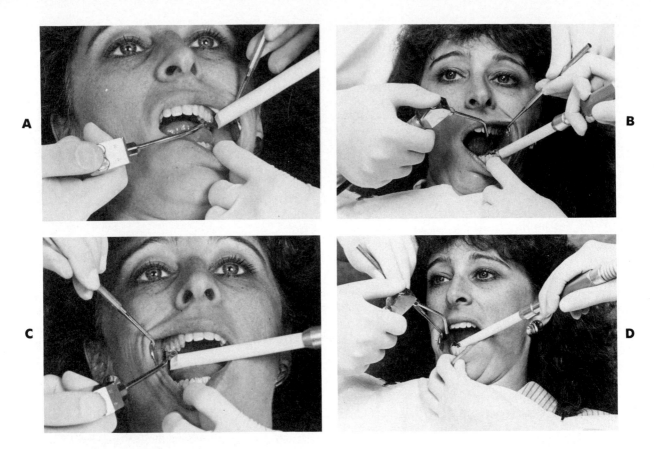

Figure 14-12 Complete-mouth rinsing sequence. **A**, Maxillary left quadrant. **B**, Mandibular left quadrant. **C**, Maxillary right quadrant. **D**, Mandibular right quadrant.

BIBLIOGRAPHY

Finkbeiner BL, Johnson CS: *Mosby's comprehensive dental assisting: a clinical approach,* St Louis, 1995, Mosby.

Robinson GE and others: *Four-handed dentistry manual,* ed 3, Birmingham, 1971, University of Alabama School of Dentistry.

Thompson EO: Clinical application of the washed field technique in dentistry, *J Am Dent Assoc* 51:703, 1955.

Thompson WR: Principles of evacuative systems, *Dent Clin North Am,* p 367, July 1967.

Torres HO and others: *Modern dental assisting,* ed 5, Philadelphia, 1995, WB Saunders.

QUESTIONS—Chapter 14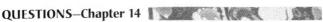

1. The bevel of the oral evacuator tip is held _____ to the tooth.
   a. Perpendicular
   b. Parallel
   c. Occlusally
   d. Mesially

2. The oral evacuator should be held in the dental assistant's _____ hand for a right-handed operator.
   a. Right
   b. Left

3. The dental assistant holds the oral evacuator in which of the following grasps:
   1. Thumb-to-nose
   2. Pen grasp
   3. Modified pen grasp
   4. Palm grasp
   a. *1* and *3*
   b. *2* and *4*
   c. *1, 2,* and *3*
   d. *4* only

4. Which of the following describe(s) the function(s) of the oral evacuator?
   1. Indirect vision
   2. Retraction of soft tissue
   3. Illumination
   4. Removal of saliva and debris from mouth
   a. *1* and *3*
   b. *2* and *4*
   c. *1, 2,* and *3*
   d. *4* only

5. If the dentist is preparing the facial surface of #8, the assistant places the oral evacuator on the _____ aspect.
   a. Facial
   b. Lingual

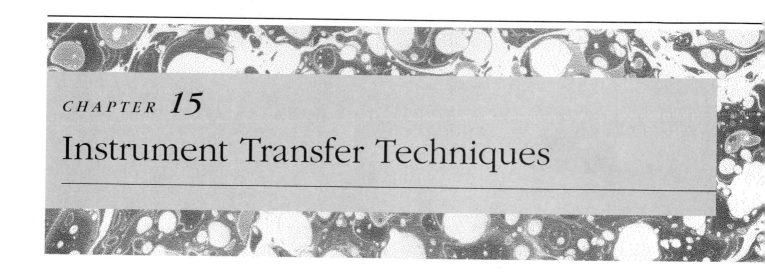

CHAPTER 15

Instrument Transfer Techniques

KEY TERMS
Crowding
Disorientation
Finger signal
Fulcrum
One-finger pickup
Recapping device
Shorting
Tangling
Three-finger pickup
Two-finger pickup

The elimination of unnecessary movement by the dentist while dental services are performed is one of the principles of work simplification. Techniques have been developed to transport instruments and materials to and from a patient's oral cavity with minimum movement by the dentist. Since hundreds of movements are required to perform dental services throughout each day, it makes sense to try to eliminate unnecessary movements and reduce the extent of movement by the operating team.

One of the principal chairside functions of a dental assistant is delivering instruments and materials to the dentist as they are needed without delay. This requires a standardization of the operating sequence so that the assistant can anticipate the operator's needs as the procedure progresses. A smooth, efficient instrument transfer technique requires coordination and communication between the dentist and an assistant. These them efforts result in less fatigue, a more continuous flow of the procedure, and a reduction in eyestrain for the dentist.

The instrument transfer techniques described in this chapter are designed to eliminate class IV and V movements and allow the dentist's eyes to remain fixed on the brightly illuminated operative field. The discussion centers on techniques used while assisting a right-handed dentist.

EFFECTIVE USE OF ASSISTANT'S LEFT HAND

Since the evacuator is handled with the right hand in most instances, the assistant's left hand is free for the following tasks during a dental procedure:

1. Retraction of soft tissue, to improve visibility and access for the dentist (Figure 15-1, *A*)
2. Retrieval and exchange of instruments as they are needed (Figure 15-1, *B*)
3. Operation of the air-water syringe to clear the operating field (Figure 15-1, *C*)
4. Wiping the working end of instruments, such as scalers, spoon excavators, and cavity-liner applicators, as they are withdrawn from the patient's mouth (Figure 15-1, *D*)

The phase of the treatment sequence and other circumstances determine how the assistant uses the left hand. A thorough knowledge of both the procedure and the dentist's established working pattern helps an assistant to be most effective with the left hand. A little common sense added to this knowledge is of value as well. For example, in difficult cases in which soft tissues are blocking visibility and access for the dentist, retraction would be the function of choice for the assistant's left hand. It is senseless for an assistant to hold the next instrument ready for exchange in the left hand if the dentist cannot even see well enough to manipulate the instrument already in use.

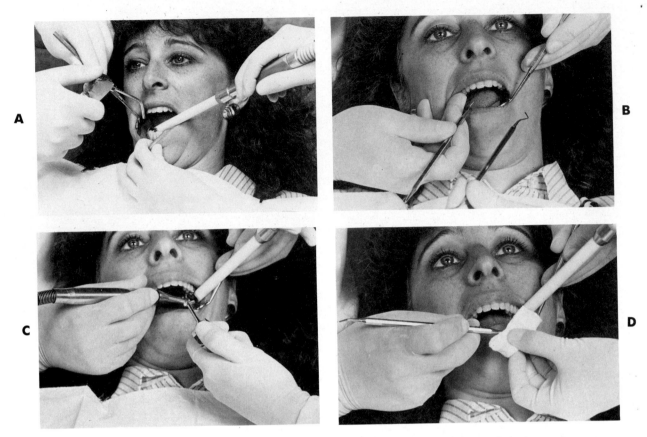

Figure 15-1 Assistant's left hand can be used for **A**, retraction of soft tissue; **B**, instrument transfer; **C**, operating air-water syringe; and **D**, debridement of instruments with 2 x 2–inch gauze sponge.

An alert assistant is mentally involved in the entire procedure along with the dentist so as to be readily aware of operator needs as treatment progresses. There is no room for daydreaming or idle minds in effective chairside assisting.

A general rule with regard to effective use of the assistant's hands is simply to remember the name of this assisting technique—*four-handed dentistry*. Not three-handed or two-handed dentistry but four-handed dentistry.

⊷ KEY POINT
- The assistant who uses only one hand during a procedure is probably not assisting the dentist enough.

COMMON INSTRUMENT TRANSFER METHODS

Following are criteria that can be used in selecting an instrument-transfer method:

1. The movement required by the operator for an instrument transfer should be limited to class III movements at the most.
2. Transfer methods used should be suitable for most common dental instruments. These include hand instruments and instruments with attached hoses.
3. Transfer methods should not require the operator's vision to shift from the operative field to execute a smooth, stable transfer.
4. Whenever possible, transfers should require the use of only the assistant's left hand (for a right-handed operator). This leaves the assistant's right hand free to do other tasks, such as maintain retraction, operate the evacuator tip, deliver materials to the oral cavity, or dry the operative field with the air-water syringe.
5. Any instrument transfer method that is selected should be easy to learn with a little practice. Stable transfers are mandatory for safety, since they are executed near the patient's face.

The three most common dental transfer methods are as follows:
- Hidden syringe transfer
- Two-handed transfer
- One-handed transfer

Hidden Syringe Transfer

Many dental patients fear the dental injection more than any other phase of dental treatment. It should be a challenge to the dental team to make injections as pleasant as possible. One important part of this task is to keep the syringe out of the patient's line of sight during its preparation and delivery to the dentist. The syringe can be prepared before patients arrive and then covered so that they cannot see it when entering the operatory.

After the injection site is prepared, the syringe should be delivered to the dentist in such a way that the patient cannot see it. Following is a method that is helpful in accomplishing the hidden syringe transfer.

Phase I: syringe preparation

1. Prepare the syringe as described in Chapter 4.
2. Orient the window located on the barrel of the syringe so it is facing the operator. The window of the syringe must be toward the operator so aspiration can be viewed.

> **KEY POINT**
> - The window of the local anesthetic syringe should face the dentist so the dentist can avoid giving an injection into a blood vessel, which could cause a local anesthetic overdose.

Phase II: patient preparation

1. Position the patient's head so that the operator has maximum access and visibility during the injection.
2. Position the operating light so that it is almost in the patient's eyes. This helps hide the syringe if the patient looks down as the syringe is transferred to the operator.
3. The injection site is prepared according to the preference of the individual dentist, but this preparation typically includes drying the mucosa with gauze and applying a topical antiseptic.

Phase III: syringe delivery

1. The dentist's left hand retracts the lips and cheeks, palpates anatomical landmarks, and holds the patient's head in the desired position.
2. The dentist continues to look at the injection site while the assistant places the syringe securely in the dentist's right hand. A shift of the operator's eyes to watch the syringe being delivered may tip off a fearful patient that the injection is about to take place.
3. The delivery of the syringe takes place over the chest below the patient's line of sight.
4. The protective needle cap is loosened before transfer to facilitate its removal during transfer to the operator.

5. The operator holds the right hand palm up with the thumb and first two fingers extended slightly to receive the syringe.
6. The assistant guides the operator's thumb into the thumb ring by holding the operator's right hand with the left hand. Stabilizing the operator's hand during the transfer eliminates the need for the dentist to watch the transfer and helps to prevent accidental needle sticks during transfer (Figure 15-2, A).
7. Once the syringe is positioned properly in the operator's hand, the window of the syringe can be oriented toward the operator by twisting the syringe barrel while still holding the operator's right hand. The assistant removes the loosened needle cap with the right hand (Figure 15-2, B and C).
8. When the assistant releases the operator's hand, it signals that the syringe is properly positioned (Figure 15-2, D).
9. As the operator performs the injection, the assistant should place the left arm over the patient's forearms as a restraint in case the patient attempts to grab the dentist's hand during the injection. When the injection is nearly complete, the assistant should have the air-water syringe and high-volume evacuator ready to rinse the patient's mouth.

> **KEY POINT**
> - A rear delivery of the anesthetic syringe is sometimes preferred by the dentist.

Phase IV: recapping the needle

It is rare to recap a needle in the medical profession because once an injection is given the needle and attached disposable syringe are immediately placed in a sharps container. Dentistry is unique because local anesthetic injections are sometimes given repeatedly and the same needle is sometimes reused on the same patient. It is necessary to recap the needle when it is not in use to avoid accidental needle sticks during the procedure.

In the past the dental assistant usually took the contaminated syringe from the dentist and recapped the needle. However, this type of syringe retrieval poses a risk of an accidental needle stick because the uncapped needle is manipulated more than necessary. Therefore the operator should recap the needle using one of the one-handed techniques described below:

1. Place the cap of the needle in a **recapping device** that will hold the cap of the needle in a perpendicular or semiperpendicular angle (Figure 15-2, E). This angle allows the dentist to recap the needle without touching the recapping device.

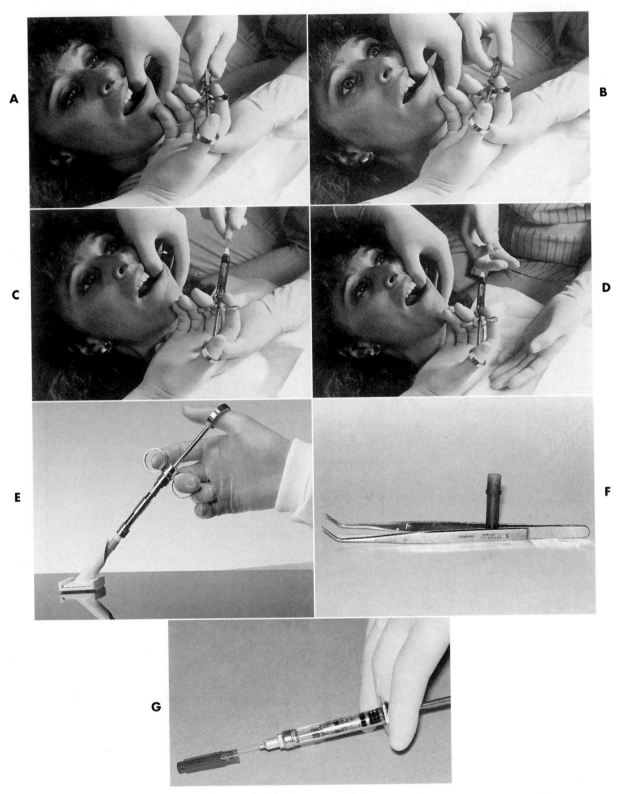

Figure 15-2 Hidden syringe transfer. **A**, Syringe placement. **B**, Window adjustment, **C**, Cap removal. **D**, Release of operator's hand. **E**, Needle capping device. **F**, Recapping needle using cotton forceps. **G**, Recapping needle using scoop technique.

2. Place the cap of the needle at a perpendicular angle between the prongs of the cotton forceps near the soldered end (Figure 15-2, *F*). Place the cotton forceps on the instrument tray. When the dentist is finished giving the injection, the needle can be recapped without handling the cap with the other hand.

3. Place the cap onto the instrument tray with the opening of the cap facing the dentist. After the dentist is finished giving the injection, the dentist can place the needle into the cap by using a scoop technique (Figure 15-2, *G*).

⚫❖ KEY POINTS
- Needle recapping should be performed with minimal manipulation of the needle.
- The operator recapping the needle should avoid placing his or her hands near the needle cap to minimize the risk of an accidental needle stick.

Two-Handed Transfer

Use of the two-handed instrument transfer technique requires both the assistant's hands. This may or may not be a disadvantage, depending on the type of treatment being rendered or the phase of the procedure in which the transfer is needed. Sometimes the assistant's right hand is not needed for other tasks when an instrument is exchanged; in this case, two-handed transfer is useful and convenient. Heavy instruments, such as surgical forceps and elevators, are easier to transfer by the two-handed method.

Essentially the technique requires use of the right hand to pick up the unwanted instrument from the operator and the left hand to deliver the new instrument (Figure 15-3). The instrument that is delivered should be oriented so that it is in the appropriate working position when placed in the operator's hand. The unwanted instrument is returned to its proper position on the preset tray so that it can be located quickly if needed again later in the procedure.

⚫❖ KEY POINT
- The two-handed transfer is often used in oral and periodontal surgery because the instruments could be quite heavy and some instruments are easier to transfer using this method.

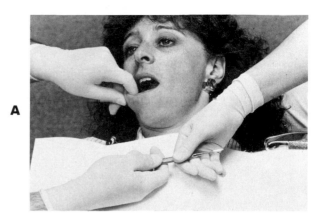

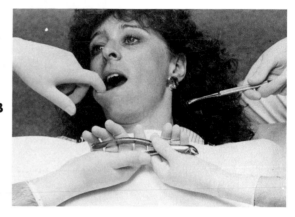

Figure 15-3 **A**, Retrieval of unwanted instrument with assistant's right hand. **B**, Delivery of desired instrument with assistant's left hand.

One-Handed Transfer (Pickup and Delivery)

The one-handed method of transferring instruments has gained popularity because it meets all the criteria stated previously. Once dental team members master this one-handed technique, they will recognize its superior convenience (Box 15-1).

The basic description of the one-handed instrument exchange applies to the transfer of hand instruments, handpieces, and air-water syringes. Forceps and scissors exchanges are made by the same fundamental method with a slight modification that is described later.

The assistant's left hand is divided into two parts, according to the function of the fingers of the hand. Those parts are as follows:

1. The thumb and first two fingers working together form the delivery part of the hand.
2. The last two fingers form the pickup part of the hand (Figure 15-4). When the dentist finishes using an instrument and wants to exchange it for another, the assistant picks up the unwanted instrument with the pickup fingers and delivers the new instrument with the delivery thumb and fingers (Figure 15-5).

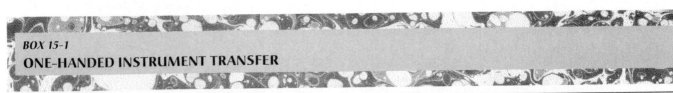

BOX 15-1
ONE-HANDED INSTRUMENT TRANSFER

PROCEDURE	RATIONALE
1. Hold instrument being delivered between tips of thumb and first two fingers. Instrument must be held close to end opposite from end operator will use after instrument is delivered.	1. To prepare instrument to be transferred.
2. Hold instrument over patient's chest approximately 8 to 10 inches away in ready position until signal is given for exchange to begin (Figure 15-6, *A*).	2. To keep instrument out of patient's line of vision and also to avoid injury to patient by keeping instrument away from patient's face.
3. Position working end of instrument so that it is in proper operating position for area being treated. Cutting edges of hand instruments and handpiece burs should be directed downward for mandibular areas and upward for maxillary areas.	3. To allow dentist to use instrument once it is transferred without having to turn instrument to use working end.
4. When the operator signals readiness to exchange instruments, position instrument close to dentist's right hand and hold it so that handle is parallel to handle of instrument in dentist's hand (Figure 15-6, *B*).	4. Dentist should not have to reach for an instrument. Also avoids tangling of instruments during transfer.

PROCEDURE	RATIONALE
5. Extend pickup fingers, and grasp instrument in operator's hand at end opposite working end (Figure 15-6, *C*).	5. To retrieve dentist's instrument.
6. Fold pickup fingers onto palm, and lift hand above operator's hand.	6. These movements lift unwanted instrument from dentist's hand and tuck it into assistant's palm (Figure 15-6, *D*).
7. Once unwanted instrument is tucked into palm, deliver new instrument by simply lowering it into operator's hand.	7. To deliver instrument that will be used next by dentist.
8. If same two instruments are exchanged again, immediately reposition retrieved instrument from pickup fingers into delivery fingers. Roll instrument between thumb and pickup fingers and shift it to delivery fingers in readiness for next exchange (Figure 15-6, *E* and *F*).	8. To prepare instrument to be exchanged again with operator.

Figure 15-6 demonstrates the entire sequence for a one-handed instrument transfer. The assistant accomplishes the entire exchange using only the left hand. The right hand is free to operate other instruments or to retract.

> ☞ **KEY POINT**
> ■ The one-handed transfer is the most common instrument transfer performed for general dental procedures.

Handpiece transfer

The handpiece can be exchanged for another instrument in the same manner (Figure 15-7). Caution should be exercised in orienting the hoses when two handpieces are exchanged to avoid tangling them during the exchange.

Air-water syringe transfer

The assistant conveniently transfers the air-water syringe to the dentist by holding the nozzle of the syringe in the delivery fingers. If the dentist is already holding a hand instrument, it can be removed with the pickup fingers as

INSTRUMENT TRANSFER TECHNIQUES

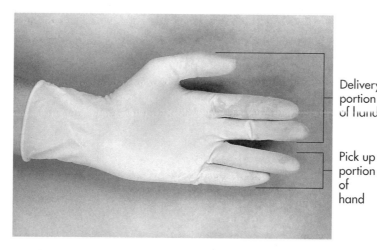

Figure 15-4   Pickup and delivery portions of assistant's left hand.

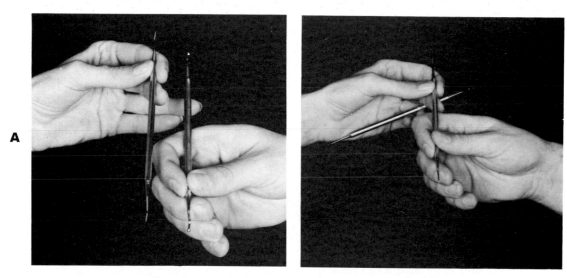

Figure 15-5   **A,** Assistant's pickup fingers in position to retrieve unwanted instrument from operator. **B,** Delivery of new instrument with delivery portion of hand.

just described. Deliver the handle of the syringe by bending the wrist slightly as the dentist positions the hand to receive it (Figure 15-8).

> **KEY POINT**
> - The assistant holds the air-water syringe tip (nozzle) to transfer the handle of the syringe directly into the operator's hand.

Scissors transfer

Scissors and hemostats are delivered in a similar fashion, except that the operator's hand must be positioned as

shown in Figure 15-9 to receive these instruments. When scissors are transferred, it is helpful to open the beaks slightly to separate the handles. This helps the dentist receive the instrument. The beaks should be closed when the assistant retrieves the scissors after use.

> **KEY POINT**
> - The assistant holds the beaks of the scissors, hemostats, and nonlocking forceps and passes the handles of these instruments into the operator's hand.

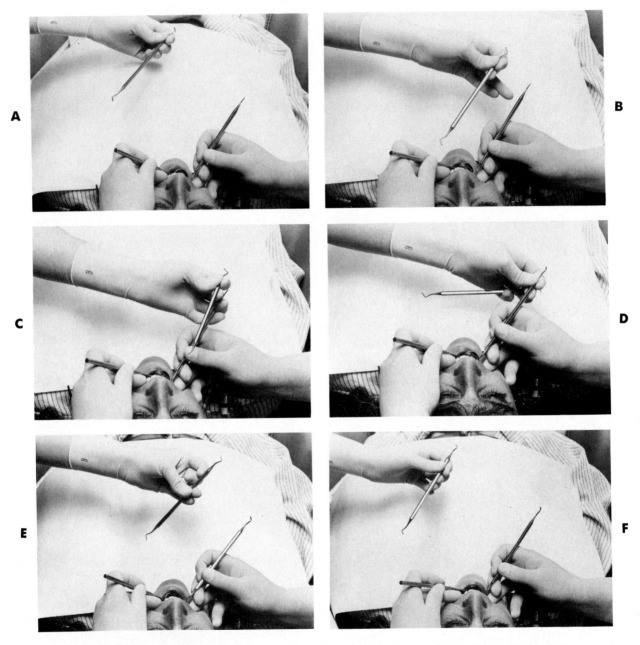

Figure 15-6   **A,** Ready position of instrument being transferred. **B,** Paralleling instrument handles. **C,** Pickup fingers grasping unwanted instrument. **D,** Tucking retrieved instrument into palm and delivery of new instrument to operator. **E,** Rolling instrument between thumb and last two fingers to reposition it in delivery portion of hand. **F,** Instrument repositioned in delivery portion of assistant's hand, in readiness for another exchange if needed.

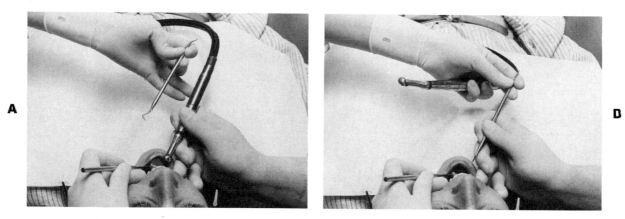

Figure 15-7 **A,** Removal of handpiece from operator. **B,** Delivery of hand instrument.

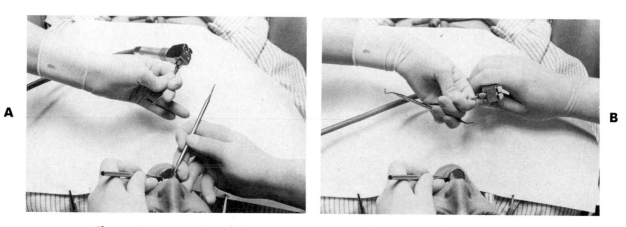

Figure 15-8 **A,** Retrieval of unwanted instrument. **B,** Delivery of air-water syringe.

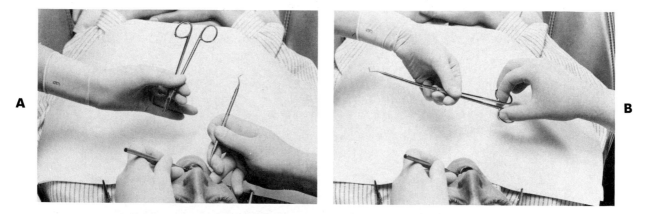

Figure 15-9 **A,** Retrieval of unwanted instrument. **B,** Delivery of scissors.

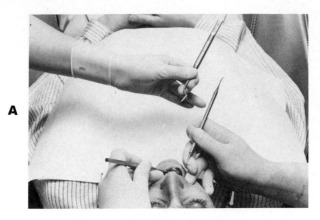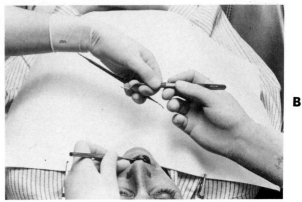

Figure 15-10 **A**, Retrieval of unwanted instrument. **B**, Delivery of cotton pliers and contents.

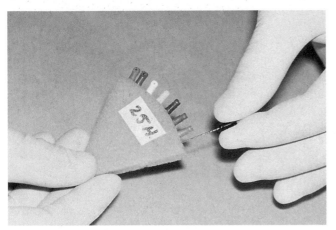

Figure 15-11 Delivery of endodontic files and reamers using foam triangle.

while pinching the beaks together with the delivery fingers and thumb to avoid dropping the paper. The pliers are delivered so that the dentist can grasp and hold the beaks together before the assistant releases them (Figure 15-10). Pickup of the same pliers is made by the pickup fingers at the working end of the pliers, again to avoid dropping the articulating paper. Many dentists prefer nonlocking cotton pliers, so this transfer method is often needed.

> **➝ KEY POINT**
> ▪ The assistant holds the beaks of the non-locking cotton forceps to keep the cotton pellet or other material between the beaks and passes the handle to the dentist.

Endodontic file and reamer transfer

Endodontic files and reamers are small instruments that are difficult to transfer without contaminating the working ends. Since sterility is essential during endodontic procedures, files and reamers can be transferred using a holding device made of a prefabricated foam triangle (Figure 15-11). After an instrument is used, the operator can reinsert it in the holding device while the assistant holds the files in the transfer zone.

Mirror and explorer transfer

At the beginning of each procedure the dentist often wishes to inspect the area being treated with a mirror and an explorer. The assistant can deliver both of these at the same time with a two-handed exchange, since no other instruments must be handled during this beginning phase. The dentist can signal readiness to receive the instruments by placing the open hands on each side of the patient's mouth. This not only tells the assistant, "I am ready," but also fixes the hands in a standard position to receive the instruments (Figure 15-12).

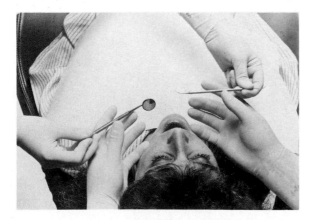

Figure 15-12 Simultaneous delivery of mirror and explorer.

Cotton pliers transfer

When nonlocking cotton pliers are used to pick up or deliver various items to and from the oral cavity, a modification in the transfer must be made. For example, if articulating paper is delivered to the dentist in nonlocking cotton pliers, the assistant must deliver the pliers to the dentist

A definite relationship exists between a well-organized preset tray and effective instrument transfer. The preset tray should be kept in order throughout a procedure, and each instrument should be returned to its proper position on the tray after it is used. This orderliness permits the assistant to select needed instruments quickly without unnecessary delays. Experienced assistants can mentally visualize the position of every instrument on the preset tray after working with the setup several times. Once the assistant has instrument positions memorized, instrument transfers become smooth and efficient.

HELPFUL HINTS
One-Handed Transfer Modifications

Alternate methods of doing the pickup-and-delivery instrument transfer are available for chairside assistants who experience difficulty using the last two fingers of the left hand for picking up an unwanted instrument. In these cases either the last finger or the last three fingers can be used to form the pickup portion of the hand (Figure 15-13). The use of the last two fingers (**two-finger pickup**) for this purpose is encouraged because of greater stability in both the pickup and delivery positions of the hand. Using the last three fingers of the hand (**three-finger pickup**) affords more dexterity, but having only the thumb and index finger available for the delivery function can be a disadvantage when transferring heavier instruments.

Use of only the last finger for pickup (**one-finger pickup**) is popular. However, to reposition a retrieved instrument into the delivery portion of the hand, the assistant has to flip the instrument (Figure 15-14). This maneuver changes the position of the working end in the assistant's hand. This may be desirable if a change of the ends is needed before returning the instrument to the operator. If a change is not desirable, a second batonlike maneuver is needed to reposition the instrument in the assistant's hand.

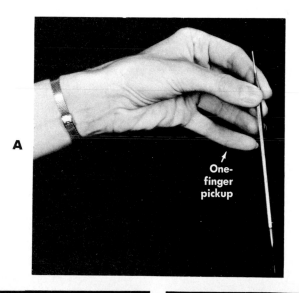

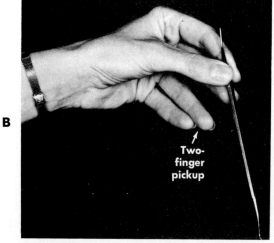
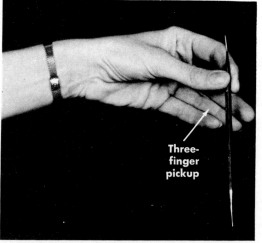

Figure 15-13   Alternative hand positions for retrieving instruments from operator. **B** is recommended.

One-Handed Transfer Practice

The chairside assistant bears most of the responsibility for executing a smooth instrument transfer. Use of the techniques requires practice to develop the necessary skill. Since the operator is not always available for practice sessions, the following practice method is recommended:

1. Hold an instrument in the delivery position of the left hand.
2. At the same time hold another instrument in the right hand with a pen grasp, simulating the operator's right hand.

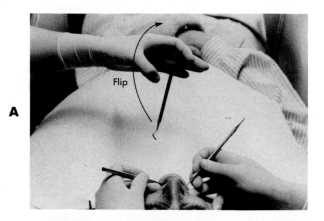

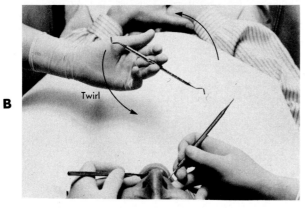

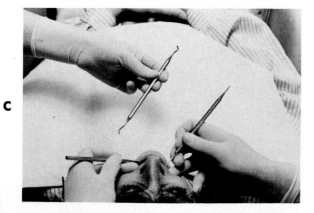

Figure 15-14 Repositioning instrument following retrieval using one-finger pickup method. **A,** Flipping instrument over into delivery portion of hand. **B,** Twirling instrument around using batonlike motion. **C,** Instrument back into delivery position.

3. Make repeated exchanges of instruments from the left hand to the right hand after repositioning the retrieved instrument in the left hand (Figure 15-15).

This exercise is designed to develop both the pickup and delivery skills of the left hand. In addition, the repositioning maneuver used to shift an instrument from the pickup fingers to the delivery portion of the left hand is developed.

Finger Signal

Repeated verbal communication can become tiring for both the dentist and assistant. A dentist can soon tire of calling for instruments as they are needed throughout a workday. The assistant can tire of unnecessary requests for instruments. Use of a standardized operating sequence helps to reduce the need for this type of communication and enhances the flow of the procedure. The operator who standardizes the sequence becomes predictable, and the chairside assistant can anticipate needs.

Once the assistant has an instrument ready to transfer, the operator can use a **finger signal** to show readiness to receive the instrument by simply withdrawing the instrument from the operative field by bending the index finger and shifting the instrument away from the oral cavity (Figure 15-16). This eliminates the need to use such verbal indicators as "ready," "now," or "OK" every time an instrument exchange is needed.

Depending on the area being treated, the dentist can help the assistant with the exchange by maintaining a **fulcrum** (finger rest) and presenting the instrument to the assistant. Maintenance of the finger rest fixes the hand in a predictable position, so that an instrument can be delivered at a fixed point without the assistant having to guess where the hand will be located as the exchange begins. This also eliminates the need for the operator to look at the instruments as the exchange is made and thus helps reduce the eye fatigue discussed previously.

If the operator's hand is located far to the patient's right side, it is helpful to present the handle portion of the instrument to the assistant during the finger-signal phase. This is accomplished by simply shifting the handle slightly toward the assistant when the signal is given (Figure 15-17). This helps the assistant to parallel the instrument handles as the exchange begins.

The operator should never present an instrument to the assistant past the patient's midline. Placing the instrument handle too close to the assistant complicates an exchange. Placing the handle at a 45-degree angle to the midline seems most favorable.

Common Problems and Solutions
Crowding

Sometimes a chairside assistant can be overzealous in having an instrument ready for transfer to the dentist by holding it too close to the operator's hand while another instrument is still being used by the operator. This **crowding**

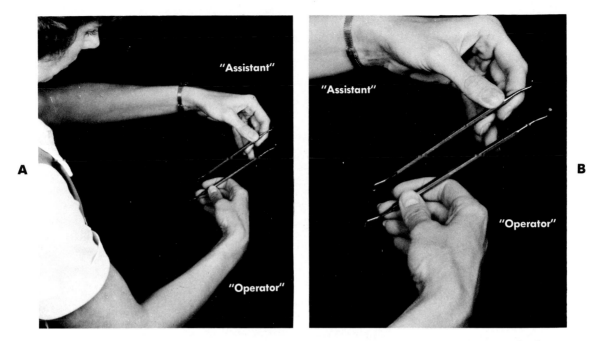

Figure 15-15 **A,** Dental assistant's hand position for practicing pickup–and–delivery method of instrument transfer. **B,** Assistant's right hand represents operator's right hand during practice session.

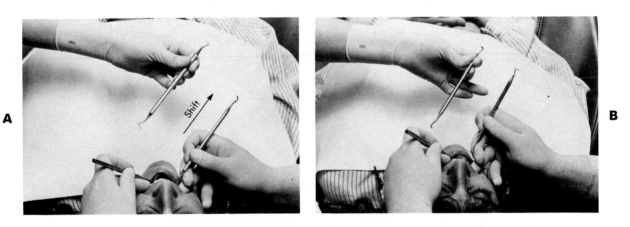

Figure 15-16 Finger signal to begin exchange. **A,** Shifting instrument away from working position. **B,** Exchange position.

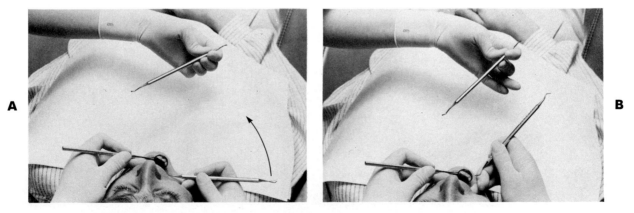

Figure 15-17 **A,** Shifting instrument handle toward assistant for improved access to handle of unwanted instrument during transfer. **B,** More convenient position for transfer.

can be distracting. In addition, it often leads to false starts of an exchange if the operator withdraws the instrument from the oral cavity, since the assistant may misinterpret this movement as a finger signal to begin the exchange. It is suggested that the chairside assistant hold an instrument ready at a distance of 8 to 10 inches from the operator's hand, in anticipation of an instrument transfer. Once a positive finger signal is given, the instrument is brought close to the operator's hand, and the handles of the instruments are then paralleled to begin the exchange.

Shorting

Shorting is the delivery of an instrument to the operator in such a way that the hand receives it too close to the working end (Figure 15-18, *A*). This usually occurs if the assistant does not hold the instrument in the delivery portion of the hand far enough from the working end (Figure 15-18, *B*). With practice the assistant should be able to judge where to grasp the instrument before delivery.

Tangling

Tangling of instruments during an exchange is usually caused by failure to parallel the handles before an exchange (Figure 15-19).

Disorientation

In **disorientation** the working end of an instrument being passed is pointed toward the wrong arch. Before delivery to the operator, instruments should be oriented in the working position that is correct for the area being treated. The operator should not have to shift an instrument in the hand after it has been delivered. The working end should be pointing upward for maxillary areas and downward for mandibular areas.

PREPARATION OF DENTAL MATERIALS

One of the challenges to an operating team is to establish favorable timing for the various phases of a procedure to promote flow. One of the most common interruptions in

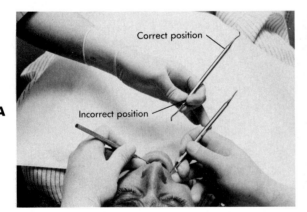
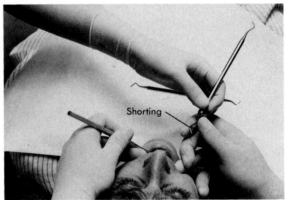

Figure 15-18　**A,** Cause of shorting. Assistant does not hold instrument far enough from working end. **B,** Delivery of instrument to operator too close to working end.

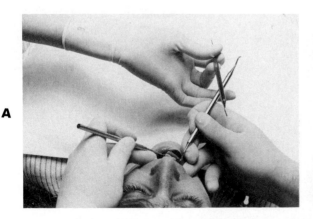
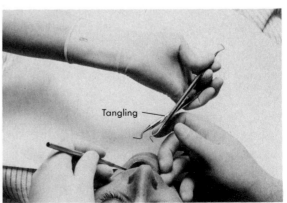

Figure 15-19　**A,** Nonparallel instrument handles may lead to tangling of instruments during exchange. **B,** Instruments tangled during transfer attempt.

flow is during the preparation of dental materials. Once a procedure has been standardized, the operating team should plan the preparation of materials so that they are ready for use when the operator needs them. This requires planning, coordination, and communication.

When the dental assistant has materials set up in advance, knows the procedure in progress, and uses a standardized sequence, all these aspects contribute to minimizing delays associated with the preparation of dental materials.

DELIVERY OF DENTAL MATERIALS

Generally materials should be delivered to the operator over the chest area of the patient.

Cements, Liners, and Composite

Cements, liners, and composite can be delivered on a mixing slab or pad, along with an insertion instrument. It is helpful for the assistant to hold the mixing pad in the right hand and a 2 × 2-inch gauze pad in the left hand. The dentist has convenient access to the material, and the

assistant can then wipe the tip of the insertion instrument when it is necessary (Figure 15-20).

↠ KEY POINT
- After mixing the dental material, the dental assistant holds the mixing pad and a 2 × 2-inch gauze pad near the patient's chin.

Impression Materials

Impression materials can be delivered directly to the operator in syringes and impression trays (Figure 15-21).

Amalgam

The question of whether the assistant should deliver dental amalgam to the operator for insertion or place it in the prepared cavity often arises. It is really a matter of convenience. The assistant who can see and reach the prepared cavity conveniently should place the material directly in the cavity, thus eliminating unnecessary instrument exchanges. However, rather than go through uncomfortable

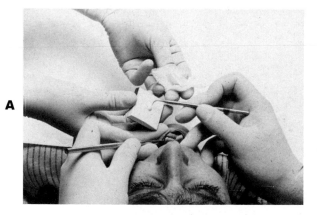 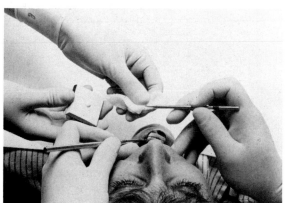

Figure 15-20 **A,** Delivery of cavity liner on mixing pad in assistant's right hand. **B,** Wiping insertion instrument with 2 x 2-inch gauze sponge between applications of liner.

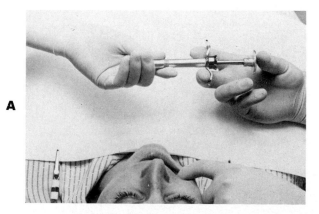 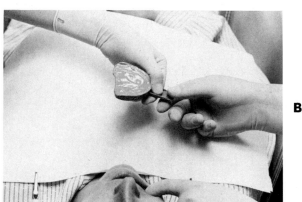

Figure 15-21 **A,** Delivery of syringe filled with impression material. **B,** Delivery of impression tray.

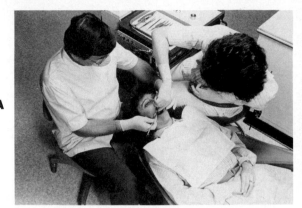
A

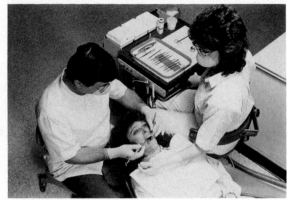
B

Figure 15-22 **A,** Dental assistant leaning excessively to insert amalgam in area of mouth that is more accessible to operator. **B,** Operator inserting amalgam in same preparation while both members of operating team remain in balanced posture.

contortions to insert the material, the assistant should deliver it to the operator for insertion (Figure 15-22).

BIBLIOGRAPHY

Ehrlich A: *Fundamentals for dental auxiliaries.* Dental hand instrument cards, Champaign, Ill, Colwell Systems, Inc.

Finkbeiner BL, Johnson CS: *Mosby's comprehensive dental assisting: a clinical approach,* St Louis, 1995, Mosby.

Robinson GE and others: *Four-handed dentistry manual,* ed 3, Birmingham, 1971, University of Alabama School of Dentistry.

QUESTIONS—Chapter 15

1. The dental assistant uses the _____ hand to pass instruments to a right-handed dentist.
   a. Right
   b. Left

2. The dental assistant uses the left hand for all of the following *except* _____.
   a. Retraction
   b. Instrument transfer
   c. Operating the air-water syringe
   d. Wiping the working end of instruments
   e. Holding the high-volume evacuator

3. After the dentist is finished giving the local anesthetic injection, the dental assistant _____ recap the needle.
   a. Should
   b. Should not

4. All of the following are recommended recapping methods *except* _____.
   a. Using a recapping device
   b. Using the prongs of the cotton forceps
   c. Holding the cap with the fingers
   d. Using a scoop technique

5. The assistant holds the _____ of the air-water syringe to pass the syringe to the dentist.
   a. Tip
   b. Nut
   c. Handle
   d. Tubing

6. The dental assistant holds the _____ of nonlocking cotton forceps to pass the forceps to the dentist.
   a. Handle
   b. Beaks

7. The dental assistant holds the _____ and the _____ when the dentist is applying a cement, liner, or composite material.
   a. High-volume evacuator, dental material
   b. Mixing pad, air-water syringe
   c. Mixing pad, dental material
   d. Cotton forceps, air-water syringe

8. If instruments become tangled during the instrument exchange, the problem is due to which of the following:
   a. The dental assistant holds the instrument too close to the instrument the dentist is using before the actual instrument transfer occurs.
   b. The dental assistant passes an instrument to the dentist and the working end is pointed toward the wrong arch.
   c. The dental assistant holds the instrument that is to be placed in the operator's hand too closely to the middle of the handle.
   d. The instrument the dental assistant is transferring is not parallel to the instrument the dentist is holding.

9. The dental assistant can use all of the following for the instrument pickup *except* _____.
   a. One-handed instrument pickup
   b. Two-handed instrument pickup
   c. One-finger instrument pickup
   d. Four-finger instrument pickup

10. For efficiency sake the operator uses a _____ to alert the dental assistant that he or she is ready for the next instrument.
    a. Hand signal
    b. Verbal signal
    c. Finger signal
    d. Foot signal

OPERATIVE DENTISTRY

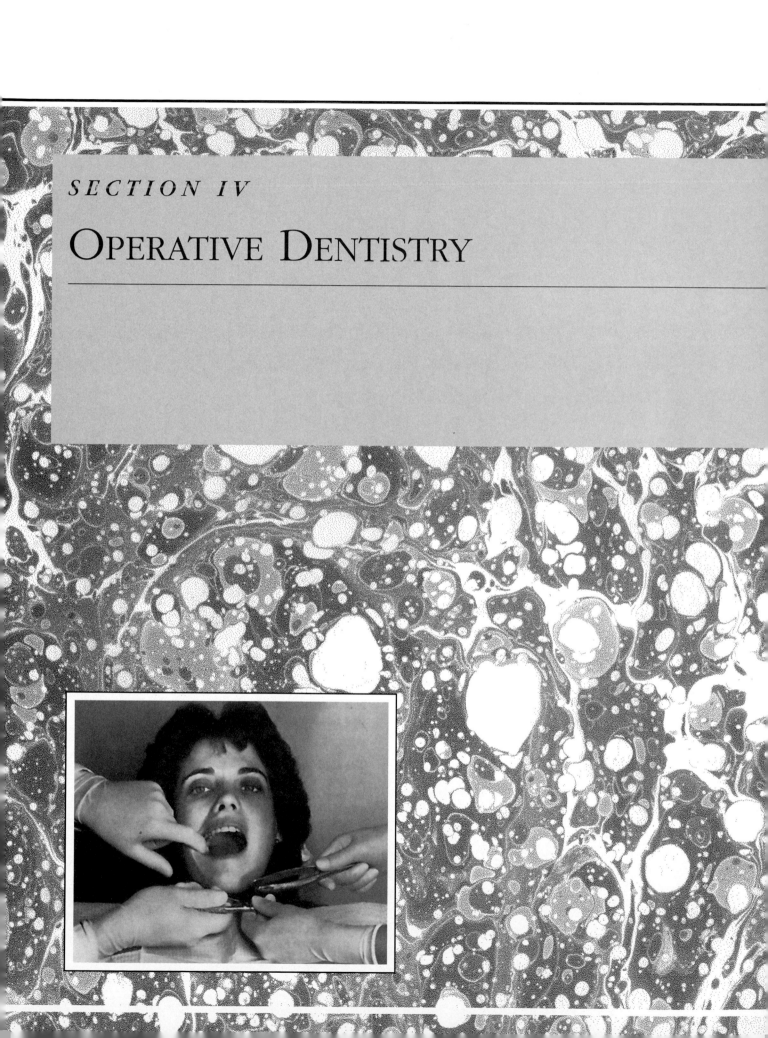

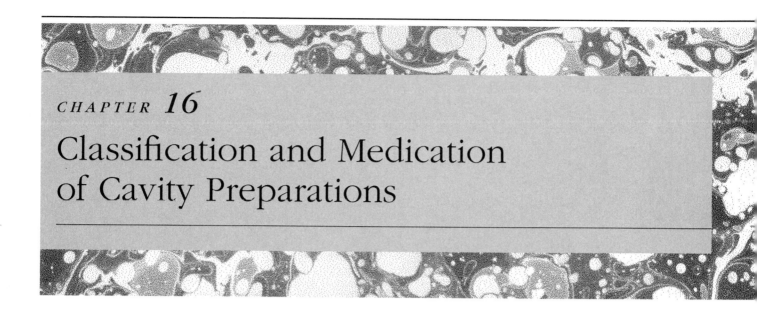

CHAPTER 16

Classification and Medication of Cavity Preparations

KEY TERMS
Black's cavity classification
Cavity liner
Cavity preparation
Cavity varnish
Cement base
Draw
Outline form
Resistance form
Retention form

Operative dentistry has traditionally been considered an area of dental practice primarily concerned with the preservation and restoration of tooth tissue. In the area of operative dentistry most carious lesions and tooth fractures are treated. Most restorations that are fabricated by operative dentistry techniques are primarily contained within the confines of the tooth itself. The public simply refers to operative restorations collectively as fillings. Restorations that serve to contain the majority of the crown area of the tooth, such as gold crowns, porcelain jackets, and fixed bridges, are often considered a part of crown and bridge prosthodontics. Crown and bridge procedures are discussed in Chapter 21.

There are several different categories of operative restorations. The methods used to fabricate these restorations vary from one dentist to another. However, each dentist must use basically the same procedures to pro-

duce a successful result. These procedures are discussed with regard to the amalgam restoration, esthetic restoration, and cast-gold inlay restoration in subsequent chapters in this section.

CAVITY CLASSIFICATION

Many years ago the dentist G.V. Black developed a system of classifying dental caries according to its location on the tooth surface. Clinical experience has demonstrated that caries occurring on tooth surfaces with developmental pits and fissures differs in its progression from caries on smooth surfaces of the teeth. As a result, the two different types of caries are treated differently and are classified by where they most commonly occur on the teeth. Table 16-1 summarizes **Black's cavity classification**.

> ◆◦ **KEY POINT**
> - G.V. Black's cavity classification uses classifications of class I to class V most frequently.

Cavity classification is useful only when teeth have a limited extension of decay on the various tooth surfaces. Teeth that are extremely decayed do not fit into Black's classification scheme. Dentists establish personal methods of referring to extensively damaged teeth.

Cavity classification is one method dentists use to assess fees for services. For example, different fees are assessed for class I amalgam restorations than for class II amalgam restorations. A basic understanding of this classification scheme is helpful to the dental assistant in business office procedures.

Table 16-1 G.V. Black's classification of cavities

Class	Description	Appearance
I	Cavities beginning in the pit and fissure areas of teeth A. Occlusal surfaces of posterior teeth	
	B. Buccal or lingual surfaces of posterior teeth	
	C. Occasional defects in either the incisal or occlusal two thirds of all teeth	
	D. Lingual surfaces of incisors	
II	Cavities on proximal surfaces of *posterior teeth*	
III	Cavities on proximal surfaces of *anterior teeth* that do not involve the incisal angle	

Table 16-1 G.V. Black's classification of cavities—cont'd

Class	Description	Appearance
IV	Cavities on proximal surfaces of *anterior teeth* that require restoration of the incisal angle	
V	Cavities on the cervical one third of all teeth that originate on a smooth surface	

MODIFICATIONS (used in various regions of the United States)

Class	Description	Appearance
II	Cavities on one proximal surface of a posterior tooth	
VI	Cavities on incisional edges or cusp tips that are not included in Black's original classification	
VI	Cavities on *both* proximal surfaces of *posterior teeth,* which when restored are joined across occlusal surface by restoration	

CAVITY PREPARATIONS

A **cavity preparation** is a systematic cutting of tooth structure in which any unwanted portion of the hard layers of the tooth is removed. These unwanted portions are usually one or more of the following:

1. Carious tooth structure
2. Fractured tooth fragments
3. Enamel not supported by dentin
4. Enamel pits and fissures considered vulnerable to carious activity

The design of the prepared cavity must provide suitable containment of the restorative material. The preparation must hold the restorative material firmly in place. Proper preparation design also helps to prevent fracture of the restorative material or of the tooth when subjected to biting forces.

All cavity preparation designs include three basic considerations:

1. Outline form
2. Resistance form
3. Retention form

Outline Form

Outline form is the overall shape of the preparation along the external surface of the enamel, or the cavosurface margin. The outline form is determined by the size and shape of the carious lesion and by the need for a suitable design that will hold a restoration firmly in place. The concept of *extension for prevention* also determines outline form. This is an extension of the preparation to eliminate deep occlusal fissures and to place the margins of the restoration in areas that are easy for the patient to keep clean (Figure 16-1).

Resistance Form

Resistance form is the internal shape of the cavity preparation. This shape is designed to protect both the restoration and the tooth from fracture when biting forces are applied to the restored tooth.

Retention Form

Retention form is the relationship that exists between different walls of the preparation. The walls of an amalgam restoration are generally parallel to slightly undercut in their relationship to each other, which creates a mechanical retention of the restorative material. Retention is also enhanced by the addition of retentive grooves in the walls of cavity preparations (see Figure 16-1). All cavity preparations that have proper outline, resistance, and retention form provide the foundation for a successful restoration.

• • •

The basic internal design of a cavity preparation is dictated by the restorative material used in it. All restorative materials placed in a prepared cavity while they are in a soft, moldable state require a different internal design from restorative materials that are placed in the prepared cavity in a completely hard state.

Moldable materials such as amalgam, acrylics, and composites require a cavity design that holds them in place by mechanical lock. Mechanical lock is provided when a soft, moldable material is packed into a cavity that has its cavity walls parallel or slightly undercut in relation to each other. The soft material hardens in the preparation after it has been properly shaped during its soft stage (Figure 16-2).

Hard substances such as cast gold and porcelain restorations (inlays) are held in place by the grasping action of the dentin and enamel walls of the cavity preparation. These restorations are hard substances at the time of insertion into the prepared cavity; thus the preparation design must not only provide a grasping action by the tooth but also allow the restoration to be conveniently

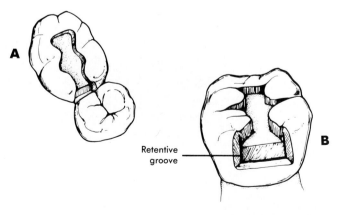

Figure 16-1 Class II amalgam preparation. **A,** Outline form. **B,** Proximal box of preparation is wider at bottom than at top and contains retentive groove.

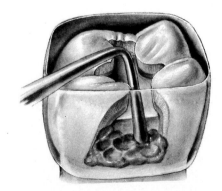

Figure 16-2 Insertion of amalgam in its moldable state into slightly undercut preparation.

(From Howard WW, Moller RC: *Atlas of operative dentistry,* ed 3, St Louis, 1981, Mosby.)

slid into place. Once the restoration is in place, it must adapt tightly to the cavity walls. Thus the internal design of a cavity preparation for a gold or porcelain inlay must have its walls tapered from the base of the preparation to the cavosurface margin. This is called **draw** (Figure 16-3). The taper should be enough to allow the insertion of the inlay into the preparation but not so much that the inlay readily falls out of the preparation. Inlays are sealed in the cavity preparation by the use of a variety of cementing agents.

Specific cavity designs for each type of restoration are shown in the discussions of each operative procedure.

MEDICATION OF THE CAVITY PREPARATION

Cavity medication is the cleaning of the cavity preparation and the placement of appropriate agents that help to maintain a healthy pulp.

Following cavity preparation it is sometimes desirable to place a base and/or liner before the final restorative material is placed. These materials are placed to accomplish one or more of the following functions:

1. To seal the dentin tubules that extend from the pulp to the surface of the prepared cavity
2. To stimulate pulpal healing
3. To sedate an irritated pulp
4. To provide thermal insulation
5. To provide a barrier between the dentin and restorative material, which may chemically irritate the pulp
6. To provide for the release of fluoride to adjacent tooth structure

No one base or lining material can provide all these functions; therefore they are often used in various combinations.

The three basic types of materials that are used to medicate the cavity preparation are as follows:

1. Cavity liners
   a. Calcium hydroxide
   b. Glass ionomer
2. Cavity varnish
3. Cement bases
   a. Glass ionomer
   b. Zinc oxide and eugenol
   c. Zinc phosphate

Placement of any of the above depends on the depth of the tooth preparation and also the type of material that will be used to fill the tooth preparation.

Definition of Cavity Depths

Cavity depths are generally defined in terms of the amount of dentin lost between the dental pulp and the outside of a tooth. These depths are typically grouped into the following categories:

1. *Ideal depth.* A cavity preparation that has ideal minimal depth to retain the restorative material (Figure 16-4, *A*).
2. *Moderate depth.* A cavity preparation that must be extended beyond the ideal minimal depth, without invading the pulp, to remove caries (Figure 16-4, *B*).
3. *Very deep preparations.* A cavity preparation that leaves only a thin layer of dentin covering the dental pulp after caries is removed or an overt exposure of the dental pulp (Figure 16-4, *C*).

Cavity Liners

A **cavity liner** is a thin, creamlike material, such as calcium hydroxide and glass ionomer materials.

Calcium hydroxide

Calcium hydroxide (Figure 16-5) is a liner designed to stimulate dental pulp cells to produce more dentin from

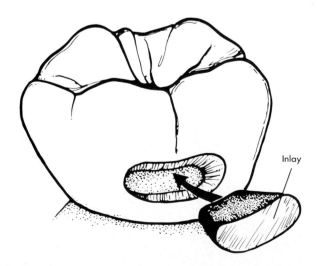

Figure 16-3   Class V inlay preparation demonstrating draw.

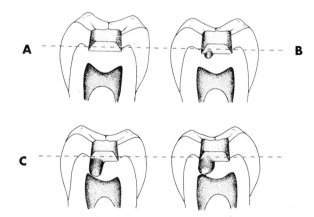

Figure 16-4   Three categories of cavity depth. **A,** Ideal depth—just beyond dentinoenamel junction. **B,** Moderate depth—extension of cavity depth slightly deeper than ideal. **C,** Very deep cavity preparations—near exposure of pulp and pulp exposure.

within the pulp chamber when the cavity preparation is near, or actually enters, the pulp. It is commonly used to stimulate healing in near and overt exposures of the pulp.

Glass ionomer lining cements

Glass ionomer lining cements (Figure 16-6) are a new material marketed in various compositions that make them suitable as cavity liners, bases, final restorations, cementation agents, or buildup materials under a crown restoration. The versatility of the various forms of glass ionomer, as well as its chemical and physical properties, has made it popular.

When used as a base or a cavity lining material, glass ionomer has a caries-inhibiting effect, since it contains fluoride. This helps to prevent decay from recurring under restorations that have glass ionomer as a liner or base.

Another advantage of this material is its ability to bond to the dentin of a cavity preparation. This characteristic helps glass ionomer maintain its position during insertion of a final restorative material, such as amalgam or composite. It should be noted that glass ionomer base and lining material bond to composite restorative material that is placed over them. As with other bases and liners, glass ionomer provides thermal insulation and a barrier between the dentin tubules and restorative materials that may irritate the dental pulp.

> ### ❧ KEY POINTS
> - Glass ionomer is caries inhibiting because it contains fluoride.
> - Glass ionomer can bond to dentin.

Cavity Varnish

Cavity varnish (copal varnish) (Figure 16-7) seals the open ends of the dentin tubules with a glazelike covering. Dentin tubules are microscopic "tunnels" that extend from the pulp to the prepared cavity. The varnish closes the end of each tubule within the cavity preparation and prevents further irritation from penetrating foreign substances. Such substances may be irritating chemicals from cement bases or other restorative materials or simply oral fluids that seep under the final restoration as a result of microleakage. Varnishes may also prevent mercury and corrosive products of amalgam restorations from penetrating the tubules and discoloring the tooth. Copal varnishes interfere with the setting of acrylic and composite materials and should not be used as a liner unless a compatible cement base is placed over the liner.

> ### ❧ KEY POINT
> - Cavity varnish should not be used with acrylic or composite materials because it interferes with the setting of the material.

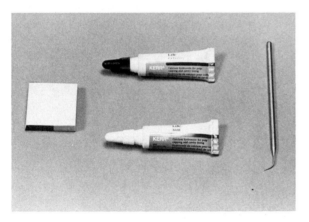

Figure 16-5   Calcium hydroxide liner with mixing pad and liner applicator.

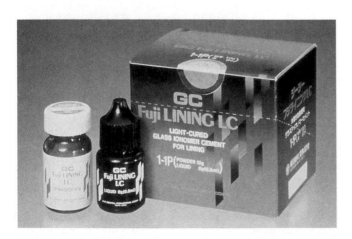

Figure 16-6   Glass ionomer lining cement.

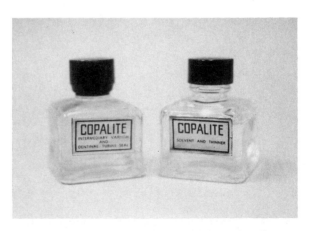

Figure 16-7   Cavity varnish and thinning solvent.

Cement Base

A **cement base** is a thick, doughlike material that hardens in the cavity preparation and replaces lost dentin. Bases are made from a variety of dental cements that can be mixed to a thick consistency (Figure 16-8). The specific role of these materials is discussed in conjunction with the treatment of specific cavity depths described below.

The following general principles regarding use of cement bases must be observed:

1. They must be compatible with the restorative materials that are placed over them. Like cavity liners, cement bases containing zinc oxide and eugenol (ZOE) interfere with the setting of resin restorative materials, such as acrylic and composite, if they come in contact with them.

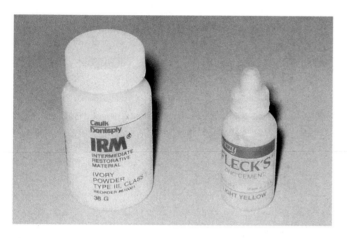

Figure 16-8   Dental cements used for cement bases. *Left,* Zinc oxide and eugenol; *right,* zinc phosphate.

2. They should be compatible with the dental pulp. ZOE cements soothe teeth and are often used as a sedative temporary filling, as well as a cement base. On the other hand, zinc phosphate, polycarboxylate, and glass ionomer cements are initially acidic when they are inserted and are not kind to the pulp if handled improperly.

3. They must be a poor conductor of thermal change. This insulating quality protects the pulp from changes in temperature associated with hot and cold foods and beverages, as well as cold air. Thermal changes can be painful if they are transmitted through a metal restoration deep into the tooth and may eventually damage the delicate dental pulp. Placing a nonmetal material, such as a cement base, under a metal restoration provides proper insulation.

4. They must be strong in terms of resisting compressive forces. This *compressive strength* is essential to support any restoration placed over the base. If a cement base collapses under pressure, the restoration over it fractures.

Amalgam Cavity Preparation
Treatment of the ideal-depth cavity preparation

The ideal-depth cavity preparation is medicated by rinsing and drying the tooth with the air-water syringe succeeded by one of the following:

1. With metal restorations, two thin coats of cavity varnish are placed over the dentin using tiny cotton pellets held in cotton forceps (Figure 16-9, *A*).

2. An alternative is one thin layer of glass ionomer liner over the exposed dentin.

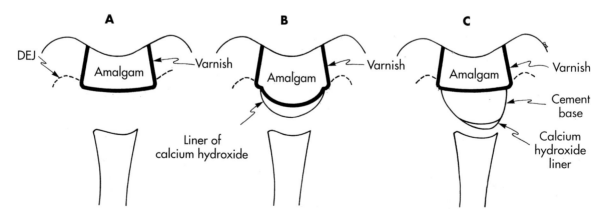

Figure 16-9   Use of liners and bases for amalgam restorations. **A,** For shallow amalgam cavity preparations, varnish is applied to walls of preparation before insertion of restoration. **B,** For moderate-depth cavity preparations, liners may be placed for thermal protection and pulpal medication. **C,** In very deep preparation, calcium hydroxide is placed in deepest region in which infected dentin was excavated, and then a base is inserted.

(From Sturdevant CM and others: *The art and science of operative dentistry,* ed 3, St Louis, 1995, Mosby.)

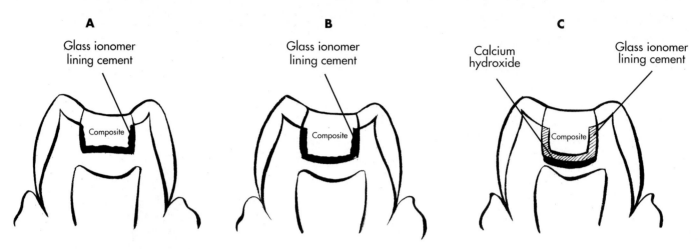

Figure 16-10 Use of liners and bases for composite restorations. **A,** Ideal-depth preparation uses liner of glass ionomer. **B,** Unless cavity preparation is very deep, moderate-depth cavity preparations use a liner of glass ionomer. **C,** Very deep cavity preparations use a calcium hydroxide liner in deepest portion of cavity preparation and then a glass ionomer liner or base is applied.

Treatment of the moderate-depth cavity preparation

After the preparation is rinsed and dried, a cavity liner may be placed for thermal protection and pulpal medication (Figure 16-9, *B*).

Treatment of the very deep cavity preparation

Whenever so much dentin is lost that the pulp is nearly exposed, additional precautions must be taken to protect this delicate tissue. Near-exposure cavity preparations are rinsed and then dried with cotton pellets. Drying with cotton pellets prevents overdrying, or desiccation.

A common approach to medicating cavity preparations for *metal restorations* is the placement of a calcium hydroxide liner over the dentin in the deepest part of the preparation. Once the calcium hydroxide liner is placed, a cement base is inserted followed by two layers of cavity varnish over the remaining dentin (Figure 16-9, *C*). With the development of stronger reinforced ZOE cements, it is also common to place a calcium hydroxide liner followed by a ZOE cement base and then cavity varnish. The dentist chooses the regimen.

Composite Cavity Preparation
Treatment of the ideal-depth cavity preparation

The ideal-depth cavity preparation is medicated by rinsing and drying the tooth with the air-water syringe. With composite and acrylic restorations, glass ionomer liner is then placed over the exposed dentin (Figure 16-10, *A*).

Treatment of the moderate-depth cavity preparation

After the preparation is rinsed and dried, the lost dentin is replaced up to the ideal depth by a cement base. Unless the cavity preparation is very deep a glass ionomer lining cement is used under moderate-depth cavity preparations for composite and acrylic restorations (Figure 16-10, *B*).

Treatment of the very deep cavity preparation

Whenever so much dentin is lost that the pulp is nearly exposed, additional precautions must be taken to protect this delicate tissue. Near-exposure cavity preparations are rinsed and then dried with cotton pellets. Drying with cotton pellets prevents overdrying, or desiccation. Cavity preparations for composite restorations are treated with calcium hydroxide in the deepest portion of the cavity, a glass ionomer base, and then the final composite material (Figure 16-10, *C*).

COMMON METHODS OF MIXING CEMENT BASES AND CAVITY LINERS

Whenever possible the dental assistant should follow the manufacturer's instructions to mix bases and liners. All brands of some products have identical mixing instructions. These are described here.

Cavity Varnish

For cavity varnish no mixing is required (Box 16-1). The product is used directly from the bottle. However, evaporation of the solvent can cause the varnish to thicken, and new solvent must be added from time to time to maintain the preferred viscosity.

> **↤ KEY POINT**
> ▪ Common trade names for cavity varnishes are Copalite and Varnal.

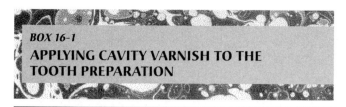

BOX 16-1

APPLYING CAVITY VARNISH TO THE TOOTH PREPARATION

ARMAMENTARIUM
- Sterile cotton forceps
- Cotton pellets
- Cavity varnish

PROCEDURE	RATIONALE
1. Grasp a cotton pellet with sterile cotton forceps and dip cotton pellet in bottle of cavity varnish.	1. Using cotton forceps that have been inserted inside patient's mouth or have been placed on instrument tray with contaminated instruments will cross contaminate bottle of cavity varnish.
2. After dentist applies a coat of varnish to tooth preparation, blow air with air-water syringe into tooth preparation.	2. To dry coat of varnish.
3. Another coat of varnish is applied by dentist and dried by dental assistant.	3. Two coats of cavity varnish are necessary to completely seal dentinal tubules.

Calcium Hydroxide

Calcium hydroxide is generally marketed in small pairs of dispensing tubes. One tube contains the base material, and the other tube contains an accelerator to cause the liner to harden or set. Equal volumes of each are squeezed onto a small mixing pad, mixed with a liner applicator, and delivered to the operative field (Box 16-2). Small quantities (droplet size) are required for typical cavity preparations.

> ◆ **KEY POINT**
> - **Common trade names for calcium hydroxide are Life and Dycal.**

Glass Ionomer Cement Bases and Liners

Glass ionomer cement bases and liners are available as one bottle of powder and one bottle of liquid. One scoop of powder is mixed with one drop of liquid (Box 16-3).

BOX 16-2

APPLYING CALCIUM HYDROXIDE TO THE TOOTH PREPARATION

ARMAMENTARIUM
- Calcium hydroxide liner
  One tube of base
  One tube of accelerator
- Liner applicator instrument
- Small paper mixing pad
- Gauze sponge

PROCEDURE	RATIONALE
1. Place small amount of equal proportions from each tube of calcium hydroxide on mixing pad. Place material from each tube next to but not touching material from the other tube.	1. Only small amount of material will be needed to line tooth preparation. Equal amounts from each tube will ensure correct mix.
2. Wipe excess material from openings of each tube.	2. To maintain material in clean and neat manner. Separate gauze sponge must be used for each tube to avoid cross-contaminating tubes.
3. Place appropriate color cap onto tubes of material.	3. To avoid cross-contaminating tubes of calcium hydroxide.
4. With liner applicator instrument, mix calcium hydroxide liner together until mix becomes all one color.	4. To ensure a homogeneous mix.
5. Wipe liner applicator with clean gauze sponge and place small amount of mixed material on end of applicator instrument.	5. To prepare instrument for application of calcium hydroxide into preparation.
6. Apply material to deepest portions of tooth preparation.	6. Refer to your practice act to determine who is legally allowed to perform this duty.
7. If dentist applies material to tooth preparation, assistant should hold paper pad with left hand and gauze sponge with right hand under patient's chin (for right-handed operator).	7. To allow dentist to wipe instrument clean and reapply material if necessary.

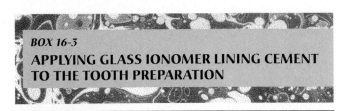

BOX 16-3
APPLYING GLASS IONOMER LINING CEMENT TO THE TOOTH PREPARATION

ARMAMENTARIUM

- Glass ionomer lining cement
  One bottle of powder
  One bottle of liquid
- Cement spatula
- Liner applicator instrument
- Small paper mixing pad
- Gauze sponge

PROCEDURE	RATIONALE
1. Place one scoop of powder and one drop of liquid on mixing pad. Place materials next to but not touching each other on mixing pad.	1. Glass ionomer lining cement consists of one bottle of liquid and one bottle of powder.
2. With spatula, quickly mix powder and liquid together until powder is completely incorporated in liquid.	2. Glass ionomer lining cement should be mixed quickly.
3. Wipe spatula.	3. Glass ionomer is very hard to remove from spatula if allowed to set.
4. Place small amount of mixed material on end of liner applicator instrument.	4. To prepare instrument for application of lining cement into tooth preparation.
5. Apply material to deepest portions of tooth preparation.	5. Refer to your state practice act to determine who is legally allowed to perform this duty.
6. If dentist applies material to tooth preparation, assistant should hold paper pad with the left hand and gauze sponge with right hand under patient's chin (for right-handed operator).	6. To allow dentist to wipe instrument clean and reapply material if necessary.

BOX 16-4
APPLYING A ZINC OXIDE AND EUGENOL CEMENT BASE TO THE TOOTH PREPARATION

ARMAMENTARIUM

- ZOE cement
  One bottle of powder
  One bottle of liquid
- Cement spatula
- Paper mixing pad
- Gauze sponge
- Plastic instrument or small amalgam plugger (condenser)
- Explorer

PROCEDURE	RATIONALE
1. Place one scoop of powder and one drop of liquid on mixing pad. Place materials next to but not touching each other on mixing pad.	1. ZOE cement base consists of one bottle of liquid and one bottle of powder.
2. Place small amount of powder aside on mixing pad.	2. Operator applies powder on plastic instrument or amalgam plugger to prevent base from sticking to instrument when applying material into tooth preparation.
3. Quickly mix powder into liquid in three or four increments until material is flaky and can be rolled into a small and slightly tacky ball.	3. To prepare material for placement in cavity preparation.
4. With explorer, place ball of cement base into appropriate area in tooth preparation.	4. Refer to your state practice act to determine who is legally allowed to perform this duty.
5. With amalgam plugger, lightly condense material into place.	5. Refer to your state practice act to determine who is legally allowed to perform this duty.
6. If dentist places cement base into tooth, then assistant holds mixing pad and remaining powder with left hand. With right hand, hold a gauze sponge under patient's chin (for right-handed operator).	6. To allow dentist to wipe instrument clean and use excess powder to prevent cement base from sticking to instrument.

> **→◦ KEY POINT**
> ▪ A common name for glass ionomer lining cement is GC Fuji Lining Cement.

Zinc Oxide and Eugenol Cement Base

ZOE cement base is available as one bottle of liquid and one bottle of powder (Box 16-4). Premeasured capsules have been recently introduced, and the capsules can be inserted into the amalgamator for mixing. The liquid contains eugenol, which gives the material an aromatic odor that in the past was often associated with dental offices. Although glass ionomer materials are becoming popular, ZOE is still used in many dental offices.

> **→◦ KEY POINT**
> ▪ A common name for ZOE is IRM.

Zinc Phosphate Cement Base

Instructions for mixing zinc phosphate cement base are presented on pp. 287-288, since it is an extension of the process of mixing cement that is used in the cementation of crowns and bridges.

• • •

Once cavity medication procedures are completed, the final restorative material can be prepared and placed in the cavity preparation.

BIBLIOGRAPHY

Charbeneau GT and others: *Principles and practice of operative dentistry,* ed 2, Philadelphia, 1981, Lea & Febiger.

Craig RG and others: *Dental materials review,* Ann Arbor, 1977, The University of Michigan School of Dentistry.

Craig RG and others: *Dental materials: properties and maniipulation,* ed 6, St Louis, 1996, Mosby.

Craig RG and others: *Restorative dental materials,* ed 9, St Louis, 1993, Mosby.

Ferrocane JL: *Materials in dentistry: principles and applications,* Philadelphia, 1995, JB Lippincott.

Grundy JR, Jones JG: *A colour atlas of clinical operative dentistry: crowns and bridges,* ed 2, London, 1992, Wolfe Publishing Ltd.

Sturdevant CM and others: *The art and science of operative dentistry,* ed 3, St Louis, 1995, Mosby.

Swift EJ: An update on glass ionomer cements, *Quin Intern* 19:125, 1988.

QUESTIONS—Chapter 16

1. Cavities that are located on the proximal surface of posterior teeth are class _____ cavities.
   a. I
   b. II
   c. III
   d. IV
   e. V

2. Cavities that are located on the cervical third of all teeth and originate on a smooth surface are class _____ cavities.
   a. I
   b. II
   c. III
   d. IV
   e. V

3. Cavities beginning in the pit and fissure areas of teeth are class _____ cavities.
   a. I
   b. II
   c. III
   d. IV
   e. V

4. The overall shape of the preparation along the external surface of the enamel is called the _____ form.
   a. Resistance
   b. Retention
   c. Outline

5. Which of the following material(s) can be used as cavity liners?
   1. Calcium hydroxide
   2. Zinc oxide and eugenol
   3. Glass ionomer
   4. Zinc phosphate
   a. 1 and 3
   b. 2 and 4
   c. 1, 2, and 3
   d. 4 only

6. Which of the following material(s) can be used as a cement base?
   1. Calcium hydroxide
   2. Zinc oxide and eugenol
   3. Glass ionomer
   4. Zinc phosphate
   a. 1 and 3
   b. 2 and 4
   c. 1, 2, and 3
   d. 4 only

7. Which of the following is the correct sequence for placement of medication in an amalgam cavity preparation?
   a. Cement base, cavity liner, varnish
   b. Cavity liner, cement base, varnish
   c. Varnish, cavity liner, cement base
   d. Cavity liner, varnish, cement base

8. Which of the following should not be used for a composite cavity restoration?
   1. Calcium hydroxide
   2. Varnish
   3. Glass ionomer
   4. Zinc oxide and eugenol
   a. 1 and 3
   b. 2 and 4
   c. 1, 2, and 3
   d. 4 only

9. How many layers of cavity varnish must be applied to the tooth preparation?
   a. One
   b. Two
   c. Three
   d. Four

10. Which of the following would be the correct measurement of powder to liquid for a zinc oxide and eugenol cement base?
    a. Two scoops powder to one drop of liquid
    b. Two scoops powder to three drops of liquid
    c. One scoop powder to one drop of liquid
    d. One scoop powder to two drops of liquid

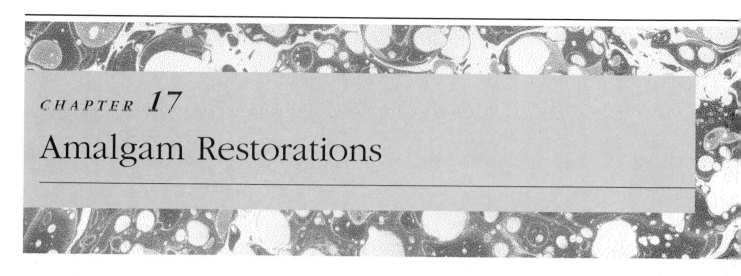

CHAPTER 17

Amalgam Restorations

KEY TERMS

Abrasive rubber polishing points
Amalgam
Amalgam carrier
Amalgam carvers
Amalgam condenser
Amalgam overhang
Amalgam well
Amalgamator
Articulating (carbon) paper
Autoclutch
Automatrix band
Burnisher
Capsule
Condensation
Contouring pliers
Dappen dish
Double-shear pins
Interproximal wedge
Matrix band
Pestle
Premeasured amalgam capsules
Retention pins
Spill
Tofflemire retainer
Trituration
Twist drill
Universal circumferential matrix band

Silver amalgam is the most common restoration used to-day. **Amalgam** is defined as an alloy of an element or a metal with mercury as one of its components. Since most dental amalgam contains approximately 40% to 70% sil-

ver, it is referred to as silver amalgam. The public refers to these restorations as silver fillings.

The amalgam restoration has been used since 1833. Its widespread use is primarily the result of the fact that it is a highly successful restoration. In addition, it is a relatively easy material to manipulate and is a relatively inexpensive restoration for the patient.

Silver amalgam has its limitations. It must not be subjected to excessive biting forces, and it must be well supported by tooth structure.

Teeth that have been subjected to massive damage through fracture or dental caries cannot be adequately restored for long periods with amalgam. These teeth are candidates for gold and/or porcelain restorations if maximum success is to be achieved.

COMMON AMALGAM INSTRUMENTS AND SUPPLIES

Certain instruments and accessories are specifically required for the fabrication of an amalgam restoration (silver filling). These, along with some of the general operative instruments already discussed, are assembled on a preset tray or placed in the operatory for use during the procedure.

Amalgam Restorative Material

Disposable **premeasured amalgam capsules** are the most popular form in which amalgam is dispensed (Figure 17-1). Each color-coded **capsule** contains a preweighed amount of silver alloy powder separated from a preweighed amount of mercury. It may also contain a small mixing device called a **pestle** that assists in the mixing process.

This type of packaging is safe, convenient, and accurate. Since the ingredients are preweighed and packaged by the manufacturer, minimal handling is required before the mixing process.

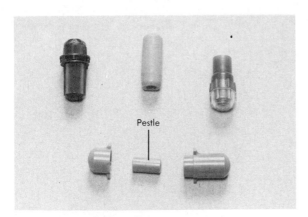

Figure 17-1   Amalgam capsules. *Top,* Various styles of pre-measured capsules. *Bottom,* conventional style of capsule and pestle used with bulk or tablet forms of amalgam

Premeasured capsules are available in three to five various weights, called a **spill** of material. One of the most popular spill weights, a single-spill capsule is used for small cavity preparations, and double and triple spills are used for larger ones.

> ☙ **KEY POINTS**
> - Premeasured capsules are usually color coded to indicate single, double, and triple spills.
> - A dentist may use premeasured capsules with different spills to fill a tooth preparation.

A less common form of dispensing amalgam is the use of a nondisposable mixing capsule and pestle that use a tablet form of silver alloy. An amalgam-dispensing device is used to place one or two tablets in the capsule (with the pestle) and the appropriate amount of mercury.

> ☙ **KEY POINTS**
> - Excess amalgam must be removed from nondisposable mixing capsules and pestles to avoid contaminating the next mixture of amalgam.
> - Nondisposable mixing capsules should be tested for leakage by placing transparent tape over the seal, mixing a normal spill, and then observing the tape for any leakage.

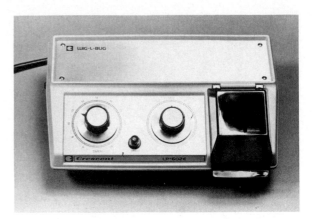

Figure 17-2   Amalgamator.

Amalgamators

An **amalgamator** (Figure 17-2) is a machine that mixes mercury with silver alloy to produce amalgam. A disposable premeasured capsule is prepared for mixing by squeezing or twisting the ends. This breaks the foil barrier separating the alloy powder from the mercury in the capsule. The prepared capsule is inserted in the amalgamator, which shakes the capsule back and forth rapidly and mixes the mercury and alloy together. Amalgamators are equipped with a timer to control the mixing time. This mixing process is called **trituration.** The trituration time increases proportionately to the amount of amalgam mixed. Exact trituration times must be determined according to the manufacturer's recommendations. All mixing of mercury should be done over a lipped tray to prevent spilling of this hazardous material.

Amalgam Carriers

After the amalgam material is mixed (triturated) in the amalgamator, it must be transferred to the cavity preparation in small increments to ensure proper filling of the preparation. An **amalgam carrier** (Figure 17-3) is convenient for this purpose.

Carriers are filled with amalgam by pressing the opening of the instrument into the mix. This forces the material into the barrel of the carrier. After transfer to the prepared tooth the material can be expelled from the barrel by pressing a lever or a plunger that activates a small piston in the barrel. The piston pushes the material out of the barrel into the preparation. The carrier is refilled repeatedly until the preparation is completely filled with amalgam.

Both syringe and lever-action carriers are available. The lever style is available in both single- and double-ended models. Some manufacturers offer carrier models with different barrel sizes.

A **dappen dish** or a special amalgam holding dish sometimes called an **amalgam well** can be used to consolidate the mixed material and facilitate filling the amalgam carrier (Figure 17-4).

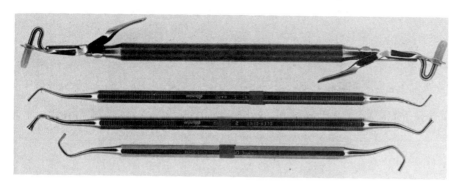

Figure 17-3 Amalgam instruments. *Top to bottom*: Amalgam carrier, No. 1 Ward condenser, No. 2 Ward condenser, No. 6B Clev-Dent back-action condenser.

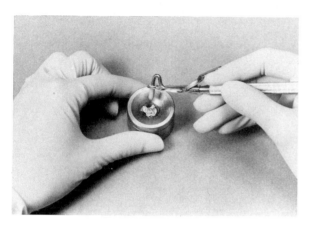

Figure 17-4 Amalgam well used to consolidate amalgam mix while carrier is filled.

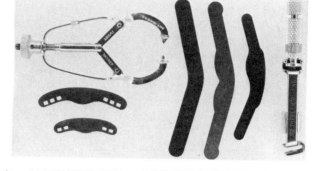

Figure 17-5 Matrix retainers and bands. *Left to right*: Ivory retainer with bands, Tofflemire retainer with assorted bands.

◆ KEY POINTS
- Carefully transfer the amalgam carrier to the dentist because the amalgam could fall out of the carrier if the instrument or assistant's hand is suddenly jarred.
- The dentist usually uses the smaller end of the carrier first to fill the interproximal spaces.

Amalgam Condensers

An **amalgam condenser** (see Figure 17-3) is an instrument with a flat surface on the working end that is used to press amalgam against the cavity walls and floors.

Both automatic and hand-operated condensers are available. Hand instruments are more popular by far. They are usually double ended, with one end smaller than the other. Hand condensers are available in different styles and sizes. They are generally considered superior to automatic condensers, which tend to bring too much mercury to the surface too quickly.

Dentists usually prefer to condense with a small condenser until the preparation is one half to two thirds full. The remaining additions of amalgam material are condensed with a larger condenser. This ensures excellent adaptation of the restorative material to cavity walls and in retentive areas.

Matrix Bands

A **matrix band** (Figure 17-5) is a thin strip of stainless steel sheet metal that is used to create a form around a prepared tooth. Matrix bands are needed only for cavity preparations that are not completely surrounded by tooth structure. Examples of such preparations are classes II, III, and VI and those for teeth that are even more extensively damaged. Class I and V cavity preparations are completely surrounded by tooth structure and do not require matrix bands.

A matrix band serves a dentist in the same manner that a form for concrete serves a construction worker. It contains the restorative material in a desired place and gives it shape. After the restorative material acquires its desired shape, the matrix, or form, can be removed.

Amalgam is inserted into the cavity preparation with an amalgam carrier. Then it is pressed into place to adapt the material tightly against the cavity walls and the matrix band. This process is called condensation. **Condensation** provides a good seal to prevent excessive leakage of the restoration in the future. Condensation also improves the strength of the amalgam to resist fracture. To achieve adequate condensation in cavity preparations that have open aspects, the dentist uses the matrix band as a metal wall to pack the amalgam against. Without the matrix band, the amalgam material would simply flow out of the open aspect of the preparation when con-

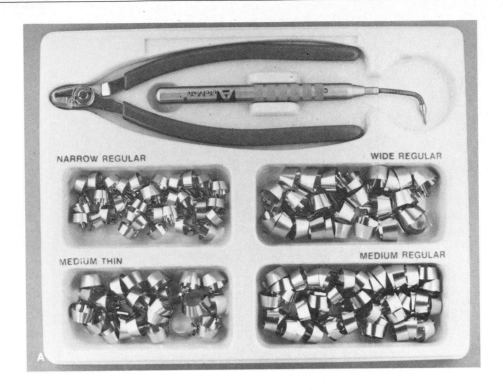

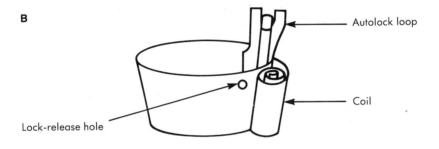

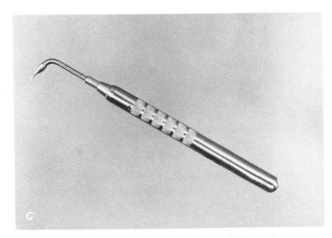

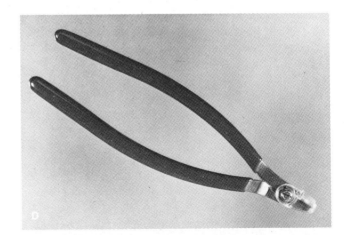

Figure 17-6 **A,** Automatrix retainerless system. **B,** Automatrix band. **C,** Automate II tightening device. **D,** Shielded nippers.

(**A** Courtesy L.D. Caulk Co., Milford, Del. From Sturdevant CM: *The art and science of operative dentistry,* ed 3, St Louis, 1995, Mosby.)

densation pressure is applied to the material (see Figure 17-17).

Matrix bands are available in many different types and brands. The two most common types are the **universal circumferential matrix band** and the **Automatrix band.**

The universal circumferential matrix band has two ends that must be held together to form a loop with a special device called a matrix retainer.

The Automatrix retainerless system is shown in Figure 17-6, *A*. The Automatrix band (Figure 17-6, *B*) is already formed into a loop and does not need a matrix retainer. The Automatrix band uses an automatic tightening device (Figure 17-6, *C*) to close the matrix loop so that it is secure around the tooth. A special cutting device called shielded nippers (Figure 17-6, *D*) is used to cut the Automatrix band for removal.

Matrix Retainers

Matrix bands are held in place around a prepared tooth either by an adjustable clamp called the matrix retainer or a preformed retainerless (Automatrix) band is tightened around the tooth using a special tightening device. Figure 17-5 shows two styles of retainers. The **Tofflemire retainer** is by far the most popular retainer today. It is used with various styles of circumferential matrix bands.

Contouring Pliers

Contouring pliers (Figure 17-7, *A*) can shape matrix bands to conform to a prepared tooth. The matrix band is squeezed in the beaks of the pliers, which press it into the desired shape.

Interproximal Wedge

Although the matrix band is held tightly against the tooth by the retainer, a small amount of amalgam can still escape, under condensation pressure, from the preparation between the tooth and the band. This is not of major significance except in cervical areas of preparations on proximal surfaces. These areas are rather inaccessible to carving, and the potential for excess amalgam to become lodged interproximally is great. Excess amalgam along the cervical margin is commonly referred to as an **amalgam overhang**. Overhangs are damaging to surrounding tissues if they are allowed to remain (see Chapter 22). All other areas of the restoration can easily be trimmed with carving instruments because the operator has access to them.

The best way to treat an overhang is to prevent it in the first place. This can be done with an **interproximal wedge** (Figure 17-7, *B*). The wedge is usually a triangular wooden or plastic stick that is inserted between the teeth after the matrix band is placed. The wedge is forced tightly into place between the teeth (Figure 17-7, *C*). The wedge then acts as a brace to hold the matrix band tightly against the tooth to ensure that amalgam cannot escape into the interproximal area during condensation.

Another benefit of the wedge is that when it is in place, it separates the teeth slightly to compensate for the thickness of the matrix band. The amalgam is then inserted and condensed. When the matrix band is removed, there is a space the thickness of the matrix band between the new restoration and the adjacent tooth, which is closed as the separated teeth move back together. Dentists use their own judgment in determining the amount of separation that is desirable.

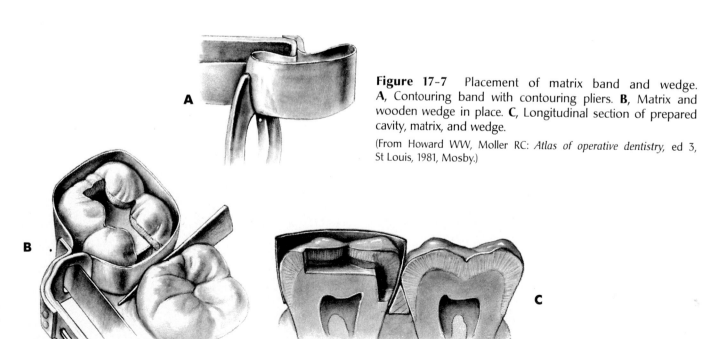

Figure 17-7 Placement of matrix band and wedge. **A**, Contouring band with contouring pliers. **B**, Matrix and wooden wedge in place. **C**, Longitudinal section of prepared cavity, matrix, and wedge.

(From Howard WW, Moller RC: *Atlas of operative dentistry*, ed 3, St Louis, 1981, Mosby.)

Table 17-1 Indications for use of interproximal wedge

Amalgam preparation cavity classification	Matrix band needed?	Number of wedges
Class I	No	None
Class II	Yes	1
Class III	Yes	1
Class V	No	None
Class VI	Yes	2
Larger than class VI	Yes	2 if both mesial and distal aspects are involved
Exceptions: Preparations with cervical margins on distal aspect of last molars or on teeth with adjacent teeth missing	Yes	Wedge only cervical margin adjacent to another tooth

A wedge is needed in an interproximal space only where there is a prepared cervical margin. Hence a class II amalgam preparation requires one wedge, and a class VI mesioocclusodistal (MOD) requires two wedges. Wedges cannot be used when there is no adjacent tooth to wedge against, as on the distal aspect of the last molars and in areas of missing teeth. Overhangs that might occur in these regions are readily accessible to carvers for removal.

> **⇒ KEY POINTS**
> - An interproximal wedge prevents over-hangs.
> - An interproximal wedge can only be placed between two teeth.

Table 17-1 reviews the need for matrix bands and interproximal wedges in amalgam preparations.

Preparation of the Tofflemire Matrix Assembly

Since the Tofflemire, or circumferential, matrix assembly is the most common amalgam matrix used, an explanation of how to assemble it for use in various quadrants of the oral cavity is warranted.

Figure 17-8 demonstrates the parts of the Tofflemire retainer. These parts function as follows:

Frame The main body of the retainer to which the vise, spindle, and adjustment knobs are attached.
Vise A clamplike device that holds the ends of the matrix band in the retainer.
Spindle A screwlike rod used to lock the ends of the matrix band in the vise.
Outer knob An adjustment knob used to tighten the spindle against the band in the vise.

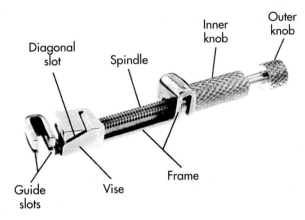

Figure 17-8 Tofflemire matrix retainer.

Inner knob An adjustment knob used to slide the vise along the frame to either increase or decrease the size of the matrix band loop.
Guide slots Slots that enable matrix band loop positioning in the direction of choice.

For purposes of orientation, two important aspects of the retainer must be recognized (Figure 17-9):

Occlusal aspect The openings of the guide slots on the end of the retainer, as well as the diagonal slot in the vise, are not visible.
Gingival aspect The openings of the guide slots on the end of the retainer, as well as the diagonal slot in the vise, are visible.

Once the dental assistant can identify the parts of the retainer and their functions, as well as recognize the occlusal and gingival aspects of the retainer, the preparation of the matrix assembly is simplified.

The procedures for preparing the Tofflemire retainer and the matrix band are described in Box 17-1.

If the loop is positioned above the retainer, it is prepared for use in either the patient's lower left or upper right quadrant (Figure 17-10, *D*). On the other hand, if the loop is positioned below the retainer, it is prepared for use in either the patient's lower right or upper left quadrant (Figure 17-10, *E*).

> **⇒ KEY POINTS**
> - A Tofflemire retainer and matrix band setup for the upper right quadrant will fit the lower left quadrant.
> - A Tofflemire retainer and matrix band setup for the upper left quadrant will fit the lower right quadrant.

Another and perhaps more convenient way to identify the correct orientation of the band is to hold the retainer so that the guide-slot end is away from you. If the retainer

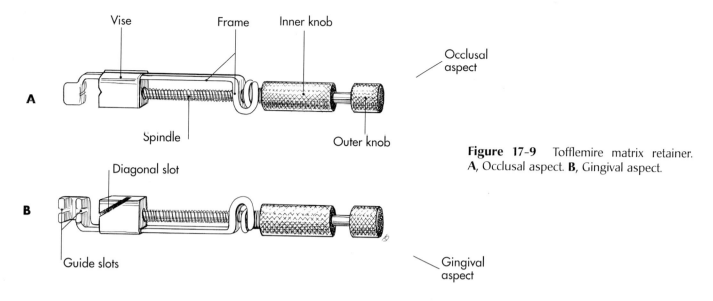

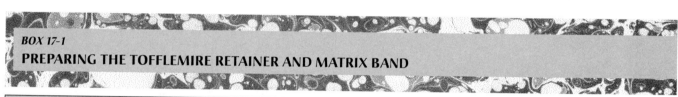

Figure 17-9 Tofflemire matrix retainer. **A**, Occlusal aspect. **B**, Gingival aspect.

BOX 17-1

PREPARING THE TOFFLEMIRE RETAINER AND MATRIX BAND

PROCEDURE	RATIONALE	PROCEDURE	RATIONALE
1. Hold retainer by vise in left hand so that gingival aspect is visible.	1. To prepare retainer for insertion of matrix band.	8. At same time, thread joined band through guide slot next to vise.	8. To prepare retainer to secure two ends of matrix band.
2. Turn outer knob clockwise until end of spindle is visible in diagonal slot in vise (Figure 17-10, *A*).	2. To engage spindle in diagonal slot.	9. Continue threading joined band so that it emerges from between prongs of guide slots. Once loop is positioned, seat band completely in slots.	9. To ensure that both ends will be secured in retainer.
3. Turn inner knob until vise moves to within approximately 3/16 inch of guide slots at end of retainer.	3. This moves vise close to guide slots to make it easier to insert matrix band.		
4. Turn outer knob counterclockwise until tip of spindle just disappears from view in diagonal slot in vise. Retainer is now ready for insertion of matrix band (Figure 17-10, *B*).	4. To move spindle out of diagonal slot so that matrix band can be placed.	10. Turn outer knob clockwise to clamp band in vise.	10. To secure both ends of matrix band in retainer.
5. Hold matrix band so it forms shape of a smile (Figure 17-10, *C*).	5. To obtain correct orientation of matrix band for insertion into retainer.	11. If loop has been flattened somewhat by placement in retainer, handle end of mouth mirror can be used to make loop round again (see Figure 17-12). Once loop is rounded, size of loop can be made larger or smaller by turning inner knob as needed. Diameter of tooth being restored dictates approximate size of loop.	11. To reshape matrix band if loop has become flattened.
6. Bring ends of band together so loop is formed.	6. Both ends of matrix band must be inserted into retainer.		
7. With gingival aspect of retainer toward you, slide joined ends of band, occlusal edge first, into diagonal slot of vise.	7. To prepare retainer to secure two ends of matrix band.		

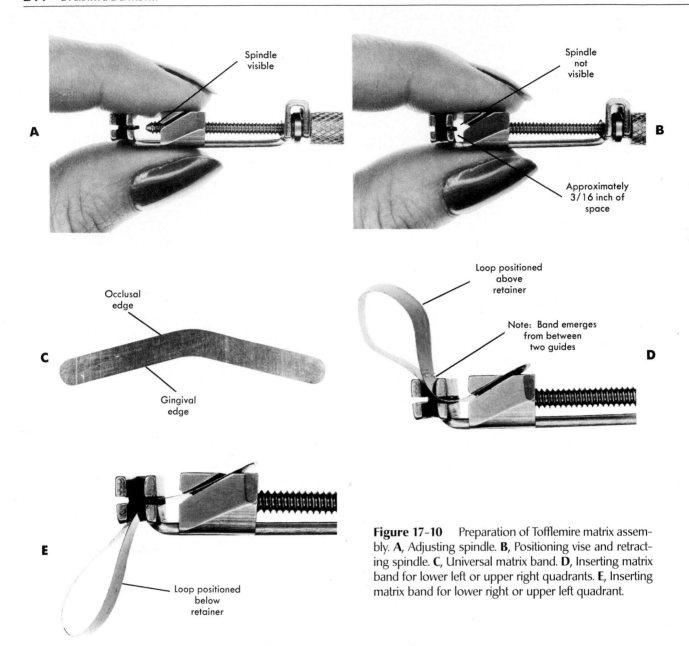

Figure 17-10   Preparation of Tofflemire matrix assembly. **A,** Adjusting spindle. **B,** Positioning vise and retracting spindle. **C,** Universal matrix band. **D,** Inserting matrix band for lower left or upper right quadrants. **E,** Inserting matrix band for lower right or upper left quadrant.

and band assembly are used for lower teeth, the guide-slot openings are positioned downward toward the gingiva. The band loop is positioned to the right of the retainer if it is used on the patient's right side (Figure 17-11, *A*). If the retainer is used on the patient's left side, the band loop is positioned to the left of the retainer (Figure 17-11, *B*).

If the retainer is used on upper teeth, the guide-slot openings are positioned upward toward the gingiva. Again, the band loop is positioned to the right of the retainer for use on the patient's right side (Figure 17-11, *C*) and to the left of the retainer for use on the patient's left side (Figure 17-11, *D*). If the loop has been flattened by placement in the retainer, use the handle end of a mouth mirror to make the loop round again (Figure 17-12).

When the assembly is placed, the retainer is located on the buccal aspect of the tooth being restored. Further, the gingival aspect of the retainer is always placed toward the

gingiva to facilitate removal once the amalgam has been inserted in the tooth.

> ◆❖ **KEY POINTS**
> - The Tofflemire retainer is usually placed on the buccal aspect of the teeth.
> - The retainer should be placed onto the tooth so that it can be lifted easily off the tooth in the occlusal direction.
> - The assistant should prepare the matrix assembly as part of the operatory preparation sequence so that delays can be avoided when the matrix is needed during the procedure. (In many states dental assistants are now allowed to place matrix.)

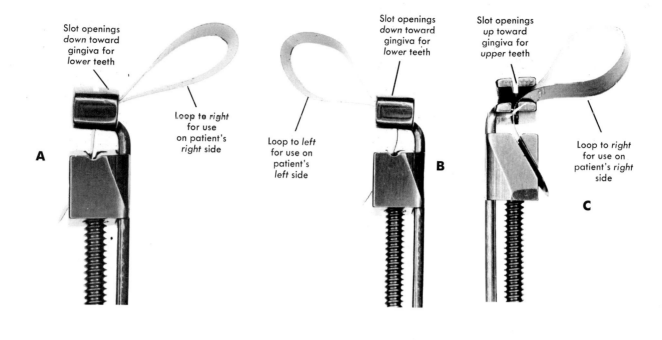

Slot openings *down* toward gingiva for *lower* teeth

Loop to *right* for use on patient's *right* side

A

Slot openings *down* toward gingiva for *lower* teeth

Loop to *left* for use on patient's *left* side

B

Slot openings *up* toward gingiva for *upper* teeth

Loop to *right* for use on patient's *right* side

C

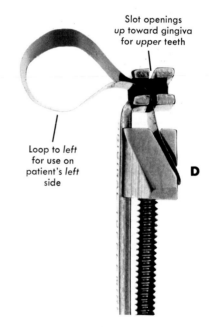

Slot openings *up* toward gingiva for *upper* teeth

Loop to *left* for use on patient's *left* side

D

Figure 17-11 Common configurations of Tofflemire matrix assembly. **A,** Used in lower right quadrant. **B,** Used in lower left quadrant. **C,** Used in upper right quadrant. **D,** Used in upper left quadrant.

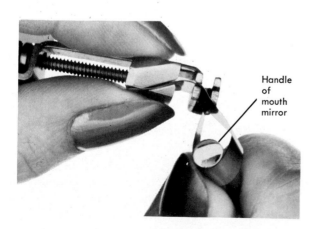

Handle of mouth mirror

Figure 17-12 Rounding loop using handle end of mirror.

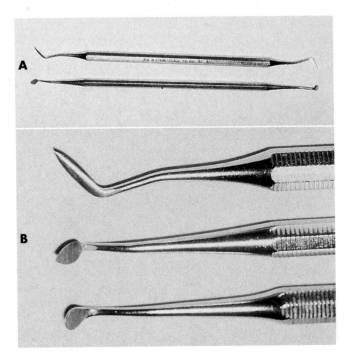

Figure 17-13 Amalgam carvers. **A**, *Top,* Hollenbeck carver; *bottom,* discoid-cleoid carver. **B**, *Top to bottom:* Hollenbeck, cleoid, discoid.

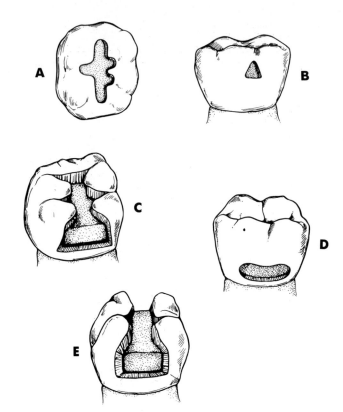

Figure 17-14 Common classes of cavity preparations used for amalgam restorations. **A** and **B**, Class I. **C**, Class II. **D**, Class V. **E**, Class VI (MOD). (See also Table 16-1.)

Amalgam Carvers

Every dentist has favorite **amalgam carvers**. Two of the more popular designs are shown in Figure 17-13, *A*.

The cleoid-discoid and half Hollenbeck carvers facilitate the carving of the occlusal aspect of a restoration. Their design permits easier establishment of cusp inclines and occlusal grooves and fossae in the restoration (Figure 17-13, *B*).

> **KEY POINT**
> ▪ During the carving process the assistant should be using the oral evacuator to pick up excess amalgam.

Burnishers

A **burnisher** is a smooth-tipped hand instrument used to smooth and enhance the occlusal anatomy of an amalgam restoration (see Chapter 6). Burnishers are used immediately after the carving phase if the dentist chooses to employ them. Their use is not mandatory.

> **KEY POINT**
> ▪ The acorn carver is a very commonly used burnisher.

AMALGAM RESTORATIVE PROCEDURE
Amalgam Cavity Preparations

Amalgam cavity preparation designs incorporate the principles discussed previously with regard to outline, retention, and resistance forms. Figure 17-14 shows some conventional cavity preparation designs.

Armamentarium

The instrument selection and arrangement vary considerably between operators. The armamentarium in Figure 17-15 is an example of a typical setup for any amalgam procedure. Any materials that cannot be processed on the preset tray should be kept in an immediate-access area for auxiliary items.

If rubber dam isolation is used, a separate preset tray is required in addition to the armamentarium shown in Figure 17-15. Strict adherence to infection control measures is essential.

Fabrication of an Amalgam Restoration: Class II Example

Although the specific technique used in the fabrication of an amalgam restoration may vary from one dentist to another, virtually all techniques follow the same fundamental steps. When a dentist restores a tooth with a class

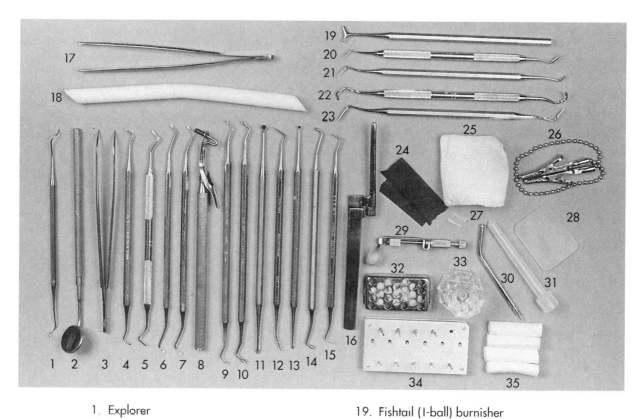

Figure 17-15   Amalgam restoration armamentarium.

(From Finkbeiner BL, Johnson CS: *Mosby's comprehensive dental assisting: a clinical approach,* St Louis, 1995, Mosby.)

1. Explorer
2. Mirror
3. Cotton pliers
4. Spoon excavator
5. Enamel hatchet
6. Mesial gingival marginal trimmer
7. Distal gingival marginal trimmer
8. Amalgam carrier
9. #1 Condenser
10. #2 Condenser
11. #7 Cleoid-discoid carver
12. Ward's carver
13. #5 Cleoid-discoid carver
14. #21B Anatomical burnisher
15. Ball burnisher
16. Articulating paper holder
17. Thumb forceps
18. HVE tip

19. Fishtail (1-ball) burnisher
20. Hollenback carver
21. Smooth and anatomical carver
22. Back-action condenser
23. Wesco 25
24. Articulating paper
25. 2 × 2 gauze
26. Patient napkin chain
27. Wedges
28. Plastic film divider to mix liners
29. Tofflemire matrix band and retainer
30. Air/water syringe tip
31. Air/water syringe tip cover
32. Cotton pellets
33. Dappen dish
34. Assorted burs
35. Cotton rolls

II amalgam restoration, the following fundamental steps are employed:

1. Anesthetic administration
2. Isolation
3. Cavity preparation
4. Cavity medication
5. Matrix placement
6. Insertion
7. Initial carving
8. Matrix removal
9. Final carving
10. Polishing
11. Postoperative instructions

Anesthetic administration

The appropriate area is anesthetized, and the standard anesthetic setup and technique, as described in Chapter 4, are used.

The dental assistant hands the dentist the topical anesthetic for application. In some states the dental assistant is allowed to place the topical anesthetic. The dental assistant assembles the anesthetic syringe and passes it to the operator for administration. Following local anesthetic administration, the dental assistant rinses the patient's oral cavity.

Isolation

The area treated is isolated with one of the isolation techniques described in Chapter 8. Good isolation technique is extremely important because it provides maximum visibility and access to the operating area. In addition, the quality of the finished restoration is enhanced because proper isolation prevents contamination of the restorative material.

The dental assistant places the rubber dam clamp on the rubber dam forceps and passes the forceps to the operator. The rubber dam is placed by the assistant and the dentist. The dentist usually places the septal portion between the teeth, and the dental assistant uses dental floss to push the dam between the teeth. The assistant uses the air-water syringe to blow air on the rubber dam while the dentist inverts or tucks the rubber dam around the teeth. In most states the dental assistant is allowed to place the rubber dam.

Cavity preparation

Most dentists follow a pattern in cavity preparation. The first phase is cutting through the hard enamel layer—*opening the cavity*. This is often done with a No. 35 in-

verted cone bur, a round bur, a diamond fissure bur, or a No. 245 bur. These burs are efficient instruments for cutting through the very hard enamel layer. After being opened, the cavity is enlarged to gain the necessary outline, retention, and resistance forms. This is accomplished very well with any of the side-cutting burs, such as a No. 56 plain fissure bur or a No. 171 plain tapered fissure bur (Figure 17-16, *A* and *B*).

The refinement of the cavity preparation is accomplished by scraping the walls and floors with enamel hatchets, chisels, and gingival margin trimmers.

If the carious lesion extends beyond the desired form of the cavity preparation, the caries is removed with slow-speed round burs and spoon excavators. This is a precautionary measure to avoid removing more tooth structure than absolutely necessary.

After the cutting and refining procedures have been completed (Figure 17-16, *C*) the cavity medication phase begins.

During the cavity preparation stage the dental assistant changes the burs on the dental handpieces and uses an instrument transfer technique to pass the hand instruments to the dentist.

Cavity medication

Cavity medication is discussed in detail in Chapter 16. If caries has extended beyond the normal cavity prepara-

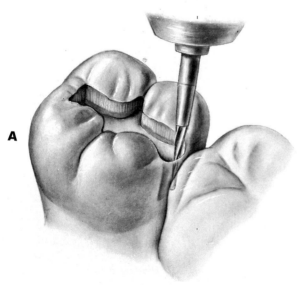
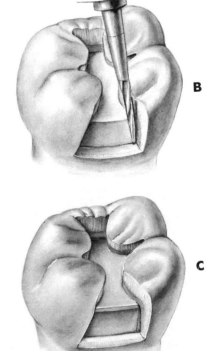

Figure 17-16 Preparation of class II amalgam cavity. **A,** Gaining outline form. **B,** Creating retention and resistance form. **C,** Finished preparation.

(From Howard WW, Moller RC: *Atlas of operative dentistry,* ed 3, St Louis, 1981, Mosby.)

tion depth, cement bases are used to replace destroyed dentin.

During the cavity medication stage the dental assistant mixes the appropriate bases and liners. The assistant passes the liner applicator and other hand instruments to the dentist. At least three gauze sponges are held to wipe off excess material from the instruments. In some states the dental assistant is allowed to place the base and/or liner.

Matrix placement

Matrix bands are placed around the prepared tooth to create a form, or mold, into which the soft amalgam is placed.

Once the band is in place around the tooth, it must be forced against the cervical margin of the proximal box with an interproximal wedge. The retainer is placed along the buccal surfaces of the teeth when it is in position. The wedge is usually inserted from the lingual aspect. (It should be noted that if a cavity preparation has both mesial and distal proximal boxes to be restored, two wedges are needed.)

The dental assistant assembles the matrix band and passes the interproximal wedge to the dentist. In some states the dental assistant is allowed to place the matrix band and wedge or wedges.

Insertion

Once the matrix band and wedge are in place, the amalgam is triturated (mixed) and placed in the cavity preparation with an amalgam carrier.

The dental assistant can place the amalgam directly in the preparation while the dentist condenses it in place, or the assistant can alternately exchange the carrier and condenser with the dentist as the amalgam is placed and condensed in the preparation. The amalgam is placed in the deepest portion of the cavity preparation first.

Condensation of the amalgam has two basic purposes:
- To adapt the material to the cavity walls
- To eliminate excess mercury from the mix to strengthen the restoration

Condensation is usually done by hand with a condenser or plugger. Amalgam is added in small increments and condensed until the cavity is slightly overfilled. Figure 17-17 demonstrates this process.

During the condensation phase the dental assistant may alternate transferring the amalgam carrier and different-sized condensers to the dentist.

Initial carving

Before the matrix band is removed, the excess amalgam on the occlusal surface can be carved away with a

Figure 17-17 Insertion and condensation of amalgam in prepared cavity. Small increments of amalgam are inserted and condensed in cavity until it is overfilled.

(From Howard WW, Moller RC: *Atlas of operative dentistry*, ed 3, St Louis, 1981, Mosby.)

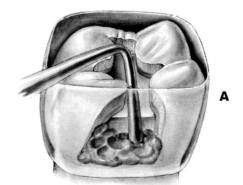

A

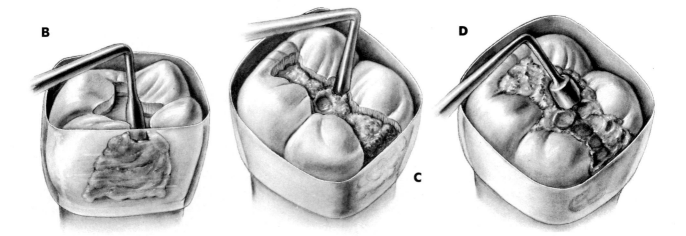

B

C

D

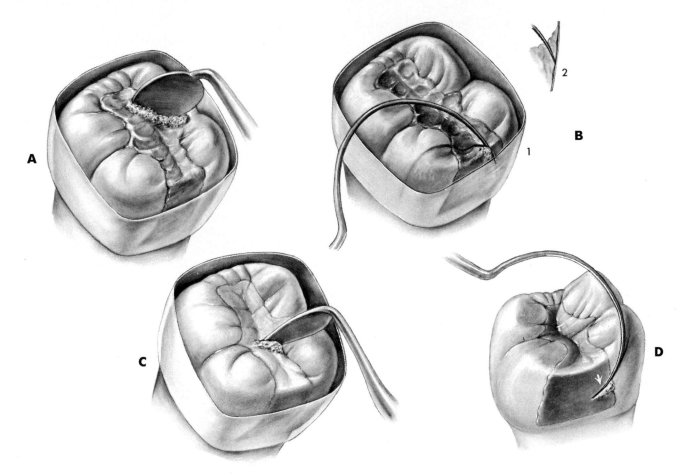

Figure 17-18   Carving amalgam. **A**, Carving away excess amalgam. **B**, Relieving marginal ridge. *1* and *2*, Relationship of explorer tip to matrix band. **C**, Carving occlusal anatomy. **D**, Carving smooth–surface margins.

(From Howard WW, Moller RC: *Atlas of operative dentistry*, ed 3, St Louis, 1981, Mosby.)

cleoid-discoid carver (Figure 17-18). A popular instrument often used for initial carving is the acorn burnisher. In addition, a small portion of amalgam must be removed between the matrix band and the marginal ridge of the restoration (Figure 17-18, *B*). This minimizes the possibility of fracturing the new restoration during band removal.

During all carving procedures the assistant should keep the evacuator tip close to the restoration so that amalgam shavings are removed as soon as they are carved away. This is especially important when rubber dam isolation is not used.

Matrix removal

The matrix band retainer and wedge assembly are usually removed in the following order: retainer, wedge, and band. The wedge and the band can be removed with cotton pliers or a small hemostat. The band must be removed in a bucco-occlusal direction to avoid fracturing the still-soft amalgam restoration.

Final carving

While the amalgam is still soft, it is advisable to carve the less accessible areas first to remove any amalgam that may have squeezed out of the cavity preparation during condensation. These areas are the buccal and lingual proximal margins, as well as the cervical margins. A smooth surface carver such as the Ward C carver or the explorer is used for this purpose (Figure 17-18, *D*).

The occlusal portion of the restoration is then carved so that it contacts the opposing tooth properly when the jaws are closed together. If a rubber dam is used for isolation, it must be removed before the occlusion (bite) is established. The cleoid carver is an excellent choice for this procedure. The various anatomical grooves and cusp inclines can be formed very nicely with this instrument.

The dentist checks proper occlusion by having the patient close the jaws while holding a piece of **articulating (carbon) paper** on the biting surface. A heavy blue

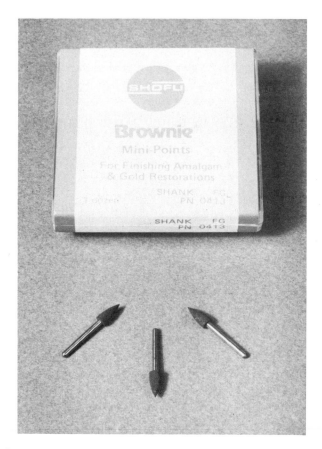

Figure 17-19 Abrasive rubber points used to polish metal restoration.

or red mark on the restoration indicates that the restoration is "high" and that it must be reduced to blend into the normal biting pattern of the patient.

Some dentists prefer to wipe the completed restoration with a moist cotton roll after carving. This helps to leave a smooth surface on the restoration.

The dental assistant may pass the carvers and burnishers to the dentist for the carving of the occlusal anatomy. The oral evacuator is used to help take away excess amalgam particles. The assistant also passes the articulating paper to the dentist or the assistant may hold the articulating paper between the patient's teeth to check the occlusion.

Polishing

The amalgam restoration can be polished after placement. Polishing smooths the surface of the metal so that plaque does not adhere to it readily and makes the restoration more attractive.

Polishing is accomplished by using a series of **abrasive rubber polishing points** and rubber cups. The points and cups fit into the handpiece. These points and cups are available in different grades of abrasiveness. The dentist usually uses the points and cups in this color order (Figure 17-19):

- Brownie (brown) abrasive rubber point/cup
- Greenie (green) abrasive rubber point/cup
- Super greenie (green with yellow stripe on shank) abrasive rubber point/cup

Postoperative instructions

Amalgam requires several hours to reach its maximum hardness. During this time the patient should be cautioned to protect the new restoration during meals. Hard-textured foods should be avoided.

Because amalgam conducts hot and cold much more quickly than normal tooth structure the patient should be warned that the tooth may be sensitive to hot and cold foods and drinks. This sensitivity may last for weeks to months but should gradually go away.

If the patient's mouth is still numb, caution should be taken with eating or drinking while still anesthetized. There is a risk of injuring the soft tissues or causing trauma with hot or cold foods.

This precaution is not as critical in small occlusal restorations or in class V restorations.

Class I, V, and VI Restorations

The class VI mesioocclusodistal (MOD) restoration (see Box 16-1) is fabricated in the same manner as the class II except that two wedges are required to adapt the cervical aspect of the band on both the mesial and distal surfaces of the preparation.

Class I and V restorations do not require use of a matrix band, since the entire cavity preparation is surrounded by walls of tooth structure. The preparation can be filled with amalgam and condensed into place by simply forcing it against these cavity walls.

Any restorations placed entirely on smooth surfaces require only the use of a smooth surface carver (Ward, Wall, or Hollenbeck carver) to shape the restoration properly.

BONDED AMALGAMS

A newer method of placing amalgam restorations is the use of a bonding material that acts as an adhesive between the amalgam and the tooth.

The following procedure describes the placement of amalgam bonding after the tooth has been prepared:

1. *Place calcium hydroxide base or glass ionomer lining cement (if needed).* If the cavity preparation is near the pulp a calcium hydroxide base can be placed for pulpal protection.
2. *Place matrix band and wedges (if needed).*
3. *Place acid conditioner.* Etch according to the manufacturer's recommendations, usually 15 to 30 seconds. Rinse and lightly dry.

4. *Place primer.* Mix primer and apply.
5. *Place bond agent.* The bond agent is applied over the primer. Usually a dual-cure bond agent is used.
6. *Place amalgam.* The amalgam is quickly mixed and condensed into the cavity preparation before the bond agent can set.

PIN-RETAINED AMALGAM RESTORATIONS

On occasion the dentist is confronted with a restorative problem that requires use of amalgam in substantially damaged teeth. For amalgam to be successful, it must be retained within the confines of the remaining tooth. When retention is reduced by loss of tooth structure, the amalgam can be retained by the use of **retention pins** along with the remaining tooth tissue.

All the pin techniques used today involve drilling holes into the dentin using a special **twist drill** provided by manufacturers of pin kits. Starter holes must be drilled between the pulp and the external portion of the root (Figure 17-20). After the starter holes are drilled, the appropriate type of twist drill is used to complete the holes.

While several types of pins have been used over the years, the threaded pin is the most widely used today. These pins are held in place by twisting the threaded pin into a slightly smaller hole made by a twist drill. The pin acts like a tiny screw and holds itself in place. The upper portion of the pin extends into the cavity preparation (Figure 17-21) so that amalgam can be condensed around it and thus retained.

Threaded pins are twisted into the pinhole using either a small hand wrench or a special handpiece chuck (**autoclutch**) for the conventional-speed handpiece. Pins that are placed using this instrument are mounted by the manufacturer in a plastic burlike shank, which holds the pin in the contra-angle. The pin is designed to shear off when it reaches the desired depth in the pinhole (Figure 17-22).

Some manufacturers make retainers that have two pins attached end to end and mounted in one plastic shank (Figure 17-23). These retainers are used when multiple pins are placed at the same time. The first pin shears off when the proper depth is reached; then the second pin can be placed in the next pinhole without reloading the contra-angle. These are referred to as **double-shear pins.** Threaded pins are available in a variety of diameters and are made from either stainless steel or titanium.

After the pins are inserted in a prepared tooth the matrix band and retainer are placed, and amalgam is condensed around the retention pins to restore the tooth. The matrix band is then removed, and the amalgam is carved with conventional instruments.

It should be noted that use of retention pins is not limited to amalgam restorations alone. If a tooth is extensively damaged as a result of caries or fracture, a center

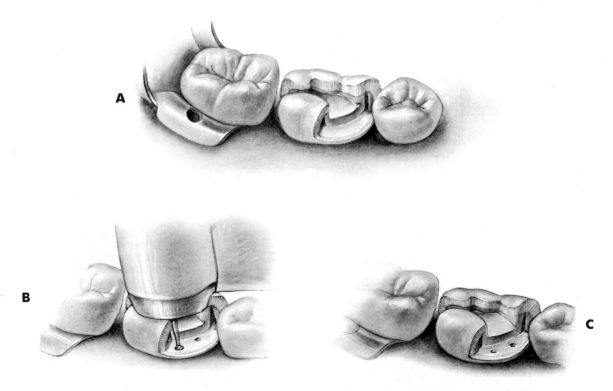

Figure 17-20   Retention pin placement. **A**, Prepared cavity. **B** and **C**, Placing starter holes.
(From Howard WW, Moller RC: *Atlas of operative dentistry*, ed 3, St Louis, 1981, Mosby.)

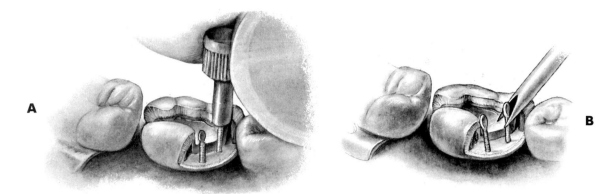

Figure 17-21   Threaded pins (Whaledent). **A,** Placing threaded pins using special wrench. **B,** Bending pins with special instrument provided with kit.

(From Howard WW, Moller RC: *Atlas of operative dentistry,* ed 3, St Louis, 1981, Mosby.)

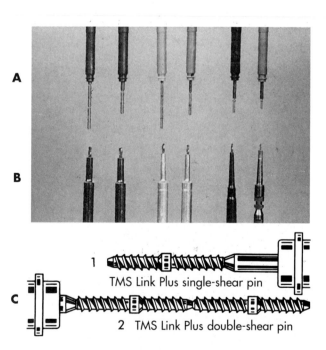

Figure 17-22   Threaded pins mounted in plastic shanks for use in autoclutch (high-torque) contra-angle. **A,** Various sizes of single- and double-shear threaded pins. **B,** Matching sizes of twist drills. **C,** Single- and double-shear pin styles.

(Courtesy Whaledent International, New York.)

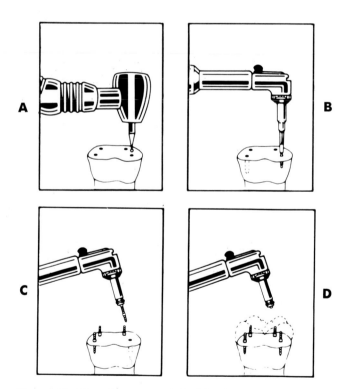

Figure 17-23   Placement of double-shear pin using high-torque contra-angle. **A,** Starter holes. **B,** Drill pin holes. **C,** Insert pins. **D,** Restored tooth.

(Courtesy Whaledent International, New York.)

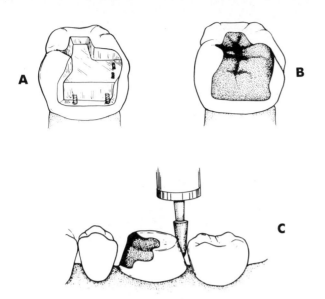

Figure 17-24 Amalgam core. **A,** Pin placement. **B,** Amalgam in place. **C,** Forming crown preparation.

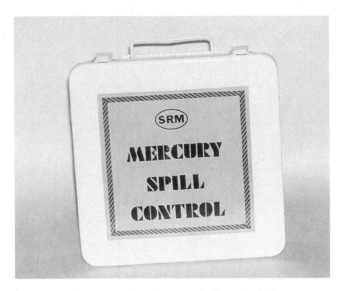

Figure 17-25 Mercury spill control kit.

core of amalgam can be placed, shaped properly after setting with burs and diamond stones, and then covered by a cast gold crown. The *amalgam core* is held in place by several pins, and the gold crown covering provides the necessary strength (Figure 17-24). Such cores are also fabricated from special composite core materials, as well as silver-impregnated glass ionomer cements.

AMALGAM OVERHANGS

It is possible to remove an amalgam overhang on an amalgam filling that has already hardened. Two methods follow:

1. *Use of a hand instrument such as a curette or gold knife.* The dentist or hygienist may use a curette or gold knife in a scalinglike action to shear off excess amalgam. The excess amalgam is removed a little at a time rather than in one large piece. Many scaling strokes may be needed for large overhangs; therefore a handpiece and the appropriate burs may be more efficient.
2. *Use of handpiece and appropriate burs.* Because of their thin shape, flame-type burs can be used to remove excess amalgam in the interproximal area. If possible, sandpaper disks may also be helpful.

SAFETY PRECAUTIONS

Research has shown there is a potential hazard to the health of dental personnel who come in contact with mercury or mercury-containing substances, such as amalgam. Dental assistants are vulnerable, since they mix mercury with the silver alloy and dispose of the excess amalgam material.

Although mercury can be absorbed through the skin, poisoning commonly results from aspiration of mercury vapors in the lungs. Mercury poisoning results in a wide variety of signs and symptoms depending on the total accumulation of mercury in the body.

The vulnerability of dental personnel in general practice is significant because the amalgam restorative procedure is the predominant service provided by the general practitioner. As a result the following measures are recommended to minimize the risk of mercury poisoning:

1. Use premeasured amalgam capsules to reduce the contact with mercury and to minimize the risk of mercury spillage.
2. Use an amalgamator with a protective cover to confine any capsule leakage to a limited area. Placement of the amalgamator in a covered area of a cabinet also helps to confine contamination to a small area.
3. Store scrap amalgam left over from a procedure in a tightly sealed plastic container. Previous recommendations suggested placing amalgam scrap in glycerin, water, or x-ray fixer. However, newer regulations recommend storing the scrap by itself because any solution that the amalgam scrap is placed in will also become a hazardous waste.
4. Purchase a mercury spill kit to clean up any accidental mercury spills (Figure 17-25).
5. Do not allow scrap amalgam and spilled mercury to accumulate in cabinetry, in the crevices of the dental chair, or on the floor of the operatory. Always mix mercury over a lipped tray.
6. Use water spray and central evacuation during the removal of an existing amalgam restoration to avoid creation of mercury dust in the breathing zone of the operating team.

7. Exclude all food, drink, and smoking materials from the work area.
8. Consider using monitoring devices periodically to assess the contamination level of the work area.
9. Analyze urine samples of dental personnel periodically.

It should be noted that no evidence of danger of mercury poisoning exists for patients who have amalgam restorations placed in their teeth.

BIBLIOGRAPHY

Craig RG: *Restorative dental materials,* ed 9, St Louis, 1993, Mosby.

Craig RG, O'Brien WJ, Powers JM: *Dental materials: properties and manipulation,* ed 6, St Louis, 1995, Mosby.

Finkbeiner BL, Johnson CS: *Mosby's comprehensive dental assisting: a clinical approach,* St Louis, 1995, Mosby.

Grundy JR, Jones JG: *Colour atlas of clinical operative dentistry: crowns and bridges,* ed 2, London, 1992, Wolfe.

Johnson KF: Mercury hygiene, *Dent Clin North Am* 22:3, 1978.

May KN, Heymann HO: Depth of penetration of Link Series and Link Plus pins, *Gen Dent* 34(5):359, 1986.

McLean JW, Gasser O: Glass-cermet cements, *Quint Intern* 16(5):333, 1985.

Rao GS, Hefferen JJ: Toxicity of mercury. In Smith DC, Williams DF, editors: *Biocompatibility of dental materials,* vol 3, Boca Raton, Fla, 1982, CRC Press.

Sturdevant CM and others: *The art and science of operative dentistry,* ed 3, St Louis, 1995, Mosby.

QUESTIONS–Chapter 17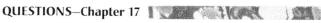

1. The mixing process of amalgam is called _____.
   a. Condensation
   b. Trituration
   c. Burnishing
   d. Carving

2. The term used for the packing of the amalgam in a tooth preparation with a plugger type of instrument is _____.
   a. Condensation
   b. Trituration
   c. Burnishing
   d. Carving

3. Which of the following can be used to carve the amalgam restoration after it has been placed?
   1. Discoid-cleoid
   2. Explorer
   3. Half Hollenbeck
   4. Rubber abrasive point
   a. *1* and *3*
   b. *2* and *4*
   c. *1, 2,* and *3*
   d. *4* only

4. The device that mixes the mercury and silver alloy powder to form amalgam is called _____.
   a. Amalgamator
   b. Capsule
   c. Amalgam carrier
   d. Condenser

5. Which of the following will prevent an amalgam overhang?
   a. Matrix band
   b. Contouring pliers
   c. Interproximal wedge
   d. Burnisher

6. The _____ edge of the matrix band must be inserted first into the Tofflemire retainer.
   a. Gingival
   b. Occlusal

7. An adjustment knob used to slide the vise along the frame to either increase or decrease the size of the matrix band loop is called the _____.
   a. Inner knob
   b. Outer knob
   c. Spindle
   d. Vise

8. A Tofflemire retainer and matrix band that are set up for the lower right quadrant will also fit the _____ quadrant
   a. Lower left
   b. Upper right
   c. Upper left

9. A matrix band is indicated for which of the following tooth preparations:
   1. Class I
   2. Class II
   3. Class V
   4. Class VI
   a. *1* and *3*
   b. *2* and *4*
   c. *1, 2,* and *3*
   d. *4* only

10. A matrix band is placed on a lower left third molar for a MOD cavity preparation. An interproximal wedge is placed on which of the following surfaces.
   a. Mesial only
   b. Distal only
   c. Mesial and distal

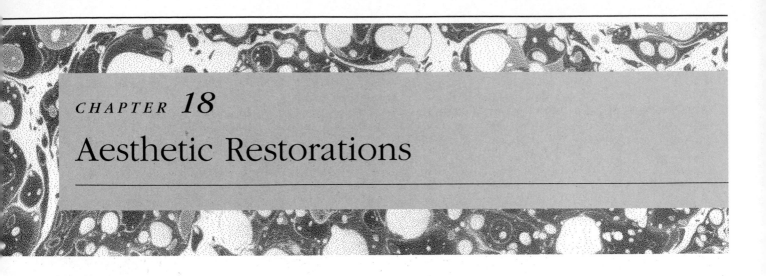

CHAPTER 18

Aesthetic Restorations

KEY TERMS

Acid etching
Celluloid crown forms
Composite resin inlay
Composite restorative materials
Conditioner
Cure
Dentin smear layer
Dual-cure bond agent
Enamel tags
Etchant
Etched porcelain veneers
Finishing disks
Finishing stone
Flash
Light-activated composite systems
Matrix strip holder
Matrix strips
Paste-paste composite material
Pistol grip composite syringe
Polishing strips
Primer
Surgical scalpel
Veneering

The restoration of tooth surfaces that are readily visible during normal oral functions presents an interesting challenge to the dental team. There is an increasing demand for aesthetics in dental restorations placed in these visible surfaces. Few patients will tolerate an unsightly metal restoration placed in a visible surface of an anterior tooth

or in the facial aspect of the maxillary premolars. Although metal restorations would function well in these teeth, their poor aesthetic quality discourages their use.

Continuous dental research projects have been devoted to the development of a restorative material that has a favorable appearance, lasts a reasonable length of time under the influence of the oral environment, and is not harmful to the tooth. Although a perfect material has not yet been developed, three types of restorative materials are currently being used, with varying degrees of success—composite resins, glass ionomers, and porcelain.

Because of the unique environment in which these materials are placed, they all ultimately fail for one reason or another. Dental restorations are subjected to chemicals produced by oral bacteria, chemical substances found in saliva, and various foods and beverages. The alternate heating and cooling of these restorations, along with the chemical substances just listed, have a damaging effect on aesthetic restorative materials. The restorations slowly disintegrate, begin to leak oral fluids into the cavity preparation, or discolor.

In the past such materials as silicate cements and unfilled resins (acrylic) were the principal aesthetic restorative materials. Today composite resins (minifilled resins and microfilled resins) and glass ionomer cements are predominantly used. These materials seem to resist the undesirable effects of the oral environment better than silicate cement or acrylic.

The following discussion represents the basic instrument and supply items needed to fabricate these restorations.

COMPOSITE RESTORATIVE MATERIALS

Three major categories of **composite restorative materials** are used in aesthetic restorations: fine, microfine, or hybrid (a combination of fine and microfine) resins.

The primary differences among them are the type and size of the filler particles used. All are referred to as composite resins because they are a combination of resin material and filler particles. Some products contain a catalyst that initiates hardening. Other products placed in a prepared cavity harden after exposure to visible light.

Light-Activated Systems

Another form in which composite materials are marketed is single-paste **light-activated composite systems** that are simply placed in a prepared cavity and hardened by exposure to visible light (Figure 18-1). No mixing is required when these materials are used.

> **•❖ KEY POINT**
> - The assistant should not dispense the material on the paper pad until it is needed. This prevents prolonged exposure to room light and subsequent inadvertent setting of the material.

Composite materials are usually placed in the cavity preparation one layer at a time and cured before the next layer is added. The advantage of this technique is discussed later. Special light shields and glasses are available to protect the eyes from the intense light used during the curing process.

Paste-Paste System

Composite materials are marketed in different forms. A less common form of composite than the light-activated systems is the **paste-paste composite material** system (Figure 18-2). In fact, light-activated systems have virtually replaced paste-paste systems. However, paste-paste systems are still used for core buildup procedures. The manufacturer provides two different pastes in small jars. One is usually called universal or base paste. The other is the catalyst paste. The base paste is usually available in different shades to facilitate a color match with the tooth being restored. However, the universal shade is satisfactory for most patients.

An equal volume of each paste is dispensed on a small paper mixing pad with a disposable spatula that is supplied with the material. One end of the spatula is used to stir and dispense the base material, and the other is used for the catalyst. This prevents contamination of the remaining material left in the jars. The two equal portions are kept separated on the pad until the mixing begins.

Once the cavity preparation is finished, the dental assistant uses either end of the spatula to mix the two pastes together for 20 to 30 seconds. The mixed material can be delivered to the dentist on the mixing pad for placement

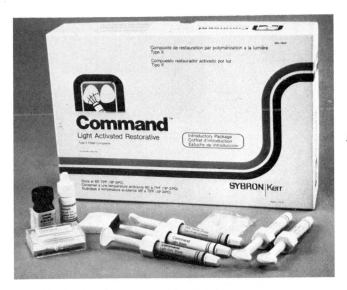

A

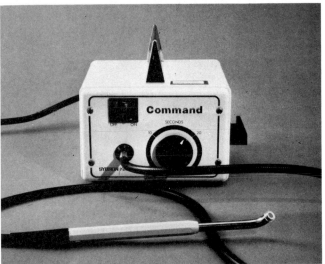

B

Figure 18-1   Light-accelerated composite system. **A**, Composite materials. **B**, Visible light source.

into the preparation with a filling instrument, or the material can be loaded into a composite syringe that the dentist uses to inject the material into the cavity preparation.

Characteristics of Composite Resins

Some characteristics of composite resins determine the technique used to place them in prepared teeth as final restorations. These characteristics include the following:

1. Ability to bond to the surface of enamel, glass ionomer, and, to a lesser extent, the dentin, given the proper chemical preparation of these surfaces
2. Shrinkage after hardening (curing)
3. Ability to bond to itself, which allows layering
4. Greater strength of the larger particle size (fine) composite

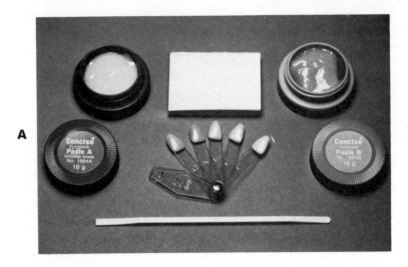

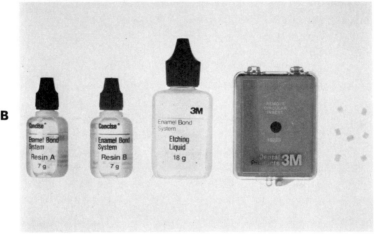

Figure 18-2 Paste–paste composite material. **A**, Materials for mixing composite. **B**, Materials for etching and bonding procedures.

5. Greater color stability and stain resistance and smoother surface finish of the smaller particle size (microfine) composite
6. Ability to harden (cure) under light or the need of a catalyst to harden

The insertion techniques that depend on these characteristics are discussed here.

Acid Etching and Enamel Bonding

Both the paste-paste system and the light-activated systems incorporate the following technique of **acid etching** in the restorative procedure.

1. The cavity of the prepared tooth is gently bathed with a mild acid (30% to 50% phosphoric acid) for at least 15 seconds. The acid is available in either liquid or gel form. Cotton pliers and cotton pellets are used to apply the liquid form of the acid. Etching gels are usually applied directly to the tooth from a syringe.
2. Following etching, the acid is rinsed away using only the air-water syringe and oral evacuator for at least 15 to 20 seconds. The etching procedure roughens the tooth, which helps to bond the composite resin material to it (Figure 18-3). This not only enhances retention of the material in the tooth, but also forms a better seal around the margins of the final restoration.
3. The etched cavity preparation is lightly air dried. The newly etched area should not be wiped dry with a cotton pellet. Wiping burnishes the tiny **enamel tags** created by the etching process, which destroys the retention potential.

> ➤ **KEY POINT**
> - If an etched tooth is contaminated with saliva, the etched area must be reetched for 10 seconds. An etched tooth should have a frosty white appearance.

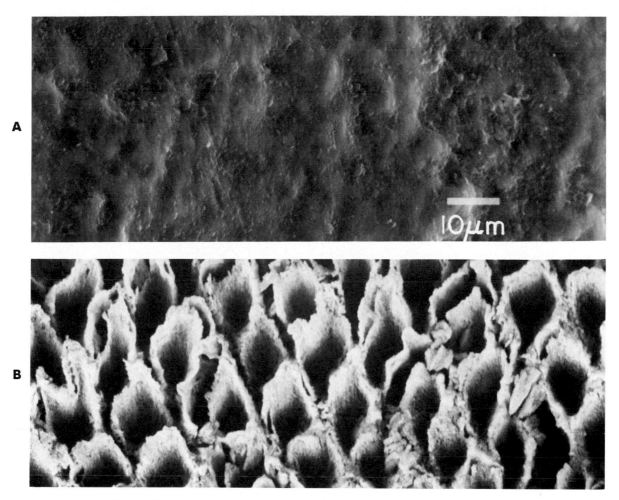

Figure 18-3 Effect of acid etching of enamel at approximate magnification of X2000. **A**, Normal enamel. **B**, Etched enamel.

(Courtesy Leon Silverstone, DDS, School of Dentistry, University of Colorado, Denver.)

Before the composite material is placed in the preparation, a bonding agent and composite material are applied to the etched area and allowed to **cure.** The composite material bonds to the bonding agent as it cures. Light-activated materials are exposed to the curing light for 20 seconds.

Bonding Agents

Cavity preparations that involve the dentin pose a special problem because dentin differs from enamel. The dentin consists of hard tooth structure and soft organic material from the dentin tubules. When the dentin is cut with a bur, an organic film of debris is produced by the frictional heat of the bur rotating against the dentin surface. This film is called the **dentin smear layer**. The smear layer must be removed to allow bonding to dentin.

Many types of bonding agents are available today. Earlier bonding agents were usually designated for enamel bonding or dentin bonding. These bond agents have been replaced by universal bonding agents that bond to both enamel and dentin. Most bonding agents consist of three or more components, which are described below:

1. *Dentin surface cleaner/acid etch.* The dentin surface cleaner is also called **conditioner** or **etchant**. This material is a weak acidic solution used to remove the smear layer on dentin. Some dentists use a regular acid-etch solution (30% to 50%) in lieu of the dentin surface cleaner. The dentin surface cleaner is rinsed from the tooth after application.
2. *Primer.* The **primer** is a wetting agent used to improve the bond of the composite to the tooth.
3. *Bonding resin.* Bonding resin wets and flows onto the primed dentin surface, which acts as an adhesive to the composite that will be placed directly over it. Bonding resins are available as either light-cure type or dual-cure type. A dual-cure type of bonding resin can either be cured under visible light or chemically cured.

Glass ionomer bonding

Glass ionomer lining cement can bond to dentin to some degree. When a cement base or liner is needed, calcium hydroxide and/or glass ionomer can be placed over the dentin and allowed to set. Both the glass ionomer base and the enamel are acid etched and covered with bonding resin and cured with visible light for 15 seconds between coats. The glass ionomer provides some dentin bonding and a source of fluoride for caries prevention under the composite restoration. The composite material bonds to the etched enamel and the glass ionomer base when it is inserted.

> **⇨ KEY POINT**
> ▪ Glass ionomer lining cements are the liner of choice for composite restorations because of their ability to bond to composite.

Insertion of Restorative Materials

Composite resins shrink when they are cured. This phenomenon can result in microleakage of the restoration. Incremental packing of the composite material into the cavity preparation is designed to compensate for shrinkage. Several small increments of material are placed in layers into the preparation until it is filled. Pliable composite resin bonds to the hardened form, and thus each layer can be cured with the light source before the next layer is added. This method compensates for the shrinkage of the previously cured layer.

A modification of this technique is the veneering of composites during the filling process not only to reduce shrinkage, but also to modify the shade and surface quality of the restoration. Minifill composite resin is used to fill two thirds of a large cavity preparation, since it has superior strength. The surface one third of the preparation is filled with microfill composite, since it has superior shade quality and improved surface smoothness. This helps to prevent staining from foods and beverages. A similar principle is used in creating a natural appearance in labial composite veneers on maxillary anterior teeth. Different shades of composites can be blended as the layers are added during the restorative process. Typically a more yellow shade is placed near the cervical one third of the tooth, whiter shades are placed in the middle third, and translucent shades are placed along the incisal edges.

The dental assistant must know the characteristics of composite resins so that proper insertion techniques are used. This issue is significant, since the assistant prepares the armamentarium and assists during each step of the procedure.

INSTRUMENTS AND SUPPLIES FOR COMPOSITE RESTORATIONS

Filling Instruments

Plastic or Teflon-tipped filling instruments (Figure 18-4) are frequently used to place composite material in the cavity preparation. The instruments shown in Figure 6-15, *B*, are used to place and shape composite material during a composite veneering procedure. The various shapes, sizes, and blade angles provide dentists with a choice of instruments and facilitate the placement and shaping of large areas of composite on the tooth surface.

Composite syringe

One problem dentists often encounter in the fabrication of a composite restoration is the placement of restorative material in rather small preparations. The material is a thick, sticky paste. It tends to be pulled out of the preparation because it sticks to filling instruments. Because it is a thick paste, the material is difficult to force into retentive areas of a preparation to ensure adequate adaptation and retention of the restoration.

The **pistol grip composite syringe** (Figure 18-5, *A*) has solved both of these insertion problems. The syringe dispenses composite from a unidose (one-dose) composite applicator. The material can be slowly injected into the preparation.

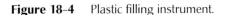
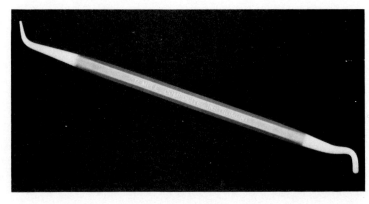

Figure 18-4 Plastic filling instrument.

Scalpel

The **surgical scalpel** (Figure 18-5, *B*) is a popular instrument for finishing composite restorations. The 12B style of blade is a common choice for this procedure because of its curved shape and double cutting edge. The scalpel blade is disposable; therefore new blades ensure maximum instrument sharpness and sterility.

The scalpel blade is specifically used to trim away excess composite along the margins of the restoration after the matrix is removed.

Matrix Strips

Matrix strips (Figure 18-6, *A*) act in a similar way to the matrix bands used in amalgam restorations. They serve to shape the proximal aspect of the restoration.

Matrix strips are made of either clear plastic (Mylar) or celluloid. A matrix strip holder can be used to hold them in place before the material is inserted, or the matrix can be held in place by the contact of the adjacent teeth (see Figure 18-13). An interproximal wedge is sometimes advisable to hold the matrix in place, prevent overhangs, and separate teeth.

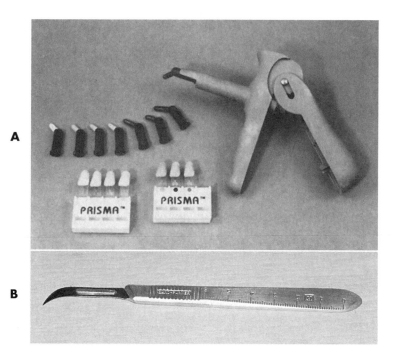

Figure 18-5 **A,** Pistol grip composite syringe and unidose composite applicator. **B,** No. 12B scalpel.

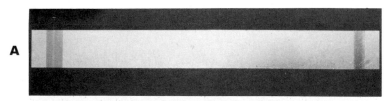

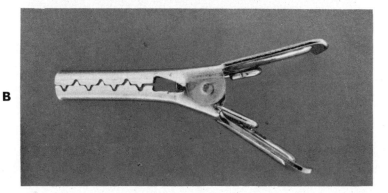

Figure 18-6 **A,** Matrix strip. **B,** Mylar strip holder.

Matrix Strip Holder

The **matrix strip holder** (Figure 18-6, *B*) is a clamplike device that can be used to hold the matrix in place after the composite material has been inserted into the cavity preparation and the matrix is wrapped around the tooth to form the proximal surface.

Celluloid Crown Forms

Celluloid crown forms are designed to act as molds to reconstruct a part of or the entire crown of a prepared tooth. The crown forms are available in various sizes of canines, lateral incisors, and central incisors. These crowns are fitted to the prepared teeth and filled with acrylic or composite. The filled crown form is placed over the prepared tooth and allowed to harden (Figure 18-7, *A*). Then the crown form is removed and discarded, and the aesthetic restorative material is left on the prepared tooth. This type of crown is also used as a temporary covering for a prepared tooth until a permanent crown can be made.

Portions of the celluloid crown form can be cut away and used to shape portions of teeth. It is common for dentists to use the incisal portion of a crown form to shape the incisal edge of a composite restoration or to use one half of a crown form to shape a class IV composite restoration (Figure 18-7, *B*).

Finishing Stones

The best finish on a composite restoration is that which is left by the matrix strip. However, minor finishing is usually required to achieve smooth margins and proper occlusal contact.

Composite restorations can be finished nicely with a **finishing stone** such as fine diamond stones, finishing burs, and white stones in a conventional-speed handpiece. Stones, finishing burs, and white stones are available in both HP and RA types and in various shapes.

Finishing Disks and Strips

Finishing disks (Figure 18-8) are small, abrasive disks of sandpaper that are used to contour and polish various restorations, including composites. They are available with paper, plastic, or rubber backing. Disks vary in diameter from ½ to 1 inch. Various grits, ranging from coarse to extremely fine, are offered by manufacturers. They are used on the conventional-speed handpiece with a mandrel.

Polishing strips are used to contour the proximal surface of a composite restoration and to smooth margins that cannot be reached by a disk. Strips are available in various widths and grits.

A strip can be inserted interproximally by either of the following methods:

1. It is inserted like dental floss into the interproximal area (Figure 18-9, *A* and *B*). Some manufacturers provide strips with a smooth area on the strip to help ease the strip between the teeth.
2. A long diagonal on the end of the strip is cut to create a point that can be threaded into the interproximal area from the facial aspect of the teeth (Figure 18-9, *C*).

Lubricant

When rotary instruments such as burs and stones are used to grind composite materials, a water-soluble lubricant is recommended (Figure 18-10). The lubricant reduces frictional heat and prevents the instrument from being clogged with debris.

COMPOSITE RESTORATIVE PROCEDURES

Since the composite resin is the most common restorative material used in aesthetic restorations today, this procedure is described in detail. Figure 18-11 provides an overview of the composite restorative procedure.

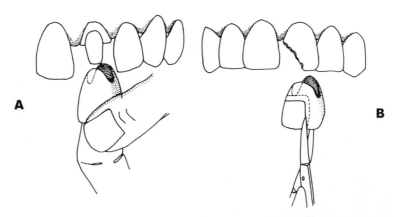

Figure 18-7 **A,** Transparent celluloid crown trimmed and fitted to prepared tooth. **B,** Incisal angle of celluloid crown can be cut from rest of crown and used as a form to shape restorative material in class IV restoration.

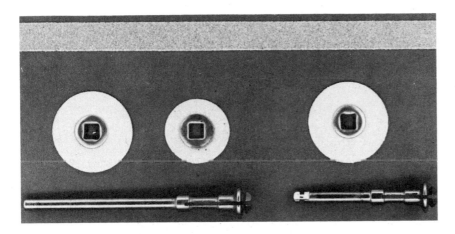

Figure 18-8 Finishing strip and disks with mandrels.

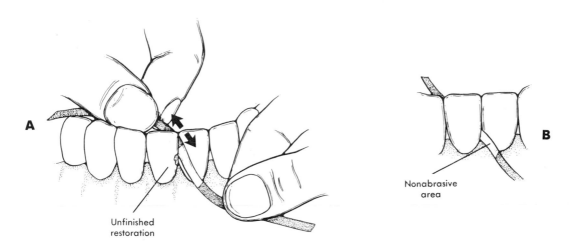

A

Unfinished
restoration

Nonabrasive
area

B

Figure 18-9 Use of interproximal finishing strip. **A,** Back and forth motion of strip used to smooth proximal surface of restoration. **B,** Strip is inserted between teeth at nonabrasive area of strip. **C,** Inserting polishing strip under contact area.

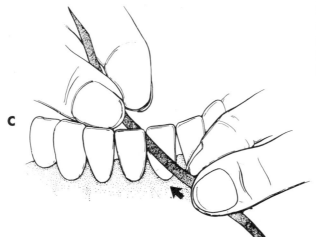

C

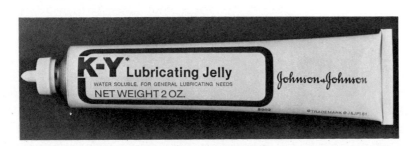

Figure 18-10 Water-soluble lubricant.

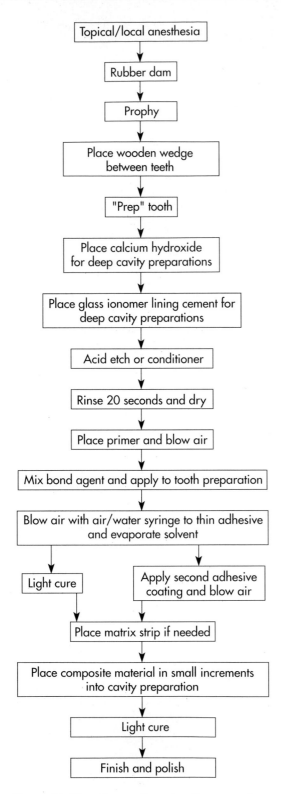

Topical/local anesthesia

↓

Rubber dam

↓

Prophy

↓

Place wooden wedge between teeth

↓

"Prep" tooth

↓

Place calcium hydroxide for deep cavity preparations

↓

Place glass ionomer lining cement for deep cavity preparations

↓

Acid etch or conditioner

↓

Rinse 20 seconds and dry

↓

Place primer and blow air

↓

Mix bond agent and apply to tooth preparation

↓

Blow air with air/water syringe to thin adhesive and evaporate solvent

↓

Light cure | Apply second adhesive coating and blow air

↓

Place matrix strip if needed

↓

Place composite material in small increments into cavity preparation

↓

Light cure

↓

Finish and polish

Figure 18-11 Composite restoration procedure.

Armamentarium

A suggested armamentarium for the aesthetic (composite) restoration is shown in Figure 18-12.

Composite Cavity Preparations

The restorations discussed here are indicated for use in class III, IV, and V cavity preparations in which aesthetics is a primary consideration. Whenever possible, the labial aspect of a tooth should be preserved to enhance the aesthetic quality of the final restoration. It is for this reason that class III restorations are usually prepared from a lingual approach. Class IV and V preparations should be kept as conservative as possible to improve the appearance of the final restoration.

The designs of cavity preparations for aesthetic restorations are shown in Figure 18-13.

Composite restoration: a class III example

The class III is the most common cavity preparation used for aesthetic restorations. The fabrication of this restoration follows the scheme listed:

1. Anesthetic administration
2. Isolation
3. Cavity preparation
4. Cavity medication
5. Matrix strip placement
6. Insertion
7. Finishing

Anesthetic administration. Local anesthesia is used to anesthetize maxillary teeth and mandibular teeth. The dental assistant hands the dentist the topical anesthetic for application. In some states the dental assistant is allowed to place the topical anesthetic. The dental assistant assembles the anesthetic syringe and passes it to the operator for administration. Following local anesthetic administration, the dental assistant rinses the patient's oral cavity.

Isolation. Rubber dam isolation is considered the best isolation method for any restoration when it can be used. Careful use of cotton roll isolation is also acceptable.

The dental assistant places the rubber dam clamp on the rubber dam forceps and passes the forceps to the operator. The rubber dam is placed by the assistant and the dentist. The dentist usually places the septal portion between the teeth, and the dental assistant uses dental floss to push the dam between the teeth. The assistant uses the air-water syringe to blow air on the rubber dam while the dentist inverts or tucks the rubber dam around the teeth. In some states the dental assistant is allowed to place the rubber dam and the rubber dam clamp.

Cavity preparation. The entire cavity preparation for a class III composite restorative procedure can be accomplished with round burs and a Wedelstaedt chisel. A lingual approach is used to maximize aesthetics.

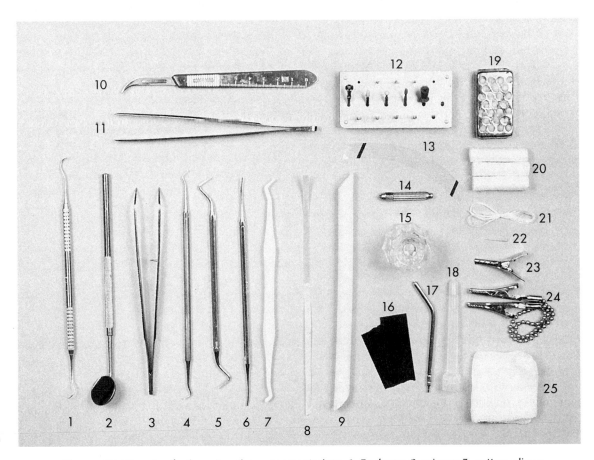

Figure 18-12 Aesthetic restoration armamentarium. *1*, Explorer; *2*, mirror; *3*, cotton pliers; *4*, spoon excavator; *5*, binangle chisel; *6*, Wedelstaedt chisel; *7*, plastic Teflon instrument; *8*, linen strip; *9*, HVE tip; *10*, #12B scalpel blade and handle; *11*, thumb forceps; *12*, bur block, with assorted burs and stones; *13*, Mylar/celluloid matrix strip; *14*, bur tool; *15*, dappen dish; *16*, articulating paper; *17*, air/water tip; *18*, air/water tip cover; *19*, cotton pellets; *20*, cotton rolls; *21*, floss; *22*, wedge; *23*, matrix strip holder; *24*, napkin chain; *25*, 2 × 2 gauze.

During the cavity preparation stage the dental assistant changes the burs on the dental handpieces and uses an instrument transfer technique to pass the hand instruments to the dentist.

Cavity medication. Cavity medication can be accomplished as described previously. Acid etching and bonding resins can be applied at this time.

> **⊸ KEY POINT**
> ▪ Cavity varnish and zinc oxide and eugenol are not compatible with composite materials.

The dental assistant mixes the appropriate cavity medications and holds the mixing pad and 2 × 2-inch gauze pad near the patient's chin as the dentist applies the medication to the tooth preparation.

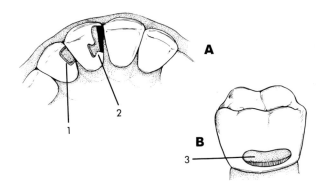

Figure 18-13 Common preparations in which aesthetic restorative materials are used. **A,** From palatal view of the maxillary anterior teeth, class III (*1*) and class IV (*2*). **B,** From buccal view of mandibular molar, class V (*3*).

Matrix strip placement. The matrix strip is placed through the contact area in a faciolingual direction. A wooden wedge can be placed cervically to adapt the strip against the tooth surface and to separate the teeth slightly (Figure 18-14, *A*).

Insertion. Once the matrix strip is in place, the composite resin can be inserted in the cavity preparation. Chemically activated composites must be mixed according to the manufacturer's directions. Light-cured composites are simply placed in the preparation in small increments and cured between layers.

A filling instrument and/or a pistol grip composite syringe can be used to place the composite resin. Care must be taken to avoid trapping air in the material during insertion. Air bubbles appear as opaque spots in the finished restoration.

After the material is inserted in the preparation, the matrix strip is pulled tightly around the tooth to form the proximal aspect of the restoration (Figure 18-13, *B* and *C*). The strip is held in place until the material reaches its initial set. This can be determined by holding a sample of the excess material in the hand to feel when it has achieved initial hardness. If a light-cured composite is used, the dental assistant holds the light probe against the matrix strip near the prepared cavity and activates the light.

The strip and wedge are removed when the initial hardness is reached. The restoration can now be trimmed and polished during the finishing phase.

Finishing. Excess material that squeezes out of the cavity preparation when the strip is pulled is called **flash.** Flash is trimmed away from the cervical and facial margins with a scalpel (and polishing disks if needed). The lingual flash is removed with a large, round finishing bur or a fine-grain diamond stone that is lubricated with water-soluble lubricant. The lingual contour of the restoration is also formed with these cutting instruments. Polishing strips are used to refine the proximal contour of the restoration.

Many experts in composite materials believe that restorations requiring a small amount of finishing resist staining more than restorations that require much finishing.

Fabrication of a class IV composite restoration

The class IV restoration is used to restore teeth with missing incisal angles as a result of fracture or extensive caries (Figure 18-15, *A*).

The armamentarium for this procedure is the same as for a class III restoration.

The fabrication of this restoration employs the following scheme:

1. Anesthetic and isolation methods
2. Cavity preparation
3. Cavity medication
4. Matrix placement
5. Insertion
6. Finishing

Anesthetic and isolation methods. Anesthesia and isolation methods are the same as for the class III restoration.

Cavity preparation. After the outline form has been completed, the preparation is often so extensive that additional retention is needed to hold the restorative material in place. This can be accomplished using acid-etch enamel bonding supplemented with pin retention (Figure 18-15, *B* and *C*). The same types of pins used for the pin-retained amalgam can be used for this purpose.

Cavity medication. Cavity medication follows the scheme outlined in Chapter 16. Preparations that are deeper than normal can be lined with glass ionomer cement on the axial wall.

Matrix placement. Matrix strips can be used to form the proximal aspect of the restoration in less extensive cases. The operator can properly shape the incisal aspect by grinding the excess material with a polishing disk.

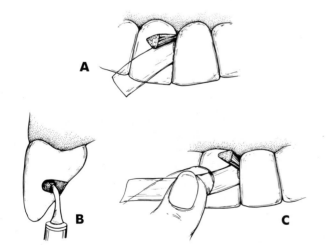

Figure 18-14 Insertion of composite restorative materials. **A,** Matrix strip and wedge in place. **B,** Injection of composite into preparation. **C,** Pulling strip into position to form proximal surface of preparation.

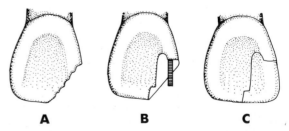

Figure 18-15 Restoration of a class IV cavity with aesthetic material. **A,** Fractured incisor. **B,** Prepared tooth with retention pin. **C,** Finished restoration.

In more extensive cases a celluloid crown form is trimmed with scissors so that the appropriate incisal angle is removed from the rest of the crown (see Figure 18-7). This celluloid "incisal angle" is used as a matrix to shape the proximal and incisal aspects of the restoration.

Insertion. When the celluloid crown form method is used, the form is partially filled with composite resin. The dentist builds up the bulk of the restoration with individual layers of cured resin. The filled crown form is then placed over freshly cured resin in the preparation to form the incisal angle of the restoration. A small hole is punched in the incisal angle portion of the crown form to prevent air entrapment during the filling process.

Once the celluloid crown is in place, any excess composite resin is removed and the restoration is hardened with the curing light.

Finishing. After the material is cured, the crown form is removed and the restoration is shaped and polished with polishing disks, strips, and large finishing burs lubricated with a lubricant.

Fabrication of class V composite and glass ionomer restorations

The only difference in the fabrication of a class V composite restoration is that a matrix band is not needed in the procedure. The restorative material can be easily inserted into the preparation, shaped with a filling instrument, and light cured. Finishing should be kept to a minimum, using only a scalpel and polishing disks.

In cases where exposed root surfaces need restoration, not much cavity preparation can be done, since there is not much tooth structure between the pulp and the outside of the tooth. Consequently dentists rely on dentin bonding agents to hold such a restoration in place. The following is a typical procedure for the placement of a glass ionomer or composite restoration:

1. The tooth is conditioned with polyacrylic acid (10%), which is applied to the surface of the area to be restored for 20 seconds.
2. The cavity preparation is rinsed and lightly dried.
3. A calcium hydroxide liner is applied if it is a deep cavity preparation.
4. The glass ionomer material is mixed and applied to the tooth surface, or a composite material is applied to fill the tooth preparation.

Fabrication of posterior composite restorations

Posterior composite restorations (Figure 18-16) continue to grow in popularity because of their aesthetic quality and, to a lesser extent, because of patients' unfounded fear of mercury poisoning associated with amalgam restorations.

The restorative technique is similar to that of the amalgam restoration. Once the cavity preparation is finished, one of the cavity medication strategies described previously is carried out. Deeper cavity preparations are usually treated with a calcium hydroxide liner, and then a glass ionomer lining cement is placed. The glass ionomer lining cement is then acid etched with the enamel margins. A matrix band and wedge are placed when proximal surfaces are being restored. Some dentists prefer clear, nonmetal matrix bands to facilitate the transmission of light to the cervical margins during curing.

A bonding resin and then a composite resin are placed in the cavity preparation in layers, and each layer is cured before the next is added until the preparation is filled. The matrix is removed, and the restoration is finished with fine diamond stones and finishing burs.

Composite Inlays

A new technique for placing posterior composite restorations is the laboratory-processed **composite resin inlay** (Figure 18-17). This restoration is made using a replica (die) of the tooth being restored. The impression-taking technique used to obtain a die is discussed in Chapter 19. Like the porcelain inlay discussed later in this chapter, the composite inlay is fabricated in a dental laboratory and returned to the dentist for cementation into a prepared tooth.

In the laboratory a high filler content composite is heat and pressure cured in the shape of the inlay. This results in a strong, wear-resistant restoration that does not shrink in the mouth since it is cured in the laboratory.

At the cementation appointment, the prepared tooth is acid etched, and bonding resin is placed on both the etched enamel and the inside of the inlay. A thin layer of a combination light- and chemical-cure composite cement (**dual-cure bond agent**) is applied to both the inlay and the preparation. The inlay is seated in the preparation and light cured. The cement is designed to self-cure if it is not completely exposed to the curing light.

The occlusion and margins can be adjusted using the instruments and devices described previously. This restoration can be repaired by adding regular composite resin to it if necessary.

> ### ➻ KEY POINT
> - Zinc oxide and eugenol temporary cements should not be used in temporary fillings during the laboratory phase, since residual eugenol may interfere with the set of the composite resin used to cement the inlay in place. An acrylic resin temporary filling is recommended.

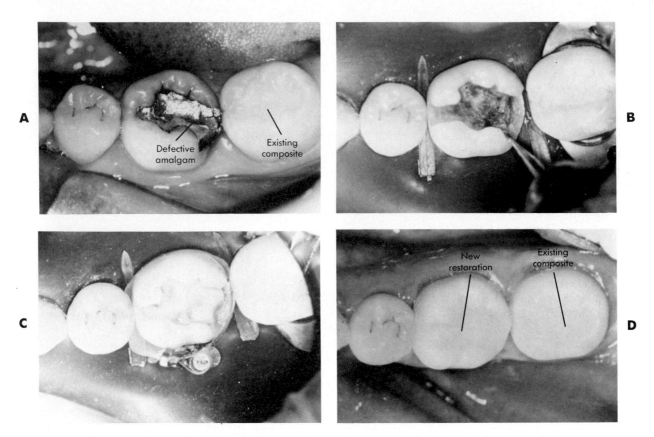

Figure 18-16 Fabrication of MOD posterior composite restoration. **A,** Defective amalgam being replaced with composite. **B,** MOD cavity preparation. **C,** Clear matrix and clear plastic wedges in place along with glass ionomer lining. **D,** Finished restoration.

(Courtesy Michael Goldfogel, DDS, Englewood, Colo.)

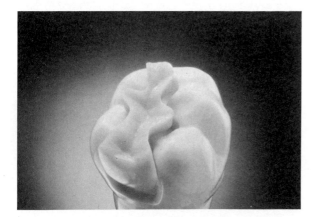

Figure 18-17 Laboratory-processed composite inlay.

(Courtesy Williams Dental Company, Inc, Buffalo, NY.)

Composite and Glass Ionomer Cores

Special composite resins and silver-impregnated glass ionomers are available for use as core materials that are placed around retention pins, such as the pin-retained amalgam described in Chapter 17. A popular type of silver-impregnated glass ionomer is available in a unidose capsule that can be activated and mixed in an amalgamator (Figure 18-18). The capsule has a dispensing spout that can be used with a special applicator to place the material directly into the tooth preparation. It should be noted that these materials are also used with special prefabricated posts. These posts are cemented in the pulp canal of an endodontically treated tooth to form a strong retentive core over which a crown can be placed. This technique is discussed in Chapter 21 in conjunction with special crown fabrication techniques.

Composite Veneers

The ability to bond composite resin to enamel, as well as the development of the more aesthetic microfine resins, has contributed to the extensive use of veneering tech-

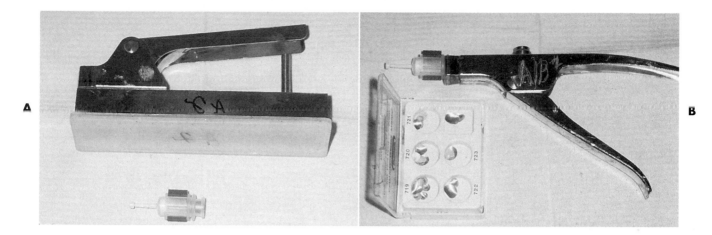

Figure 18-18   Silver-impregnated glass ionomer material. **A,** Unidose applicator. **B,** Applicator with capsule.

niques to achieve aesthetic results. **Veneering** is simply the bonding of layers of composite resin to the enamel surface of teeth to reshape them to improve the patient's appearance. The results can be dramatic. Often when teeth are restored in this manner, the need for more costly crown restorations and orthodontic treatment is eliminated.

The basic steps in the procedure are as follows (Figure 18-19):

1. Surfaces being restored are polished with nonfluoridated or oil-free pumice and rinsed to remove any surface debris.
2. The teeth being restored are isolated using either a rubber dam or cotton rolls.
3. Teeth are acid etched for 15 seconds with 30% to 50% phosphoric acid gel on surfaces that are covered by the composite. The gel is rinsed away using the air-water syringe and oral evacuator simultaneously for at least 15 seconds, and the preparation is air dried.
4. The etched areas on the enamel are painted with two thin coats of bonding resin and cured with visible light between coats.
5. When appropriate, a Mylar matrix strip is placed between the mesial and distal contact areas of the tooth being restored. The matrix assists with the shaping of the proximal surfaces of the restoration.
6. Layers of composite resin are applied to the tooth surface using flat-bladed instruments such as a plastic filling instrument or the Goldfogel insertion instruments. The layers are light cured for 40 to 60 seconds each as they are added and shaped.
7. An opaque agent may be applied in thin layers to mask any natural discoloration of the teeth and light cured.
8. The cured restoration is finished with finishing disks and polishing strips. A lubricant is used to prevent clogging of the abrasive and to reduce frictional heat.

Indirect composite veneers

Because it is time consuming and fatiguing to place direct composite veneers on several teeth, an indirect method may be more desirable. Indirect composite veneers are usually fabricated at a dental laboratory and then are placed on the prepared tooth at a separate cementation appointment.

Indirect composite veneers are similar to other composite materials and can be bonded to the tooth with a bonding agent as described in the following procedure:

1. The tooth is cleaned with a pumice slurry.
2. A priming agent is applied to the tooth side of the veneer.
3. A bonding agent is applied to the tooth side of the veneer, but it is not light cured.
4. The veneer is seated onto the tooth for an initial try-in.
5. The shade of the bond agent is checked and the veneer removed. The bond agent is removed if a different shade is desired, or the veneer is set aside if the bond agent color initially placed on the veneer is acceptable.
6. A matrix strip is placed on either side of the tooth. Indirect veneers are usually placed one at a time.
7. The tooth is acid etched.
8. A thin layer of bond agent is applied to the etched enamel and lightly blown with air but not light cured.
9. A different shade of bond agent or more of the initial bonding agent is applied to the tooth side of the veneer.
10. The veneer is placed onto the tooth.
11. A disposable brush or explorer is used to remove the excess.
12. The veneer is light cured for 40 to 60 seconds on the facial and lingual sides.
13. The excess bond agent is removed with a scalpel.
14. The veneer is finished with the appropriate finishing burs and stones.

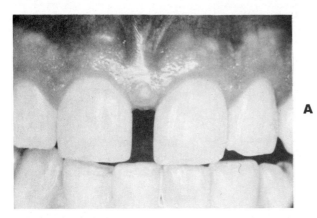

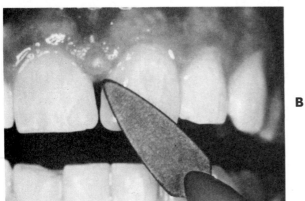

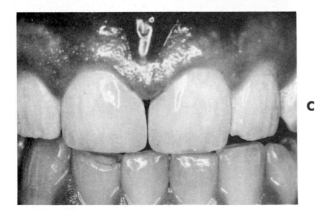

Figure 18-19 Elimination of midline diastema (space) using composite veneers on adjacent teeth. **A,** Before treatment. **B,** Placing composite on etched surfaces. **C,** Finished restoration. (Courtesy Michael Goldfogel, DDS, Englewood, Colo.)

PORCELAIN RESTORATIONS

Porcelain has been used as a restorative material for many years. For a time porcelain restorations were used less frequently when porcelain-fused-to-metal restorative techniques were developed. The fused restorations were both aesthetic and strong; but recent developments in porcelain technology have resulted in stronger materials and innovative techniques. An all-porcelain restoration is one

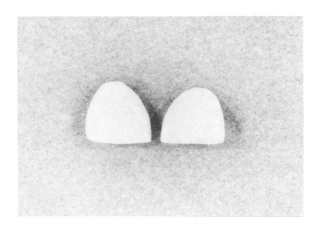

Figure 18-20 Porcelain veneers.

of the most aesthetic restorations available to dentistry. The types of porcelain restorations in use include veneers, inlays, and jacket crowns. Porcelain jacket crowns are discussed in Chapter 21.

Etched Porcelain Veneers

Etched porcelain veneers (Figure 18-20) are thin shells of porcelain that are custom made to fit over the labial surfaces of maxillary anterior teeth to improve a patient's appearance. Patients who have stained or mottled teeth are prime candidates for this service.

The basic technique involves use of a rounded-end diamond stone in a high-speed handpiece to remove some of the labial enamel of the teeth being restored. A rubber impression is taken of the upper arch using the impression technique described in Chapter 19. A stone model is made from the impression and sent with an appropriate shade selection to the dental ceramist for the fabrication of the veneers. Temporary veneers can be made from composite by acid etching and bonding only a few small areas of the enamel to hold the material.

When the patient returns for insertion of the veneers, the composite temporaries are removed and the tooth surface is cleared of any debris. The veneers are dipped in water and placed on the tooth surface to test the fit. Care should be taken during the handling of the veneers, since they are etched and conditioned with a silane primer that promotes a chemical bond between the resin and the porcelain. The veneers are usually etched and conditioned with silane at the dental laboratory. If the veneers are tried in, then the veneer must be reetched and reconditioned with silane. Therefore some dentists prefer not to try in the veneer and to go directly to the cementation phase of the procedure.

1. The prepared teeth are polished with pumice and water.
2. A matrix strip is placed between the teeth.
3. The enamel is etched.

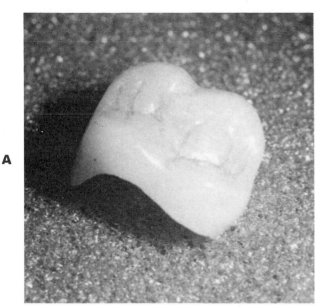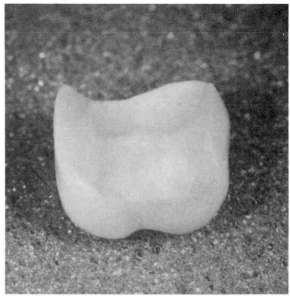

A   **B**

Figure 18-21 All-ceramic restoration. **A**, Occlusal view. **B**, Internal view. (Courtesy Robert Trombly, DDS, Aurora, Colo.)

4. A resin bonding agent is applied to the etched enamel and the tooth side of the silane-primed veneer.
5. A thin layer of a selected shade of light-cured resin bonding medium is placed on the tooth side of the veneer.
6. The veneer is placed on the tooth.
7. The excess bonding agent is applied with a disposable brush or a scalpel.
8. The veneer is light cured for 40 to 60 seconds on the facial and lingual sides.
9. The excess cured bonding agent is removed with a scalpel.
10. The veneer is finished with the appropriate finishing burs and stones.

All-Ceramic Restorations

All-ceramic restorations (Figure 18-21) are aesthetic and reasonably strong. They can be fabricated for occlusal as well as for two- and three-surface restorations. They are fabricated in the dental laboratory, as is the composite inlay, and cemented in the prepared tooth with composite resin.

There are currently three types of all-ceramic restorations in use:
1. Porcelain
2. Castable glass (Dicor)
3. CEREC system

All-porcelain restorations are fabricated in the dental laboratory from finely ground ceramic powders that are wetted and shaped in the desired form. The fabricated in-

lay is heated in a special oven that transforms the inlay into a translucent toothlike material.

All-ceramic restorations are etched on the cavity side of the restoration and treated with a silanating agent to improve the bond.

All-castable-glass restorations are made from glass that is transformed into a ceramic type of material. Castable glass restorations are fabricated in a method similar to cast gold inlays and onlays, which are described in Chapter 19. Special equipment is used to cast the inlay and instead of using a gold ingot a special glass ingot is used.

CEREC system restorations are fabricated at chairside using a CAD/CAM (computer aided design/computer aided manufacturing) system. The advantage of a CEREC system is that the patient does not have to return for a cementation appointment because the tooth is prepared and the restoration is fabricated in one appointment. The disadvantage of this system is the cost of purchasing the computer and equipment to fabricate the restoration.

All-Ceramic Restoration Procedure

The cavity preparation is similar to that of a gold inlay or onlay in that it is tapered to provide draw. Once the cavity medications are in place, a final impression is taken of the prepared tooth. An alginate impression is taken of the opposing arch, as well as a bite registration. The role of these items is discussed in greater detail in Chapter 19. Models and dies made from the impressions are sent along with an appropriate shade to the dental ceramist

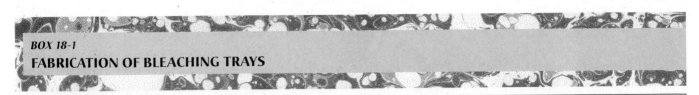

BOX 18-1
FABRICATION OF BLEACHING TRAYS

ARMAMENTARIUM

- Study model (upper and lower)
- Resin sheet
- Block out (light cured)
- Light cure unit
- Vacuformer
- Scissors
- Alcohol
- Gauze 2 × 2–inch sponge
- Microtorch or alcohol torch
- Matches

PROCEDURE	RATIONALE
1. Trim study model; keep quantity of stone to a minimum by trimming within a few millimeters of gingival margin.	1. Trimming study model close to gingival margin will ensure that resin sheet will adapt well to teeth.
2. Let dry at least 2 hours.	2. Wet stone or plaster will create air bubbles in resin sheet.
3. Apply 0.5 mm of block out to facial surface of study model (Figure 18-22). Light cure block out; then wipe off top oily layer with alcohol and 2 × 2–inch gauze sponge.	3. Block out will create a reservoir for bleaching gel when tray is inserted in mouth.
4. Follow instructions for Vacuformer and resin sheet to make bleaching tray.	4. Resin sheet is heated and placed on top of study model. A suction pulls resin sheet to fit snugly around study model.
5. Cut bulk of tray material away with scissors.	5. To make trimming of tray easier.

PROCEDURE	RATIONALE
6. Carefully and precisely trim tray just short of gingival margin. Take care to scallop around interdental papilla.	6. Bleaching tray should be trimmed so there is minimal contact with gingiva. Bleaching solution placed in bleaching tray is irritating to gums. Tray is trimmed just short of gingiva because there will be small amount of shrinkage when edges are heat flamed for smoothing.
7. Return tray to study model and check margins.	7. To avoid a tray that touches gingiva.
8. Light microtorch or alcohol torch and adjust to low setting. Gently flame edges of tray while it is still on study model.	8. To smooth edges of bleaching tray. *Note:* Some shrinkage of tray will occur along edges.
9. Readapt heated edges or margins with wet finger by pressing tray against study model.	9. When tray is heated it may pull away from study model.

for the fabrication of the restoration. An acrylic temporary filling is placed in the prepared tooth until the next appointment.

There are also several resinlike materials that can be used to temporize an inlay preparation. Protemp II (ESPE-Premier), Unifast LC (GC America), and Luxatemp (Zenith) are several brands on the market. Some of these materials are available in an Automix cartridge. Another type of dispensing that is available includes a base and catalyst syringe. The plunger on the syringe is screwlike and must be turned a complete rotation to dispense a unit of material. The plunger will click when turned a complete rotation. The base and catalyst material are

mixed and placed inside a lubricated cavity preparation. The preparation is lubricated to aid in removal of the temporary filling after it is cured. The occlusion is adjusted, and after polishing the temporary filling can be placed in the tooth with a mixture of calcium hydroxide.

> ### ◆ KEY POINT
> - Zinc oxide and eugenol cements should not be used since they interfere with the setting of composite, which is used for the cementation of the permanent restoration.

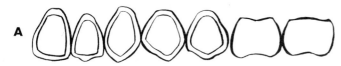

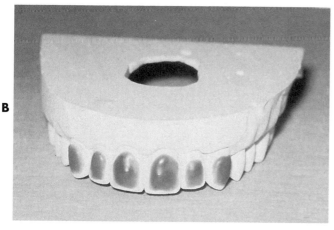

Figure 18-22 Study model preparation for bleaching tray fabrication. **A** and **B,** Block-out placement.

Composite, porcelain, and CEREC inlays are treated before insertion into the tooth. Composite can be etched, sandblasted, or softened with a solvent. Porcelain is etched and treated with a silanating agent that improves the bond to the composite cement. These procedures are sometimes performed at the dental laboratory. The following procedure describes the cementation appointment after the temporary filling is removed and the tooth is cleaned thoroughly:

1. A clear plastic matrix strip and wedge or wedges are placed between each affected proximal surface.
2. The tooth is acid etched.
3. A bonding agent is applied to the cavity side of the preparation.
4. A dual-cure composite cement is placed into the cavity preparation and on the cavity side of the veneer.
5. The restoration is inserted.
6. The excess cement is removed with a disposable brush or a scalpel.
7. The restoration is light cured from the occlusal, facial, and lingual surfaces for 40 to 60 seconds (each surface).
8. The restoration is finished with diamond burs and finishing stones. Abrasive strips are used for the interproximal areas.
9. The occlusion is checked and adjusted with a finishing bur.
10. The restoration is repolished where adjustments were made. The dentist may use finishing burs, rubber abrasive points, and porcelain polishing paste that is applied with a bristle brush.

BLEACHING

Home bleaching of the teeth has recently become popular. Home bleaching techniques are safe and quite successful for patients who are dissatisfied with the color of their teeth. A bleaching gel made of a strong hydrogen peroxide solution (Carbamade peroxide) is placed on custom bleaching trays. The bleaching trays are placed on the upper and lower arches for several hours to overnight for 1 week. Results can be seen after 1 day and are more or less permanent. Patients should be cautioned about tooth sensitivity to hot and cold that can occur with the bleaching process. Box 18-1 describes the process for the fabrication of bleaching trays.

BIBLIOGRAPHY

Craig RG: *Restorative dental materials,* ed 9, St Louis, 1993, Mosby.

Ferracane JL: *Materials in dentistry: principles and applications,* Philadelphia, 1995, Lippincott.

Garcia-Godoy F, Malone WFP: Microleakage of posterior composite resins using glass ionomer cement bases, *Quin Intern* 19:13, 1988.

Gordon AA, von der Lehr WN, Herrin HK: Bond strength of composite to composite and bond strength of composite to glass ionomer lining cements, *Gen Dent* 34(4):290, 1986.

Grundy JR, Jones JG: *Colour atlas of clinical operative dentistry: crowns and bridges,* ed 2, London, 1992, Wolfe.

Phillips RW, Moore BK: *Elements of dental materials for dental hygienists and dental assistants,* ed 5, Philadelphia, 1994, Saunders.

Schulein TM, Chan DCN, Reinhardt JW: Rinsing times for a gel etchant related to enamel/composite bond strength, *Gen Dent* 34(4):296, 1986.

Strassler HE, Litkowski LJ: Dentin bonding with composite resin: an update on materials and techniques, *Compendium* 8(5):318, 1987.

van de Voorde A, Gerdts GJ, Murchison DF: Clinical uses of glass ionomer cement: a literature review, *Quin Intern* 19:53, 1988.

QUESTIONS—Chapter 18

1. The term used to describe the process of making a composite turn into its hardened state is called:
   a. Flash
   b. Cure
   c. Etch
   d. Bonding

2. If etched enamel is accidently exposed to saliva, the tooth must be reetched for _____ seconds.
   a. 5
   b. 10
   c. 30
   d. 60

3. Which of the following removes the dentin smear layer?
   a. Conditioner
   b. Primer
   c. Bond agent
   d. Varnish

4. All of the following materials are compatible with composite materials *except:*
   a. Glass ionomer
   b. Calcium hydroxide
   c. Zinc oxide and eugenol
   d. Primer

5. Which of the following describes the correct placement of cavity medications and bonding agents in a composite restoration?
   a. Calcium hydroxide, glass ionomer, conditioner, primer, bond agent
   b. Glass ionomer, calcium hydroxide, primer, conditioner, bond agent
   c. Calcium hydroxide, primer, glass ionomer, conditioner, bond agent
   d. Glass ionomer, primer, calcium hydroxide, conditioner, bond agent

6. A(n) _____ can be used to remove excess composite material or flash from the margins of the restoration.
   a. Explorer
   b. Floss
   c. Scissors
   d. Scalpel

7. Small class V cavity preparations can be restored with which of the following:
   a. Glass ionomer
   b. Composite
   c. Porcelain
   d. *a* and *b*
   e. *a* and *c*

8. An aesthetic restoration that is actually a facing placed on the anterior teeth to correct crowding or tooth discoloration is called a(n) _____.
   a. Inlay
   b. Veneer
   c. Onlay
   d. Core

9. Porcelain inlays ideally require _____ appointment(s), and CEREC system CAD/CAM inlays ideally require _____ appointment(s).
   a. One, one
   b. One, two
   c. Two, one
   d. Two, two

10. Light-cured composites are placed in the cavity preparation in which of the following manners:
    a. All at once
    b. In small increments

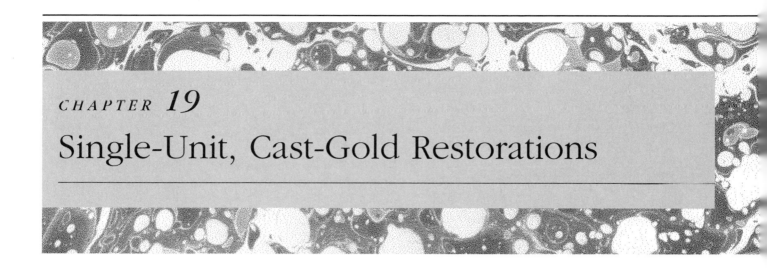

CHAPTER 19

Single-Unit, Cast-Gold Restorations

KEY TERMS

Automix system
Bite registration
Boiling bath
Cast-gold crown
Cementation appointment
Cooley peg
Draw
Dual-arch tray
Full crown
Gingival retraction cord
Gold inlay
Hemostatic agent
High/heavy viscosity
Hyperocclusion
Impression trays
Low/light viscosity
Medium viscosity
Mixing tip
Occlusal clearance wax
Onlay
Opposing teeth
Orangewood stick
Preparation appointment
Putty-wash technique
Storage bath
Tempering bath
Three-quarter crown
Two-viscosity impression technique
Vacuformer
Wash

Some gold restorations are fabricated by casting molten gold alloy into a mold and allowing it to harden. Restorations made from cast gold include crowns, bridges, and inlays. For convenience, a gold restoration used to restore or replace a tooth is referred to as a *unit* of gold work. A single-unit, cast-gold restoration is one used to restore a single tooth. Single-unit, cast-gold restorations discussed in this chapter include various types of crowns and inlays. Cast-gold bridges and aesthetic crowns made of porcelain and gold are discussed in Chapter 20.

COMMON CAST-GOLD RESTORATIONS

Pure gold and alloys of gold have properties that make them extremely useful as restorative materials. The following properties make gold and gold alloys desirable from a dental point of view.

1. Gold can be easily melted and accurately cast into various shapes.
2. Gold alloys are extremely strong and resist the crushing forces generated during mastication far better than amalgam.
3. Gold has superb edge strength. The margins of a gold restoration do not fracture, which often occurs with an amalgam restoration.
4. Gold does not corrode or discolor in the presence of oral fluids.
5. Gold is compatible with the surrounding tissues of the tooth and usually (except in rare cases) does not cause irritation or allergic reactions.

Gold Inlays and Onlays

A **gold inlay** is a restoration made from gold alloy that has been cast to fit a cavity preparation made by the dentist. The term *inlay* implies that the bulk of the restoration is contained within the confines of a tapered cavity

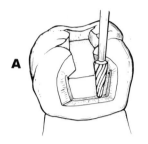
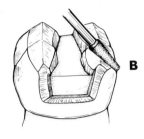

Figure 19-1 Onlay preparation. **A,** Tapered fissure bur used to develop internal form. **B,** Diamond stone used to reduce cusp height.

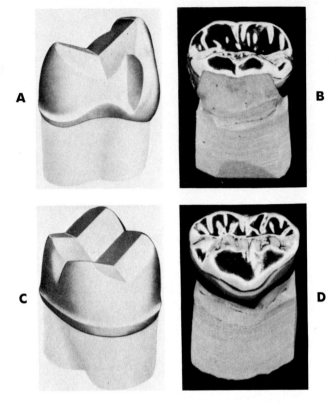

Figure 19-2 Cast-gold crowns. **A,** Three-quarter crown preparation. **B,** Cast three-quarter crown. **C,** Full crown preparation. **D,** Cast full crown.

(**A** and **C** courtesy JM Ney Co, Hartford, Conn. **B** and **D** courtesy Precision Dental Arts, Inc, Jackson, Mich.)

preparation. Various types of inlays are fabricated for class I, II, III, IV, V, and VI preparations.

A modification of the cast-gold inlay is the protected cusp or **onlay** restoration (Figure 19-1). These restorations extend over the cusps of posterior teeth to prevent fracture of the teeth when biting forces are applied.

•● KEY POINTS
- An inlay is a restoration that is contained within the confines of a tapered cavity preparation.
- An onlay is a restoration that covers mainly the cusps and occlusal surfaces of posterior teeth.

Cast-Gold Crowns

The **cast-gold crown** is one of the most common restorations in restorative dentistry. The term *crown* implies that a substantial portion of the natural crown of the tooth is reconstructed with gold, porcelain, or a combination of both. Cast-gold crowns are most often made either to rebuild three fourths of the crown portion of a tooth, which is known as a **three-quarter crown,** or to cover the entire crown of a tooth, which is known as a **full crown** (Figure 19-2, *B*).

If a three-quarter crown is done on a tooth, the facial aspect of the tooth is usually left intact. This type of restoration provides the strength needed for proper function of the tooth and preserves the natural appearance of the facial surface for aesthetics.

A full cast-gold crown (Figure 19-2, *D*) completely encases the remaining tooth structure and provides both maximum retention of the restoration on the tooth and strength to resist the forces created during mastication. Since this type of restoration is not aesthetically pleasing, it is usually placed on posterior teeth that are not readily visible when the patient speaks or smiles.

•● KEY POINTS
- A three-quarter crown covers almost the entire crown of the tooth except for the facial surface.
- A full crown covers the entire crown of the tooth.

The procedure for the fabrication of either type of restoration is basically the same. Two appointments are required. During the first appointment the tooth is prepared, and impressions are taken from which models of the patient's teeth are made. The gold restoration is fabricated in the dental laboratory using these models. The patient wears a temporary restoration while this laboratory procedure is accomplished. On the patient's return for the second appointment the temporary restoration is removed, and the restoration is fitted to the cavity preparation, the adjacent teeth, and the patient's occlusion. After all refinements are completed, it is cemented in place.

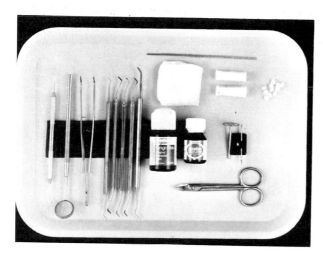

Preset tray

Cowhorn explorer, No. 3
Mouth mirror, No. 4
Cotton pliers
Spoon excavator
Enamel hatchet 8E
Gingival margin trimmers, No. 12 and No. 13
Plastic filling instrument, F P No. 1
Gingival retraction cord
Hemostatic agent
Gauze sponges, 2 × 2 inch
Lightning strip
Cotton rolls
Cotton pellets
Lightning disk
Burs, No. 171 and straight tapered diamond
Scissors (crown and collar)

Add-on items

Temporary cement
Final impression material setup
Impression trays
Alginate impression setup
Occlusal registration material

Figure 19-3 Gold restoration armamentarium (preparation appointment).

The following instruments and supplies are required for the preparation and the cementation appointments for all gold restorations.

COMMON INSTRUMENTS AND SUPPLIES
Items for Preparation Appointment
Rotary and hand instruments

Most cast-gold instrument setups consist of the common rotary and hand instruments discussed in Chapter 6. A sample armamentarium is shown in Figure 19-3.

Occlusal clearance wax

Occlusal clearance wax is a thin sheet of wax with a 28-gauge thickness. When a 1½ × ½-inch strip is folded three times to form a ½-inch square, it can be used as a gauge to determine if the dentist has removed enough tooth structure from the occlusal surface in onlay and crown preparations (Figure 19-4). The tooth structure removed from the occlusal surface will be replaced with gold.

After the ½-inch square is prepared, it is placed over the prepared tooth, and the patient is instructed to close the teeth together in a normal bite relationship. If there is proper clearance between the occlusal surfaces of the prepared tooth and the opposing teeth, there will be no indentations in the wax square. If there is inadequate clearance, more tooth structure will have to be removed.

Gingival retraction cord

Gingival retraction cord is often soaked in a hemostatic agent before placement to control bleeding. After the gold cavity preparation is completed, one or two

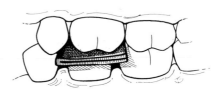

Figure 19-4 Evaluation of occlusal clearance.

pieces of this card are tucked into the gingival sulcus along any cervical margins. The cord temporarily pushes the gingiva away from the tooth and allows the impression material to be easily injected into the gingival sulcus. This ensures the dentist of a good impression of the cervical margin of the preparation, which is critical to the fabrication of a properly fitting gold restoration.

> ↩ **KEY POINT**
> - In the past epinephrine was placed on the retraction cord to help control bleeding. It is no longer recommended because epinephrine can cause heart problems in some patients.

Hemostatic agents

After the preparation of a tooth for a gold restoration, there is often some gingival bleeding caused by minor abrasion of the gingiva by preparation instruments. Control of gingival bleeding during impression-taking is essential to obtain maximum accuracy. Bleeding can be controlled by wetting the retraction cord with an astringent or a **hemostatic agent** (Figure 19-5). These agents induce clotting of blood in the small capillaries of the gingiva.

Newer types of hemostatic agents are available in a syringe form. The syringe may come with disposable tips and plastic sleeves that can by replaced for each patient to avoid cross-contamination of the syringe.

Impression trays

Impression-taking is a duplication process whereby accurate replicas of the teeth and surrounding tissues can be made. Accuracy is essential in duplicating a prepared tooth for a cost-gold restoration. Since gold inlays are fabricated in the laboratory on a replica of the patient's tooth, called a *die*, it must be an exact copy of the real tooth.

An important step in the impression-taking procedure is the selection of **impression trays** that fit the patient's dental arches. Various manufacturers make stock single-arch trays of different sizes. Metal trays (Figure 19-6, *A*) or plastic trays (Figure 19-6, *B*) can be used with a final impression material to make the die. Plastic trays are disposable, and metal trays are sterilizable. Both types of trays are usually perforated to allow impression material to ooze out of the perforations. This provides mechanical retention of the impression material in the tray after it sets. A tray adhesive may also be used to enhance this retention. The adhesive can be applied to the interior surface of the single-arch tray well in advance of the impression procedure. The retention of the impression material in the tray is critical to the making of an accurate impression. Considerable force is generated during removal of the impression from the patient's teeth. This force is in the form of a pull on the material and tends to pull it out of the tray. Tray perforation and tray adhesives prevent this from occurring.

Another type of tray, called a **dual-arch tray** (Triple Tray), can take the upper and lower quadrants and the accompanying biting relationship of the teeth all at once. The Triple Tray eliminates the need to take an impression of the teeth that oppose the tooth being restored and also eliminates the need for a bite registration.

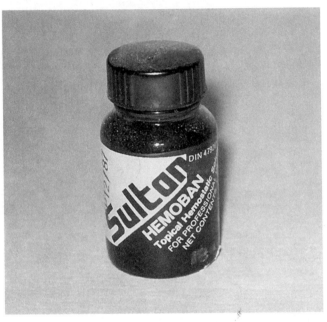

Figure 19-5   Hemostatic agent in a bottle.

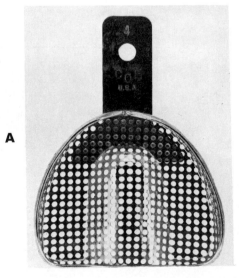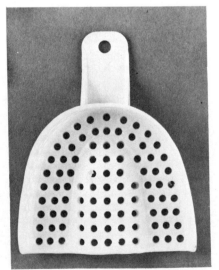

Figure 19-6   Impression trays. **A**, Perforated metal. **B**, Perforated plastic.

Regardless of which types of trays will be used, they must be a part of the setup during the preparation appointment.

Final impression materials. Although alginate impressions are used quite often in dentistry, alginate is not used to make the replica of the prepared tooth (die) because it does not produce fine detail as accurately as other impression materials that are now available.

Three common types of impression materials can be used to take an impression of a prepared tooth. They are agar hydrocolloid, polyether, and polyvinylsiloxane impression materials. Each material is accurate. Selection of the material to be used for impression-taking is the personal preference of the dentist. A text on dental materials should be consulted for the particular chemical and physical properties of these materials.

All three of these materials can be used in the syringe-tray technique of impression-taking discussed on p. 283. These impression materials and the syringe-tray technique are routinely used in restorative procedures. The same basic impression-taking technique is used in the fabrication of inlays, crowns, and fixed bridges.

◆● KEY POINT
- Three common final impression materials are polyether, polyvinylsiloxane, and agar hydrocolloid.

POLYETHER IMPRESSIONS. The items required for the preparation of polyether impressions are shown in Figure 19-7. Polyether impressions are available in **low/light**, **medium**, and **high/heavy viscosities.** The viscosity of the material refers to its flow qualities. A low-viscosity material has a more runny consistency than a medium- or heavy-viscosity material.

The following procedure is commonly used to prepare medium-viscosity polyether impressions:

1. *Dispensing.* Dispense the polyether material on the mixing pads as shown in Figure 19-7. Dispense the material so that equal lengths of base and catalyst paste lie side by side on the mixing pad. Be careful not to allow the base material to contact the catalyst until the mixing process is ready to begin. The actual amount dispensed is determined by the number of teeth included in the impression. The dentist should be consulted to guide the assistant in this regard.

2. *Mixing the material.* The assistant mixes the base and catalyst rapidly, using the spatula with a circular movement (Figure 19-8, *A*). Continue the mixing process using the flat surface of the spatula blade until the mix is rather uniform in color. This completes the blending of the materials and eliminates air bubbles in the mix.

3. *Loading the syringe.* The impression syringe consist of four parts: plunger, barrel, hub, and tip. Impregum (Reliance Dental Manufacturing, Chicago), a polyether impression material, is provided with a red loading cap and loading cap plunger. To use this syringe the red loading cap is placed on the top of the barrel, and the loading cap plunger is removed. The syringe with the loading cap is back filled from the paper pad (Figure 19-8, *B*). The red plunger is inserted and pushed down. Pushing down on the plunger will load the barrel of the syringe with the impression material (Figure 19-8, *C*). The red loading cap is removed, and the impression syringe is loaded with the regular plunger and tested (Figure 19-8, *D*). The syringe is ready for use. Transfer the syringe to the dentist who will express the material in the syringe over the crown preparation (Figure 19-8, *E*).

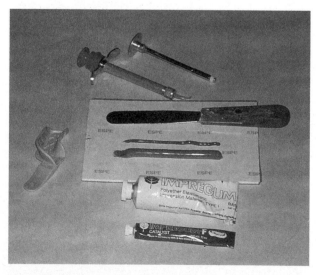

Polyether impression material
Paper pad
Spatula
Impression tray
Syringe and red loading cap

Figure 19-7 Polyether impression armamentarium. Shows equal lengths of impression material dispensed from each tube.

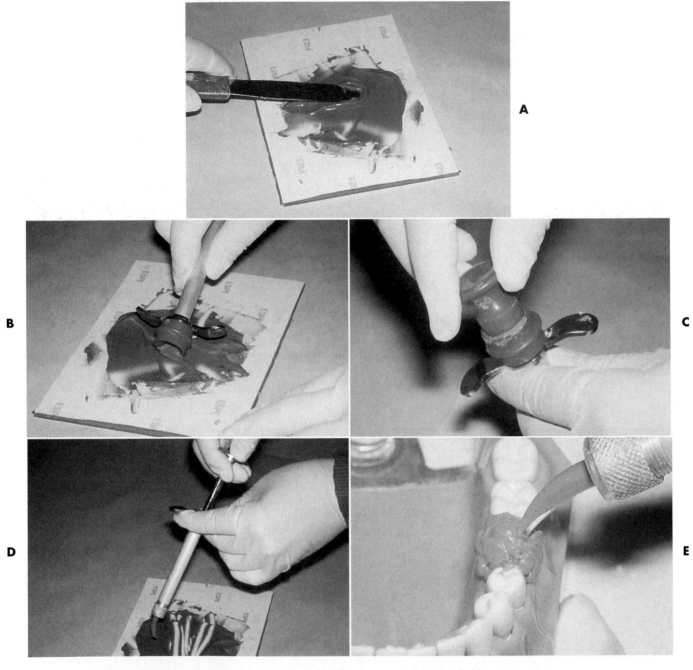

Figure 19-8 Mixing syringe type of polyether impression material. After impression material has been dispensed in equal lengths (see Figure 19-7), it is mixed with spatula (**A**). **B,** Syringe with red loading cap is back filled. **C,** Material is plunged into barrel of syringe with loading cap plunger. **D,** Loading cap and plunger are removed and syringe plunger is inserted. **E,** Remainder of material is placed into impression syringe.

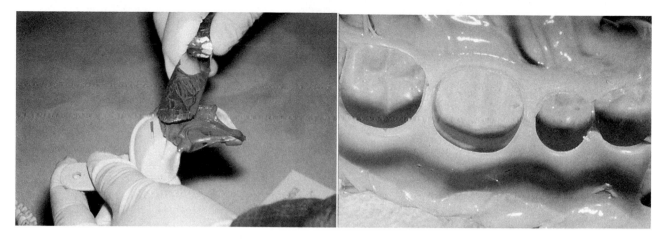

Figure 19-8, cont'd **F,** Assistant loads excess impression material into impression tray. **G,** Final impression of prepared tooth.

4. *Loading the tray material.* Load the remainder of the material on the paper pad into an impression tray (Figure 19-8, *F*). If a dual-arch tray is used, the polyether material must be placed on both the upper and lower areas of the tray. Transfer the impression tray to the dentist who will seat the tray in the patient's mouth. Figure 19-8, *G*, shows the final impression of a prepared tooth.

5. *Disinfecting the impression.* After the impression is removed from the patient's mouth, it should be rinsed with running water. The impression can be disinfected by spraying with an iodophor or chlorine dioxide disinfectant.

A medium-viscosity material can be used for both the impression syringe and the impression tray. An alternative method that is preferred by some dentists is to use a low-viscosity material for the syringe and a high-viscosity material for the impression tray. The dental assistant would have to mix the two different viscosities on separate mixing pads. The low viscosity is mixed first for the impression syringe, and the high viscosity is mixed to fill the impression tray while the dentist is applying the material from the impression syringe on the crown preparation.

The mixing scheme just outlined describes the technique for mixing polyether.

POLYVINYLSILOXANE IMPRESSIONS. Polyvinylsiloxane impression material is available in many forms. A light-bodied impression material, sometimes referred to as a **wash,** can be used as a syringe material. A medium-bodied consistency can also be used as a syringe material, and a very heavy-bodied, or thick, consistency can be used to fill the impression tray. A putty is also available that can be substituted for the very heavy-bodied material to fill the impression tray.

Polyvinylsiloxane syringe material is now available in an **Automix system** (Figures 19-9 and 19-10) that is very popular. The base and catalyst material come in an Automix cartridge that holds equal amounts of the base and catalyst side by side (Figure 19-11). The cartridge is placed in a special dispensing gun. A **mixing tip** is placed at the tip of the cartridge, and when the trigger of the dispensing gun is pulled, the base and catalyst are extruded out into the mixing tip. As the material flows through the mixing tip it is mixed thoroughly.

Box 19-1 describes the procedure for taking a polyvinylsiloxane impression with either a **two-viscosity impression technique** or a **putty-wash technique.**

AGAR HYDROCOLLOID IMPRESSIONS. Agar hydrocolloid impressions require more bulky and expensive equipment than any of the other impression-taking systems. The required items are shown in Figure 19-12.

Agar hydrocolloid is packaged in a gel state. A great deal of this material is water (up to 85%); therefore care must be exercised to store and handle it according to the manufacturer's directions to prevent evaporation.

The basic method used to take a hydrocolloid impression is to convert the solid (gel) state to a semiliquid (sol) state by heating the material in a hot-water conditioner. Once the material is in a semiliquid form, it can be inserted in the patient's mouth via an injection syringe and a special impression tray and then cooled to convert the material back to the solid state (gel). When the material is back in the solid state, the impression can be removed.

The conversion of the hydrocolloid from the gel to the sol state involves the use of three hot-water baths. The tray material is placed in all three baths during processing. The syringe material is placed only in the first two baths.

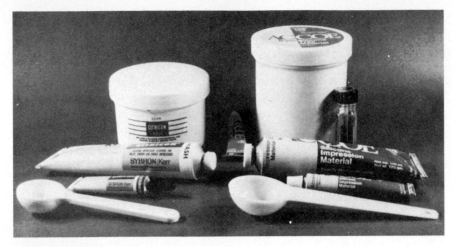

Figure 19-9 Polyvinylsiloxane impression armamentarium for syringe–tray technique.

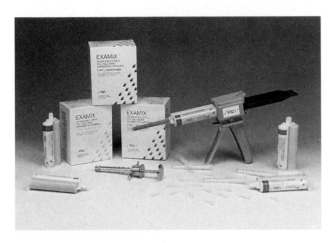

Figure 19-10 Polyvinylsiloxane impression armamentarium for two-viscosity technique.

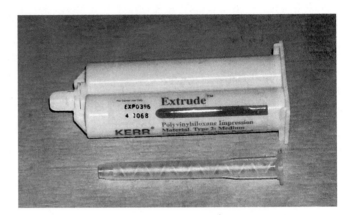

Figure 19-11 Polyvinylsiloxane Automix cartridge and mixing tip.

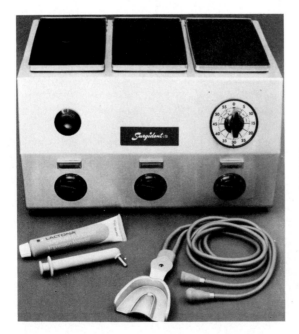

Agar hydrocolloid material (syringe and tray types)
Hydrocolloid conditioner
Injection syringe
Water-cooled trays
Water-coolant tubes

Figure 19-12 Agar hydrocolloid conditioner armamentarium. *Left to right:* Tray material (tube), syringe, impression tray, cooling tubes.

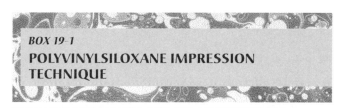

BOX 19-1

POLYVINYLSILOXANE IMPRESSION TECHNIQUE

TWO-VISCOSITY TECHNIQUE	PUTTY-WASH TECHNIQUE
1. Fit impression tray.	1. Fit impression tray.
2. Load dispensing gun with light-bodied or wash material and screw in mixing tip. Place intraoral tip on end of mixing tip.	2. Load dispensing gun with light-bodied or wash material and screw in mixing tip. Place intraoral tip on end of mixing tip.
3. Load another dispensing gun with medium-bodied or very heavy-bodied material. Screw in mixing tip.	3. Take equal scoops of base and catalyst putty material and place on mixing pad.
4. Dentist removes retraction cord.	4. Dentist removes retraction cord.
5. Dental assistant transfers light-bodied or wash material to dentist, who will apply it on crown preparation.	5. Dental assistant transfers light-bodied or wash material to dentist, who will apply it on crown preparation.
6. Dental assistant loads impression tray with other dispensing gun with medium-bodied or very heavy-bodied material.	6. Dental assistant uses hands to mix and smash base and catalyst putty together with fingers until it is a uniform color. Putty is rolled between hands and placed in impression tray.
7. Dental assistant transfers loaded impression tray to dentist, who will seat tray on top of wash.	7. Dental assistant transfers loaded impression tray to dentist, who will seat tray on top of wash.
8. Impression tray is held in place until impression material hardens.	8. Impression tray is held in place until impression material hardens.
9. Impression tray is removed and inspected for accuracy.	9. Impression tray is removed and inspected for accuracy.
10. Impression is disinfected by immersion in 2% glutaraldehyde.	10. Impression is disinfected by immersion in 2% glutaraldehyde.

> **↦ KEY POINT**
> ■ Agar hydrocolloid does not require mixing.

The preparation and technique of impression-taking with agar hydrocolloid are described in Box 19-2 and Figure 19-13.

Agar hydrocolloid had diminished in popularity since the development of the polyether and polyvinylsiloxane materials. However, it should not be overlooked because it is a very accurate impression material if handled properly.

Bite registration material

After the impression-taking procedure is finished, some dentists prefer to fabricate a device to orient the upper and lower models in the proper bite relationship during the laboratory phase. This device is commonly referred to as a **bite registration.** Various materials are frequently used for this purpose. Some of the more common ones include pink baseplate wax, silicone, or polyvinylsiloxane bite registration materials.

Pink baseplate wax. Pink baseplate wax is carved with a laboratory knife into the shape of the patient's arch. The wax is heated in warm water to soften, and the patient is instructed to bite into the wax (Figure 19-14, *A*). Air from the air-water syringe is lightly blown onto the wax to cool and harden it as the patient keeps the wax between the teeth.

Silicone and polyvinylsiloxane materials. Silicone and polyvinylsiloxane materials (Figure 19-14, *B*) are available in Automix cartridges. The Automix cartridge is placed in a dispensing gun, and a mixing tip is attached to the cartridge. The material is expressed out of the mixing tip directly on the occlusal surfaces of the teeth in one quadrant or an anterior sextant depending on the location of the prepared tooth or teeth. The patient is instructed to bite down on the registration material until it reaches a hardened state and can be removed from the mouth.

The imprints of the biting surfaces of the teeth are then used as guides to orient the upper and lower laboratory models of the teeth together (see Figure 19-22).

> **↦ KEY POINT**
> ■ A bite registration is not needed when a dual-arch tray is used.

Temporization materials

After the preparation and impression procedures have been completed, the prepared tooth must be protected (temporized) until the patient's next appointment.

BOX 19-2

IMPRESSION-TAKING WITH AGAR HYDROCOLLOID

PROCEDURE	RATIONALE
1. *Loading the syringe.* Insert one small stick of syringe hydrocolloid into barrel of syringe. It is advisable to remove protective cap from needle of syringe and insert plunger into syringe barrel, forcing out excess air around hydrocolloid stick. Replace cap over needle.	1. This method prevents expansion of air in syringe during heating process, which could force plunger out of syringe and let hydrocolloid escape into water bath.
2. **Boiling bath** (212° F [100° C]). Place loaded syringe and tube of tray-type hydrocolloid in boiling-water bath for 10 to 15 minutes.	2. This step converts gel to sol state.
3. **Storage bath** (149° F [65° C]). Both syringe and tray materials can be transferred to this bath if materials are not used immediately. They can remain in storage bath for several hours before material is used.	3. This method is used to store hydrocolloid material if it is not going to be used immediately.
4. **Tempering bath** (115° F [39° C]). When cavity preparation is completed and gingival retraction cord is placed, remove tube of tray material from storage bath. Fill hydrocolloid impression tray with soft, semiliquid material. Place filled tray in tempering bath for 5 minutes.	4. This step cools material within tolerable limits and prevents burning patient. It also causes tray material to thicken slightly. Syringe material is not tempered. Tempering would thicken material inside syringe so that it would be too thick to inject through thin syringe needle.

PROCEDURE	RATIONALE
5. *Impression procedure.* After removal of retraction cord, hydrocolloid syringe is removed from storage bath and needle cap is removed. Material is injected around prepared tooth. Dentist places syringe material around prepared tooth before seating of loaded impression tray.	5. Coolant tubes that are attached to tray provide water supply and exhaust for circulating water. One tube can be connected to a water source once impression tray is seated. Exhaust tube can be draped into nearby sink or large plastic container to collect exhausted water. Cooling usually requires 3 to 5 minutes at water temperature of 55° F (12.7° C). Loaded impression tray is seated over syringe material.
6. Filled impression tray is removed from tempering bath, and cooling tubes are attached quickly. Tray is placed in patient's mouth over prepared and adjacent teeth.	6. Impression tray contains small tubes that allow water to be circulated around impression material to cool it, thus converting it back.
7. *Disinfecting the impression.* After impression is removed from patient's mouth it should be disinfected with iodophor spray or diluted bleach solution.	7. If impression cannot be poured immediately, it should be gently wrapped in moist paper towel while die stone material is being prepared for pouring model.
8. Care must be taken because distortion can result from prolonged immersion.	8. Agar hydrocolloid is very delicate material. It loses its dimensional accuracy rapidly because of water loss. In contrast; if it is placed in water for any length of time, it absorbs water and swells. Either condition must be prevented to ensure maximum accuracy.
9. *Pouring the model.* After poured impression is in solid state, it is carefully removed.	9. To prepare for fabrication of permanent restoration.

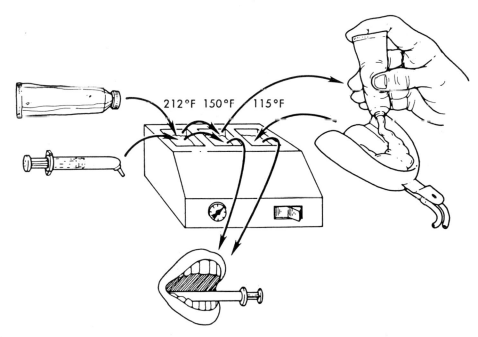

Figure 19-13   Preparation of agar hydrocolloid impression material. Boiling bath (212° F). Storage bath (150° F). Tempering bath (115° F).

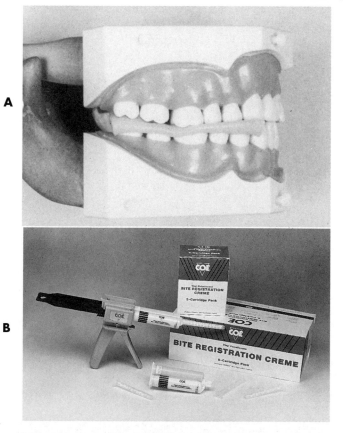

Figure 19-14   Bite registration materials. **A,** Pink baseplate wax. **B,** Polyvinylsiloxane bite registration.

There are several ways to temporize a prepared tooth. The specific method selected depends on the type of preparation and, to some extent, the personal preference of the dentist.

Inlay temporization is usually accomplished by filling the prepared cavity with a semisoft material that is easy to remove at the next appointment, when the restoration is fitted to the tooth and cemented in place. A zinc oxide and eugenol (ZOE) cement (IRM, Dentsply International, Milford, Del.) can be used for gold inlay preparations. A few strands of cotton fibers from a cotton pellet can be incorporated into the mix for added strength. The material is placed in the preparation, and the patient is asked to bite down on the material. The excess filling material is carved away, and the material is allowed to harden before the patient is dismissed (Figure 19-15). Other temporization materials include acrylic and a newer resinlike temporary material explained in Chapter 18.

Items for Cementation Appointment of Gold Inlays
Armamentarium

A suggested armamentarium for cementation of gold inlays is shown in Figure 19-16.

At the appointment for inserting the gold restoration (the seating appointment) a few instruments should be added to the armamentarium. Some of these instruments and devices are described here.

Seating devices

To check the fit of a gold restoration properly, it must be seated completely on the tooth. A convenient way to accomplish this is to concentrate biting forces onto the occlusal surface of the restoration. This drives the restoration to its final position on the tooth. Figure 19-17 shows the use of the three most common devices for this purpose.

After all adjustments have been made on the restoration, the final cement is prepared and placed on the tissue

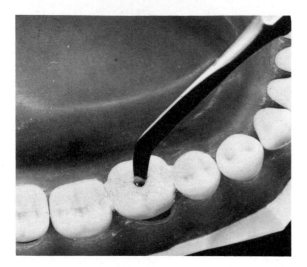

Figure 19-15 Temporization of an inlay preparation with IRM.

surface of the restoration. The restoration is placed on the tooth and initially seated with finger pressure. Then it is finally driven into place with one of the seating devices. Next it is burnished, and any minor adjustments can be made.

Burnishers

Burnishers are available in hand types and straight-handpiece types. They are used to bend the fine margins of a gold restoration down on the tooth surface immediately after cementation. The margins frequently are bent in the handling of the gold restoration. The burnisher is rubbed across the gold margin from the gold toward the tooth structure. This perfects the fit of the margin to the tooth structure.

Finishing stones, burs, and disks

Various shapes and styles of fine-grit grindstones and finishing burs are available to make minor adjustments on gold restorations. They are used to correct occlusion, finish margins, and reduce heavy contact between a gold restoration and an adjacent tooth. Sandpaper disks are used to finish proximal margins.

Dental cements for final cementation

Three types of cement (zinc phosphate, polycarboxylate, and glass ionomer) are popular as final cementation agents for gold and porcelain restorations. A text on dental materials should be consulted for the properties and characteristics of these cements.

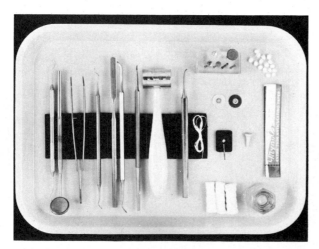

Figure 19-16 Gold restoration cementation arma–mentarium.

Preset tray

Cowhorn explorer, No. 3
Mouth mirror, No. 4
Cotton pliers
Spoon excavator
Cement spatula, No. 324 or No. 24
Plastic filling instrument, F.P. No. 1
Gold foil condenser, straight
Gold foil mallet
Hand burnisher, 5S
Dental floss
Craytex polishing wheels
Moore's mandrels
Green stone, wheel shaped
Green stone, knife edge
Ball burnishers, H.P.
Cotton pellets
Moore's disks
Articulating paper
Bur, R.A. No. 4
Cooley peg
Cotton rolls
Dappen dish

Add-on items

Finel cement material
Cavity varnish
Isopropyl alcohol
Mixing slab or pad

Two critical characteristics of any dental cement are film thickness and strength. Cement must be thin so that it can ooze out between the tooth structure and the gold restoration when the crown is seated. A cement that is too thick can prevent the restoration from seating completely during cementation procedures. On the other hand, the strength of a cement is important to retain the restoration and to maintain a proper seal between the tooth and restoration. If the cement is mixed so that it is too thin, strength is markedly reduced.

Zinc phosphate cement. Zinc phosphate cement is one of the oldest cementation agents used in dentistry today. Proper mixing of this material is accomplished by mixing it to a specific consistency within a time limit. Several methods can achieve the proper consistency of zinc phosphate for use in the cementation of a gold restoration. The method described uses the following materials (Figure 19-18, *A*):

- Zinc phosphate (powder and liquid)
- Glass slab
- Cement spatula
- Stopwatch

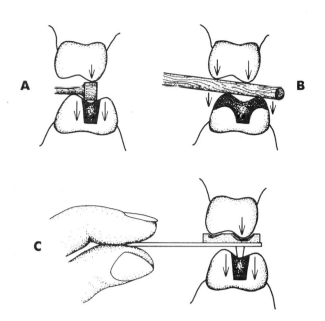

Figure 19-17   Gold restoration seating devices. **A,** Cooley peg. **B,** Orangewood stick. **C,** Inlay seating device.

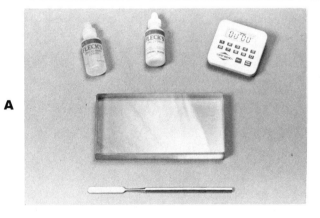
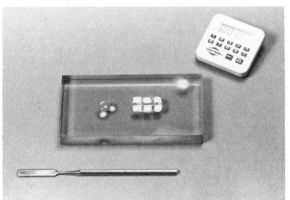
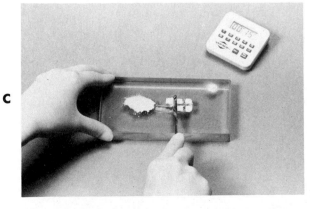
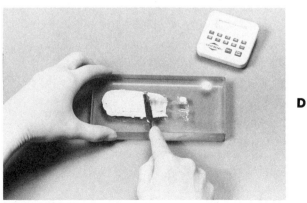

Figure 19-18   Preparation of zinc phosphate cement. **A,** Armamentarium. **B,** Dispensed materials. **C** and **D,** Increment of powder added to liquid every 15 seconds and mixed, using broad spatulations.

Continued.

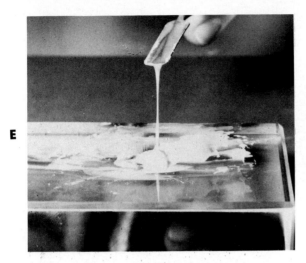

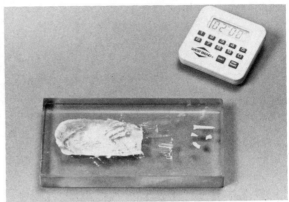

Figure 19-18, cont'd   E, Testing mix. F, Cement base consistency.

The mixing procedure is as follows:

1. *Dispensing the materials.* Zinc phosphate cement produces heat when the powder and liquid components are combined. Therefore a glass slab is required as a mixing surface to absorb the heat and cool the mix. The liquid/powder ratio that works well is a ½-inch pile and a ¼-inch pile of powder to be mixed with six to seven drops of liquid. After the powder is dispensed, divide all the powder into six equal sections. Then dispense six to seven drops of liquid onto the surface of the slab to the left of the divided powder (Figure 19-17, *B*). An additional ½-inch pile of powder can be placed in the upper right-hand corner of the slab in case it is needed.

2. *Incremental mixing.* The object of this mixing technique is to mix the powder and liquid together slowly to minimize heat production. However, if the mixing time is excessive, the mix will begin to set. Trial mixes have demonstrated that a favorable mixing pace calls for adding and mixing one of the six sections of powder every 15 seconds. Thus it will take 90 seconds to mix all six sections into the liquid. However, all six sections may not be needed to reach the proper consistency for cementation. Add each section of powder to the liquid, and apply it with broad strokes over an area the size of a silver dollar (Figure 19-17, *C* and *D*).

3. *Testing the mix* (Figure 19-17, *E*). After the addition and mixing of the fourth section, it is good to test the mix for proper consistency. Proper consistency is determined by gathering the mixed cement into a small puddle on the slab. Dip the broad surface of the spatula into the puddle, and raise the spatula slowly from the slab. The cement should string out approximately 1 to 1½ inches between the slab and the spatula blade before it drops off the spatula back into the puddle. If it strings out longer than 1½ inches, the mix is too

thick. If it is less than 1 inch, more powder must be added. Continue testing as the fifth and sixth sections of powder are added. Sometimes it is necessary to add some of the extra powder stored in the upper right-hand corner of the slab to achieve the proper consistency. *Consistency* is a key word. Mixing zinc phosphate cement is not just a matter of combining six or seven drops of liquid with one large and one small pile of powder every time a mix is made. The temperature and humidity of the day will influence how much powder can be added to the liquid before the ideal consistency is reached.

4. *Application of the cement.* When the proper consistency of the cement has been reached, cover the tissue surface of the restoration with a thin coat of cement. Deliver the restoration to the dentist on the slab, with the restoration resting on the coated surface. A filling instrument should accompany the delivery of the restoration so that the dentist can add some additional cement to the preparation before seating the restoration in place.

⇨ KEY POINTS

- A glass slab must be used to mix zinc phosphate cement.
- When zinc phosphate is mixed to the proper consistency as a permanent cement, the material should lift 1 to 1½ inches from the glass slab.

ZINC PHOSPHATE CEMENT BASE. Zinc phosphate cement is used not only for final cementation purposes but also as a cement base under various restorations. A cement base is

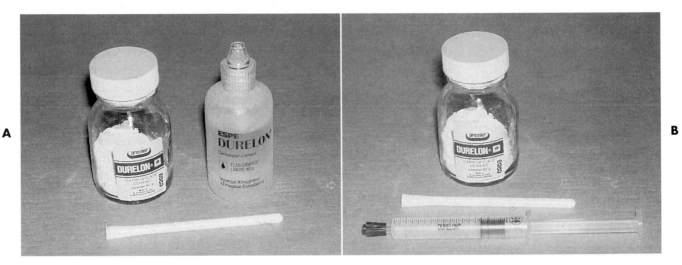

Figure 19-19   Polycarboxylate final cementation materials. **A,** Polycarboxylate liquid in bottle. **B,** Polycarboxylate liquid in syringe.

a strong dental cement that has been mixed to a doughlike consistency and used as artificial dentin in deep cavity preparations (see Chapter 16).

To prepare zinc phosphate cement for use as a cement base, the basic mixing technique just described is used, except that three ½-inch piles of powder are placed in the upper right-hand corner of the slab instead of the large and small piles recommended for cementation purposes.

Once the cement base is mixed to the consistency described for cementation, the extra powder from the upper right-hand corner of the slab is brought into the mix, one-half pile or less at a time, until the cement is well blended into a thick, doughlike consistency. Gloved fingers can be coated with powder from the slab, and the doughlike cement can be rolled into a rope. Small pieces can be cut off the "rope" and delivered to the operator for use in the prepared cavity (Figure 19-17, *F*). The entire mixing time should not exceed 2½ minutes to allow enough working time for the operator to place the cement base.

Polycarboxylate cement. Polycarboxylate cement possesses some of the desirable characteristics found in zinc phosphate cement, but it does not cause the pulpal irritation produced by the acidic zinc phosphate. A big plus from the dental assistant's viewpoint is the ease of mixing compared with that of zinc phosphate cement. The following materials are needed to prepare polycarboxylate cement:
- Polycarboxylate cement (powder and liquid)
- Paper mixing pad
- Measuring scoop
- Spatula
- Stopwatch

Following is a description of the preparation of Durelon (Premier Dental Mfg., Philadelphia), a brand of polycarboxylate cement:

1. *Dispensing the ingredients.* Place one scoop of powder in the center of the mixing pad. The special measuring scoop is provided by the manufacturer. The polycarboxylate liquid is available in two forms. If the polycarboxylate liquid is in a plastic bottle, place three drops of the liquid component adjacent to the powder (Figure 19-19, *A*). If the polycarboxylate liquid is in a dispensing syringe provided by the manufacturer, push the plunger until three increments (or markings on the syringe) are dispensed (Figure 19-19, *B*).

2. *Mixing technique.* Combine the liquid and powder all at one time. The powder must be completely wetted by the liquid. Use a folding action with the spatula to accomplish this. For a smooth mix, spread the mix over an area the size of a silver dollar with the broad surface of the spatula. The mixing should be completed within 30 seconds.

3. *Coating the restoration.* Place the cement on the restoration in the same manner as described for zinc phosphate cement. Durelon cement sets rather quickly, so care must be taken to avoid delay in delivering the restoration to the dentist.

> ➥ **KEY POINT**
> - The correct ratio of polycarboxylate cement powder to liquid is one scoop of powder to three drops of liquid or three increments from the dispensing syringe.

Glass ionomer cements. Glass ionomer cements are a relatively new type of cement used in dentistry. They are nonirritating to the pulp and also have anticariogenic properties. Glass ionomer cements contain fluoride that is slowly released over time and helps to prevent recurrent decay around the margins of the restorations.

The following materials are needed to prepare a typical glass ionomer cement (Figure 19-20):

- Mixing pad
- Glass ionomer cement (powder and liquid)
- Measuring scoop
- Spatula
- Stopwatch

Following is a description of the preparation of Ketac Cem (Buffalo Dental Manufacturing Co., Brooklyn, N.Y.), a type of glass ionomer cement:

1. *Dispensing the ingredients.* Dispense one level scoop of powder with the measuring scoop provided by the manufacturer on the mixing pad with two drops of liquid.
2. *Mixing technique.* Combine half of the powder into the liquid using a folding action of the spatula. Once the powder is completely wetted, press the mix against the pad with the broad surface of the spatula. Mix the last half of the powder into the liquid, and use repeated strokes over the mix with the spatula, in a barber's stropping motion, to produce the proper film thickness in the mix. The mix should be completed quickly.

➡ KEY POINT
- The correct ratio for the glass ionomer powder and liquid is two drops of liquid and one scoop of powder.

CAST-GOLD INLAY PROCEDURE

Having completed an overview of the more common instruments and supplies used in the cast-gold restoration procedure, the following is a step-by-step description of how the procedure is accomplished. The mesioocclusodistal (MOD) inlay has been selected as an example.

Inlay Preparation Appointment: MOD Example

As mentioned previously, fabrication of an inlay usually requires two appointments. One appointment is devoted to the preparation of the tooth and impression taking. The second appointment is used for cementation of the finished restoration. The time between these two appointments must be sufficient to allow for the casting of the inlay in the laboratory. The patient wears a temporary dressing in the prepared tooth between the two appointments.

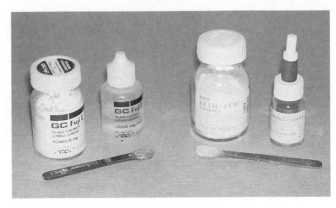

Figure 19-20   Glass ionomer final cementation materials.

The sequence of events that takes place at the **preparation appointment** is as follows:

1. Opposing model impression
2. Bite registration
3. Anesthetic administration
4. Isolation
5. Cavity preparation
6. Gingival retraction
7. Impression-taking
8. Temporization

Opposing model impression

A model of the **opposing teeth** is needed by the laboratory technician to fabricate the occlusal portion of the inlay. If an inlay is being made on a lower tooth, then a model of the upper teeth is needed to determine how the lower inlay fits the anatomy of the upper teeth when patients close their teeth together. The dental assistant uses alginate to take impressions of the opposing teeth. It is most efficient to perform this part of the procedure at the beginning of the appointment.

Alginate impressions require use of the items shown in Figure 19-21.

The mixing procedure is as follows:

1. Prepare the material by adding premeasured alginate powder to the rubber mixing bowl, which contains a premeasured amount of water. Manufacturers provide the proper measuring devices with their product.

➡ KEY POINT
- Always place the water in the mixing bowl and add the powder to the water. This method will ensure minimal bubbles in the resulting mix.

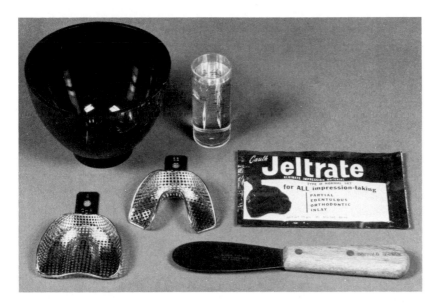

Rubber mixing bowl
Wide-bladed spatula
Water measure
Powder scoop (unless premeasured packets are used)
Alginate material
Alginate impression trays

Figure 19-21   Alginate impression armamentarium.

2. Mix the powder and water together with the wide-bladed spatula within 1 minute. The mix must be smooth and creamy. To accomplish this, press the alginate against the sides of the rubber bowl with the spatula while mixing.

3. Load the material in the tray and place in the patient's mouth. (A description of the alginate impression technique is presented at the end of this section.) Setting times range from 1½ to 3 minutes, depending on whether regular-set or fast-set alginate is used. The temperature of the water also influences setting time. Most manufacturers recommend a temperature of 70° F (21.1° C) for maximum accuracy and ample working time.

4. After the impression is removed from the patient's mouth, rinse it with water and place it in an iodophor disinfectant for 10 minutes. After 10 minutes in the disinfectant, the model can be poured with plaster or dental stone. For maximum accuracy a model should be made from the impression within the first 30 minutes after removal.

A handy tip for the assistant is to use premeasured bags of alginate powder that are available from the manufacturer or to premeasure the alginate from a bulk container and store it in plastic sandwich bags. This is a good way to save valuable chairside time.

This model is made from an impression of the opposing teeth. An impression tray is filled with a rapid-setting impression material called alginate. The tray is placed over the opposing teeth and allowed to set. The impression is removed, and the opposing model can be made. The syringe-type technique is not necessary to make this impression.

> **➙ KEY POINT**
> ▪ An opposing model is not necessary when a dual-tray technique is used.

Bite registration

For the fabrication of an inlay that will properly fit the bite of the patient, the laboratory technician must have the following four elements:

1. A model of the opposing teeth
2. A model containing the prepared tooth
3. A registration of the patient's biting relationship to guide the technician as to how the two opposing models fit together
4. A device, called an articulator, to hold the models in the proper biting relationship and simulate the movement of the jaws

The opposing model can be fitted in the appropriate sides of the bite registration and then mounted on the articulator with plaster used to hold them in place (Figure 19-22). The dental assistant may take the bite registration before local anesthetic is administered because it may be easier for the patient to close in a normal way.

Anesthetic administration

See Chapter 4 for a discussion of anesthetic techniques.

Isolation

Cotton roll isolation works well during gold preparation procedures. If a rubber dam is used, it must be removed before gingival retraction and impression-taking.

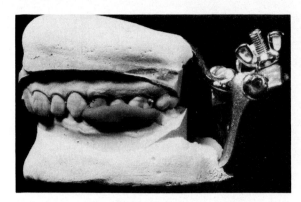

Figure 19-22   Bite registration used to mount models on articulator. Plaster is used to fasten models to articulator.

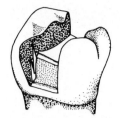

Figure 19-23   MOD inlay preparation.

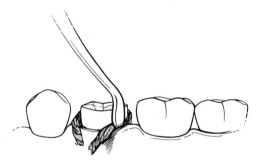

Figure 19-24   Gingival retraction cord in place.

Cavity preparation

Gold inlays are fabricated for all classes of cavity preparations. All these cavity preparations have internal draw built into their design.

Draw is a term used to describe the relationship of the cavity walls from the floor of the cavity preparation to the cavosurface margins. The walls must be slightly tapered so that the gold restoration can slide into place (Figure 19-23). Excessive taper would result in loss of retention of the restoration in the tooth. Dentists use tapered burs (No. 171) and straight tapered diamonds to establish the proper amount of taper.

Most dentists prefer to place small bevels on the cavosurface margins of the preparation. It is easier to fit gold casting to a beveled surface than to a butt joint. A flame-shaped diamond stone and gingival margin trimmers are useful for this purpose.

Inlay preparations must have smooth cavity walls to achieve a proper fit of the inlay inside the tooth. Enamel hatchets are often used to plane the cavity walls.

Cement bases are placed at this time if they are needed (see Chapter 16).

The dental assistant works closely with the dentist to transfer instruments to the dentist. If necessary, the dental assistant also changes the burs on the dental handpiece before transferring the handpiece to the dentist.

Gingival retraction

After the preparation is finished, the gingiva must be retracted away from the cervical margins of the preparation. The purpose is to create a space between the cervical portion of the tooth and the gingiva to allow impression material to record the cervical margin accurately.

This retraction is accomplished by gently tucking gingival retraction cord in the gingival crevice in the region of the cervical margin of the preparation (Figure 19-24). A special cord-packing instrument or a plastic filling instrument can be used for this purpose. A common practice is to place two strands of the cord to gain adequate retraction. The cord must remain in place for 3 to 4 minutes. Hemostatic agents are sometimes used to stop gingival bleeding that may occur.

The impression material can be dispensed and mixed while the operator is waiting for the retraction to take place.

The dental assistant is often responsible for cutting the appropriate length of retraction cord and wetting the retraction cord in the hemostatic agent. After transferring the cord-packing instrument to the dentist the dental assistant either places the retraction cord loosely around the crown preparation or gives the retraction cord to the dentist for placement. In some states a dental assistant with expanded functions may be allowed to place the retraction cord around the tooth preparation.

Impression-taking

Impression-taking is a method used by dentists to make a duplicate of the patient's teeth and surrounding tissues. The laboratory technician makes an exact model of the patient's teeth and the prepared cavity from this impression. The gold inlay is made on this model and returned to the dentist for cementation in the patient's prepared tooth.

The most common method of impression-taking employs the syringe-tray technique. This technique requires the use of two consistencies of the same impression material. One thinner consistency of material is mixed and loaded in a special injection syringe. A second, thicker material is mixed and loaded in any impression tray that will fit over the patient's teeth.

Following is the sequence of events in taking the impression:

1. The gingival retraction cord is removed.
2. The preparation is air dried.
3. The injection syringe is used to squirt impression material into the widened gingival crevice and into the cavity preparation (Figure 19-25, *A*). The procedure eliminates entrapment of air bubbles in the impression.
4. The tray filled with the thicker impression material is placed over the prepared tooth and the adjacent teeth (Figure 19-25, *B*). This records the relationship of the prepared tooth to the adjacent teeth.
5. After the material reaches its final set, the impression is removed from the patient's mouth.

The three most common types of material can be used for this syringe-tray type of impression: agar hydrocolloid, polyether, and polyvinylsiloxane. Each dentist has a personal preference for one material for impression-taking. All the materials mentioned are accurate.

For this portion of the procedure the dental assistant will most likely dispense and mix the final impression materials. In some states a dental assistant with expanded functions may be allowed to seat the final impression in the patient's mouth.

Temporization

After cavity preparation, impression-taking, and bite registration are completed, a temporary filling material is placed in the cavity preparation. This material is usually a temporary ZOE cement or a flexible plastic filling material.

The temporary restoration accomplishes the following:

1. Prevents sensitivity in the prepared tooth
2. Aids in preventing fracture of the prepared tooth
3. Prevents the prepared tooth from drifting out of position between appointments

In some states the dental assistant is allowed to fit and cement the temporary filling material.

Inlay Cementation Appointment: MOD Example

After the preparation appointment the patient wears the temporary restoration while the inlay is fabricated in the laboratory. The patient then returns for a **cementation appointment** to have the inlay cemented in the prepared tooth.

The sequence of events in the completion of the inlay restorative procedure is as follows:

1. Anesthetic administration
2. Isolation
3. Removal of the temporary restoration

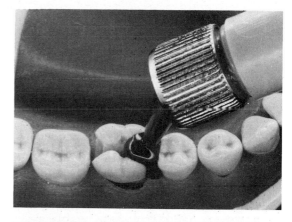

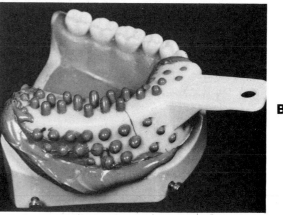

Figure 19-25 **A,** Injection of syringe-consistency impression material into cavity preparation and gingival crevice. **B,** Impression tray with heavier tray-consistency material in place.

4. Contact adjustment
5. Occlusal adjustment
6. Polishing
7. Cementation
8. Margin finishing

Anesthetic

The same type of local anesthetic is administered as was required during the preparation appointment. It should be noted that some patients do not require anesthetic during seating appointments. In such instances it is desirable not to use an anesthetic, since it may inhibit the patient's ability to bite normally.

Isolation

Cotton roll isolation is probably the most popular isolation method used for this procedure because the patient is required to close the teeth together several times during the seating process. The rubber dam clamp prevents closure if a rubber dam is used for isolation.

Removal of temporary restoration

The temporary filling material can be removed from the cavity preparation with the spoon excavator or with a slow-speed round bur (No. 4). This must be done carefully so that the preparation is not damaged in the process. The cavity preparation must be absolutely free of any of the temporary material or other debris. Any debris left in the preparation prevents the inlay from seating completely in the tooth. Cotton pellets are helpful in removing debris. A thorough rinsing of the preparation with the air-water syringe completes the cleaning process.

In some states a dental assistant is allowed to remove the temporary restoration and also to remove the temporary cement around the tooth preparation.

Contact adjustment

The contact areas of an inlay are the areas on the inlay that contact the proximal surfaces of the adjacent teeth (Figure 19-26). These areas are often excessively contoured by the laboratory technician. If this is the situation, the excessive gold is ground away until the inlay will seat completely in the tooth.

After the inlay is seated in the tooth, the amount of contact between the inlay and adjacent teeth can be checked by passing dental floss through the contact areas. The contacts must be snug but not so tight that it is difficult to pass floss between the inlay and the adjacent teeth. On the other hand, the floss should not pass through freely. A contact that is not tight enough will allow food to be forced between the teeth, which can damage the interproximal gingiva.

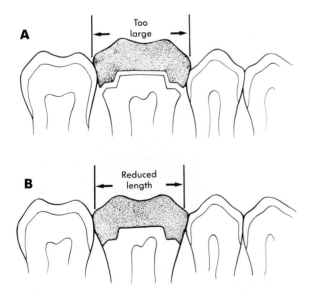

Figure 19-26 Adjustment of contact areas. **A,** Mesiodistal dimension is too large, and inlay does not seat completely. **B,** Corrected mesiodistal dimension allows inlay to seat completely.

It is a good policy for the dental assistant to hold a filling instrument on the occlusal surface of the inlay during the check with the dental floss. This prevents the inlay from being dislodged from the tooth, which could result in the patient swallowing or aspirating the restoration.

To check the contact fit of the inlay, it is necessary to have the inlay completely seated in the cavity preparation. The wooden **Cooley peg,** orangewood stick, cotton roll, or other bite device is used to force the inlay all the way into the preparation (see Figure 19-17).

After the contacts are checked and adjusted, the cervical areas are checked with the explorer to determine the fit of the inlay along the cervical margins. If the gold is too bulky in this area, the inlay is removed, and the excessive gold is ground away with a finishing stone or disk until the fit is perfected.

If the inlay is difficult to remove from the preparation, a straight gold foil condenser can be tapped gently on a proximal surface of the inlay to drive it out of the preparation. The assistant must keep a finger on the inlay to prevent it from dropping out of the tooth.

Occlusal adjustment

After the inlay is completely seated, the fit of the occlusal surface of the inlay to the opposing teeth must be assessed. This is done by having the patient bring the teeth together on a piece of articulating paper. If the inlay is too high, or in **hyperocclusion,** heavy marks will show on the occlusal surface of the inlay when the paper is removed. In addition, the patient can usually sense even the slightest hyperocclusion in a restoration.

If the inlay is in hyperocclusion, the excessive gold on the occlusal surface is ground away until the inlay fits the occlusal surfaces of the opposing teeth. This often requires repeated try-ins and corrections until the occlusion is perfected.

A correct bite registration and mounting of the laboratory models during the fabrication of the inlay greatly reduces or even eliminates the need for occlusal adjustment.

Polishing

When all corrections have been made on the inlay, the external surface of the inlay is polished with a fine abrasive rubber wheel (Craytex). It is then taken to the dental lathe and polished with various abrasive polishes to impart a high shine to its surface. The inlay can be cleaned in an ultrasonic cleaner or hand scrubbed to remove all polish residue. It is then placed in a dappen dish and disinfected with an appropriate disinfectant.

Cementation

The inlay is now ready to be seated in the prepared tooth permanently with a final cement material. Figure 19-15 and 19-16 show several of the popular brands available for this purpose. If zinc phosphate cement is used, it is necessary to varnish the dentin before the inlay is cemented in place. This prevents the acidic cement from irritating the prepared tooth. Varnish is not necessary if the other cements are used.

The prepared tooth is rinsed thoroughly and dried. The operative field must be well isolated and kept dry until the inlay is cemented in the preparation. The cavity varnish is applied at this time if it is needed.

Zinc phosphate cement is mixed with the cement spatula on a mixing slab (see Figure 19-18), and the tissue surface of the inlay is coated with cement. The cement slab can be brought to the operative site with the inlay turned down on the slab. The operator can then coat the preparation with cement, using the plastic filling instrument. The inlay is placed in the preparation and seated with finger pressure. The Cooley peg, orangewood stick, cotton roll, or other bite device is then placed over the inlay, and the patient is instructed to bite on the peg to drive the inlay to seat completely into the preparation. The patient is asked to maintain biting pressure until the cement reaches its initial set (see Figure 19-17, *A*).

In some states the dental assistant is allowed to remove the excess cement from the cemented restoration.

Margin finishing

After the cement has reached its initial set, the peg is removed. Excessive cement can be removed from the site with a spoon excavator and explorer.

All margins can be checked for fit with the explorer. Any margins that are bulky on the occlusal and proximal surfaces can be polished with finishing stones or a disk in a conventional-speed handpiece.

Next the margins are burnished with ball burnishers in the straight handpiece and with the hand burnisher. Burnishing is a procedure of pressing the malleable gold tightly against the tooth margin by slight stretching of the metal. This improves the seal of the inlay and smooths the junction between the tooth structure and the gold.

After the cement has reached the final set, the mouth can be rinsed, and the patient can be dismissed.

FULL CAST-GOLD CROWN

The same sequence of steps is used to fabricate a full gold crown as was described for the gold inlay. Differences within each step are described here.

Crown Preparation

Crown preparations (Figure 19-27, *A* and *B*) are done with the high-speed handpiece and either tapered fissure burs or diamond stones. These instruments permit rapid removal of tooth structure. Minor refinements can be made with the conventional-speed handpiece and fine grindstones and sandpaper disks.

The preparation for the full crown involves a reduction of the entire circumference of the tooth, as well as its oc-

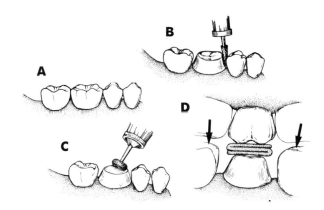

Figure 19-27 Preparation of tooth for a full cast-gold crown. **A,** Tooth before preparation begins. **B,** Reduction of circumference of tooth, creating a draw. **C,** Reduction of occlusal surface. **D,** Checking occlusal clearance with three thicknesses of occlusal indicator green wax.

clusal height (Figure 19-27, *C*). The three-quarter crown is done similarly except that the facial surface is left intact.

The occlusal height of the tooth must be reduced enough to allow for adequate thickness of the gold crown on the occlusal surface. It is quite common for dentists to determine adequate occlusal clearance by having the patient bite into a ½-inch square of 28-gauge occlusal wax that has been folded into three thicknesses (Figure 19-27, *D*).

The relationship of the vertical aspects of the prepared tooth is such that draw is established (see Figure 19-27, *B*). Excessive tapering of the vertical portion of the preparation must be avoided to prevent loss of the retention quality of the preparation.

After the preparation is completed, the gingiva is retracted, and an impression is made with agar hydrocolloid, polyether, or polyvinylsiloxane impression materials with the syringe-tray technique or the two-viscosity technique. If necessary, the bite registration is taken at this time, and an alginate impression is made of the opposing teeth.

Posterior Crown Temporization Methods

The prepared tooth can be covered with a temporary crown such as the aluminum shell type, with an acrylic crown made using the vacuum adaptation technique, or with a resinlike temporary material as described in Chapter 18.

Temporary crowns are usually cemented in place with a temporary cement.

Aluminum shell crown method

Stock aluminum shell crowns have been used for years as temporary crowns. They are available in either anatomical or nonanatomical forms and in a variety of sizes to fit molar and premolar teeth. They are all "a mile too long" and must be trimmed with crown-and-collar scissors to the proper length and cervical shape.

The cervical margin is smoothed with a fine green grinding stone. Proper crown contour can be achieved with contouring pliers. (The preparation of an aluminum shell crown is identical to that of the stainless steel crown. After the crown has been properly fitted to the tooth, it is filled with a temporary cement and seated on the prepared tooth. Excess cement is removed, and the patient is dismissed.

Vacuum adaptation method

Vacuum adaptation is an accurate method of making full-crown and three-quarter-crown temporary dressings for both anterior and posterior teeth. The procedure is as follows:

1. An alginate impression is taken of the area of the dentition to be treated. A plaster model is made from this impression. The impressions must be taken before the tooth is prepared.
2. The model is placed on the platform of a **Vacuformer** with the teeth upright (Figure 19-28, *A*).
3. A sheet of plastic coping material is mounted in the holding frame.
4. The heating element is turned on, and the coping material is softened. When it sags in the middle approximately 1 to 1¼ inches (Figure 19-28, *B*), the vacuum motor is turned on, and the holding frame is quickly lowered to place the softened material over the model (Figure 19-28, *C*). The vacuum will draw the material onto the model and tightly adapt it to the shape of the teeth.

5. The machine is turned off after 15 seconds of adaptation, and the model is removed.
6. The coping material can be cut away from the model with a scalpel blade (Figure 19-28, *D*) or an abrasive disk on a slow-speed handpiece. The tooth to be prepared plus at least half of each adjacent tooth should remain intact to create the mold or matrix for the temporary restoration.
7. The plastic mold should be added to the gold preparation setup at the time of the preparation appointment after it has been placed in disinfectant solution and washed.
8. At the preparation appointment after the crown preparation has been completed and the necessary impressions are obtained, the temporary crown can be made. The crown is made from self-curing acrylic such as Duralay. Self-curing acrylics are mixed into a thick paste and placed in the plastic mold (Figure 19-28, *E*). The filled mold is placed over the prepared tooth, and the patient is instructed to bite down to hold it in place (Figure 19-28, *F*). The mold should be removed and replaced repeatedly during the set of the acrylic to prevent it from locking on the teeth. As the temporary crown starts to harden, a chemical reaction produces heat. The acrylic temporary crown can become quite warm and should not be left on the tooth because it could produce pulpal damage. The temporary crown is placed in warm water to accelerate the setting reaction.
9. After the acrylic has hardened completely, the mold can be removed from the mouth. The acrylic is separated from the mold, and the excess acrylic is ground away.

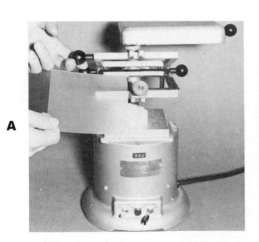
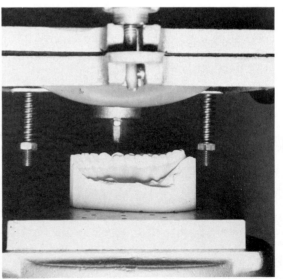

Figure 19-28 Temporary crown construction using vacuum–adapted mold. **A,** Model positioned on Vacuformer. **B,** Coping material sags 1 inch when softened enough to adapt.

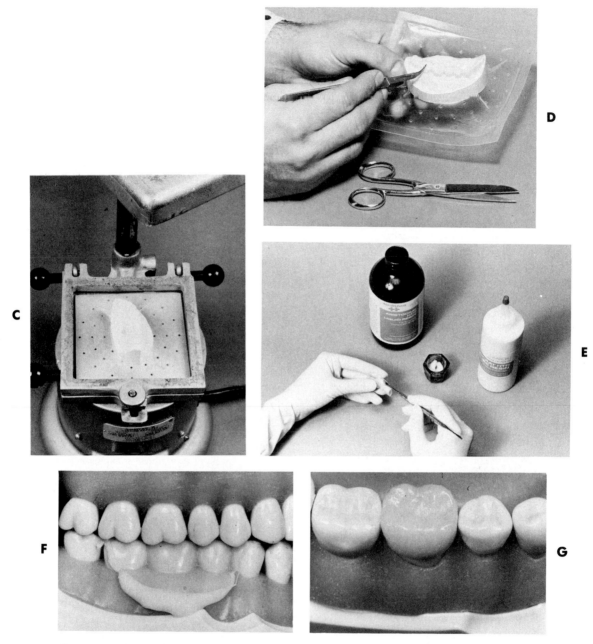

Figure 19-28, cont'd **C,** Holding frame drawn over model with vacuum turned on. **D,** Adapted coping material and model are removed from Vacuformer. Mold is cut from model with scalpel and scissors. **E,** Filling the mold. **F,** Filled mold in place. **G,** Finished crown.

10. The acrylic temporary crown is polished and seated temporarily with temporary cement (Figure 19-28, *G*).

The vacuum adaptation method has gained popularity because the same basic process can be used to make temporary bridges, bite splints, mouth guards, baseplates, and custom impression trays. The vacuum adaptation method is very convenient, and the result is excellent.

Cementation

The cementation appointment for placement of a crown involves the same procedure as for inlay cementation. The temporary crown is removed, and the preparation is cleaned thoroughly. The proximal contact, occlusion, and cervical margins must all be checked, and necessary adjustments made before the crown is cemented with a per-

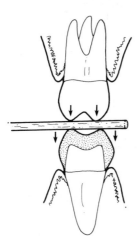

Figure 19-29 Final seating of cast–gold crown using orangewood stick.

manent cementation material. If zinc phosphate cement is used, the preparation must be coated with cavity varnish before cementation.

The assistant should not fill a crown completely with cement but rather place a coat of cement over the entire internal surface. Excessive cement makes it more difficult to seat the crown completely on the prepared tooth.

The crown can be delivered to the dentist on the mixing slab with its occlusal surface up. The dentist can then coat the prepared tooth with cement from the slab and easily grasp the upright crown for quick placement on the preparation. The crown is initially seated with hand pressure. Then the patient is instructed to bite down on an **orangewood stick** or a Cooley peg that is placed over the crown to drive it into place (Figure 19-29). This pressure is maintained until the cement sets. If any cervical burnishing is required, it is done with a hand burnisher after the cement reaches its initial set. Excess cement is removed, and the patient can be dismissed.

BIBLIOGRAPHY

Craig RG and others: *Restorative dental materials,* ed 9, St Louis, 1993, Mosby.

Malamed SF: *Medical emergencies in the dental office,* ed 4, St Louis, 1993, Mosby.

Rosenstiel SF, Land MF, Fujimoto J: *Contemporary fixed prosthodontics,* ed 2, St Louis, 1994, Mosby.

QUESTIONS–Chapter 19

1. A restoration that extends over the cusps of posterior teeth but leaves the facial and lingual aspects of the tooth intact is called a(n) _____.
   a. Inlay
   b. Onlay
   c. Three-quarter crown
   d. Full crown

2. All the following are used as final impression materials for crown and bridge procedures *except:*
   a. Alginate
   b. Agar hydrocolloid
   c. Polyether
   d. Polyvinylsiloxane

3. The _____ bath is used to cool the agar hydrocolloid material in the impression tray before it is inserted in the patient's mouth.
   a. Storage
   b. Boiling
   c. Tempering

4. Which of the following permanent cements requires a glass slab for mixing?
   a. Polycarboxylate
   b. Zinc oxide and eugenol
   c. Glass ionomer
   d. Zinc phosphate

5. Which of the following permanent cement(s) has/have anticariogenic qualities?
   a. Polycarboxylate
   b. Zinc oxide and eugenol
   c. Glass ionomer
   d. Zinc phosphate

6. Which of the following describes the correct consistency when zinc phosphate is mixed as a permanent cement?
   a. Until it is smooth and creamy
   b. When the cement is doughlike
   c. When a homogeneous mix is reached
   d. When the material strings out 1 to 1½ inches

7. Which of the following is the correct ratio of powder to liquid for glass ionomer cement?
   a. 1:1
   b. 1:2
   c. 2:1
   d. 1:3

8. All the following can be used to seat a gold restoration *except:*
   a. Orangewood stick
   b. Cooley peg
   c. Cotton roll
   d. Gauze, 2 × 2 inch

9. All the following are permanent cements *except:*
   a. Zinc phosphate
   b. Zinc oxide and eugenol
   c. Glass ionomer
   d. Polycarboxylate

10. Which of the following may be used to determine if the dentist has removed enough of the occlusal surface of a full crown or onlay preparation?
    a. Bite registration material
    b. Impression material
    c. Occlusal indicator wax
    d. Orangewood stick

DENTAL SPECIALTIES

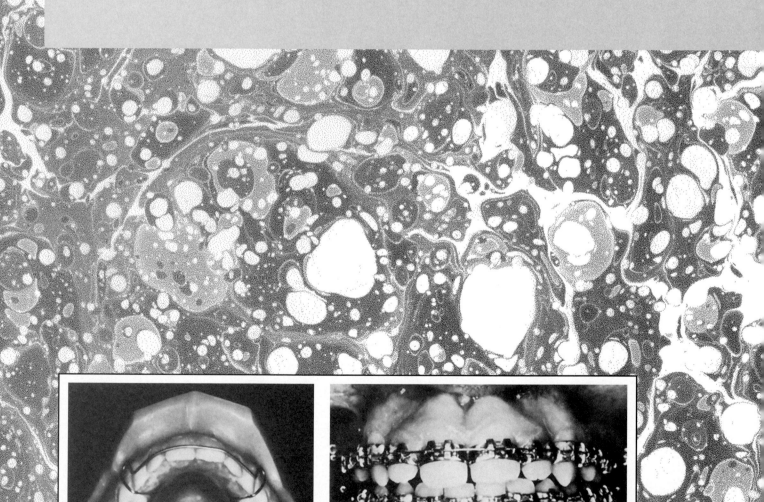

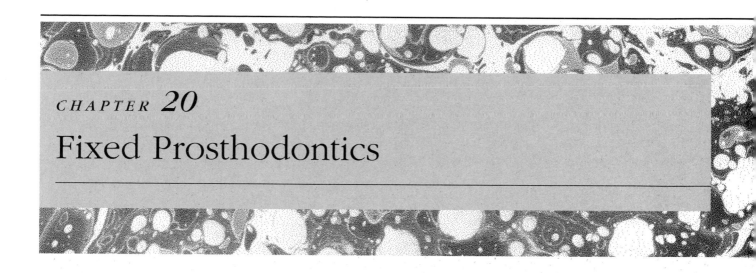

Fixed Prosthodontics

Abutment
Aesthetic crown
Aesthetics
All-ceramic crowns
Bruxism
Cast-gold post and core
Coping material
Draw
Drifting
Extrusion
Fixed bridge
Fixed prosthodontics
Maryland bridge
Overeruption
Pontic
Porcelain-bonded-to-metal crown
Resin luting cements
Retention core
Retention pins
Retention post
Shade
Shade guide
Tipping

Fixed prosthodontics is the area of dental practice that involves extensive restoration of teeth using a variety of crowns and replacement of missing teeth with bridges. These are prosthodontic restorations that are cemented onto prepared teeth and cannot be removed by the pa-

tient, hence the term *fixed*, as opposed to *removable*, prosthodontics.

The basic procedures used to fabricate a bridge are similar to those used for a single-unit cast restoration. To avoid repetition of the principles already presented, a review of Chapter 19 is suggested.

No attempt is made here to discuss all fixed prosthodontic procedures, but a few of the more common restorations are presented to expose the reader to the principles involved in the restorative process. The dentist's tasks vary considerably from one restorative procedure to another, but the assistant's role changes very little. Therefore the restorations selected for discussion here should provide the assistant with enough background to assist the dentist regardless of which restorative procedure is being done. The cast-gold crown, the aesthetic crown, and the fixed bridge are the basic fixed prosthodontic services commonly performed today.

Not only are the basic steps the same for the fabrication of each of these types of restoration, but also the armamentarium is similar if not identical. It is common for dentists to have a crown and bridge preset tray for inlays, crowns, and bridges and another for the cementation appointment. Chapter 19 reviews the armamentarium needed for single-unit cast-gold restoration appointments. Additions to these basic instrument setups are mentioned during discussions of each restorative procedure.

AESTHETIC PREFERENCES IN CROWNS

Aesthetics is a matter of personal preference of each patient. Some patients do not object to the appearance of gold in highly visible areas of the mouth, but others find it most objectionable. In fact, some patients even favor the appearance of gold teeth in their mouths. These preferences are based on the background of the individual with regard to ethnic differences, social habits, and occupational influences. Beautiful models would probably not want their maxillary central incisors restored with full gold crowns, but some individuals believe that this not only is attractive but also represents wealth. Of course, these are two extremes of aesthetic preference, yet the dentist is frequently confronted with the choice of restoration that will meet the aesthetic needs of the patient. Other influences in the choice are the strength requirements of the tooth to be restored and the economic situation of the patient.

❖ KEY POINT

▪ An **aesthetic crown** is a full crown that has at least the facial aspect covered with a tooth-shaded material. There are two basic types of aesthetic crowns:
1. The all-ceramic crown
2. The porcelain-bonded-to-metal crown

All-Ceramic Restoration

All-ceramic crowns (Figure 20-1, *A* and *B*) are the most aesthetically pleasing restoration because they can resemble the natural tooth better than a porcelain-bonded-to-metal crown. This is due mostly to the absence of the metal substructure. Light can pass through the porcelain in much the same way that it passes through actual tooth structure, giving the restoration a very natural appearance. This type of crown is not as strong as a porcelain-bonded-to-metal crown and is susceptible to fracture under heavy occlusal forces; however, newer resin-bonding techniques have improved the fracture resistance of these crowns. All-ceramic restorations are usually placed on individual teeth and are used on a limited basis for fixed bridges because of the brittle nature of the restoration.

Porcelain-Bonded-to-Metal Crown

The **porcelain-bonded-to-metal crown** (Figure 20-1, *C* and *D*) is made for teeth that need full coverage, but for aesthetic purposes a gold crown cannot be used. The porcelain can be bonded to various types of metal such as

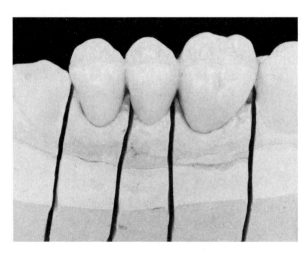

Figure 20-2 Posterior porcelain–veneered restorations. Porcelain is fused over entire surface of gold.

(Courtesy Precision Dental Arts, Inc, Jackson, Mich.)

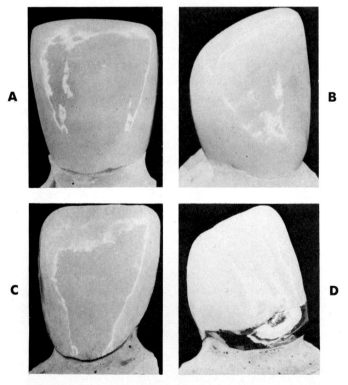

Figure 20-1 Anterior aesthetic crowns. **A** and **B**, All-ceramic crown. **C** and **D**, Porcelain-fused-to-metal crown.

(Courtesy Precision Dental Arts, Inc, Jackson, Mich.)

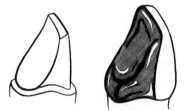

Figure 20-3 Cast crown with porcelain that is fused to one or more surfaces.

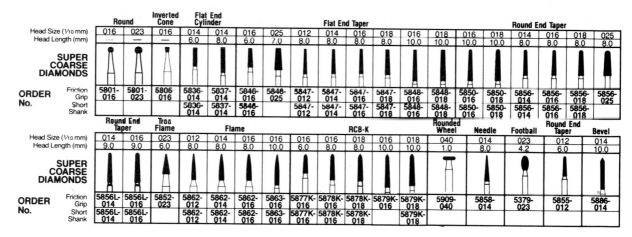

Figure 20-4 Assortment of shapes of diamond stones.

(Courtesy Brasseler, Inc, Savannah, Ga.)

precious gold or other metal alloys. When the porcelain is bonded to gold, it may be called a porcelain-bonded-to-gold crown. When the porcelain is bonded to metal, it may be called a porcelain-bonded-to-metal or porcelain-fused-to-metal crown. The dentist usually has a preference for one name over the others, but regardless of which name is used, these crowns have a natural appearance because porcelain can be fused to the metal substructure in areas with aesthetic considerations.

Porcelain can be fused in various areas depending on the aesthetic need. For example, porcelain can cover the entire metal substructure, resulting in a crown with porcelain margins (Figure 20-2), and some crowns are fabricated with porcelain only on the facial surface because the incisal and lingual surface is normally not visible during oral functions (Figure 20-3).

The porcelain-bonded-to-metal crown is probably the most popular aesthetic crown in use today. Modern laboratory technology has created and improved this restoration so that it is strong and attractive. It resists fracture, abrasion, and discoloration. It can be used in all areas of the mouth as a single restoration, or it can be joined with other restorations to form splints and bridges to replace missing teeth.

A disadvantage to this restoration is that the tooth is reduced significantly to provide sufficient thickness of the porcelain to mask the metal substructure. Another disadvantage is that porcelain is abrasive in nature and can wear down natural teeth or metal restorations.

Aesthetic Crown Preparations

Like cast-gold crown preparations, the aesthetic crown preparation is done principally with the high-speed handpiece and tapered fissure burs and diamond stones. Various shapes of available diamond stones are shown in Figure 20-4.

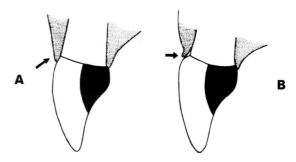

Figure 20-5 Anterior veneered crown. **A,** Properly contoured crown. **B,** Poorly contoured crown.

Since these restorations involve full coverage of the prepared tooth, the circumference and vertical height of the tooth are reduced.

> **KEY POINT**
> - An aesthetic crown preparation requires more reduction than the cast-gold crown preparation in areas that will be replaced by porcelain.

The additional reduction required by an aesthetic crown allows the necessary space to accommodate the thickness of the porcelain on that surface. If additional reduction of tooth structure is not done, the finished restoration will be too bulky by the time a layer of gold and a layer of porcelain are added. This bulk detracts from the natural appearance of the restoration (Figure 20-5). Figure 20-6 illustrates some common crown preparations.

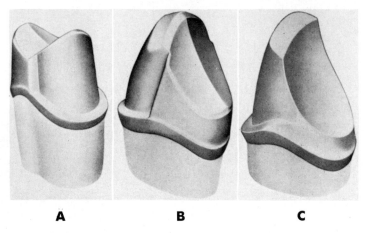

A   **B**   **C**

Figure 20-6   Common aesthetic crown preparations. **A,** Posterior veneer preparation. **B,** Anterior veneer preparation. **C,** Porcelain jacket preparation.

(Courtesy JM Ney Co, Hartford, Conn.)

Before beginning an aesthetic crown preparation, the dentist should select a shade so that the completed restoration matches the adjacent teeth. **Shade** is the combination of color and translucency of a tooth. The correct shade is obtained by comparing samples of various colors and translucencies, contained in a **shade guide,** with the tooth to be prepared and with adjacent teeth (Figure 20-7). The shade guide must be added to the standard cast-gold preparation setup when aesthetic crowns are done. The shade samples are number coded so that the dentist can record the selection on the patient's record for future reference. Often teeth are combinations of shades, and the dentist will record these combinations. When the patient's models and dies are sent to the laboratory technician, the shade is included in the written instructions.

The shape of the tooth is also important to achieve proper aesthetics. A preoperative study model is of considerable value to the technician in constructing the crown to a shape and contour that blend with the rest of the dentition. The impression for study models can be taken at the diagnostic appointment.

After the crown is prepared, an impression is taken with polyether (Impregum), vinyl polyvinylsiloxane (Extrude or Express), or agar hydrocolloid impression materials. Occlusal registration and an alginate impression are taken of opposing teeth if a single-arch tray is used before a temporary crown is placed.

Temporization of Aesthetic Crowns

Aesthetic crown preparations require the use of a reasonably aesthetic temporary crown. Therefore the aluminum shell crown is not frequently used.

Anterior teeth are temporized with preformed polycarbonate crowns (Figure 20-8), custom acrylic crowns

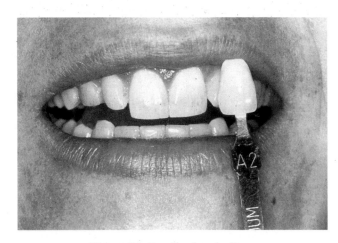

Figure 20-7   Shade selection.

made with the vacuum-molding technique, or a newer type of composite resin temporary material, such as Protemp (Figure 20-9). The custom acrylic crown and newer type of custom resin temporary material have the advantage of a greater range of shade selection for the temporary crown. The polycarbonate crown is available in only one shade.

Polycarbonate crowns are available in various sizes for each anterior tooth. Some companies even offer maxillary premolar crowns. Polycarbonate crowns can be fitted on a prepared tooth by limited grinding with a diamond bur to contour the cervical area.

The crown can be filled with a temporary cement and seated on the tooth. If extensive alteration of the crown is anticipated, it is filled with a self-curing acrylic and placed on the prepared tooth. As the acrylic hardens, the crown

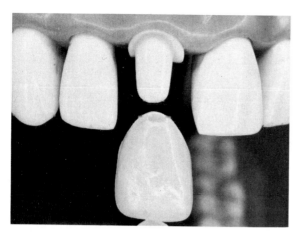

Figure 20-8 Preformed polycarbonate crown.

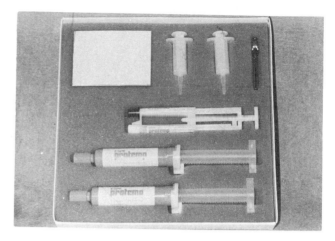

Figure 20-9 Custom resin temporary material.

should be removed and seated repeatedly to prevent the acrylic from adhering to the preparation. After the acrylic is completely hard, any alterations necessary to fit the crown properly can be made by grinding the filled crown. The crown can be polished and temporarily cemented to the prepared tooth with a thin layer of temporary cement.

Posterior teeth are generally temporized with a custom acrylic crown. Some manufacturers provide polycarbonate crowns for premolars, which are helpful. The vacuum-molding process has made fabrication of suitable, aesthetic temporary crowns much easier.

Cementation of Aesthetic Crowns

Box 20-1 describes a cementation procedure for a porcelain-bonded-to-metal crown or an all-ceramic crown.

Resin luting cements can be thought of as a runny composite material. The mixing techniques differ depending on which brand of resin cement is used. Therefore it is best to consult the manufacturer's instructions for the proper mixing procedure.

FIXED BRIDGE

A **fixed bridge** is a restoration that is used to replace missing teeth. The term *fixed* means that the restoration is cemented in place and therefore not removable by the patient. The term *bridge* has been adopted to designate this restoration because of it similarity in design to a bridge that spans a river (Figure 20-10). The supports at the ends of the bridge, called **abutments,** are the teeth that support the fixed bridge at each end. As the river bridge spans the river, the fixed bridge spans edentulous spaces that were once occupied by teeth (Figure 20-11).

The basic parts of a fixed bridge are the abutments and the pontic. The **pontic** is the artificial tooth that replaces the missing natural tooth. Each individual abutment or

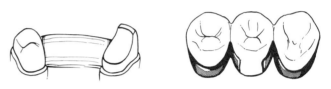

Figure 20-10 Fixed bridge.

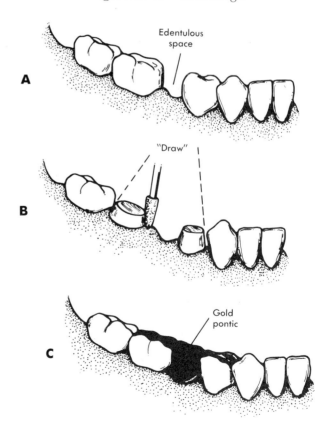

Figure 20-11 Preparation of a three-unit fixed bridge. **A,** Edentulous space. **B,** Full-crown preparations that draw with each other. **C,** Seated bridge with an all-gold pontic held in place with veneer crowns on abutment teeth.

BOX 20-1

CEMENTATION PROCEDURE FOR PORCELAIN-BONDED-TO-METAL CROWN OR ALL-CERAMIC CROWN

PROCEDURE	RATIONALE	PROCEDURE	RATIONALE
1. Temporary crown is removed, and preparation is cleaned thoroughly.	1. To prepare tooth for cementation of permanent crown.	6. Permanent cement is mixed. Crown can be cemented with zinc phosphate, polycarbonate, resin cement, or glass ionomer cement. If zinc phosphate is used, tooth should be coated with cavity varnish.	6. Permanent cement is usually mixed when crown is ready to be cemented on tooth, thus giving operator sufficient working time.
2. Crown is placed on preparation; and proximal contacts, occlusion, and cervical margins are checked and adjusted as needed.	2. To check fit of permanent crown.	7. Both preparation and internal surface of crown are covered with cement.	7. To avoid any voids or incomplete seal of permanent crown to tooth.
3. If adjustments are necessary, they are done with special porcelain grinding wheels (Dedeco). Various sizes and grits are available.	3. To adjust fit of permanent crown before permanently cementing crown into tooth. Any area of porcelain that is ground should be smoothed by fine-grit Dedeco wheel on conventional-speed handpiece and then polished with alumina paste on laboratory lathe. Porcelain jackets have glaze on outer surface that creates fine finish on crown and protects restoration from staining.	8. Crown is seated with orangewood stick or cotton roll.	8. Pressure must be maintained on permanent crown until cement is set.
		9. Excess cement is removed.	9. Excess cement will accumulate plaque and debris and be irritant to periodontium.
4. If extensive grinding is done during adjustments, crown should be sent back to dental laboratory.	4. To reglaze crown before final cementation.	10. Patient is given postoperative instructions.	10. Patient should be advised to: • Brush and floss area • Call office if there are any problems
5. Tooth preparation is cleaned and dried. Air-abrasion device may be used to clean internal surface of crown.	5. To clean and dry tooth preparation and permanent crown before cementation. Glass ionomer cement is especially sensitive to moisture contamination.	11. Procedure is documented in chart, including type of crown and permanent cement used.	11. To document for treatment records and also for medicolegal purposes.

---

pontic is commonly referred to as a unit of the bridge. The bridge shown in Figure 20-11, *C,* is an example of a three-unit bridge (two abutments and one pontic). Other bridges are designed to replace several missing teeth; therefore more units are joined to form these bridges. For example, if the four maxillary incisors are missing, and a fixed bridge is fabricated to replace them, the bridge is

six units long. There are four pontics to replace the missing teeth and two abutments to attach the bridge to the two canines.

It is common for a patient to have abutment teeth that are in need of extensive restoration as well as needing a bridge to replace a missing tooth between them. Abutments usually are either three-quarter crowns or full crowns. Depending on the aesthetic demands of the patient, full-crown abutments are either all-gold or porcelain-bonded-to-metal crowns.

Pontics are either all gold or porcelain bonded to metal. The pontic is connected to the abutments by joints on the proximal surfaces. An example of an anterior porcelain fused to metal bridge is shown in Figure 20-12.

> ## ➥ KEY POINTS
> - Abutments are the supporting teeth in a fixed bridge.
> - A pontic is the part of the fixed bridge that replaces the missing tooth.

Need for Fixed Bridge

The fixed bridge is an excellent way to replace missing teeth if the abutment teeth are strong and well supported by alveolar bone. These restorations are far more comfortable and aesthetic than a removable partial denture that could be used for the same purpose. Aside from aesthetics, the need for a bridge is based on the fact that most of the teeth in the mouth depend on the presence of adjacent and opposing teeth to maintain their proper

position in the dentition (Figure 20-13). When a tooth is lost, **drifting** of the surrounding teeth out of position can occur, and **overeruption (extrusion)** of the tooth opposing the empty space can occur into the space. The result of this phenomenon is that **tipping** of the teeth out of position occurs with the following undesirable effects:

1. The patient not only loses the biting function of the missing tooth, but also the abutment teeth are less efficient in chewing because they do not contact the opposing teeth properly.
2. The biting relationship of the teeth is changed to abnormal chewing patterns, which can result in injury to the temporomandibular joint.
3. The malaligned teeth can trigger clenching and **bruxism** (tooth-grinding habits). These habits can injure the temporomandibular joint and cause muscle spasms in the muscles of mastication.
4. Teeth that are tipped cannot resist the forces placed on them as well as they could when they were upright. Biting forces on a tipped tooth usually cause it to tip farther.
5. Abnormal force applied to tipped teeth often causes loss of the bone support of the tooth, resulting in its eventual loss.
6. Extrusion or overeruption of an opposing tooth over the edentulous space can create an interfer-

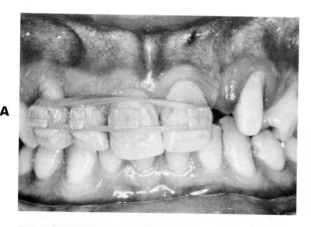
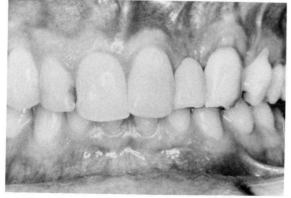
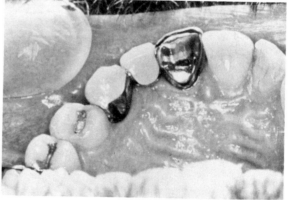

Figure 20-12 Porcelain-fused-to-metal anterior bridge. **A,** Orthodontic appliance in place to move central incisors into favorable position before bridge fabrication. **B,** Palatal view of finished bridge. **C,** Labial view of seated bridge.

(Courtesy Robert Lorey, DDS, Ann Arbor, Mich.)

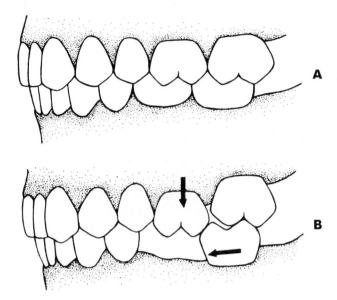

Figure 20-13 Effects of loss of mandibular first molar. **A,** Dentition before loss. **B,** Changes that can occur after loss of tooth.

ence in the normal biting pattern, which can result in temporomandibular joint damage.

7. Drifting and tipping of teeth cause contacts between teeth to open, which allows food to become trapped between the teeth. This food impaction injures the gingiva.

Despite the negative effects of losing a tooth or teeth, not all patients are candidates for fixed bridges. Some are better treated with a removable partial denture. Still others may be better off with no treatment under certain circumstances. The best time to fabricate a bridge for a patient is as soon as healing is complete after an extraction and before drifting occurs. The supporting teeth must be reasonably sound with favorable bone support before this type of treatment is pursued.

Fabrication of Three–Unit Mandibular Posterior Bridge

Although specific designs of fixed bridges vary considerably according to the individual needs of the patient, the basic format used to construct the bridge is the same. The mandibular three-unit posterior bridge has been selected as an example because it is a common restoration in general dental practice. This example will demonstrate the replacement of a missing mandibular right second premolar with the bridge.

For discussion purposes the bridge design used in this example will have a full-crown abutment on the first molar. The premolar retainer will also be a full crown. This retainer and the pontic will be porcelain bonded to metal for aesthetic reasons.

Treatment planning

Treatment planning is a major part of bridge construction. The dentist must have the essential information provided by the patient history, oral examination, radiographs, and study models to plan the appropriate treatment. All this information can be obtained in one diagnostic appointment and analyzed before the patient returns for treatment. The diagnostic information guides the dentist's decision as to whether a fixed bridge is an appropriate form of treatment. If a bridge is appropriate, the information is helpful for the dentist in designing the restoration to meet the patient's aesthetic and functional needs.

Preparation of abutment teeth

The abutment teeth are prepared for the full crown in a similar manner to that described previously. The exception to this is that these preparations must not only have **draw** within each preparation, but also must draw with each other (see Figure 20-11, *B*). The finished bridge needs to slide onto the prepared abutments and be cemented into place. Establishing draw between individual preparations for a bridge is one of the more difficult tasks for the dentist, especially in bridge designs that involve more than two abutments.

Taking the impression

After preparations are finished and draw has been established between them, the gingiva is retracted and an impression is taken using the syringe-tray technique. A bite registration is needed, along with an alginate impression of the opposing teeth. Full-arch impressions are more favorable than quadrant-sized impressions because the occlusion of the patient can be more accurately determined during the laboratory phase of the bridge fabrication.

Temporization

Temporization is a very important part of bridge construction. A temporary bridge needs to be constructed so that the abutment teeth cannot shift position in any direction. The opposing teeth must contact the temporary bridge when the jaws are closed to prevent extrusion. Any shifting of teeth during the interim laboratory phase results in loss of fit of the permanent bridge on the abutment teeth and improper occlusion. Patients should be instructed to contact the dentist immediately if a temporary bridge becomes dislodged or fractured. If a patient must wear the temporary bridge for more than 2 weeks, it is wise to have the patient return periodically to check on the occlusal wear of the bridge.

An exceptionally favorable way to construct a temporary bridge is with the vacuum-adaptation method (Figure 20-14). The technique that follows is similar to the one used to fabricate a temporary crown.

1. The edentulous space is filled with a denture tooth that has been ground to fit, with a special high-heat

clay material, or with a piece of wax that can be formed into the shape of a tooth. This will represent the pontic in the temporary bridge (see Figure 20-14, *A*).

2. The study model with the pontic attached to it is placed in the Vacuformer, and a thin sheet of plastic **(coping material)** is vacuum adapted to it to form the mold for the bridge (see Figure 20-14, *B*).

3. The coping material is cut away from the model and trimmed (see Figure 20-14, *C* and *D*).

4. After the preparations are finished, the mold is filled with temporary acrylic (see Figure 20-14, *E*) and placed on the preparations. The patient is instructed to bite on the filled mold to hold it in place (see Figure 20-14, *F*).

5. After the initial set of the acrylic, the filled mold is removed and the excess acrylic is trimmed away. The bridge is returned to the mouth for final setting. (The bridge should be lifted off the preparations periodically as the material hardens to prevent fusion to the preparations.)

6. When the temporary bridge has completely hardened, it can be trimmed, polished, and cemented with a temporary cement (see Figure 20-14, *G* and *H*).

Cementation

The basic procedure used for the cementation of a fixed bridge is the same as that for the gold crown and inlay. However, since the bridge spans a greater part of the occlusion than does a single crown, it is common to find

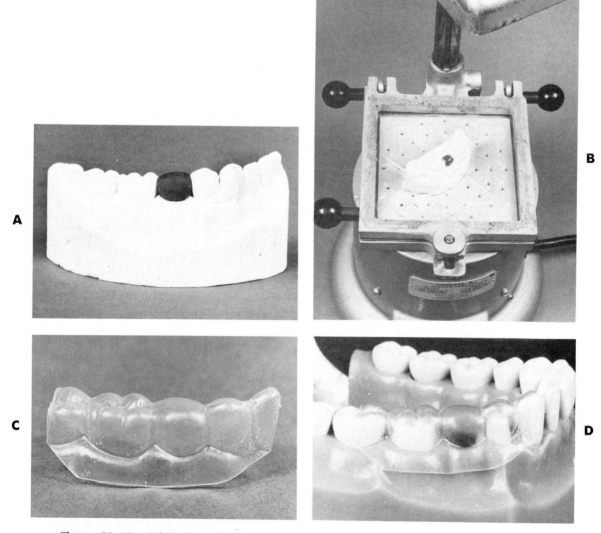

Figure 20-14 Fabrication of temporary bridge by vacuum–adaptation mold technique. **A,** Clay pontic is placed in edentulous space on preoperative study model. **B,** Coping material is adapted to model. **C,** Mold of area of bridge is cut away from rest of coping material. **D,** Mold and its relationship to prepared teeth.

Continued.

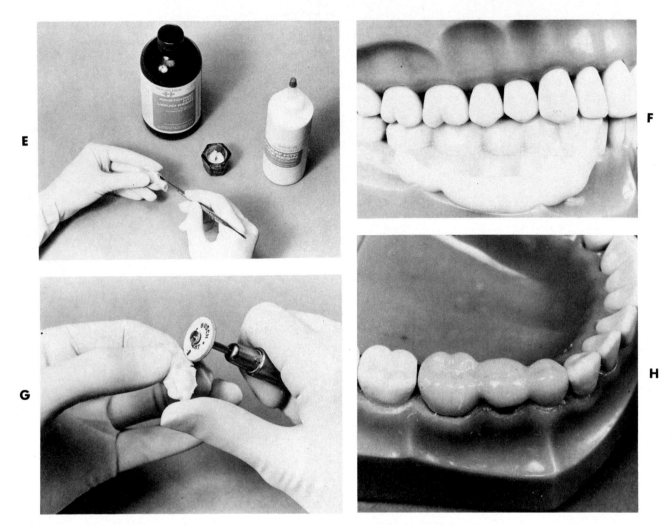

Figure 20-14, cont'd   **E,** Filling mold with acrylic. **F,** Placement of filled mold over prepared teeth. **G,** Trimming temporary bridge. **H,** Finished bridge.

more time spent on refining the biting relationship of the bridge to the opposing teeth. An additional consideration in the cementation of the bridge is the adjustment of the relationship of the pontic to the edentulous ridge. The pontic must permit easy cleaning under the bridge during oral hygiene procedures. It must also contact the ridge so that it looks like a natural tooth in cases in which aesthetics is a major concern.

Fixed bridges are cemented with any of the final cementing materials discussed previously. After the cement has set, the excess is removed with a spoon excavator, explorer, and dental floss from around the retainers and under the pontic. The patient should be instructed to clean the bridge using normal toothbrushing techniques and dental floss with a floss threader (see Chapter 10).

Resin-Retained Fixed Bridge (Maryland Bridge)

An alternative bridge design emerged in 1973 for the abutment teeth that cannot be prepared in the traditional manner. These bridge designs are usually used on anterior teeth to avoid reducing sound tooth structure of the abutment teeth needed for traditional bridge designs. Maryland bridges work well when occlusal forces are minimal. The bridge has one pontic supported by thin metal retainers that are located both proximally and lingually on the abutment teeth (Figure 20-15). The retainers are specially designed metal extensions held in place with composite-resin bonding material. Both anterior and posterior designs are used.

Preparation

Teeth are prepared by removing just enough enamel thickness on the abutment teeth to make room for the metal retainers. Since retention of the bridge depends entirely on the bond of composite to etched enamel, the dentist cannot remove all of the enamel in the prepared areas.

Impressions

The same impression methods described in Chapter 19 for a single-unit, cast-gold restoration are used for this bridge technique. Bite registration and shade selection are also described in Chapter 19.

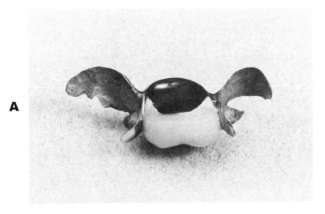

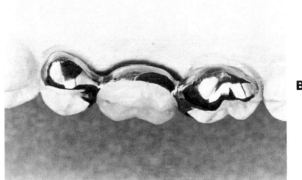

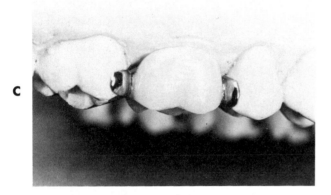

Figure 20-15 Posterior Maryland bridge. **A,** Retainers extending from pontic. **B,** Palatal view on model. **C,** Buccal view on model.

(Courtesy Robert Trombly, DDS, Aurora, Colo.)

Temporization

Self-curing, acrylic, temporary coverings are placed over the prepared areas of abutment teeth to prevent drifting and extrusion of teeth between appointments.

Cementation

The bridge is fabricated in the dental laboratory with the tooth tissue surface of the retainers roughened by electrolytic etching to enhance the bond of composite to the metal. Since this etching technique was developed at the University of Maryland School of Dentistry, the restoration is often referred to as a **Maryland bridge.** The cementation process is done using rubber dam isolation. After the temporary acrylic coverings are removed, the abutment teeth are cleaned with pumice and water and then dried. Prepared areas on the abutments are acid etched with phosphoric acid for 30 to 60 seconds, rinsed thoroughly, and dried. A dual-cure composite designed specifically for use as a cementing agent is applied to the etched surfaces of the bridge retainers and positioned properly on the tooth. Excess composite material is removed, and the patient is dismissed.

RETENTION CORES AND POSTS

Most teeth restored with crowns are significantly altered as a result of fracture, extensive caries, or large, worn-out

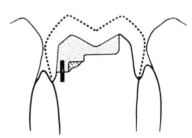

Figure 20-16 Pin-retained amalgam.

restorations. Before a preparation for a crown or bridge can be done, a dentist must decide whether the remaining tooth structure is sufficient to retain the restoration after it is made. If a tooth being restored will not be sufficiently intact to retain the restoration on its own, the dentist must enhance the retention capability of the tooth.

Retention Cores

If a significant amount of tooth structure will be lost, the dentist may buildup the tooth to replace the lost tooth structure. This buildup is called a **retention core.** In this type of procedure the dentist removes the caries or defective restoration and then builds the tooth back to its ideal contour. The tooth can then be prepared as if it were intact.

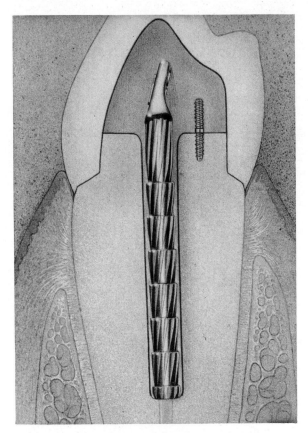

Figure 20-17 Para-Post Plus prefabricated post.
(Courtesy Whaledent, Inc, New York.)

BOX 20-2
PROCEDURE FOR PLACEMENT OF AMALGAM CORE

PROCEDURE	RATIONALE
1. Tooth is isolated.	1. For moisture control and optimum visibility.
2. Tooth is prepared with high-speed handpiece and low-speed hand-piece	2. To remove defective restorations or caries.
3. If necessary, retention pins are placed.	3. To augment retention of amalgam core.
4. If necessary, place base, varnish, and liner.	4. For pulpal protection.
5. Matrix band is placed on prepared tooth and sta-bilized.	5. To allow amalgam to be properly condensed; also facilitates carving of amalgam.
6. Mix and condense amal-gam.	6. To fabricate amalgam core.
7. Amalgam is contoured and finished.	7. To create a smooth amal-gam-tooth interface for better plaque control and to make it easier for dentist to prepare margins of crown preparation.

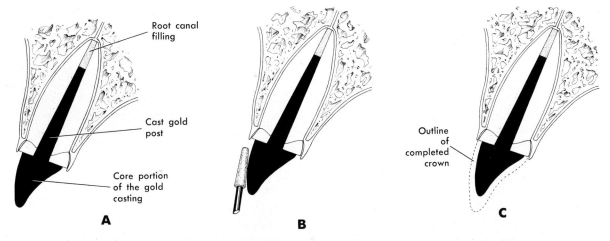

Figure 20-18 Gold post and core cast to fit into prepared root canal of endodontically treated tooth. **A**, Gold post cemented in root canal. **B**, Final adjustments can be made on core portion of casting if necessary. **C**, Anterior crown can now be made to fit over cast post and core.

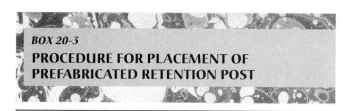

BOX 20-3

PROCEDURE FOR PLACEMENT OF PREFABRICATED RETENTION POST

PROCEDURE	RATIONALE
1. Root canal filling material is removed. Gutta-percha is removed with either warmed endodontic plugger or bur such as Gates Glidden bur.	1. Before post can be placed, root canal filling material must be removed to make room for post.
2. Root canal is enlarged.	2. Root canal of tooth must be widened to create snug-fitting post.
3. Prefabricated post is selected and tried in root canal.	3. To find appropriately fitting post.
4. Post is cemented.	4. To hold post firmly into place.

A retentive core can be made of amalgam, composite, or silver-impregnated glass ionomer in conjunction with **retention pins** (Figure 20-16), as described in Chapter 17. The dentist often places pins to hold the cores in place. The pins hold the core in place, and the core helps to hold the finished restoration in place.

Cores made with amalgam are still regarded as the strongest. Box 20-2 describes the procedure for the placement of an amalgam core. Composite and silver-impregnated glass ionomer (Ketac Silver) are also strong core materials and less thermoconductive than amalgam. These materials also provide the advantage of an immediate set, which allows the dentist to proceed with the crown preparation immediately after placement.

Post-Retained Cores

When the tooth is so badly damaged that a pin-retained core does not provide sufficient retention, a **retention post** must be placed before proceeding with the final restoration. Posts occupy the hollow pulp chamber and root canal of the tooth for anchoring. An endodontic procedure called a pulpectomy, which removes the dental pulp and replaces it with a soft rubber filling material called gutta-percha, must be performed. This procedure is commonly referred to as a root canal and is described in detail in Chapter 22. When the endodontic treatment is finished, the coronal part of the gutta-percha is removed. This leaves a hollow space for the placement of the retention post (Figure 20-17).

Prefabricated retention posts are popular, since they can be fitted at chairside and cemented during one appointment. Box 20-3 describes placement of a prefabricated retention post. Once a prefabricated post is cemented, it can be surrounded by any of the core materials mentioned previously to fabricate the core itself.

Cast-Gold Post and Core

Another approach to the fabrication of a post and core is the time-honored **cast-gold post and core** combination. The hollow root canal is prepared so that it has a long, tapered shape. An impression is made of the canal and remaining tooth structure and sent to the dental laboratory where both the post and core portions are cast as one unit in gold. On return the post and core unit is cemented into place and refined in shape as needed during the crown-preparation phase. The final restoration is then cemented over the gold post and core (Figure 20-18).

BIBLIOGRAPHY

Grundy JR, Jones JG: *Colour atlas of clinical operative dentistry: crowns and bridges*, ed 2, London, 1992, Wolfe Publishing Ltd.

Rosenstiel SF, Land MF, Fujimoto J: *Contemporary fixed prosthodontics*, St Louis, 1995, Mosby.

QUESTIONS—Chapter 20

1. Porcelain is _____ abrasive than a natural tooth.
   a. More
   b. Less

2. Aesthetic crowns are usually temporized with all of the following *except:*
   a. An aluminum shell temporary
   b. A polycarbonate temporary
   c. A custom acrylic temporary
   d. A custom resin temporary

3. The part of the fixed bridge that is used to replace a missing tooth is called _____.
   a. An abutment
   b. A retention core
   c. A pontic
   d. A retention pin

4. A buildup of material on the natural tooth to create better retention of the permanent restoration is called _____.
   a. An abutment
   b. A retention core
   c. A pontic
   d. A retention pin

5. When a tooth is lost from the dentition, all the following can occur *except:*
   a. Drifting
   b. Tipping
   c. Extrusion
   d. Intrusion

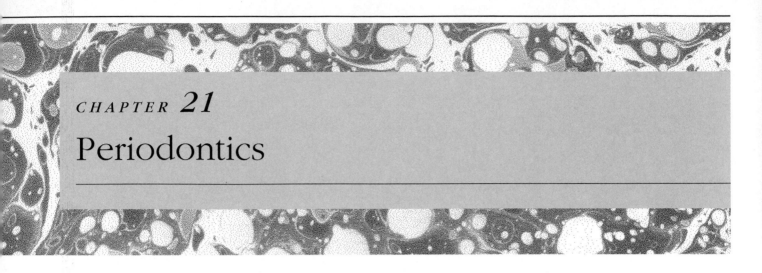

CHAPTER *21*

Periodontics

KEY TERMS

Bone resorption
Bone surgery
Curettage
Curette scalers
Distal wedge procedure
Electrosurgery
Flap surgery
Gingival grafts
Gingival pocket
Gingivectomy
Gingivitis
Guided tissue regeneration
Hoe scalers
Occlusal equilibration
Osseous surgery
Osteoclasts
Periodontal dressing
Periodontal file scalers
Periodontal knives
Periodontal pocket
Periodontal probe
Periodontal scaling and root planing
Periodontitis
Periodontium
Plaque
Pseudopocket
Root planing
Scalers
Scaling
Sickle scalers
Surgical scalpel
Surgical suction tips

Periodontics is the branch of dentistry that deals with the diagnosis and treatment of diseases that destroy the supporting tissues of the teeth. These supporting tissues are collectively referred to as the periodontium (Figure 21-1). Diseases that damage the periodontium are called periodontal diseases.

It is estimated that three of four adults will have some form of periodontal disease during their lifetime. Periodontal disease is not age specific; therefore children as well as adults are susceptible. Box 21-1 describes a widely used classification recommended in 1991 by the American Academy of Periodontists.

Dental caries and periodontal disease together are the most common conditions that the dentist must deal with in practice. The prevention and treatment of these diseases can ensure that patients will be able to preserve their teeth for a lifetime.

> ↦ **KEY POINT**
> - Periodontal disease is not one specific disease; rather the term is used to describe a variety of diseases that affect the supporting structures of the teeth.

ETIOLOGY OF PERIODONTAL DISEASE

Plaque, a white to brown sticky substance that consists of bacteria and bacterial by-products, is the primary factor in the development of periodontal disease. In addition, local factors such as malocclusion, overhanging restorations, poorly fitting appliances or prostheses, and cigarette smoking have been implicated as etiological factors in periodontal disease. Genetic, nutritional, hormonal, and metabolic factors may modify the progress of periodontal disease but have not been found to contribute as primary etiological factors.

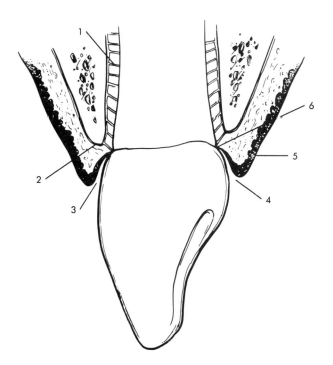

Figure 21-1 Periodontium. Periodontal ligament (*1*), alveolar crest (*2*), gingival crevice (sulcus) (*3*), free gingival margin (*4*), gingiva (*5*), epithelial attachment (*6*).

Progress of Periodontal Disease

Periodontal disease consists of two types of diseases: gingivitis and periodontitis. Box 21-2 shows the several types of gingivitis and periodontitis. Two existing theories concerning the relationship of gingivitis to periodontitis exist. One theory suggests that gingivitis is a less severe form of periodontitis and gingivitis progresses to periodontitis. An alternative theory suggests that gingivitis is a separate disease entity from periodontitis. Regardless of the relationship, periodontal disease has been found to be episodic, in which the disease can alternate between periods of remission and active disease.

Case Type I: Gingival Disease

Case type I periodontal disease is often termed *gingivitis.* There are many types of gingivitis. A positive aspect of this disease is that it is reversible without permanent destruction of the alveolar bone.

In gingivitis the tissue becomes inflamed. Inflammation is an attempt by the body to ward off physical and chemical injury and bacterial invasion of the tissues. The injured area becomes engorged with blood to provide an abundance of nutrients, oxygen, and white blood cells. The white blood cells destroy invading bacteria and remove debris from the site of injury. The accumulation and congestion of blood in the injured tissue result in a change in color, shape, and texture of the gingival tissue.

BOX 21-1

CLASSIFICATION OF PERIODONTAL DISEASE BY CASE TYPES

CASE TYPE I—GINGIVAL DISEASE

Inflammation of the gingiva characterized clinically by changes in color, gingival form, position, surface appearance, and presence of bleeding and/or exudate.

CASE TYPE II—EARLY PERIODONTITIS

Progression of the gingival inflammation into the deeper periodontal structures and alveolar bone crest, with slight bone loss. There is usually a slight loss of connective tissue attachment and alveolar bone.

CASE TYPE III—MODERATE PERIODONTITIS

A more advanced stage of the preceding condition, with increased destruction of the periodontal structures and noticeable loss of bone support, possibly accompanied by an increase in tooth mobility. There may be furcation involvement in multirooted teeth.

CASE TYPE IV—ADVANCED PERIODONTITIS

Further progression of periodontitis with major loss of alveolar bone support usually accompanied by increased tooth mobility. Furcation involvement in multirooted teeth is likely.

CASE TYPE V—REFRACTORY PERIODONTITIS

Includes those patients with multiple disease sites that continue to demonstrate attachment loss after appropriate therapy. These sites presumably continue to be infected by periodontal pathogens no matter how thorough or frequent the treatment provided.

From American Academy of Periodontology: *Current procedural terminology for periodontics and insurance reporting manual, ed 7, Chicago, 1995, The Academy.*

Inflammation of the gingiva, or **gingivitis**, is diagnosed by examining the gingiva for changes in color, form, and density (texture). Normal gingiva is a firm, pale pink tissue with sharp, free gingival margins and pointed interdental papillae (Figure 21-2). Inflamed gingiva has a reddish color, with rounded swollen gingival margins and blunt interdental papillae (Figure 21-3). The density changes from firm to spongy. The tissue may bleed readily when it is pressed or during toothbrushing. The gingival crevice may deepen slightly as a result of swelling of the gingiva (Figure 21-4). The extent of these changes depends on the severity of the inflammatory process.

BOX 21-2

CLASSIFICATION OF PERIODONTAL DISEASES

I. GINGIVAL DISEASE

A. *Gingivitis*—Inflammation of the gingiva characterized clinically by changes in color, gingival form, position, surface appearance, and presence of bleeding and/or exudate. The most common cause of gingivitis is bacterial plaque.

1. Nonspecific gingivitis—The most common form of gingivitis. It is caused by dental plaque bacteria and their products.
2. Acute necrotizing ulcerative gingivitis (ANUG)—an infection which first affects the interdental papillary area and is characterized by necrosis and pseudomembrane formation.

B. *Manifestations of systemic diseases and hormonal disturbances*—Associated with viral diseases including acute herpetic gingivostomatitis, blood dyscrasias including leukemia, autoimmune diseases such as pemphigus, and metabolic diseases such as diabetes. In some types of gingival disease modification of the sex hormones is considered to be either the initiating or complicating factor.

C. *Drug associated*—Gingival inflammation and/or enlargement resulting from plaque-associated gingivitis complicated by systemic drug administration. Dilantin hyperplasia is a common example.

D. *Miscellaneous gingival changes associated with various etiologies*—Includes all other pathologic and physiologic alterations in the gingival tissue. Changes include atrophy, cyst formation, hyperplasia, neoplasia, and degeneration and may be due to heredity, growth and development, infection, irritation, or trauma.

II. MUCOGINGIVAL CONDITIONS

Changes in the position and relationship of the gingiva and gingival margin to the alveolar mucosa. It includes gingival recession and aberrant frena and/or muscle attachments.

III. PERIODONTITIS

A. *Adult Periodontitis*

1. Slight—Progression of the gingival inflammation into the deeper periodontal structures and alveolar bone crest, with slight bone loss. The usual periodontal probing depth is 3 to 4 mm with slight loss of connective tissue attachment and slight loss of alveolar bone.
2. Moderate—A more advanced state of the above condition, with increased destruction of the periodontal structures and noticeable loss of bone support possibly accompanied by an increase in tooth mobility. There may be furcation involvement in multirooted teeth.

3. Advanced—Further progression of periodontitis with major loss of alveolar bone support usually accompanied by increased tooth mobility. Furcation involvement in multirooted teeth is likely.
4. Rapidly progressive—Includes several unclassified types of periodontitis characterized either by rapid bone and attachment loss, or slow but continuous bone and attachment loss, and resistance to normal therapy. It is usually associated with gingival inflammation and continued pocket formation.

B. *Juvenile periodontitis* (JP)—Found in children and young adults. All forms usually progress at a rapid rate.

1. Prepubertal—An uncommon disease manifested by the formation of pockets and destruction of the alveolar bone around some, but not all, of the deciduous teeth. Onset may occur during, or immediately after, the eruption of the primary teeth. This disease may be present in either a generalized or localized form.
2. Generalized (GJP)—Circumpubertal or post-pubertal. An inflammatory process of the connective tissue and the bone surrounding the teeth, leading to progressive destruction of these tissues. Destruction may be cyclical with exacerbations and remissions. Increased pocket probing depth and loss of attachment are found.
3. Localized (LJP)—A specific periodontitis thought to be associated with one or more of the following: infection with *Actinobacillus actinomycetemcomitans*, heredity, or abnormalities in white blood cell function. Bone loss pattern has a predilection for the permanent central incisors and first molars.

C. *Periodontal abscess*—The result of the closure of the orifice of a deep periodontal pocket with the development of a localized acute infection, often accompanied by severe bone destruction.

IV. PATHOLOGY ASSOCIATED WITH OCCLUSION

Trauma from occlusion—Tissue injury to the periodontal attachment apparatus caused by excessive occlusal forces. The most recognized etiologic factor is bruxism (clenching and grinding of the teeth). It may be associated with disorders of the temporomandibular joints.

V. OTHER CONDITIONS OF THE ATTACHMENT APPARATUS

Includes all pathologic processes of the periodontium including infection, abrasion, trauma, and cystic, degenerative, or neoplastic changes.

From American Academy of Periodontology: *Current procedural terminology for periodontics and insurance reporting manual*, ed 6, Chicago, 1991, The Academy.

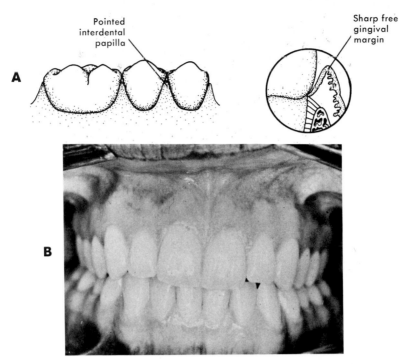

Figure 21-2   Normal gingiva. **A**, Sketches. **B**, Photograph.

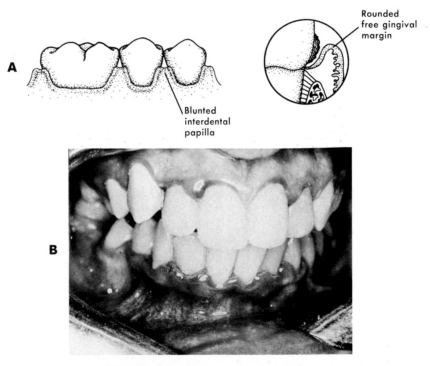

Figure 21-3   Changes in gingival form associated with gingivitis. **A**, Sketches. **B**, Photograph.

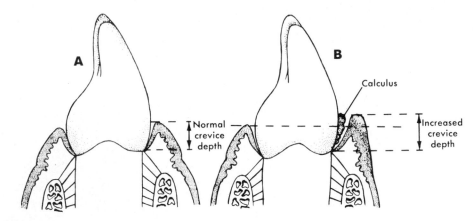

Figure 21-4 **A**, Normal gingival crevice depth. **B**, Deepened gingival crevice resulting from swelling.

The treatment for gingivitis is a thorough dental prophylaxis coupled with meticulous home oral hygiene procedures. Dental restorations that are contributing to local irritation should be replaced. Once the local irritants are removed and prevented from recurring, the gingiva will return to normal.

Case Types II Through V: Periodontitis

Case types II, III, IV, and V are different forms of periodontitis. **Periodontitis** is generally associated with loss of alveolar bone that surrounds and supports the tooth. Accompanying the loss of bony support is the migration of the epithelial attachment toward the apex of the tooth and inflammation of the deeper periodontal structures. Mobility, furcation involvements, and tooth loss can also occur with the more severe forms.

Because the cells of the epithelial attachment become repositioned apically on the root surface (Figure 21-5) the result is a deeper gingival crevice. When the gingival crevice deepens because of enlargement of the gingiva as in gingivitis, the deepened crevice is called a **gingival pocket**, or a **pseudopocket**. The epithelial attachment remains stationary. Deepening of the gingival crevice resulting from migration of the attachment apically is called a **periodontal pocket**.

Unfortunately, once a periodontal pocket forms, the accumulation of irritants in the deep gingival crevice makes it more difficult for the patient to remove plaque. Thus the destructive process continues. As the inflammation reaches the alveolar bone, it stimulates cells called **osteoclasts** to increase resorption of bone. **Bone resorption** is also stimulated by occlusal trauma on the tooth. It is normal for bone to be continually formed and then to be removed (resorbed) by cells located on the surface of bone. Inflammation and occlusal trauma together accelerate bone resorption to a rate faster than it can be reformed. As a result, there is a net loss of bone around the

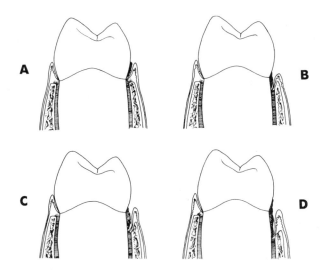

Figure 21-5 Migration of epithelial attachment and destruction of alveolar bone, resulting in periodontal pocket. **A**, Accumulation of irritants. **B**, Apical migration of epithelial attachment in response to irritant. **C** and **D**, Continued migration of attachment and accumulation of irritant on root surface.

root of the tooth, and the tooth becomes hypermobile. If the periodontitis continues to destroy sufficient bone, the tooth will eventually be lost.

The treatment of periodontitis depends on the severity of the disease. Nonsurgical or surgical methods may be employed. One of the initial nonsurgical steps in treatment is the thorough removal of all local irritants from the periodontal pockets and around the teeth. This extensive scaling procedure is often called a **periodontal scaling and root planing**, to differentiate it from the routine dental prophylaxis that does not involve the scaling of deep periodontal pockets. Additional procedures may include the following:

1. Surgery to eliminate periodontal pockets (gingivectomy, gingivoplasty)

BOX 21-3

DENTAL ASSISTANT DUTIES DURING INITIAL EXAMINATION STAGE

PROCEDURE	DUTIES
Medical-dental history	Assist patient in filling out medical-dental history form. Observe patient for physical or psychological limitations or conditions that could affect treatment.
Oral examination	Record probe readings, gingival assessments, mobility, furcation involvements, occlusion and malocclusion, existing restorations, and oral hygiene observations.
Study models and photographs	Take and pour study models. Assist dentist with intraoral photographs.
Dental laboratory tests	Assist dentist with taking and sampling for laboratory tests.
Treatment plan presentation	Review financial arrangements with patient.

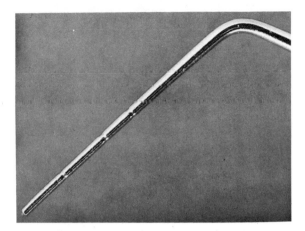

Figure 21-6   O-style periodontal probe.

2. Occlusal adjustment to eliminate excessive occlusal trauma
3. Restorative procedures (splints, bridges, and crowns) to establish proper contacts, occlusion, and contours of teeth
4. Orthodontic procedures to establish proper contacts and occlusion

PERIODONTAL DIAGNOSTIC PROCEDURES

The same diagnostic procedures described in Chapter 2 are used in periodontics. Box 21-3 describes duties of the dental assistant during this initial examination period. The specific information the dentist is looking for with regard to periodontal status will be discussed here.

Medical-Dental History

The patient's medical-dental history should reveal systemic conditions such as chronic illness, nutritional deficiencies, and personal habits that may influence the progress of periodontal disease or its treatment.

The dental portion of the history provides valuable information regarding the dental status of the patient. The frequency of brushing, flossing, and dental prophylaxis procedures is a good indication of the patient's effort to prevent periodontal disease. Knowledge of missing teeth, dates of extractions, orthodontic treatment, and restorative procedures is of value to the dentist.

The history should also reveal the patient's attitude toward the preservation of his or her teeth. Successful periodontal treatment depends greatly on a positive attitude by the patient.

Oral Examination

A visual inspection of the gingiva is essential to detect the changes that are associated with the inflammatory process. Changes in the color and shape of the gingival tissue are critical to the diagnosis. Palpation of the gingiva with the side of an explorer will reveal the texture, or density, of the tissue.

Periodontal probing is essential to diagnose the existence of periodontal pockets. The **periodontal probe** is a thin dipstick-like device that is used to measure the depth of the gingival crevice and to determine the relationship of the epithelial attachment to the cementoenamel junction. The O-style probe (Figure 21-6) is marked in increments of 3, 6, and 8 mm from the tip toward the shank of the instrument. Probing is often recorded at six points on a tooth, three on the buccal aspect and three on the lingual aspect (Figure 21-7). The probe is inserted in the gingival crevice to the depth of the epithelial attachment. The distance between the attachment and the gingival margin is recorded (Figure 21-8). If apical migration of the attachment is suspected, the probe tip can be used to locate the cementoenamel junction. The distance from here to the gingival margin is recorded. The two recordings can be compared to determine the amount of apical migration or true periodontal pocket formation.

Accumulation of plaque, stains, and calculus on the teeth should be noted and recorded. This is helpful in correlating areas of tissue damage with the areas of accumulation of local irritants. A general assessment of the pa-

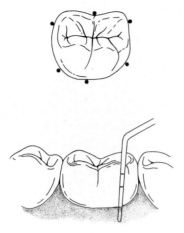

Figure 21-7 Common sites for measuring gingival crevice.

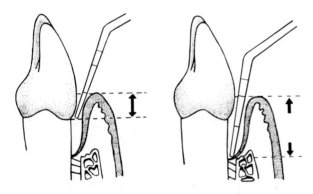

Figure 21-8 Measuring crevice depth. Probe is inserted into crevice to level of epithelial attachment. Depth of crevice is noted. Probe tip can be used to locate cementoenamel junction on tooth. If epithelial attachment is located apically to junction, periodontal pocket exists.

tient's oral hygiene should also be noted. Use of disclosing agents is a valuable method of detecting the more subtle accumulations of plaque.

Each tooth should be tested for mobility by pushing it with the opposite ends of a mouth mirror in a buccolingual direction and pressing on the occlusal or incisal surface. A simple scale of +, 1, 2, or 3 is often used to describe mobility:

- +: slight mobility
- 1: mobility of 1 mm in the facial-lingual direction
- 2: mobility of 2 mm in the facial-lingual direction
- 3: mobility of 3 mm in the facial-lingual direction and the tooth is depressible

These figures can be recorded on the dental chart for reference. Drifted teeth, missing teeth, malposed teeth, and open contacts should all be recorded, since they make up the dysfunctional factors in the progress of periodontal disease.

Existing restorations and prosthetic devices should be assessed to determine their possible contribution to periodontal problems.

Analysis of the patient's occlusion, or bite, is an integral part of a periodontal examination. It is well known that improper contacting of upper and lower teeth when the jaws are closed can create undesirable traumatic forces on teeth, which can contribute to the progress of periodontal destruction.

Study Models and Photographs

Diagnostic study models and photographs are useful to document oral findings. Models provide the dentist with a three-dimensional view of the patient's teeth, jaws, and gingiva. Malposed teeth, undesirable occlusal relationships, and poor gingival contours can be examined thoroughly on the models. Excessive-wear areas (facets) on teeth are easily detected on the study models. These are often good indications of excessive occlusal forces on a tooth.

Photographs provide a color recording of the gingiva and plaque and calculus accumulation for reference. Models and photographs should be kept as permanent records to document the progress of periodontal treatment. The dates on which study model impressions and photographs are taken should be recorded on the patient's record, the models, and the photographs.

Radiographs

Radiographs are useful in determining the degree of periodontal involvement. The loss of bone around teeth can be seen on the radiograph, although it cannot be relied on completely (Figure 21-9). Periodontal probing is the most accurate method of assessing the location and extent of bone loss. Overhangs on restorations are readily seen on bite-wing radiographs (Figure 21-10).

Dental Laboratory Tests

Several dental laboratory tests have been developed to assist in the diagnosis of periodontal disease. Although the tests are not used routinely, newer and simpler techniques continue to be developed and may become a regular part of a periodontal examination in the future. Examples of currently available tests include sampling and identification of plaque bacteria, flow rate of gingival fluid, and white blood cell activity.

Treatment Plan Presentation

Following the periodontal diagnostic procedures, the dentist decides the appropriate treatment for the patient based on the information gathered during the examination. The dentist presents the treatment plan to the patient by explaining the periodontal chart using educational diagrams and three-dimensional models to demonstrate the patient's current periodontal status. The

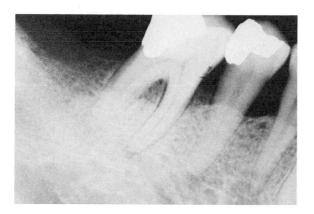

Figure 21-9   Radiograph revealing extensive loss of alveolar bone resulting from periodontitis.

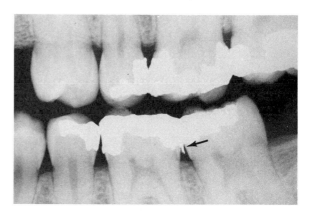

Figure 21-10   Bitewing radiograph demonstrating existence of cervical overhang of amalgam restoration.

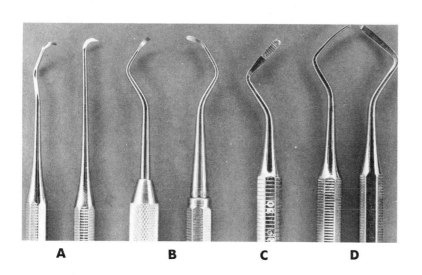

Figure 21-11   Common periodontal hand instruments. **A**, Sickle scalers. **B**, Curette scalers. **C**, Periodontal file scaler. **D**, Hoe scalers.

dentist and the patient cooperate to arrive at a carefully planned treatment satisfactory to both the patient and dentist. The dentist may or may not discuss the financial aspects of the treatment.

> **KEY POINT**
> - Financial arrangements are often delegated to the financial assistant, who often has a dental assisting background. It is frequently necessary for the financial assistant to explain or review aspects of the patient's treatment that require a dental background.

COMMON PERIODONTAL INSTRUMENTS

Figure 21-11 shows examples of commonly used periodontal instruments.

Scalers

Scalers are hand instruments used to remove local irritants from the tooth surface and to plane roughened root surfaces. They are available in a variety of shapes and styles. Most styles fit into one of three categories: sickles, hoes, and file scalers.

Sickle scalers derive their name from their sicklelike shape. The narrow, tapering tip of the instrument makes it convenient for use in scaling proximal surfaces of teeth. Sickles are especially useful in scaling proximal surfaces of anterior teeth because of the limited size of the interproximal space. They are available in straight or modified (Jacquette) designs.

Hoe scalers are less popular than the sickle and curette types. The sharp corners on the cutting edge create a risk in using it for subgingival scaling. The corners of the blade can gouge grooves in the soft root if the instrument is not handled carefully. Hoe scalers are most frequently used to remove heavy accumulations of supragingival calculus on the buccal and lingual surfaces of teeth.

Periodontal file scalers are miniature files that can be inserted into interproximal areas and periodontal pockets. They are used with a pull motion to remove small residual calculus particles after scaling and to smooth roughened tooth surfaces. The periodontal file and curette scaler are often used together in root-planing procedures.

Curette scalers are available in a number of designs. Each design seems to vary the relationship of the blade to the handle of the instrument. The basic design features in all of them are a rounded tip, a rounded back of the blade, and a cutting edge along two of the edges of the blade. Curette scalers are used to scale all surfaces of the teeth. They are particularly favorable instruments for removing subgingival calculus without damaging the root surface. Root planing and subgingival curettage can also be done with the curette scaler.

Periodontal Probe

The periodontal probe (see Figure 21-6) is a measuring device that is used to determine the depth of the gingival crevice. The O-style probe has markings on the instrument that serve as references to determine pocket depth.

Scalpels

The **surgical scalpel** is commonly used for oral surgical procedures, including gingivectomy. A standard scalpel handle is used with replaceable blades of various shapes (Figure 21-12). The Bard-Parker No. 12B blade is convenient for removing gingival tissue on the facial aspect of the alveolar process. Because of the double cutting edge of this blade, it can cut with pulling and pushing motions. The sharp tip of the blade can be used to remove interproximal soft tissue.

Periodontal Knives

Gingival surgery involves not only the removal of unwanted gingiva, but also the contouring of remaining soft tissue, which is necessary to reestablish the normal function of the gingiva.

Periodontal knives (see Figure 21-12) were developed to give the operator access to areas of the mouth that could not be reached with standard scalpel blades. The lingual aspect of the alveolar process is a typical area that is inaccessible for gingivectomy procedures using a scalpel blade.

Periodontal knives have the necessary angles in the shank of the instrument, making them convenient to use in resecting and contouring the gingiva. The Orban No. 1 and No. 2 style knives are excellent choices for removing interproximal soft tissue because of their narrow blade design. The disadvantage of periodontal knives is that they require precise sharpening after each use to keep them functional.

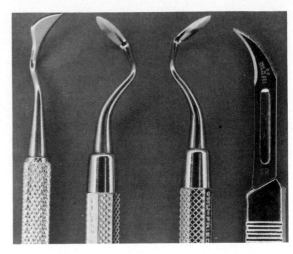

Figure 21-12 Periodontal surgical knives. *Left to right*: Kirkland knife, No. 1 and No. 2 Orban knives, and No. 12B scalpel.

Electrosurgery Setup

Electrosurgery is a useful surgical method that employs the use of a tiny arc of electrical current to make the incision in the gingiva. In electrosurgery, not only is soft tissue cut but also blood is coagulated, which limits bleeding during the procedure.

The electrosurgery device consists of a control box, a foot-operated on-off switch, and two terminals (Figure 21-13). One terminal is held by the patient or placed in contact with the patient in some way. Some manufacturers use a metal plate that the patient may sit on or lie on during the surgical procedure as one terminal. The other terminal, in the form of a probe with a wire-end, is held in the dentist's hand.

When the dentist touches the patient's gingiva with the tip of the probe and activates the foot switch, current flows through the wire tip and burns the incision in the gingiva. The assistant must keep the oral evacuator near the surgical site to remove the odor of burning tissue. Various cutting tips are available for better access to difficult working areas of the mouth (Figure 21-14).

> **KEY POINT**
> - It is wise to use nonmetal evacuator tips and mouth mirrors during electrosurgery procedures in case the cutting probe inadvertently contacts these instruments.

Evacuator Tip

Oral surgical procedures require constant removal of blood from the surgical site to maintain visibility for the operator. The smaller **surgical suction tips** are better

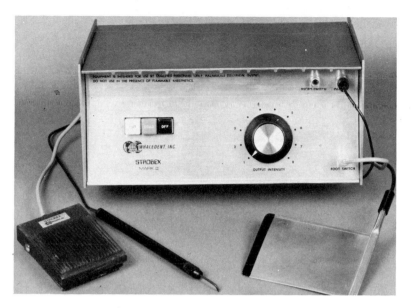

Figure 21-13   Electrosurgery unit.

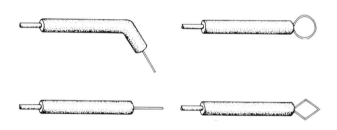

Figure 21-14   Various cutting tips for electrosurgery unit.

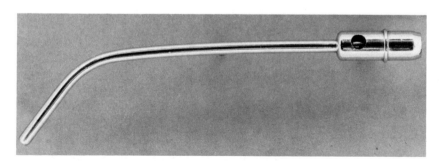

Figure 21-15   Surgical evacuator tip.

for this purpose (Figure 21-15). They remove small quantities of blood from the incision effectively, since the smaller tip can be directed specifically to smaller areas in the surgical field.

The tip should be dipped in sterile saline solution occasionally during the surgery to aspirate some fluid through the tip and hose. This clears away clotted blood that accumulates in the tip and evacuation hose. Nonmetal tips should be used during electrosurgery.

COMMON NONSURGICAL PERIODONTAL TREATMENT PROCEDURES
Scaling and Root Planing

Scaling and root planing procedures eliminate plaque and calculus from the surfaces of the teeth. The armamentarium for a periodontal scaling procedure is shown in Figure 10-5.

Periodontal scaling and dental prophylaxis share the same ultimate goal—to remove irritants to prevent peri-

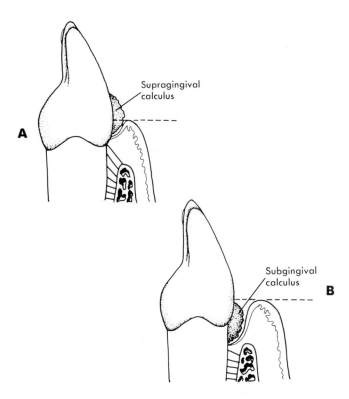

Figure 21-16 Location of calculus. **A,** Supragingival. **B,** Subgingival.

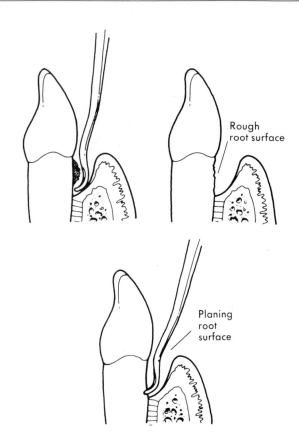

Figure 21-17 Exaggerated sketch of scaling and root planing.

odontal injury. The difference is in the location of the irritants being removed. The routine prophylaxis usually involves removal of irritants such as calculus above the gingival margin (supragingival calculus) or located just below the gingival margin (subgingival calculus) (Figure 21-16). Periodontal scaling implies more extensive scaling procedures to remove subgingival calculus located in deep periodontal pockets.

Scaling must be done with sharp scalers and curettes to ensure complete removal of the very adherent calculus. Once calculus is removed from a root surface, the underlying cementum is often rough from the damaging effects of the calculus. This roughness must be removed to prevent the gingiva from being continually irritated. Voids in the cementum become ideal areas for the rapid accumulation of plaque and subsequent calculus formation again. These voids are removed by root planing, a process of planing or shaving the root surface with a curette to remove surface roughness (Figure 21-17).

> **⊶ KEY POINT**
> ▪ A smooth root surface will minimize plaque adherence and assist the patient in adequate plaque control.

Gingival Curettage

One method of eliminating minor pocket formation is through the use of gingival curettage. This procedure involves the removal of the delicate lining (epithelium) of the periodontal pocket. Not only the lining is removed but also some underlying damaged tissue (Figure 21-18, *A*).

Once the calculus and other debris have been removed and the pocket lining curetted, there will be a reduction in edema that will also reduce the pocket depth. Slight reattachment may also occur, thus eliminating the pocket (Figure 21-18, *B*). The entire procedure can be accomplished with standard curette scalers. The success of subgingival curettage depends on the extent of pocket formation and the healing capabilities of the patient.

Antibacterial Therapy

Scaling, root planing, and **curettage** are traditional treatment methods for periodontal disease. In recent years antimicrobial mouthrinses and antibiotic regimens have supplemented these traditional therapies. The control of bacterial growth in dental plaque and in the gingival crevice is the focus of this therapeutic strategy.

Two mouthrinses, Listerine and chlorhexidine, have been approved by the American Dental Association (ADA)

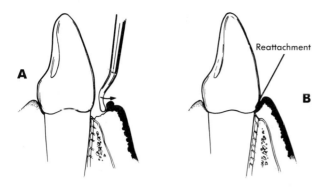

Figure 21-18 **A**, Subgingival curettage of lining of gingival crevice. **B**, Reattachment of gingiva to root surface.

to control plaque through general oral rinsing and by local irrigation of the gingival crevice. Irrigation devices are discussed in Chapter 10.

In selected cases the dentist may prescribe a systemic antibiotic such as tetracycline to control bacteria that are harbored in periodontal pockets and are associated with periodontal disease.

A fairly new treatment modality is the insertion of tetracycline-impregnated fibers into the gingival sulcus. The fibers are similar to retraction cord used for crown and bridge procedures and are inserted in a similar manner. The fibers are left in the gingival sulcus for a limited time and removed. Much research is being conducted in this approach to periodontal therapy.

At present the use of antibiotics, antibiotic-impregnated fibers, and antimicrobial mouthrinses is viewed as adjunctive to scaling, root planing, curettage, and vigorous home care by the patient.

COMMON SURGICAL PERIODONTAL TREATMENT PROCEDURES

The objectives of periodontal surgery are to preserve the periodontium by making it easier for the patient to perform adequate plaque control, to make it easier for the dentist or dental hygienist to perform proper scaling and root planing, and possibly to promote gingival reattachment.

Role of Surgical Dental Assistant in Periodontal Surgery

The role of the surgical dental assistant during periodontal surgery is to assist the dentist in such a manner that treatment is administered smoothly and efficiently. Box 21-4 outlines characteristics of an excellent surgical assistant.

The preparations for periodontal surgery are often delegated to the dental assistant. The assistant should per-

---

BOX 21-4

CHARACTERISTICS OF A SURGICAL ASSISTANT

1. Is professional and efficient, yet relaxed. The assistant's good nature will help relax the patient at a time when the patient may be nervous and insecure. An excellent assistant inspires confidence in the physician and the office.
2. Has a genuine interest in the health care of the patient and a genuine desire to help.
3. Keeps patient records neat and orderly and sets the x-ray films on the view box before surgery.
4. Sharpens surgical instruments to perfection before each surgery, sterilizes all instruments, and prepares the tray of surgical instruments before surgery.
5. Prepares and stores the periodontal pack (when used) before or after the surgery as needed.
6. Protects the patient's lips by applying petroleum jelly before surgery.
7. Scrubs hands clean before surgery. Wears surgical rubber gloves and a face mask. Wears a cap to restrain the hair.
8. Knows both how to position mirrors and how to take photographs.
9. Knows all the surgical instruments by name and appearance.
10. Is aware of each stage of the operation and the sequence of operating.
11. Adjusts the intraoral light to provide access and vision for the surgeon.
12. Hands the instruments to the surgeon in proper sequence and replaces them to precise position on the surgical tray.
13. Is responsible for keeping the patient's face clean and for keeping instruments clean and in order during surgery.
14. Communicates with the surgeon without speaking, if at all possible, and certainly without alarming the patient.

From Grant DA and others: *Periodontics in the tradition of Gottlieb and Orban*, ed 6, St Louis, 1988, Mosby.

---

form the following preoperative surgical preparations:

- Be aware of any antianxiety medications or preoperative instructions given to the patient before the surgical appointment.
- Prepare, sterilize, and set out the surgical instrument tray.
- Perform a surgical scrub.
- Place the chart and patient x-rays in plain sight.
- Drape the patient to prepare for the surgery.

During the surgery, the assistant is responsible for the following:

- Retracting the soft tissues
- Evacuating oral fluids
- Debridement of the surgical site
- Delivering instruments or materials to the operator
- Preparing the surgical sutures and trimming the suture if necessary
- Adjusting the lighting
- Mixing the periodontal dressing
- Placing the periodontal dressing if permitted by state regulations

The postsurgical duties of the assistant include the following:

- Giving postoperative instructions both orally and in written form
- Giving the patient gauze and an ice pack to control bleeding and postoperative inflammation
- Explaining antibiotic or pain-relieving prescriptions if prescribed by the dentist

Gingivectomy

Once periodontal pockets are formed, they must be eliminated, since they have the following undesirable effects on the patient:

1. They accumulate assorted debris and bacteria, which can lead to local and systemic infection.
2. Root caries can develop quickly as a result of debris accumulation in the pocket.
3. Putrefaction of pocket debris can create bad tastes and foul mouth odors.
4. Untreated pockets continually collect debris, which results in a deepening of the pocket as alveolar bone is destroyed. This results in hypermobility and eventual loss of the tooth.

One method of eliminating periodontal pockets is by surgically removing the diseased gingival tissue. This procedure is called a **gingivectomy**. Besides eliminating the ill effects of periodontal pockets listed previously, the gingivectomy procedure benefits the patient in the following ways:

1. Diseased gingival tissue is removed.
2. Favorable gingival contour can be reestablished, within limits.
3. The surgical removal of the wall of the pocket gives the operator direct access to remove calculus (Figure 21-19) and plane rough root surfaces.
4. The patient gains access to clean the root surfaces previously inaccessible because of the existence of the pocket.

Armamentarium (Figure 21-20)

Gingivectomy procedures are usually performed with a scalpel, periodontal knives, surgical scissors, or electrosurgery. The choice is made according to the preference of the dentist.

There is some difference of opinion as to whether a patient requiring gingival surgery should have a periodontal scaling before the surgery. Dentists who wish to prescale before surgery will schedule a separate appointment for that purpose. A typical appointment scheme is shown in Box 21-5.

At the surgery appointment the patient is premedicated if necessary and anesthetized with local anesthetic. Box 21-6 describes the steps of a sample gingivectomy surgical procedure.

For an illustration of the preoperative and postoperative appearance of a periodontitis patient, see p. 330 (Figure 21-25).

Flap Periodontal Surgery

Flap surgery is used for very deep periodontal pockets, when the alveolar bone has become rough and irregularly shaped or when there are furcation involvements. There are many types of flap surgical procedures; however, the same goal is achieved. A modified Widman flap is described in detail.

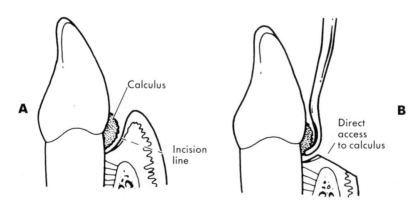

Figure 21-19 Surgical elimination of periodontal pocket, **A**, gives direct access to subgingival calculus, **B**.

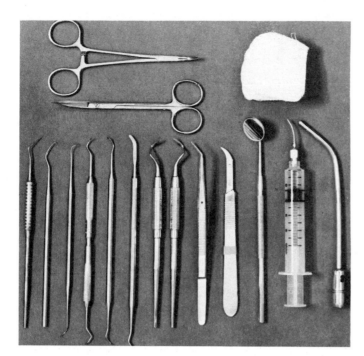

Hemostat
Suture scissors
Sterile gauze sponges, 2 × 2 inch
Periodontal probe
Explorers, No. 17 and No. 3
Curette scalers, Columbia No. 13 and No. 14
Sickle scaler, Jacquette
Plastic filling instrument, F.P. No. 1
Periodontal knives, Orban No. 1, No. 2
Cotton pliers
Bard-Parker scalpel handle
Bard-Parker scalpel, No. 12B blade
Mouth mirror
Irrigation syringe (for sterile saline solution)
Surgical suction tip

Add-on items

Sterile cup of saline solution
Surgical gloves for operator and assistant
Periodontal dressing
Cotton tip applicator
Iodine lotion
Mixing pads, paper
Cement spatula, No. 336
Petroleum jelly
Anesthesia setup

Figure 21-20 Gingivectomy armamentarium.

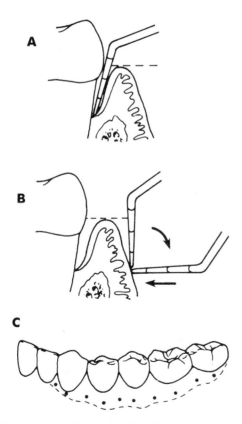

Figure 21-21 Marking periodontal pockets for gingivectomy procedure. **A**, Measuring depth of pocket. **B**, Transposing measured depth to gingival surface. Gingiva is marked by puncturing mucosa at level of pocket depth. **C**, Incising just apical to puncture marks.

BOX 21-5

APPOINTMENT SCHEDULE FOR GINGIVECTOMY PATIENT

APPOINTMENT	TREATMENT
1	Prescale the teeth
2	(1) Gingivectomy (pocket elimination)
	(2) Residual calculus removal
	(3) Root-plane rough surfaces
	(4) Placement of surgical dressing
3	(1) Remove surgical dressing after 1 week
	(2) Rinse area of surgery with hydrogen peroxide
	(3) Gently polish teeth with soft rubber cup and dental floss
	(4) Rinse thoroughly with warm water
	(5) Place new surgical dressing
4	(1) Remove final surgical dressing 1 week after placement
	(2) Repeat rinsing and polishing procedures
	(3) Patient home care instructions given
5	Recall patient 6 weeks after surgery to evaluate healing and home care effectiveness

BOX 21-6

SAMPLE GINGIVECTOMY PROCEDURE

PROCEDURE	RATIONALE
1. Area operated on may be swabbed with iodine lotion, or patient may be asked to rinse with antibacterial mouthrinse.	1. To reduce bacterial contamination in surgical field.
2. Field is isolated with sterile 2 x 2–inch gauze sponges.	2. To isolate surgical site.
3. After local anesthetic is administered, pockets are measured on facial and lingual gingiva with periodontal probe and gingiva is punctured with probe tip level of base of pocket (Figure 21-21). Pocket marker may be used as alternative method for marking gingiva (Figure 21-22).	3. To visibly mark depth of pocket by making small puncture wounds on gingiva. Dentist uses blood spots from punctures to outline contour of incision.
4. Using either scalpel or periodontal knife, dentist cuts gingiva just apical to puncture marks (Figure 21-23, *A*). Blade of instrument is positioned so that bevel is created along incised gingiva.	4. To reestablish normal tapered contour of free gingival margin.
5. Interdental papillae are incised with narrow-bladed periodontal knife (Orban No. 1 or 2).	5. To reestablish normal contour of interdental papillae.
6. Detached gingiva is removed with curette scaler and tissue forceps (Figure 21-23, *B*).	6. To remove diseased tissues.

PROCEDURE	RATIONALE
7. If residual calculus is revealed by removal of diseased gingiva, it is removed and root surface is planed with periodontal files and curettes as needed.	7. Preoperative scaling and root planing on deep periodontal pockets are difficult, and calculus may not be removed from all subgingival surfaces of tooth.
8. Surgical field is thoroughly rinsed and inspected. Refinements are then made if they are needed.	8. To clear surgical field so dentist can determine if pockets have been eliminated and proper contour of gingiva has been established.
9. Periodontal surgical dressing is prepared and placed over entire surgical area. Dressing is held in place by mechanical lock of dressing that is forced into interproximal spaces (Figure 21-23, *C*).	9. To protect surgical site from trauma while healing.
10. Patient is given postoperative instructions in oral and written forms before being dismissed (Figure 21-24).	10. To inform patient about postoperative care for surgical site and complications that could arise.

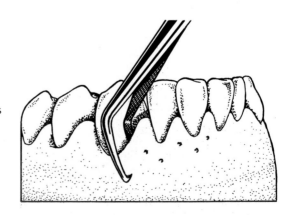

Figure 21-22 Marking periodontal pockets with a pocket marker.

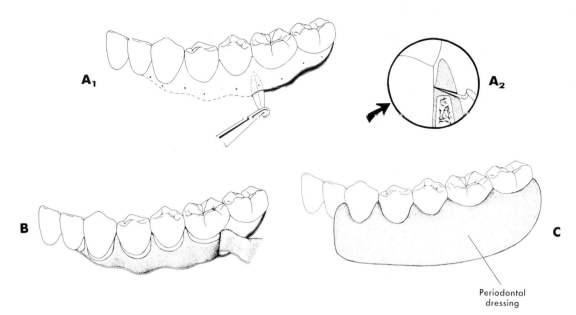

Figure 21-23   **A,** Incision and resection of gingiva during gingivectomy. **B,** Removal of excised gingiva with tissue forceps. **C,** Periodontal dressing in place.

_____ , D.D.S.   Telephone _____

POSTOPERATIVE INSTRUCTIONS TO PATIENT
AFTER PERIODONTAL SURGERY

1. Do not eat or drink for 2 hours after surgery.
2. Do not investigate dressing with tongue or fingers. This dressing serves as a bandage to protect the wound.
3. Avoid tart or spicy foods.
4. Drink fruit juices with a straw.
5. In some cases a dressing will be placed over the area. The dressing serves to protect the area of surgery and to keep you comfortable. If small pieces break off, do not be alarmed. If a large piece falls off, or if the dressing is uncomfortable, call the doctor. As an emergency measure, cover the wound with softened paraffin.
6. Some swelling may occur. This is to be expected. Place ice pack over the area that has undergone surgery and rinse frequently and gently with warm water (one glass) with one teaspoon of salt.
7. A slight amount of seepage may occur, giving your saliva a red color. Do not be alarmed. If the seepage persists, call the doctor.
8. For postoperative comfort, take pills according to instructions in prescription given to you. Take antibiotics if they are prescribed.
9. Brush parts of mouth on which surgery was not performed. Brush only the biting surfaces of the teeth where surgery was performed. Be sure to brush! When no dressing is placed, brush and use floss, but do not carry the floss under the gum line.
10. Rinse mouth carefully after eating. Clean outside of dressing with moistened cotton swab or Q-tips.

Figure 21-24   Postoperative instructions to a periodontal surgery patient.

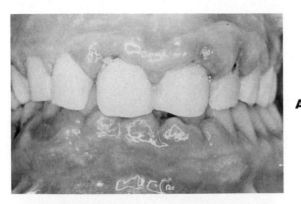

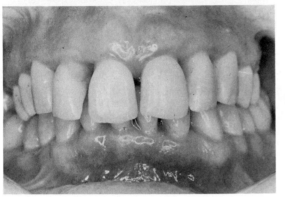

Figure 21-25 **A**, Severe periodontitis before surgery. **B**, View of same patient 6 weeks after surgery.

(Courtesy Raul D. Caffesse, DDS, Ann Arbor, Mich.)

Modified Widman Flap

For the modified Widman flap procedure, the patient is prepared for surgery with a thorough periodontal scaling, overhang removal, and instruction in oral hygiene procedures. After a 3- to 4-week period of high-level oral hygiene, the surgery is performed.

The procedure involves the removal of the lining of the periodontal pocket and some adjacent marginal gingiva (Figure 21-26). During the surgery a conservative flap is retracted on both the buccal and lingual aspects of the involved teeth. The flap retraction allows the dentist to gain access to the roots of the teeth and the surrounding alveolar bone. The damaged tissue is removed after being incised. Curettes are used to remove the incised tissue (Figure 21-27). The roots of the teeth are planed, and alveolar bone is recontoured as needed. The surgical site is flushed thoroughly with sterile saline solution, the flap is repositioned and sutured in place, and a conventional periodontal dressing is placed.

One to two weeks after surgery the dressing and sutures are removed, and the teeth are polished. Home care instructions are reviewed again with the patient.

A sample armamentarium for the Widman flap procedure is shown in Figure 21-28. The procedure is outlined below using the four-handed dentistry technique.

Box 21-7 describes the steps of a sample modified Widman flap surgical procedure. The mandibular left posterior segment serves as an example of an area of the mouth to be treated.

The advantages of the Widman flap procedure compared with the gingivectomy procedure include (1) optimal coverage of root surfaces with soft tissue after healing, which facilitates oral hygiene and improves esthetics, and (2) less exposure of root surfaces, which may help to minimize root sensitivity and root caries.

Osseous (Bone) Surgery

The operator may perform **osseous** or **bone surgery** to correct defects in the alveolar bone created by the periodontal disease process. Bone surgery may either remove the bony defect or augment the bony defect with bone (graft) or with a bone substitute.

Distal Wedge Procedure

Periodontal pockets that occur on the distal surface of the last molars can be treated by cutting and removing a triangular (wedge-shaped) piece of tissue behind the last molar (Figure 21-29, *A* and *B*). The underlying tissue is reduced (Figure 21-29, *C*), and the sides of the incision are sutured together (Figure 21-29, *D*).

Gingival Grafts

There are many types of **gingival graft** procedures. One of the most common grafts involves removing tissue from the hard palate and placing it on an area with severe gingival recession (Figure 21-30).

Guided Tissue Regeneration

Once the gingival attachment migrates toward the apex of the tooth, minimal reattachment may or may not occur following traditional periodontal therapy procedures such as scaling and root planing, gingivectomy, or flap procedures. **Guided tissue regeneration** is used as an effort to improve the reattachment mechanism by inserting special membranes to encourage growth of periodontal ligament fibers at the surgical site. This in turn encourages regeneration of new attachment above the new growth of periodontal ligament fibers.

Periodontal Dressing

A **periodontal dressing** is used to cover the surgical wound and is primarily for patient comfort postoperatively. The dressing also protects the surgical site from trauma such as eating hard or spicy foods.

The assistant prepares the periodontal dressing to be placed over the operative area. There are several preferred formulas used to make a periodontal surgical dressing.

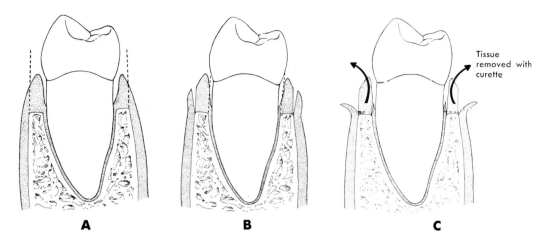

Figure 21-26   Incisions required for modified Widman flap procedure. **A**, First incision at least 0.5 to 1 mm away from free gingival margin. **B**, Second incision extends from bottom of gingival crevice to alveolar crest. **C**, Third incision releases damaged tissue, which can then be removed with curette scaler.

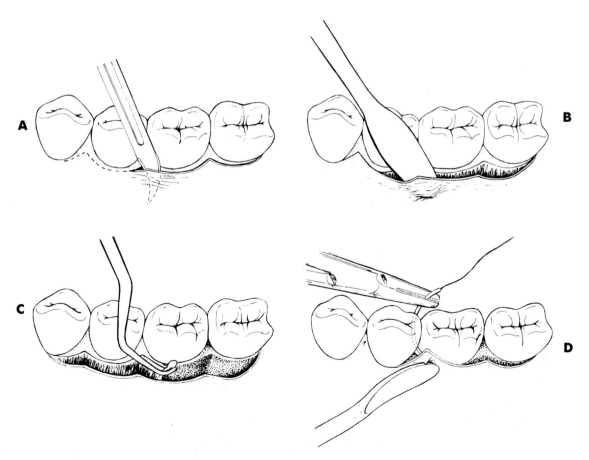

Figure 21-27   Flap procedure performed with aid of chairside assistant (buccal view). **A**, Incising buccal gingiva. **B**, Flap reflection with periosteal elevator. **C**, Use of curette to remove granulomatous tissue and accretions. **D**, Chairside assistant can support buccal gingiva with periosteal elevator to facilitate penetration with suture needle.

BOX 21-7
MODIFIED WIDMAN FLAP PROCEDURE

PROCEDURE	RATIONALE
1. Patient is anesthetized, and dentist probes gingiva throughout surgical site with periodontal probe.	1. To test for anesthesia.
2. Operator retracts tongue with mouth mirror in left hand, and assistant retracts cheek with evacuator in right hand. Assistant's left hand can also be used for additional retraction as needed. Assistant transfers No. 12B scalpel to operator in exchange for periodontal probe. Pickup-and-delivery instrument transfer can be used.	2. Soft tissue is retracted to maintain clear operating field. No. 12B scalpel is often used to make initial incision.
3. Incision is made around area to be treated (see Figure 21-27, A). Assistant evacuates as needed along incision using surgical tip.	3. As operator makes incision, blood can block operating field. Surgical tip oral evacuator is useful for clearing operating field. Note that whenever surgical tip is used to evacuate blood, it is good to aspirate sterile water or saline solution periodically from a container into tip during procedure to prevent clogging of lumen of tip with clotted blood.
4. Periosteal elevator is transferred to operator in exchange for scalpel.	4. Periosteal elevator is used to reflect gingiva from alveolar bone (see Figure 21-27, B).
5. Curette is delivered to operator in exchange for periosteal elevator. Roots can be planed as needed. Assistant continues to evacuate as necessary with right hand. A 2 x 2–inch gauze sponge is held in left hand to wipe tip of curette.	5. Curette is used to remove incised tissue from around teeth (see Figure 21-27, C). The 2 x 2–inch gauze sponge is used to wipe tip of curette as debris is removed from surgical site.

PROCEDURE	RATIONALE
6. Surgical site is flushed with sterile saline solution from irrigating syringe as assistant evacuates fluid. Surgical site is inspected.	6. To clear operating field for inspection.
7. Bone contouring can be accomplished at this point if required. Surgical site is rinsed again.	7. It is desirable to eliminate rough or irregularly shaped bone.
8. Suture needle is transferred in needle holder in proper orientation for insertion from lingual toward buccal gingiva through interproximal space. As needle is passed through interproximal space, assistant can support buccal flap with back of large end of periosteal elevator (see Figure 21-27, D).	8. Sutures are used to close surgical wound. Assistant supports buccal flap with periosteal elevator so that needle can penetrate tissue without moving it out of position.
9. While operator is securing knot in suture, assistant retrieves surgical scissors. Operator holds strands of suture material taut with needle holder as assistant cuts material approximately 1/8 inch above knot. Suturing continues until wound is closed. Surgical site is then rinsed.	9. Suturing holds tissue firmly to alveolar bone.
10. A 2 × 2–inch gauze compress moistened with saline solution is placed over surgical site for patient to bite on while periodontal dressing is prepared by assistant.	10. Gauze compress helps to stop bleeding from surgical wound.
11. Periodontal dressing is rolled into rope and delivered to operator on mixing pad. Gauze compress is removed.	11. Periodontal dressing is rolled into rope to facilitate placement over surgical site.

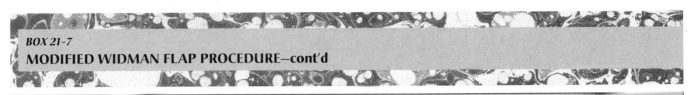

BOX 21-7
MODIFIED WIDMAN FLAP PROCEDURE—cont'd

PROCEDURE	RATIONALE	PROCEDURE	RATIONALE
12. Assistant can retract cheek with mouth mirror, using right hand. Left hand delivers filling instrument (FP No. 1) to operator. Assistant's left hand can be used to wipe tip of filling instrument with 2 x 2–inch gauze sponge.	12. Filling instrument is used to shape and trim periodontal dressing. The 2 x 2–inch gauze sponge is used to wipe filling instrument as portions of dressing are trimmed away.	13. After periodontal dressing is in place, patient's mouth is rinsed. Assistant cleans patient's face, and postoperative instructions are given before dismissing patient.	13. During surgery, blood and other oral fluids are transferred to outside of patient's face. Postoperative instructions are given both orally and in written form to warn patient about potential postoperative complications and also to inform patient about care of surgical site.

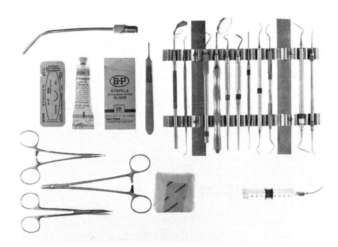

Surgical suction tip
Suture, 4-0, with needle
Achromycin ointment, 3%
Scalpel handle No. 12B blade
Mirror (operator)
Cowhorn explorer, No. 3
Periodontal probe
Mirror (assistant)
Knives, Orban No. 1 and No. 2
Periosteal elevator (wax spatula), No. 7
Curette, Columbia No. 13 and No. 14
Curette, McCall's No. 13 and No. 14
Interdental file, No. 3S and No. 4S
Hemostat
Needle holder
Suture scissors
Sterile gauze sponges, 2 × 2 inch
Irrigation syringe
Sterile saline solution (not shown)

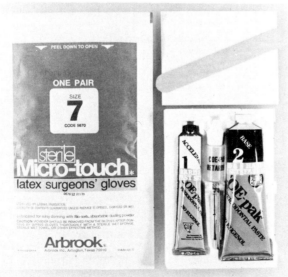

Surgical gloves (2 pair)
Mixing pad
Tongue depressor (spatula)
Periodontal dressing

Figure 21-28 Armamentarium for Widman flap procedure.

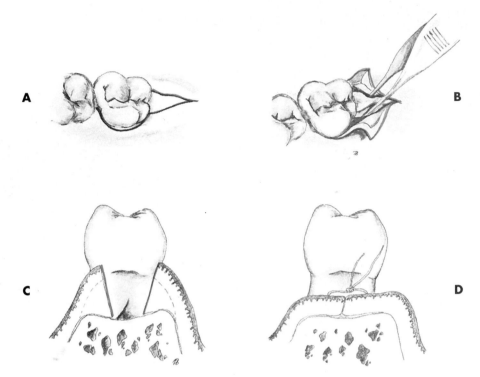

Figure 21-29 Distal wedge procedure. **A,** Buccal and lingual vertical incisions are made through retromolar pad behind mandibular second molar. **B,** Triangular wedge of tissue, prepared by vertical incisions, is dissected from underlying bone and removed. **C,** Walls of buccal and lingual flaps are reduced in thickness by undermining incisions (*broken lines*). **D,** Flaps, which have been trimmed and shortened to avoid overlapping wound margins, are sutured.

Eugenol or noneugenol types of dressings are opaque materials marketed in two tubes. One tube is a base material, and the other is an accelerator (Figure 21-31). Box 21-8 describes how the material is prepared.

A light-cured periodontal dressing is also available and requires no mixing. The material almost matches the gingival tissue in color when cured. It can be extruded onto a mixing pad, molded into a rope shape (Figure 21-32), and then placed over the surgical site, shaped, and light cured.

Occlusal Equilibration

The health of the periodontium depends not only on the constant elimination of local irritants and favorable nutrition but also on favorable forces being applied to the teeth. A healthy periodontium requires the stimulation of some occlusal force, yet excessive force can be severely damaging. A delicate balance exists between adequate forces needed for periodontal stimulation and excessive forces that cause injury. Individuals vary in resistance to excessive occlusal forces.

The **periodontium** is designed to tolerate forces applied to a tooth in the direction of its long axis. Any force that tends to tip teeth out of position is potentially trau-matic to the periodontal tissues. Teeth that are rotated, tipped, or drifted out of position are the most vulnerable. Opposing teeth that do no mesh properly are also subject to damaging forces (Figure 21-33). Any occlusal arrangement that results in trauma to the periodontium is called traumatic occlusion.

It is generally agreed that traumatic occlusion does not cause periodontal pocket formation. Traumatic occlusal forces act to accelerate pocket formation in the presence of inflammation caused by local irritants. Traumatic occlusion alone can cause hypersensitivity and hypermobility, even in the absence of periodontal pocket formation.

It should be noted that some oral habits have traumatic effects on the periodontium of the teeth. Chronic habits such as pipe smoking, tongue thrust, pencil biting, clenching, and bruxism create excessive forces on teeth that can traumatize the periodontium. These habits must be controlled to eliminate their resultant traumatic effect.

Discrepancies in a patient's occlusion are injurious not only to periodontal tissues but also to the temporomandibular joint and the muscles of mastication. Occlusal interferences and oral habits can cause a deflection of the mandible out of its normal position when the upper and

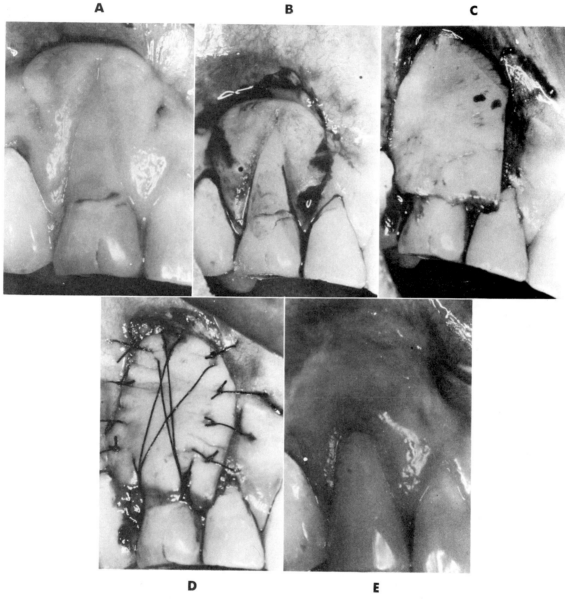

Figure 21-30 Illustration of free gingival graft to cover recession over maxillary canine. Deep area of recession exists over maxillary canine, which is broad coronally and narrow apically and extends within 1 mm of mucogingival junction. **A,** Preoperative photograph. **B,** Initial incision before removing gingiva in interproximal areas mesial and distal to area of recession to prepare recipient bed. **C,** Graft (from palatal donor site of patient) is approximately one fourth to one third larger than area taken from gingival epithelium. **D,** Free gingival graft sutured into place over recipient bed and area of recession. **E,** Two-year postoperative view showing large band of attached gingiva covering approximately one half of original area of recession, resulting in aesthetic scallop matching that of adjacent teeth.

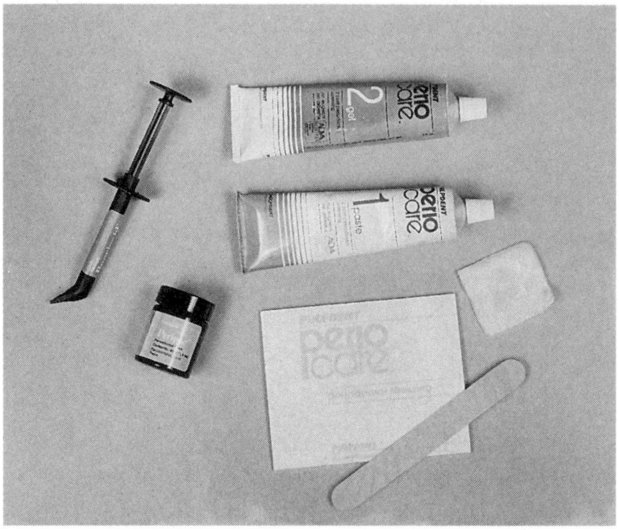

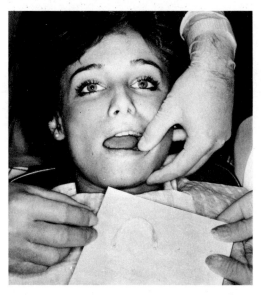

Figure 21-31 Traditional periodontal dressing.

Figure 21-32 Delivery of periodontal dressing.

BOX 21-8
MIXING AND PLACEMENT OF EUGENOL OR NONEUGENOL TYPE OF PERIODONTAL DRESSING

PROCEDURE	RATIONALE
1. Extrude equal lengths of material from tubes onto mixing pad (½ to 1 inch is usually sufficient for quadrant).	1. To achieve proper mix as recommended by manufacturer.
2. Mix material with tip of disposable tongue blade until mix is of one homogeneous color (approximately 45 seconds).	2. Tip of tongue blade is used rather than side to avoid material clinging to broad surface of tongue blade. This ensures that adequate material will stay on paper pad after mixing.
3. Wait 1 to 3 minutes before handling. Material should be consistency of old bubble gum.	3. To ensure that material is in workable stage and not too sticky.
4. Lubricate fingers.	4. To avoid material sticking to gloves.
5. Roll material into rope shape with rolling motion of fingers.	5. To prepare material for placement onto surgical site.
6. Material is placed over surgical site and pressed into interproximal areas.	6. To cover surgical site and to lock material into place between interproximal areas.
7. Material is shaped to follow normal contours and muscle attachments near surgical site.	7. To avoid soft tissue irritation or impingement on frenum attachments or vestibule.
8. Articulating paper is used to check if dressing interferes with patient's occlusion.	8. To avoid interfering with patient's occlusion.

lower teeth are brought together. This chronic shifting of the mandible during oral functions is traumatic to the joint, and muscle spasms are frequently associated with undesirable occlusion.

Favorable occlusion is an important key to periodontal health, as well as the health of the entire chewing mechanism. Therefore the establishment and preservation of a favorable occlusion are important goals in periodontal, orthodontic, restorative, and prosthetic procedures.

A periodontal treatment plan will include efforts to eliminate inflammation and periodontal pockets as well as efforts to eliminate traumatic occlusion. These efforts may include orthodontic treatment, extensive restorative dentistry, extraction of teeth, and selective grinding procedures. All these corrective procedures are directed toward the elimination of occlusal forces that tend to tip teeth and toward the distribution of occlusal forces as evenly as possible over several teeth. Any occlusal inter-

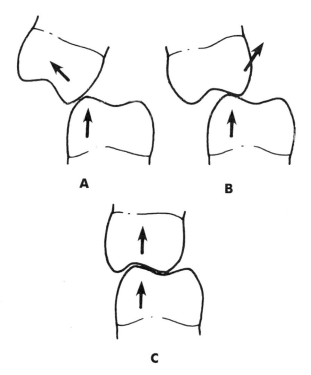

Figure 21-33 **A** and **B**, Traumatic occlusion. **C**, Favorable biting relationship between opposing teeth.

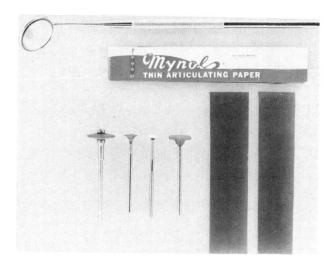

Figure 21-34 Occlusal equilibration armamentarium.

ferences that tend to force teeth out of contact with each other or deflect the mandible out of position when the jaws are closed must be eliminated. The biting surfaces of the teeth must mesh in such a manner as to allow movement of the mandible in all directions without locking on a few teeth, which would result in damaging forces on those teeth. Eliminating all occlusal interferences and establishing favorable occlusal forces on the teeth constitute **occlusal equilibration.** The armamentarium for this procedure is shown in Figure 21-34.

Procedure

Occlusal equilibration is most often accomplished by determining the location of occlusal interferences with articulating paper and occlusal wax and then removing them by selectively grinding the teeth. The grinding can be done with either the high-speed or conventional-speed handpiece. Diamond stones are used in the high-speed handpiece, and various shapes of gem stones are used in the conventional-speed handpiece. Once the grinding is complete, the ground surfaces are polished with abrasive rubber wheels. If occlusal interferences cannot be removed by selective grinding, alteration of the biting relationship must be accomplished by restorative procedures or orthodontic movement of the teeth. In some cases it is necessary to extract some undesirably positioned teeth to eliminate interferences.

ORAL HYGIENE

The success of all periodontal treatment depends on the patient's ability to maintain a high level of oral hygiene. Rigorous home care efforts coupled with routine recall visits to the dentist are absolutely mandatory.

The oral hygiene procedures and devices discussed in Chapter 10 play an important role in home care for the patient. Patients who do not meet this responsibility are vulnerable to recurrence of periodontal disease. Patient education via plaque-control programs assists periodontal patients in achieving oral hygiene skills and sustaining the necessary motivation to preserve their teeth.

BIBLIOGRAPHY

Finkbeiner BL, Johnson CS: *Mosby's comprehensive dental assisting: a clinical approach*, St Louis, 1995, Mosby.

Gencoe RJ, Goldman HM, Cohen DW: *Contemporary periodontics,* St Louis, 1990, Mosby.

Grant DA and others: *Periodontics in the tradition of Gottlieb and Orban*, ed 6, St Louis, 1988, Mosby.

Hoag PM, Pawlak EA: *Essentials of periodontics,* ed 4, St Louis, 1990, Mosby.

Lindhe J: *Textbook of clinical periodontology*, ed 2, Copenhagen, 1992, Munksgaard.

Strom T: Nonsurgical antibacterial periodontal treatment, *JADA* 116:22, 1988.

Wilkins EM: *Clinical practice of the dental hygienist*, ed 7, Malvern, Pa, 1994, Williams & Wilkins.

QUESTIONS—Chapter 21

1. All the following are used for incising or contouring the gingiva for a gingivectomy *except:*
   a. 12B scalpel
   b. Orban gingival knives
   c. Kirkland gingival knives
   d. Interproximal knife (Gold knife)

2. During the periodontal surgery, the dental assistant is responsible for all the following *except*:
   a. Mixing the periodontal dressing
   b. Preparing the surgical sutures
   c. Suturing the surgical site
   d. Retracting soft tissue

3. The periodontal probe is primarily used to measure _____.
   a. Depth of the periodontal pocket
   b. Amount of gingival recession
   c. Mobility
   d. Furcations

4. Which of the following can be used for root planing?
   a. Hoe scaler
   b. Curette
   c. 12B scalpel
   d. Electrosurgery

5. Which of the following periodontal surgical procedures involves the removal of the lining of the periodontal pocket and some adjacent marginal gingiva?
   a. Gingivectomy
   b. Osseous surgery
   c. Gingival graft
   d. Flap surgery

6. Which of the following periodontal surgical procedures takes attached gingiva from one area of the mouth and transplants it in an area with severe gingival recession?
   a. Gingivectomy
   b. Osseous surgery
   c. Gingival graft
   d. Flap surgery

7. All the following are true for mixing of a eugenol or noneugenol periodontal dressing *except*:
   a. Mix with a tongue depressor.
   b. Lubricate fingers before touching.
   c. Roll into a rope before placing it on the surgical site.
   d. It should not be placed distal to the last molar.

8. Which of the following is recommended to prevent clogging of the surgical suction during the surgical procedure?
   a. Replace frequently.
   b. Occasionally aspirate tap water.
   c. Occasionally aspirate sterile saline.
   d. Nothing is needed; the surgical suction tip rarely clogs.

9. If small pieces of the periodontal dressing fall off after the patient leaves the office, the patient should _____.
   a. Call the dental office
   b. Put it back on
   c. Do nothing
   d. Go to the dental office to get it replaced

10. The operator uses a _____ to outline the pocket depth before making the initial incision.
    a. Periodontal probe
    b. Pocket marker
    c. 12B scalpel
    d. *a* and *b*
    e. *b* and *c*

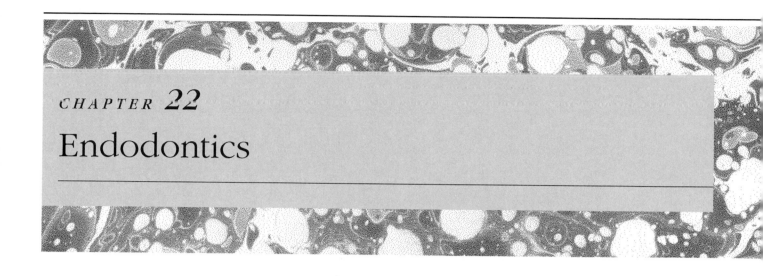

Endodontics

KEY TERMS

Acute apical
    periodontitis
Apical periodontitis
Apicoectomy
Avulsed tooth
Barbed broach
Chronic apical
    periodontitis
Electrical pulp test
Endodontic files
Endodontic storage box
Endodontics
File stops
Fistula
Galvanism
Granuloma
Gutta-percha
Gutta-percha plugger
    (condenser)
Hyperemia
Irreversible pulpitis
Mechanical pulp
    exposure

Necrosis
Nonvital pulp
Obturation
Percussion
Periapical abscess
Periapical cyst
Pulp exposure
Pulpectomy
Pulpitis
Radiolucency
Retrofill amalgam
Reversible pulpitis
Root amputations
Root canal sealer
Selective anesthesia
Spreader
Test cavity preparation
Transillumination
Trial-point radiograph
Vital pulp

One of the great advances in modern dentistry has been in the treatment of diseases of the dental pulp and the periapical tissues. **Endodontics** is the specialty that is concerned primarily with these diseases.

Before major advances in endodontics, many teeth were needlessly extracted. The demand by the public to preserve their teeth has been met in part by the dentist's ability to treat injured or infected pulpal and periapical tissue successfully. The following topics are presented in this chapter:

1. Causes of pulp injury or pulp death
2. Common diseases of the pulp and periapical tissues
3. Injury
4. Diagnostic methods used in endodontics
5. The endodontic dental assistant
6. Pulpectomy
7. Surgical endodontics

CAUSES OF PULP INJURY OR PULP DEATH

The dental pulp can be injured in several ways. Some injured pulp can be treated and returned to normal. On the other hand, some injured pulpal tissue dies after the injury. Whether a pulp survives an injury depends on many factors, such as the following:

1. *Age of the patient at the time of injury.* Younger patients usually have a greater ability to recover from any injury than older patients. The blood supply to the teeth is greater in a young patient.
2. *Extent of the injury.* A tooth that receives a mild blow has a greater chance of survival than a tooth that has its crown completely fractured by a severe blow to the mouth.
3. *Period that the tooth is left untreated after exposure to the injurious agent.* Caries that invades the pulp and remains for a long time before being treated will cause the tooth to have less chance of survival than a tooth that is treated immediately.
4. *Method of treatment.* There are many methods of treating an injured pulp. Some methods are more successful in certain patients than in others. Also, the skill of the dentist and the cooperativeness of

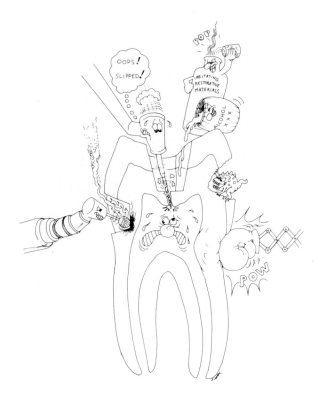

Figure 22-1   Common causes of injury to pulp.

the patient must be considered in any treatment method.

Many circumstances contribute to the survival or death of a dental pulp that has been injured, but most of them fit into the list of factors just mentioned.

The dental pulp is living tissue. Any living tissue can die, or undergo necrosis, after the slightest injury. Following are some of the most common causes of injury to the pulp (Figure 22-1):

• Traumatic blows to the teeth
• Extensive dental caries
• Mechanical pulp exposure
• Chemical irritation
• Thermal irritation
• Galvanic shock

Traumatic Blows to Teeth

All dental patients are subject to the hazards of everyday living that can result in unexpected injury to the facial area and specifically to the teeth. These hazards range from common household accidents to auto collisions and athletic injuries. It is estimated that one of three boys and one of four girls will have suffered a dental injury by the time they finish high school.

This type of injury varies from fracture of an entire jaw to a small fracture of one tooth. Any injury that disrupts the blood supply to the tooth or exposes the pulp to the environment outside the confines of the tooth can result in pulp death.

A sharp blow to one or more teeth can result in the fracture of either the crown or the root of those teeth, causing exposure or possible tearing of the pulp.

Even if the crown is only slightly fractured, or not fractured at all, as a result of a blow to the tooth, the pulp can still undergo necrosis. The reason is that the tooth is loosened in the surrounding alveolus enough to tear the blood vessels that enter the tooth through the apical foramen. These are the vessels that carry the nourishing blood to keep the pulp alive. If this pipeline is permanently damaged, the pulp cannot receive the blood supply it needs to survive (Figure 22-2).

Mild trauma to the pulp can result from a dental restoration being in hyperocclusion, in other words, a "high filling." This can result from inadequate carving of restorative materials during operative procedures. Such a pulpal trauma is easily corrected by recontouring the problem restoration.

Extensive Dental Caries

Untreated dental caries usually continues to increase in size until treatment is received or until the tooth is totally destroyed. When the size of the caries increases to the point at which it invades the pulp, this delicate tissue is severely threatened.

Dental caries is a combination of a variety of bacteria, the toxins and acids they produce, and caustic breakdown products of the destroyed dentin. The invading caries exposes the delicate pulpal tissue to these harmful substances, which destroy the cells of the pulp. If the process is not intercepted by treatment, the pulp dies.

Whether a pulp survives carious invasion, or **pulp exposure**, depends largely on the size of the exposure and the age of the patient. The larger the exposure, the less chance the pulp has to recover. A massive exposure of the pulp to the caustic caries simply overwhelms the defense mechanism of the pulp. A more abundant blood supply to the pulp increases the defensive and reparative functions of the pulp.

> ➡ **KEY POINT**
> ▪ Younger patients have a greater chance to recover from pulp exposure because of the greater blood supply to young teeth.

The reason immature teeth have a greater blood supply has to do with the large apical foramen present in such teeth. This large opening in the end of the root permits an abundant flow of blood to the pulp. The foramen gets progressively smaller with age, and thus the blood supply to the pulp also decreases with age. A small pulp exposure in a teenaged patient is expected to heal readily, whereas the same exposure in a 40-year-old patient would probably result in pulp death.

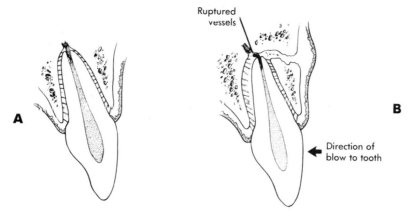

Figure 22-2 **A,** Normal tooth and its apical blood vessels. **B,** Rupture of apical blood vessels resulting from trauma to tooth.

Carious exposure of the dental pulp occurs when the invasion of caries into the dentin progresses at a rapid rate. A rapidly advancing carious lesion surpasses the defensive response of the pulp to produce reparative dentin. A slowly advancing carious lesion has less chance of exposing the pulp, since the pulp has time to produce these defensive barriers against the progressive decay.

Mechanical Pulp Exposure

In addition to dental caries, the pulp can be exposed by other means. These exposures are usually a result of dental procedures that inadvertently invade the pulp. Poor cavity preparation methods and improper pin placement procedures are two common causes of **mechanical pulp exposure** (see Figure 22-1). As unfortunate as this situation is for the patient, it does occur and must be recognized. The same principles of size of the exposure and age of the patient apply to pulp recovery after mechanical exposures. However, mechanical exposures tend to heal more favorably than carious exposures because there are no toxic substances associated with them.

Chemical Irritation

The health status of the pulp can be greatly influenced by certain chemical substances that come in contact with the dentin. Past clinical experience has clearly shown that patients can experience pulp injury or pulp death after the placement of certain chemical substances commonly used in restorative procedures. This is caused by permeability of the dentin layer, created by the presence of the dentinal tubules (Figure 22-3, *A* and *B*). Any injurious substance that is applied to the dentin makes its way into the pulp via the dentinal tubules. This is particularly true when such a substance is placed on dentin deep in the tooth near the pulp.

Several materials used in dentistry to restore teeth can harm the teeth if not handled properly. An example is incomplete removal of acid etch from a prepared tooth.

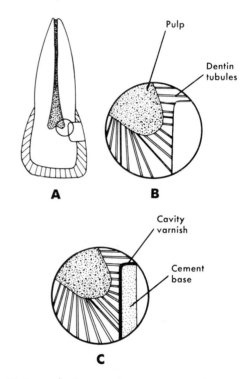

Figure 22-3 **A,** Enlargement of class III cavity preparation to show its relationship to dental pulp. **B,** Dentin tubules that form tiny passageways between cavity preparation and pulp. **C,** Open tubules sealed by cavity varnish and cement base.

The acid can penetrate the dentin and injure or even destroy the pulp. To use a material of this type in a tooth and, at the same time, prevent insult to the pulp, the tooth must be rinsed adequately. Zinc phosphate cement can also cause pulpal irritation. Proper preparation places acceptable dental varnishes and/or lining materials between the pulp and the acidic cement to prevent penetration into the pulp (Figure 22-3, *C*).

Another clinical situation that can result in chemical irritation of the pulp is a faulty restoration that allows leakage of oral fluids and bacteria between the restoration and the dentin. This can irritate the pulp. Proper replacement of such a faulty restoration easily solves this problem.

Thermal Irritation

The dental pulp, like many other tissues of the body, functions best at normal body temperature. If the temperature of the pulp varies significantly from body temperature, patients experience discomfort, and pulpal injury can occur. A common example of thermal irritation to the pulp is placement of metallic restorative materials too close to the pulp. Metals such as dental amalgam and gold are excellent thermal conductors, much more so than the natural tooth. In other words, metals transfer temperature change readily. A metal spoon in a hot cup of coffee transfers the heat from the coffee to the fingers through the handle of the spoon. The same phenomenon occurs when metal restorations are cooled. A healthy drink of a cold beverage or a bite of ice cream can be a painful experience for the patient.

> **•◊ KEY POINT**
> ▪ A patient with a metal restoration deep in the tooth can experience pulpal irritation because extreme temperature changes in the mouth are readily transferred through the metal to the pulp.

Since the depth of cavity preparations is often determined by the size of the carious lesion being treated, dentists cannot control cavity preparation depth in every instance. However, the depth at which the restorative metal is placed can be controlled. This is accomplished by the use of cement base materials. These cement bases are chosen because they insulate the tooth from thermal extremes and do not transfer heat from one point to another well. They function in the same manner as a hot pad used by cooks to handle hot cooking utensils. In other words, cement bases act as an insulating material between a metal restoration and the dentin nearest the pulp.

> **•◊ KEY POINT**
> ▪ Proper use of bases between the restoration and the dentin covering the pulp protects this delicate tissue.

A second common source of thermal irritation to the pulp can occur during the preparation of a tooth with high-speed rotary instruments. Dental burs in a modern high-speed handpiece spin at a range of 400,000 to 450,000 revolutions per minute. This creates an effective cutting instrument to remove enamel and dentin quickly. However, in the process of quickly cutting hard tooth structure, a great deal of frictional heat is generated between the bur and the tooth. If this heat is not minimized, significant heat is transferred to the pulp, and damage can result. This heat is controlled by the use of water-spray devices attached to the head of the handpiece. These water-spray devices direct water toward the cutting end of the bur to keep it cool during the cutting process. One of the chief duties of a dental assistant is to remove this water coolant continually from the patient's mouth as it sprays into the tooth being prepared. Although water-coolant sprays can be a nuisance at times because they impair visibility, they are essential to protect the pulp from becoming overheated during cavity preparation. Effective use of the dental assistant to control the water coolant has greatly reduced the inconvenience of this necessary technique.

Galvanic Shock

Although galvanic shock is an unusual cause of pulpal damage, it is worthy of a brief explanation, since it can be a temporary source of pulpal pain. **Galvanism** is the flow of electrical current between two different metals through an electrolyte. An electrolyte is a solution containing atomic substances that allow current to flow through the solution.

If a patient has two different metals present in the mouth and these metals contact each other, an electrical "battery" is created, and current flows through the electrolyte (saliva) to complete the electrical circuit. The current that flows can be of sufficient magnitude to shock the pulp. The two metals can be entirely different, such as gold and silver amalgam, or simply different compositions of the same metal alloys. (Different manufacturers use different compositions in their silver and gold alloys.)

It is fairly common for patients to complain of shock when the teeth are closed after a new amalgam restoration has been placed. This is especially true if the tooth contacts a different metal, such as gold, when the teeth are brought into contact during jaw closure. Another common example of this phenomenon is the accidental contact of an eating utensil or aluminum foil with a metal dental restoration. Galvanic shock results again, since two different metals contact in the presence of saliva (the electrolyte).

The pain the patient feels in the tooth is due to the fact that electrical current is an excellent stimulant to pulpal nerve fibers. Electrical stimulation of pulpal nerve fibers is actually used to test the vitality of a pulp. This matter is discussed in conjunction with diagnostic methods used in endodontics.

COMMON DISEASES OF PULP AND PERIAPICAL TISSUES

Hyperemia

Hyperemia means that an excessive amount of blood has collected in the blood vessels of a body part. The pulp is no exception. The first response of the pulp to injury is dilation of the arterioles in the pulp. As these vessels dilate, they become engorged with blood.

Since the soft pulp is enclosed in a hard chamber of dentin, the enlargement of the vessels creates mild pressure within the pulp. This increase in pressure squeezes the nerve fibers of the pulp. The pressure only makes the nerve fibers more sensitive to stimuli that may be added to the tooth. The tooth will not be painful unless it is further stimulated by either heat or cold. Cold temperatures elicit a painful response more often than heat. The pain will begin when the stimulus is applied and cease when it is removed.

The magnitude of hyperemia depends on the degree of injury to the tooth. Common causes of injury to the pulp are discussed in the beginning of this chapter.

> ➼ **KEY POINT**
> ▪ Since hyperemia is not actually a disease itself, but rather the first stage of the inflammatory defensive process, it can be reversed if the injury is not too severe.

Pulpitis

Pulpitis is inflammation of pulpal tissue. Any of the causes of injury mentioned previously can result in pulpitis. Many dentists differentiate among degrees of pulpitis, using descriptive terms such as acute, subacute, chronic, and suppurative. This differentiation among the various degrees of pulpitis is helpful to the dentist in determining the status of the pulp and the appropriate treatment.

The degree of pulpitis present in a tooth depends totally on the type of injurious agent, its intensity, and the time of exposure to the pulp. Pulpitis that clear up after the insulting agent has been removed is called **reversible pulpitis**. Pulpitis that has progressed to a point in which the pulp cannot recover from the insulting agent, even upon removal of the agent, is called **irreversible pulpitis**. Irreversible pulpitis must be treated by removal of the pulp.

Necrosis

Necrosis is the death of tissue. Pulpal necrosis is usually the result of severe pulpitis. This is the rationale behind treatment of severe pulpitis by removing a portion or all of the pulp in an injured tooth. Pulpal necrosis also oc-

---

> **BOX 22-1**
>
> **TYPICAL REACTIONS TO THERMAL STIMULI AND WHAT THEY INDICATE**
>
> | CONDITION | RESPONSE |
> |---|---|
> | Hyperemia | Less painful than a cold test; pain disappears when heat is removed |
> | Pulpitis | Painful response that lingers a few moments after heat is removed |
> | Abscess | Violent pain reaction to heat; relieved by application of cold |
> | Necrotic pulp | No response to heat or cold |

curs when the blood supply is halted because of traumatic injury to the tooth.

A tooth with a necrotic pulp cannot remain untreated. Dead tissue undergoes a series of chemical changes that result in a highly irritating end product. The process is called decomposition, or putrefaction. The decomposed end product consists of toxins and other irritating substances created by the breakdown of the dead fleshy pulp. This foul-smelling mixture of irritating substances seeps out of the apical foramen and irritates the periapical tissues.

A patient with a necrotic pulp may experience excruciating pain from a dead tooth because of the painful irritation of the periapical tissue by the caustic decomposition products of the dead pulp. On the other hand, a patient can experience pulp death and subsequent periapical tissue destruction with little or no pain. The variation seems to be related primarily to the rate at which these changes take place. A slower necrotic process tends to be less painful than a rapid one. Patients have been known to experience pulpal necrosis and extensive periapical destruction over several years without a trace of discomfort.

> ➼ **KEY POINT**
> ▪ A tooth with a dead pulp does not necessarily mean that the patient will not be bothered by the tooth.

Acute Apical Periodontitis

Apical periodontitis is an inflammation of the periodontal tissues near the apex of a tooth when pulpal inflammation occurs. The inflammatory response of the periodontal tissue is caused by contaminants from the pulp canal. These contaminants can be the caustic breakdown product of the necrotic pulp, bacteria that have entered the tooth via dental caries, or excessive endodontic medications used to treat the nonvital tooth. The inflammatory response begins with dilation of the blood vessels of the periodontal ligament in the apical region. If this process occurs quickly, edema results. This condition is called **acute apical periodontitis**. Pressure forms between the alveolar bone and the tooth. Two things result from this pressure. First, the tooth can be pushed slightly away from the apical part of the alveolus. The tooth will be high to the patient's bite, and pain will result when biting forces are placed on it. Second, the nerve receptors located in the periodontal ligament are squeezed as a result of the increase in pressure, so that even the slightest additional force placed on the tooth will elicit a painful response. Thus tapping on a tooth is a common test for the presence of apical periodontitis.

The pain associated with acute apical periodontitis is usually less than the pain associated with pulpitis, since the pulp canal is far more confining to swollen tissue than the space between the tooth and alveolar bone. There is usually no detectable radiolucency at the apex of the tooth in acute apical periodontitis.

Periapical Abscess

If a large number of bacteria get past the apex of the tooth, a severe inflammatory response may occur that results in a localized collection of pus called a **periapical abscess**. The patient experiences pain, varying degrees of swelling, and a high temperature. The patient will also state that the tooth feels high.

The pus can be forced through the open marrow spaces in the bone and result in widespread swelling and pain. Bone resorption can accompany this increase in pressure so that the thin facial aspect of alveolar bone can be resorbed and the pus can balloon out through the thin alveolar mucosa. If the thin mucosa ruptures, the pus can escape into the oral cavity, and the pressure is immediately relieved.

One of the emergency treatment measures commonly used to treat a periapical abscess is to establish drainage of pus from the periapical area. This can be accomplished by making an opening into the pulp chamber through the crown with a dental bur (Figure 22-4). Such an opening allows the pus to escape from the periapical area through the pulp canal to the oral cavity. Another method is to make an incision through the alveolar mucosa over the apex of the involved tooth. This allows direct drainage from the periapical region to the oral cavity. Some cases may require both drainage methods.

This process of periapical abscess can occur so quickly that it often surpasses the bone resorption process. Thus it is possible to have an extensive periapical abscess without any radiographic evidence of periapical bone loss.

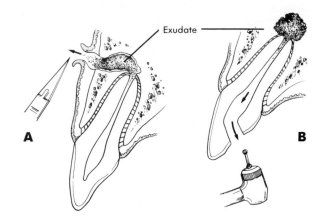

Figure 22-4 Establishment of drainage for periapical abscess. **A**, Via incision in labial mucosa. **B**, Via crown of tooth.

> ➾ **KEY POINT**
> ▪ Periapical abscesses must be drained either by opening the tooth or making a small incision in the tissue overlying the abscess.

Chronic Apical Periodontitis (Granuloma)

Chronic apical periodontitis (granuloma) occurs when the pulpal response to the bacteria and irritants is slower. Loss of bone around the apex of the tooth can occur if the inflammation is not eliminated. As long as the pressure from the inflammation persists, bone resorption will continue. It is possible for significant bone loss to occur with little or no pain (Figure 22-5). Chronic apical periodontitis is usually asymptomatic, and a radiolucency at the apex of the tooth is usually visible.

If all bacteria and decomposition products can be eliminated from the pulp canal and the apical foramen can be sealed, the granuloma may resolve. The essence of endodontic treatment is to accomplish that task.

Granuloma with Fistulation

Periapical abscesses may sometimes form a tract through the bone that drains pus from the abscess. This drainage tract is called a **fistula** and may appear as a gum boil near the apex of the tooth. The patient may complain of a bad taste in the mouth from the drainage of the pus. Sometimes it is difficult to determine which tooth formed the fistula. The dentist may need to insert a gutta-percha point into the fistula and take a radiograph. The gutta-percha point will be radiopaque and literally point to the involved tooth or root in the radiograph.

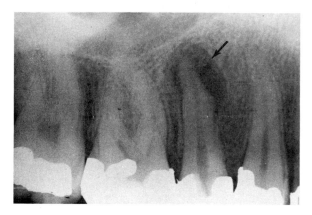

Figure 22-5   Periapical bone loss resulting from formation of granuloma (*arrow*).

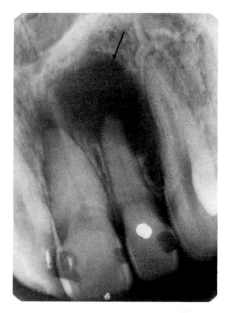

Figure 22-6   Periapical cyst (*arrow*).

Periapical Cyst

A **periapical cyst** is a fluid-filled cavity lined by epithelial cells. Some granulomas undergo a change from their original form to that of a cyst. The bordering epithelial cells form the cyst lining (Figure 22-6).

Periapical cysts can expand to considerable size. The pressure from their expansion can stimulate significant bone resorption and even cause teeth to move out of their normal position.

> **KEY POINT**
> - Once a cyst has formed, the involved tooth will need a root canal and the dentist will need to surgically remove the epithelial lining of the cyst by curettage for the abscess to resolve.

Injury: Avulsed Tooth

An **avulsed tooth** is a tooth that has been knocked out of the bony socket. An avulsed tooth should be replanted and stabilized as soon as possible. The following steps should be performed after a tooth has been avulsed:

1. Rinse tooth gently, do not scrub.
2. Gently replant the tooth back into the socket. If the tooth cannot be replanted, it should be placed in saline, milk, or saliva.
3. Immediately transport the patient to the dental office for treatment (Figure 22-7).

DIAGNOSTIC METHODS USED IN ENDODONTICS

Several mechanisms have been devised to assist the dentist in the diagnostic evaluation of the pulp and periapical tissues. Following are some of the most common diagnostic tools:

- Patient history
- Radiographs
- Thermal tests
- Electrical pulp test
- Clinical observation
- Palpation
- Mobility
- Periodontal probing
- Percussion
- Selective anesthesia
- Test cavity preparation
- Transillumination

Table 22-1 describes the reactions to common endodontic diagnostic procedures.

Patient History

A thorough medical and dental history is mandatory before any treatment is begun. The medical history reveals the patient's general health status so that precautions can be taken if necessary to prevent serious complications during dental treatment.

The medical history is a helpful guide for the dentist in the treatment regimen. The choice of pain-relieving drugs, antibiotics, and root canal medications is often dictated by the patient's history of allergies, cardiovascular condition, and numerous other conditions, including pregnancy.

The patient's dental history is a valuable aid to the dentist in that the patient can communicate a step-by-step account of signs and symptoms to the dentist. It is in this

Table 22-1 Reactions to common endodontic diagnostic procedures

Symptoms	EPT/DPT	Heat	Cold	Percussion	Radiograph	Prognosis	Treatment
REVERSIBLE PULPITIS							
Acute pain of short duration, or clinically observed in dental radiograph	Positive	Normal, indicating vitality	Normal, indicating vitality	Negative	Caries invades dentin near pulp	Good—can return to normal, develop secondary dentin	Protection with sedative dressing, e.g. zinc oxide eugenol (ZOE) cement
IRREVERSIBLE ACUTE PULPITIS							
Severe pain, increasing in duration and intensity Analgesics often provide limited relief	Positive	Positive, may react more severely or may be more prolonged than normal	Positive, may provide relief	Negative, unless inflammation spreads to periapical tissue	Negative for bone change	Pulp degenerating to potential for recovery	Pulp extirpation/endodontic treatment
CHRONIC PULPITIS							
May be asymptomatic, often occurs in older patients in teeth that have been restored	Positive, may require more electric current to react	Excess amount needed to elicit reaction	Excess amount needed to elicit reaction	Negative	May note resorption in canal; evidence of bone change	No recovery	Pulp extirpation/endodontic treatment; endodontic treatment of asymptomatic teeth as prophylactic measure
ACUTE APICAL ABSCESS							
Severe pain; no relief from analgesics Intraoral or extraoral swelling present Possible draining sinus/fistula	Negative	No response	No response	Positive, often severe reactions	If early stage, no bone change; latent stage thickening of periodontal membrane is evident	No recovery	1. Establish drainage through occlusal/lingual opening up to apex of tooth with endodontic file or incision of soft tissue 2. Prescribe antibiotic 3. Hot salt oral rinses

Diagnosis	Signs and Symptoms				Radiographs		Treatment
							4. Medication for pain; narcotic optional 5. Treat endodontically at later date
NECROSIS	May be asymptomatic or previous pain	Negative	No response	Negative	No change evident	No recovery	Pulpectomy and endodontic treatment
CHRONIC APICAL PERIODONTITIS	Mild degree of pain; sensitivity less than pulpitis Tooth may feel *high* and discomfort is evident on biting or clenching teeth	Negative	No response	Negative	Bone resorption evident; radiolucent lesion at apex	No recovery	Pulpal extirpation and endodontic treatment
ROOT FRACTURE	May be asymptomatic; paresthesia may occur after traumatic blow; dull feeling	Negative	No response	Painful	May indicate fracture, if extensive; hairline fractures may be blocked	No recovery	Extirpation and endodontic treatment; root removal or removal of tooth
CHRONIC APICAL SUPPURATIVE	Draining sinus or gingival abscess present; may be mild degree of pain	Negative	Negative	Negative	Radiolucent lesion at apex	No recovery	Pulpal extirpation and endodontic treatment

EPT, Electronic pulp test; *DPT,* digital pulp test.

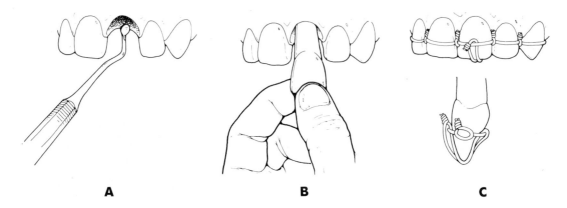

Figure 22-7   Treatment of avulsed tooth. **A,** Clotted blood is removed from alveolus with surgical curette. **B,** Avulsed tooth is inserted and positioned in alveolus. **C,** Tooth is splinted in place with wire, acrylic, or orthodontic splints.

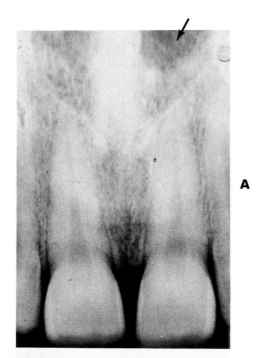

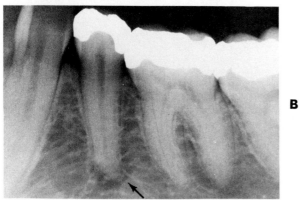

Figure 22-8   Normal anatomical radiolucencies superimposed on apices of roots (*arrow*). **A,** Nostril spots. **B,** Mental foramen.

phase of history taking that patients often reveal valuable information regarding previous injuries to the teeth, even though they may have occurred many years earlier.

There is a well-known but accurate expression among physicians and dentists with regard to history taking:"Listen to your patients, and they will tell you what is wrong with them!"

Radiographs

Radiographs, or x-ray films, of the teeth and bone are perhaps the most valuable diagnostic tool the dentist has to evaluate the structures that cannot be seen by clinical observation, that is, the pulp and periapical tissues.

Bone loss in the periapical area in response to a necrotic pulp can be detected on a radiograph. Bone loss, or resorption, appears as a dark area surrounding the apex of the root (see Figure 22-5). The presence of this dark area, or **radiolucency,** on a dental radiograph is one of the most important features used to diagnose pulp and periapical disease. Periapical cysts, granulomas, and abscesses all appear as radiolucencies on a radiograph. The differentiation among diseases as to which is actually represented by the bone resorption requires additional information that must be acquired by other diagnostic methods.

The dentist is often confronted with radiolucencies caused by normal structures located near the apices of teeth. Two common instances are the maxillary anterior and the mandibular premolar areas. When a radiograph is taken of the maxillary anterior area, the image of the nasal passages is often superimposed over the apices of the roots of the central incisors. Such "nostril spots" can easily be confused with periapical disease (Figure 22-8, *A*). Careful radiographic technique can eliminate this confusion. The second area involves the mental foramen, which is located near the roots of the mandibular premolars. If the image of the mental foramen is superimposed over

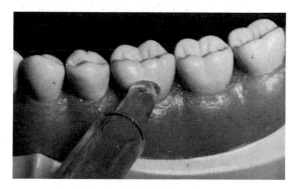

Figure 22-9 Cold test using "ice pencil."

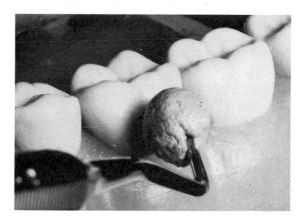

Figure 22-10 Hot test using hot gutta-percha.

the root apex of one of these teeth, it can be misinterpreted as periapical disease (Figure 22-8, *B*). These two examples emphasize the need for other information beside radiolucencies on a radiograph to make a sound diagnosis of periapical disease.

Radiographs are helpful in other ways beside detecting radiolucencies. They can demonstrate possible causes of pulpal injury before bone resorption occurs. Root fracture, deep caries, and previous pulp exposures are a few examples of possible causes of pulpal injury that can be detected on radiographs.

Root length, abnormal root curvature, and abnormal calcification can be demonstrated in an accurate radiograph. This information is helpful in determining whether the tooth can be treated endodontically. If it is determined that it can be treated, such information as extreme root curvature is helpful to the dentist in planning treatment.

One outstanding feature of the dental radiograph is its permanence. A properly exposed and processed radiograph can last forever. Thus it becomes a permanent record of the condition of the patient that can be used for future reference. Comparison of initial radiographs with postoperative films is a valuable index to determine the success or failure of treatment. Radiographs are valuable pieces of information that should be preserved for medicolegal reasons.

Thermal Tests

Subjecting a tooth to extremes in temperature is an accurate method of identifying an offending tooth as well as determining the status of its pulp.

Cold tests can be done rather easily by making an "ice pencil." Anesthetic cartridges or disposable needle covers are filled with water and frozen. These narrow sticks of ice are handy ways of applying cold to a tooth without using a bulky ice cube (Figure 22-9). The suspected tooth is isolated and dried; the ice pencil is then applied to the tooth at the cervical area. If a freezer is not available, a cotton pellet can be sprayed with ethyl chloride or Freon until it frosts. The pellet is then applied to the cervical area of the suspect tooth.

> **KEY POINT**
> - A hyperemic pulp responds readily to the decrease in temperature from a cold test.

Heat tests begin with isolating the suspect tooth and applying a thin film of lubricant at the cervical area. Out of the patient's line of sight, a piece of **gutta-percha** (⅛-inch diameter ball) is heated in a Bunsen burner while being held by a hand ball burnisher. The heating is continued until just before the gutta-percha begins to smoke, and then the material is applied to the cervical area. The lubricant keeps it from sticking to the tooth (Figure 22-10).

Typical reactions to thermal stimuli and what they indicate are described in the box on p. 343.

Teeth with extensive metal restorations often do not respond because sufficient heat is not generated by the warm gutta-percha. A rubber polishing wheel or cup can be spun on the surface of the metal restoration to create frictional heat to stimulate the tooth.

Electrical Pulp Test

The primary objective of the electrical pulp test is to determine whether a pulp is alive (**vital pulp**) or necrotic (**nonvital pulp**). Electrical current can be used to stimulate nerve fibers in the pulp via the dentin layer. If the current is applied at the cervical area of a tooth where the enamel is thin, the sensitive dentin layer is more accessible and stimulation is more effective. A battery-powered electronic instrument used to accomplish this task is shown in Figure 22-11. The instrument automatically increases the current delivered to a tooth. The dentist selects the rate of increase. A necrotic pulp does not respond to even the most intense electrical stimulation. A dying pulp can produce a variety of responses depending on the state of the pulp at the time of the test.

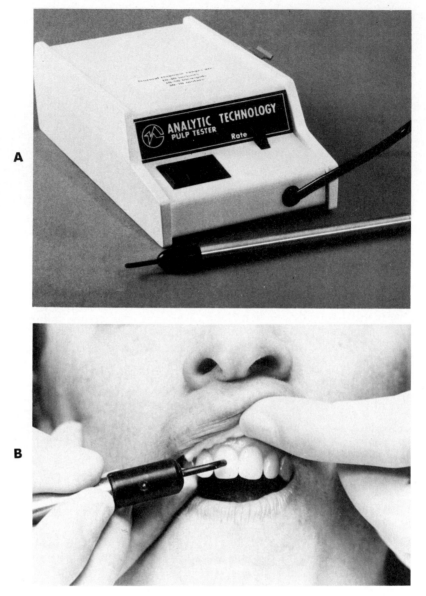

Figure 22-11 Electrical pulp test. **A**, Digital pulp tester that automatically increases intensity of electrical stimulus to tooth. **B**, Placement of test probe on isolated tooth being tested.

Endodontists caution against using only the electrical pulp test to determine the degree of vitality of a pulp. However, some general information about the status of the pulp can be obtained by comparing the response of a suspect tooth with that of a normal tooth (control tooth) of the same type on the opposite side of the mouth. For example, if the maxillary right canine is the suspect tooth, its test results should be compared with the test results of the maxillary left canine. The left canine becomes the control because it is normal. If the suspect tooth requires less current to stimulate it than the control, the suspect tooth is probably hypersensitive as a result of either pulpitis or hyperemia. These comparative tests should be re-

peated two or three times to validate the results. Since the amount of current delivered to a tooth is indicated by a numerical scale, it is simple to compare test results. Higher numbers on the scale indicate that more current is being delivered to the tooth.

The procedure for conducting an **electrical pulp test** is described in Box 22-2.

The rate of increase of current can be preset at the start of the test on some models. The level of current is shown as a digital display on a small screen. This type requires contact of both ends of the test probe with the patient. One end contacts the tooth, and the other end of the probe should be touched by the patient's fingertip dur-

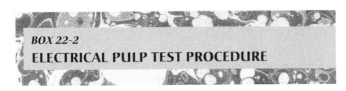

BOX 22-2

ELECTRICAL PULP TEST PROCEDURE

PROCEDURE	RATIONALE
1. Explain procedure to patient. Patient should be informed that tooth will be tested for vitality. Avoid words that suggest "electrical" or "electrical shock." Inform patient to raise left hand when tingling or pulsating sensation is felt.	1. Patient should be informed that tooth will be tested for vitality. Phrases that contain "electrical" and "shock" will alarm patient.
2. Isolate teeth to be tested with cotton rolls and dry teeth thoroughly.	2. Saliva will conduct electricity.
3. Place small dab of toothpaste on end of test probe.	3. To ensure electrical contact with tooth.
4. Set current level at zero, and apply probe to cervical one third of tooth.	4. Tooth will test better in areas that do not have thick enamel covering.
5. Increase current gradually until patient senses heat or tingling sensation in tooth.	5. To determine vitality reading.
6. Repeat test with normal tooth of same type.	6. For comparison purposes.
7. Chart results.	7. To document vitality response of control and tooth in question.

ing the test. As an alternative, an optional lip clip can be attached to the patient's lip with a wire leading to the probe handle to complete the electrical circuit. The patient can also hold the lip clip. This is necessary when the dentist is wearing rubber gloves, which prevent the completion of an electrical circuit with the patient.

> ●◦ KEY POINT
> ▪ Moisture on the tooth or directly touching the gingiva results in stimulation of the nerves in the gingiva and produces a false reading.

Electrical pulp testing is a useful tool, but it has many shortcomings that reduce its value. Some battery-operated models may give unreliable readings as the batteries weaken. Teeth with extensive restorations vary widely in their response to pulp testing. Molars with several root canals sometimes baffle dentists, since one canal may contain necrotic pulp tissue and the other canals may still have vital tissue that responds to the electrical stimulus. Control teeth may not be as normal as expected, and the test comparisons may be of little value.

The electrical pulp test is helpful in endodontic diagnosis, but it must be supported by other diagnostic findings.

Clinical Observation

As in any diagnostic procedure the value of the operator's hands and eyes cannot be underestimated. Clues to the nature of a patient's problems often lie in what the dentist can see and feel in the patient's mouth. Such clinical signs as discoloration of teeth, crown fracture, gross caries, swelling, abnormal soft tissue, and draining abscesses can be found in a clinical examination.

Clinical signs coupled with symptoms that the patient describes during the dental history are of considerable value to the dentist in arriving at an accurate diagnosis.

Palpation

The dentist applies finger pressure extraorally and intraorally over the apex of the suspected tooth. Swelling may indicate a periodontal pathological condition.

Mobility

Two mirror handles, one placed buccally and one placed lingually, are used to move the tooth in a buccal-lingual direction. Mobile teeth indicate a periodontal problem or a loose crown.

> ●◦ KEY POINT
> ▪ A tooth with severe mobility from periodontal problems would not be a good candidate for endodontic therapy.

Periodontal Probing

The dentist measures the gingival sulcus with a periodontal probe to differentiate a periodontal abscess from an endodontic abscess. The periodontal status of the tooth may also be determined to assist the dentist in treatment planning.

Percussion

Gentle tapping on the incisal edge or occlusal surface of a tooth with the end of a mirror handle is a simple test to determine the presence of acute periapical periodontitis. If a patient has an acute inflammation at the apex of the root, gentle tapping, or **percussion**, squeezes the already inflamed area, and pain results. Several normal teeth should be checked for comparison.

Selective Anesthesia

If a patient cannot accurately determine which teeth are the source of discomfort, the process of **selective anesthesia** can be of assistance. If other diagnostic tests have narrowed the choice down to two teeth, one of them can be anesthetized to see if the pain disappears. If the pain does not disappear until the second tooth is anesthetized, the second tooth is the probable offender. Selective anesthesia is most effective when the choice is between a maxillary and a mandibular tooth. The selective anesthesia process in the maxilla is reliable only when the two suspected teeth are at least two teeth apart. This method cannot be used to differentiate between two suspected mandibular teeth.

This process is often used in combination with hot and cold tests to increase the stimulus to the nonanesthetized tooth.

Test Cavity Preparation

If all other diagnostic tests fail to determine the vitality of a highly suspect tooth, the test cavity can be used as a last resort. The test consists of cutting a hole into the dentin layer of the tooth without anesthesia or water coolant, using the high-speed handpiece. The patient will readily respond if the tooth is vital. The test opening should be small and placed on a tooth surface that will minimize the disruption of the esthetic quality of the tooth.

Transillumination

Until the development of fiber-optic lighting, **transillumination** was not of any significant value in endodontic diagnosis. Fiber optics allow an intense, concentrated light to pass through the tooth from the lingual to the facial aspect. This is done most effectively on anterior teeth. Necrotic pulps cause the outline of the pulp chamber to appear darker than the surrounding tooth structure. Normal teeth show no color difference between the tooth structure and the pulp chamber.

Transillumination can also be used to detect fractures in the tooth. Although superficial fracture lines are normal, a deep fracture can result in a cracked tooth syndrome. Generally, deep fractures on the crown of the tooth can be treated by placing a fixed restoration on the tooth to hold the tooth together; however, fractures along the root of the tooth do not have a good prognosis.

• • •

Endodontic diagnosis is a result of the use of several of the aids just discussed. Skillful use and interpretation of these diagnostic methods are essential for successful endodontic practice.

ENDODONTIC DENTAL ASSISTANT

The role of the dental assistant during endodontic therapy is to assist the dentist in such a way that the treatment is administered smoothly and efficiently.

The preparations for endodontic treatment are delegated to the dental assistant. The assistant should perform the following before the endodontic therapy:

- Be aware of antianxiety medications or preoperative instructions given to the patient before the appointment.
- Allay the patient's fears concerning root canals because it is likely that the patient may have heard bad stories about endodontics from friends and relatives.
- Prepare, sterilize, and set out the endodontic tray.
- Place the chart and patient x-rays in plain sight.
- Prepare the rubber dam for isolation of the involved tooth.

During the endodontic therapy, the assistant is responsible for the following:

- Assisting with rubber dam placement
- Evacuating pus or offending odor on initial opening of the tooth
- Delivering instruments or materials to the operator
- Exposing (if licensed) and developing frequent periapical radiographs to check progress of treatment
- Measuring and marking the length with filing instruments
- Mixing or preparing medications to be placed inside the tooth
- Evacuating sodium hypochlorite disinfectant placed inside the root canal and chamber
- Adjusting the lighting

After the endodontic therapy, the assistant does the following:

- Gives postoperative instructions both orally and in written form
- May explain antibiotic or pain-relieving prescriptions if prescribed by the dentist

PULPECTOMY

The most common endodontic procedure is the **pulpectomy**, which is the removal of the entire pulp. After the removal of the pulp, the empty canal is completely filled to create a seal that eliminates further periapical irritation.

Although humans are endowed with a living pulp in each tooth, it has been found that the pulp is not absolutely necessary to preserve the tooth once it is completely formed. Most dentists would agree that for a number of technical reasons, they prefer that teeth retain their vitality. Dentists also know that a tooth with its pulp removed and the remaining structure properly treated can last a lifetime. This fact is the basis for modern endodontic therapy.

The procedures discussed in this chapter all have a common principal goal. It is essential that neither tissue fluids nor microorganisms can enter or leave the pulp canal of the nonvital tooth. An adequate seal prevents continued irritation of the periapical tissues and allows them to heal.

> ➠ **KEY POINT**
> - The principal goal of endodontic therapy is to create an absolute seal in the root portion of the tooth.

Phases of Treatment

A typical scheme of accomplishing the pulpectomy procedure involves the following phases of treatment:

1. Isolation
2. Endodontic preparations (openings)
3. Canal cleaning and filing
4. Root canal filling

Some dentists prefer to use a one-appointment procedure as described later. Some dentists prefer to use two appointments. At the end of the first appointment an antimicrobial medication is placed in the tooth opening before temporization.

Armamentarium
Basic setup

A basic armamentarium can be established for the pulpectomy procedure. This standardized setup can be used during each phase of treatment and supplemented by additional items needed for a specific phase. A typical basic armamentarium is shown in Figure 22-12.

> ➠ **KEY POINTS**
> - Some dentists may prefer to use a white rubber dam for endodontic procedures.
> - Single-tooth isolation (one hole) is used for endodontic procedures.

Rubber dam setup

Each phase of the pulpectomy is performed with a sterile technique, which requires the use of rubber dam isolation. The armamentarium and technique for applying the rubber dam are presented in Chapter 8.

Endodontic storage box

The **endodontic storage box** (Figure 22-13) is a metal compartmentalized container that can be sterilized by the dry-heat method. Various sterilizable instruments and devices are stored in the box to create a sterile endodontic kit. During a treatment procedure sterile forceps are used to retrieve items from the box to prevent contamination of the contents.

Accessory items

Various accessory items such as filling materials, irrigation solutions, measuring devices, cotton products, and cements are used in the pulpectomy procedure. These items are discussed with the procedure itself.

Procedure

The specific sequence of events for performing a pulpectomy is somewhat variable, since it largely depends on the condition of the individual patient. Since infection is present in patients with a periapical abscess, they may be

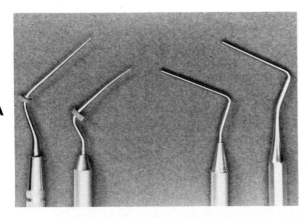
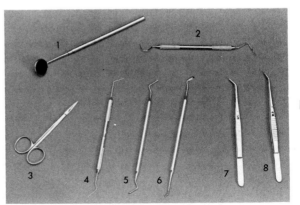

Figure 22-12 Basic endodontic armamentarium. **A,** Assorted hand instruments. Gutta–percha filling instruments. *Left,* Spreaders with stops in place. *Right,* Condensers (pluggers). **B:** *1,* Mouth mirror; *2,* explorer/periodontal probe; *3,* scissors; *4,* straight explorer; *5,* spoon excavator; *6,* plastic filling instrument; *7* and *8,* locking cotton pliers.

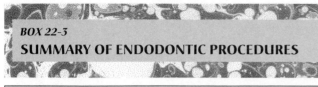

BOX 22-3

SUMMARY OF ENDODONTIC PROCEDURES

PROCEDURE	RATIONALE
1. Anesthetize tooth.	1. Tooth that is candidate for endodontic treatment may not be sensitive to treatment; however, patients differ in response to treatment.
2. Place rubber dam.	2. To maintain maximum aseptic technique and also to protect patient from chemicals used inside tooth.
3. Open tooth.	3. To access root canal or canals and chamber.
4. Remove pulp.	4. Dead or dying pulp is source of irritation and must be removed.
5. Clean and disinfect tooth with sodium hypochlorite.	5. To wash away debris and destroy bacteria in pulp chamber and canal or canals.
6. Smooth, shape, and enlarge pulp canals.	6. To ensure complete fill without voids with gutta-percha.
7. Determine root canal length with radiographs, and fit master cone.	7. To ensure complete seal at apex of tooth.
8. Mix root canal sealer, place sealer on master cone, and place into canal.	8. To ensure complete seal at apex of tooth.
9. Insert and condense additional gutta-percha points into canal.	9. To completely seal sides of canal.
10. Cut away excess length of gutta-percha with hot instrument.	10. To allow for either temporary or permanent restoration to seal canal opening.
11. Seal canal opening with temporary or permanent restoration.	11. To seal tooth from oral fluids.
12. Give patient postoperative instructions.	12. To advise patient that tooth will become brittle and permanent restoration may be indicated.

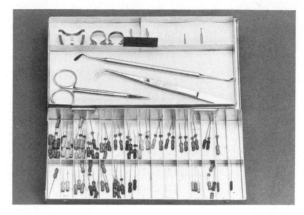

Figure 22-13 Sterile endodontic storage box with compartments for some hand instruments and smaller items such as files, rubber dam clamps, thumb-style ruler, and burs.

treated in a slightly different sequence than those with a painless granuloma. The sequence described here is an example of a single-appointment, uneventful pulpectomy with no history of infection. Box 22-3 summarizes the pulpectomy procedure.

Isolation

Pulpectomy procedures involve not only removal of the pulp and sealing of the empty canal but also sanitation of the canal as part of the procedure. Canal sanitation further ensures against future infection by eliminating bacteria before the canal is sealed. To achieve sanitation of a root canal, an absolutely dry field, free from bacteria-laden saliva, is required. This field is best kept dry with rubber dam isolation.

Endodontic preparations (openings)

After the tooth has been isolated, an opening is made through the crown of the tooth to gain access to the pulp chamber and pulp canal. The opening is made through the occlusal surface on posterior teeth or through the lingual surface on anterior teeth (Figure 22-14).

Burs or diamond stones used for this purpose are sterilized and stored in the endodontic storage box. Both friction-grip and latch-type burs are used to create the endodontic opening. Sizes vary according to the preference of the dentist. Typically a round diamond stone is used in the high-speed handpiece to penetrate the tooth structure and create an initial opening to gain access to the pulp chamber. Larger latch-type round burs as well as cross-cut, flame-shaped carbide burs are used in the conventional-speed handpiece to refine the shape of the opening.

The main objective of any endodontic preparation is to gain easy access to the pulp cavity. This permits smooth entry into the root canals during pulp removal, canal cleaning, filing, and filling.

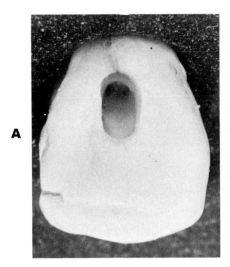
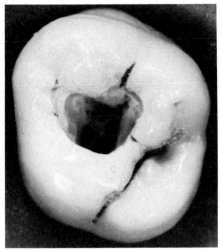

Figure 22-14   Preparation of teeth for endodontic treatment. **A**, Lingual opening on anteri-or tooth. **B**, Occlusal opening on posterior tooth.

Canal cleaning

After the endodontic opening is made, the root canal or canals must be located and cleaned. Anterior teeth usually have one root canal, whereas posterior teeth may have up to three canals of different sizes. Anatomical variations exist among patients; thus additional canals or a tooth with no canals may be found. A thin, straight explorer can be used as a probe to locate canal openings within the pulp chamber. The larger pulp canals are easy to locate, whereas smaller canals can sometimes be difficult to locate.

Once the canals are located, the pulp tissue must be removed. If the pulp tissue is still intact, a thin, flexible instrument called a **barbed broach** is used to remove it. The instrument has small barbs along its length, which are used to grip and remove (extricate) pulp tissue in the root canal (Figure 22-15). It can also be used to retrieve absorbent paper points that may become lodged in a root canal during treatment. Broaches are considered disposable and should be discarded after one use, since they are subject to fracture after repeated sterilization. If the pulp tissue has disintegrated, it is simply removed when the canal is cleaned and filed.

◆ KEY POINT
- Barbed broaches are used to remove the pulp.

With the root canals accessed and the pulp tissue removed, the root canals are cleaned biomechanically. A common method is to inject a mild solution of sodium hypochlorite (0.5%) into the canal with an irrigating sy-

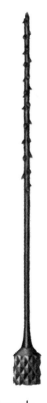

Figure 22-15   Barbed broach.

(From Cohen S, Burns RC: *Pathways of the pulp*, ed 6, St Louis, 1994, Mosby.)

ringe (Figure 22-16). A small root canal file, or reamer, is then placed into the canal and swirled in a rotary motion. The solution acts as a disinfectant to wash away debris and destroy bacteria in the canal. The rubbing of the file against the pulp canal walls has a scrubbing effect that loosens debris and bacteria. The solution is removed with a surgical suction tip on the oral evacuator. This biomechanical cleaning is essential to sanitize the canal before filing.

Canal filing

Root canal filing is a process of shaping the walls of the root canal so that they are smooth and have a specific shape and size. This is accomplished with **endodontic files** and reamers. Files and reamers are tapered instruments that fit into the root canal and are moved up and down so that the cutting edges along the length of the file remove dentin from the canal walls (Figure 22-17).

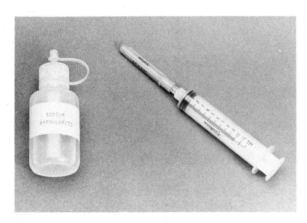

Figure 22-16 Canal irrigation syringe and solution.

They are available in a range of different diameters to accommodate different sizes of root canals. The length of the cutting portion of each instrument is the same, regardless of its diameter. They are available in hand-operated styles as well as mechanical styles. A comparison of intracanal instruments is shown in Figure 22-18. Diamond stone files are also available for use in ultrasonic instruments. File handles are color coded to facilitate size identification (Figure 22-19).

> **↦ KEY POINT**
> - Endodontic files and reamers are used to shape, smooth, and enlarge the root canal or canals.

The filing procedure begins by first establishing the approximate length of the root canal. This can be done from an accurate periapical radiograph of the tooth being treated. The file is held near the radiograph with the tip of the file at the apex of the tooth. **File stops** (markers) are tiny circular disks of silicone rubber that are placed on files and reamers to mark the length of a root canal. The file is pushed through the stop, which is slid along the cutting surface with sterile cotton pliers to a position that is even with a reference point on the crown portion of the tooth (Figure 22-20). Good reference points are the incisal edges of anterior teeth and cusps on posterior teeth (Figure 22-21). This length is measured on a small millimeter rule and transferred to the patient record for future reference and modification if necessary until a more accurate length is established as the filing process is completed (Figure 22-22).

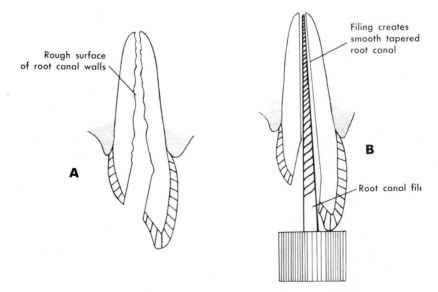

Figure 22-17   Filing root canal. **A,** Root canal before filing (exaggerated). **B,** Canal being filed.

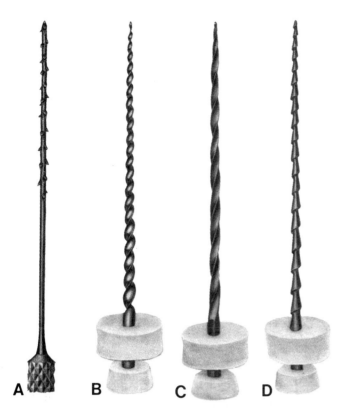

Figure 22-18 Comparison of intracanal instruments. **A,** Barbed broach. **B,** K-file. **C,** Reamer. **D,** Hedstrom file.

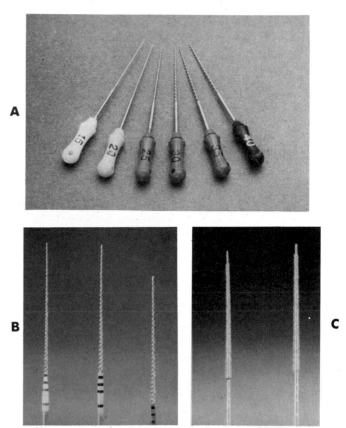

Figure 22-19 Endodontic files. **A,** Assorted sizes of hand-operated files. **B,** Files used in ultrasonic device. **C,** Diamond stones used in ultrasonic device for filing.

(Courtesy Dentsply International Inc, Milford, Del.)

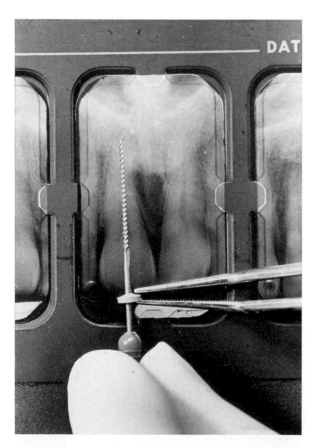

Figure 22-20 Adjusting file marker to proper length of root canal with incisal edge of tooth used as reference point.

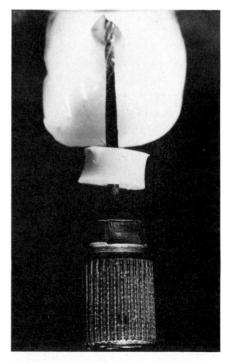

Figure 22-21 Using incisal edge as reference point to determine proper length of root canal. When preset file marker touches incisal edge, tip of file is at apex of root.

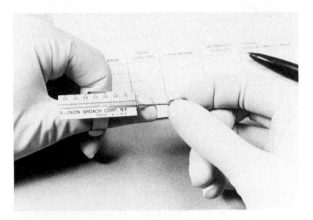

Figure 22-22 Use of thumb–style millimeter ruler to measure and record length of root canal.

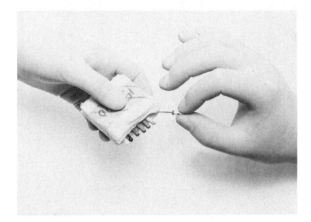

Figure 22-23 Holders for endodontic files and reamers. Use of bound stack of gauze sponges to transfer endodontic files between dentist and assistant.

As filing progresses, file sizes are increased to enlarge the size of the canal. Every time a different file is used, the rubber stop is adjusted so that the file length is the same as the reference length in the patient record. When the file is inserted into the root canal, the rubber file marker touches the reference point on the crown when the tip of the file is at the apex of the root (see Figure 22-21).

It should be noted that in teeth with more than one canal, it is essential that each canal be filed to a predetermined length. Each canal can be filed to different diameters, as well as different lengths.

The transfer of files between the dentist and the assistant can be facilitated by fabricating a sterile receptacle from a 1-inch stack of 2 × 2–inch gauze sponges that are bound together with autoclave tape (Figure 22-23) or precut triangular foam sponges and sterilized. The dental assistant retrieves the range of file sizes being used from the sterile endodontic storage box and inserts them into the edge of the stack of sponges. This device simplifies the transfer and maintains the sterility of the files during the procedure. If a file is inadvertently contaminated, another file can be used in its place, or the contaminated one can be sterilized at chairside using a glass bead sterilizer (Figure 22-24). The instrument must be immersed in the beads for 5 seconds at a temperature of 225° to 250° C (425° to 500° F).

Filing is aided greatly by flooding the root canal with a prepared mixture called RC Prep. RC Prep acts as a lubricant that keep the dentin shavings from clogging the cutting edges of the file as they are removed from the walls of the canal. After filing is complete, the canal is flushed thoroughly with sodium hypochlorite and a surgical suction tip. The canal is dried with absorbent paper points (Figure 22-25). The paper point is held in the locking pliers and inserted into the canal to absorb the solution. This is repeated with several paper points until they are completely dry when withdrawn. Paper points are available in various sizes for use in different-sized canals.

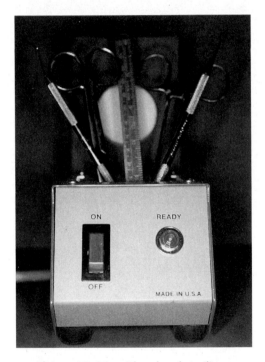

Figure 22-24 Glass bead sterilizer.

Root canal filling (obturation)

The rubber material gutta-percha used with a sealer is the most popular filling for a prepared root canal. Gutta-percha is marketed in points (cones) of various sizes (Figure 22-26). After the canal is filed to the desirable size, cleaned, and dried, an appropriate-sized point is selected and cut to the predetermined length. The proper length is verified by taking a periapical radiograph of the tooth with the gutta-percha point in the root canal and the rubber dam in place. The tip of the point should be within 1 mm of the apex of the root. This relationship should

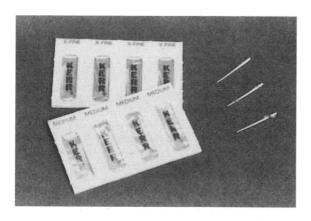

Figure 22-25   Assorted sizes of absorbent paper points.

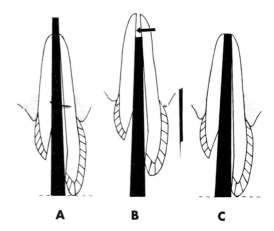

Figure 22-27   Trial-point radiographs would reveal accuracy of gutta-percha point fitting. **A**, Too long. **B**, Too short; arrow indicates space left unfilled. **C**, Accurately fitted.

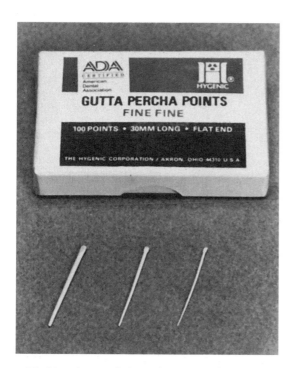

Figure 22-26   Assorted sizes of gutta–percha points (cones).

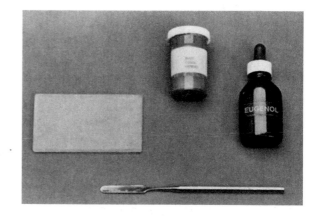

Figure 22-28   Armamentarium for mixing root canal sealer.

adequately seal the apical foramen. The radiograph is commonly referred to as a **trial-point radiograph**. If any adjustment is needed to achieve the proper length of the gutta-percha point, additional trial-point radiographs must be taken to confirm the proper length (Figure 22-27).

With the gutta-percha point properly prepared, it is ready for seating in the canal. A thin mix of **root canal sealer** (Kerr sealer, Kerr Tubliseal, Grossman's sealer) is mixed on a sterile glass slab (Figure 22-28). Some cement is placed into the canal with a reamer (Figure 22-29, *A*). The tip of the gutta-percha point is dipped in the sealer and inserted into the canal and seated to the predeter-

mined position established by the trial-point radiograph (Figure 22-29, *B*). The sealer is added assurance of a perfect seal at the apical foramen.

If any space exists between the point and the walls of either the root canal or the pulp chamber, this space can be filled with additional gutta-percha points of a smaller diameter. This is done by inserting a **spreader** beside the primary gutta-percha point and applying lateral pressure to condense the point against the walls of the canal (Figure 22-29, *D*). A smaller auxiliary point is inserted in the space occupied by the spreader just as it is removed from the canal. This is repeated until the canal is completely filled. The excess length of the gutta-percha points is cut away with a hot filling instrument or large spoon excavator (Figure 22-29, *G*). A **gutta-percha plugger (condenser)** is used to condense the warm gutta-percha vertically toward the root apex (Figure 22-29, *H*). More gutta-percha can be added if needed, and the process is

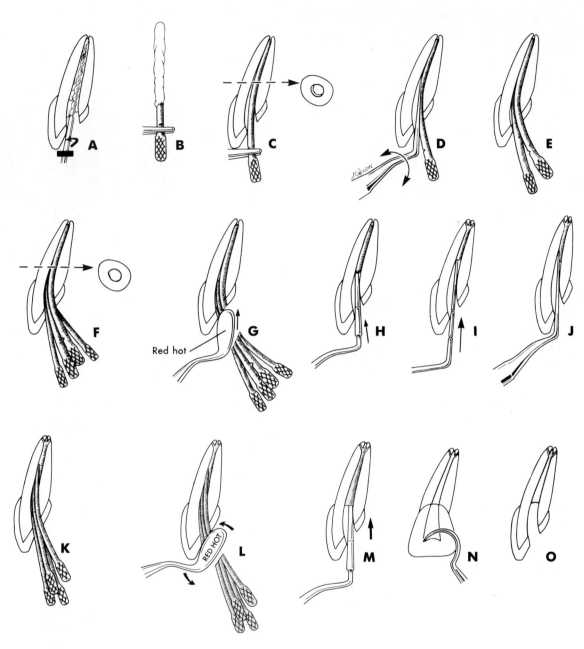

Figure 22-29   Step-by-step procedure for lateral and vertical condensation. **A,** Cement carried into canal with reamer set 1 mm short of working length. Reamer is rotated counterclockwise, spinning sealer into canal. Note constriction at apex of endodontic cavity preparation. **B,** Primary gutta-percha cone coated with cement sealer. **C,** Cone inserted into canal until mark on cone coincides with incisal edge. Arrow points to cross section of middle third of canal. **D,** Spreading to create space for additional cone. **E,** Auxiliary cone inserted into space created by spreader. **F,** Spreading process with several secondary cones added. Arrow points to cross section of middle third of canal. **G,** Butt ends of cones removed with hot instrument. **H,** Vertical condensation packing still-warm gutta-percha mass apically. **I,** After removal of gutta-percha to apical third of canal, prefitted pluggers are used to pack vertically gutta-percha mass farther apically. **J and K,** Continuation of spreading and cone addition until remainder of canal is densely filled. **L,** Butt ends of additional accessory cones removed with instrument heated red hot. **M,** Still-warm plasticized gutta-percha mass is packed vertically with prefitted cold plugger to canal orifice's level. **N,** Filling materials removed from pulp chamber and pulpal horns. **O,** Final fill after condensation.

(From Cohen S, Burns RC: *Pathways of the pulp,* ed 6, St Louis, 1994, Mosby.)

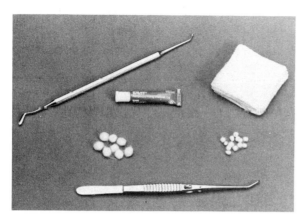

Figure 22-30 Armamentarium for placement of interim dressing. Cotton pellets prevent cement from entering root canal.

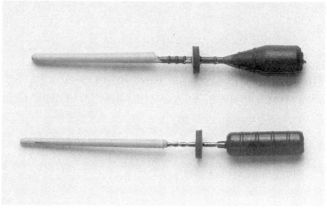

Figure 22-31 Thermal gutta–percha obturators.
(Courtesy The L.D. Caulk Division, Dentsply International Inc, Milford, Del.)

repeated until the canal is completely filled. Excess gutta-percha and any root canal sealer are removed from the pulp chamber, which is then sealed with Cavit, a temporary filling material that serves as a temporary restoration.

It should be noted that if the tooth has more than one root canal, each canal is filed individually and each requires a properly fitted trial-point gutta-percha point sealed in it.

> **⚫❖ KEY POINT**
> ▪ A perfect sealing of the apical foramen in the roots of teeth is essential to eliminate irritation of periapical tissue.

Interim dressings

Occasionally the pulpectomy procedure cannot be completed in one appointment, and a temporary filling (dressing) must be placed in the root canal opening to prevent contaminating the root canal with saliva and food debris between appointments. Cotton pellets medicated with an antimicrobial solution such as Cresatin, Formocresol, or camphorated parachlorophenol are placed in the pulp chamber, and a temporary ready-made cement such as Cavit is placed (Figure 22-30).

Thermal endodontic obturators

Thermal endodontic obturators (Figure 22-31) look like an endodontic file that has been covered with gutta-percha. The gutta-percha–covered obturator is heated in a special oven to soften the gutta-percha. The obturator is then plunged into the tooth to the desired length. A radiograph is taken to verify if the apex has been sealed,

and then the handle of the obturator is severed with a high-speed handpiece. The gutta-percha is then condensed with an endodontic plugger sometimes called a condenser. Additional auxiliary gutta-percha points are not necessary in this procedure.

SURGICAL ENDODONTICS

Not all teeth can be treated with the pulpectomy procedure just described. Anatomical and tooth developmental variables may prevent the dentist from obtaining an adequate seal at the apical foramen. As a result, surgical procedures have been developed to treat such cases.

Apicoectomy

An **apicoectomy** is the surgical removal of the apical portion of the root of a tooth. To gain access to the apex of the root, an incision must be made on the facial aspect of the alveolar ridge in the area of the tooth to be treated. After the incision is made, the soft tissue is retracted, and the bony covering of the apical portion of the tooth is removed. After the apex of the root is uncovered, it can be removed with a sterile dental bur (Figure 22-32, *A* and *B*).

When the root tip is removed, the opening into the root canal can be sealed with dental amalgam, using a procedure called a reverse filling technique. This simply means that the root canal is filled from the opposite end of the tooth instead of the approach through the crown that was described previously. A small cavity preparation is made in the end of the root, and it is filled with amalgam. This ensures that a perfect seal exists at the root end (Figure 22-32, *C* and *D*). This type of amalgam filling is sometimes called a **retrofill amalgam**.

Before the incision is closed, the periapical area is curetted (scraped) clean of any abnormal tissue that may have formed in response to the offending tooth. A special surgical curette that is larger than a scaling and root planing curette may be used.

An apicoectomy is usually performed when a standard approach through the crown cannot be done. The reason a standard approach cannot be done may be any of the following:

1. The root canal may be hypercalcified so that the canal is obstructed.
2. An extreme curvature may prevent a file from reaching the apex of the root.
3. A previous endodontic filling may have been placed in the canal but may have not achieved an adequate apical seal.
4. A coronal approach may not be possible because of the presence of a coronal restoration that would have to be sacrificed if an opening were made through it.

The apex is removed to facilitate the reverse filling procedure and to eliminate any additional foramen that might exist. Often a tooth has more than one apical foramen for each canal. These will be eliminated by the apicoectomy.

The apicoectomy procedure is usually limited to anterior teeth and some premolars because of anatomical limitations that prevent access to most posterior teeth (Figure 22-33).

Root Amputations

On occasion a multirooted tooth requiring a pulpectomy may have a root that is impossible to file completely to obtain an adequate apical seal yet the other roots of the teeth may be treatable. Instead of extracting the entire tooth, the untreatable root can be amputated from the rest of the tooth and removed from the alveolus (Figure 22-34). The remainder of the tooth can be treated by standard pulpectomy procedures. The opening to which the amputated root was attached can be sealed with amalgam in a way similar to that for the apicoectomy procedure.

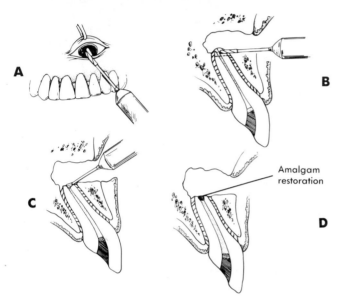

Amalgam restoration

Figure 22-32 Apicoectomy procedure. **A** and **B**, Reflection of mucoperiosteal flap and removal of end of root with bur. **C**, Forming small cavity preparation on cut end of root. **D**, Preparation is filled with amalgam to create seal in end of root. Incision is closed with silk sutures.

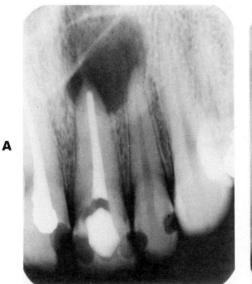
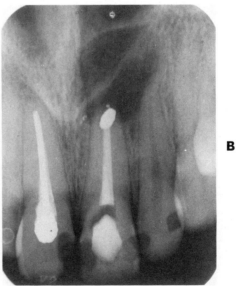

Figure 22-33 Apicoectomy. **A**, Preoperative radiograph. **B**, Postoperative radiograph.
(Courtesy JF Corcoran Jr, DDS, Ann Arbor, Mich.)

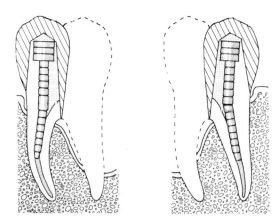

Figure 22-34 Amputation of distal root to create hemisected mandibular molar.

BIBLIOGRAPHY

Anderson RW, Pantera EA: Influence of a barrier technique on electric pulp testing, *J Endodont* 14(4):179, 1988.

Besner E and others: *Practical endodontics: a clinical atlas*, St Louis, 1994, Mosby.

Cohen S and others: *Pathways of the pulp*, ed 6, St Louis, 1994, Mosby.

Finkbeiner BL, Johnson CS: *Mosby's comprehensive dental assisting: a clinical approach*, St Louis, 1995, Mosby.

QUESTIONS—Chapter 22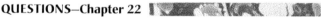

1. All the following could cause pulpal inflammation or death *except*:
   a. Blow to the tooth
   b. Dental caries
   c. Incomplete rinsing of acid etch
   d. Thumb sucking

2. Which of the following is used to lubricate the root canal during the endodontic filing procedure?
   a. RC Prep
   b. Sodium hypochlorite
   c. Formocresol
   d. Root canal sealer

3. Which of the following is used to remove the pulp once the tooth has been opened?
   a. Endodontic file
   b. Barbed broach
   c. Endodontic reamer
   d. Endodontic spreader

4. Which of the following is used to enlarge, smooth, and shape the root canal?
   a. Endodontic file
   b. Barbed broach
   c. Endodontic plugger
   d. Endodontic spreader

5. Which of the following should be avoided if a tooth is accidently knocked out of its bony socket?
   a. Replace avulsed tooth back into the socket if possible.
   b. Store avulsed tooth in water if it is not possible to replant it at the scene of the accident.
   c. See the dentist immediately.
   d. Stabilize replanted avulsed tooth.

6. A hyperemic pulp could have which of the following responses to an electric pulp test:
   a. No response
   b. Same as the control tooth
   c. Responds to a higher electrical current than that of the control tooth
   d. Responds to a lower electrical current than that of the control tooth

7. Which of the following is inflammation of the periodontal tissues near the apex of the tooth?
   a. Periodontal abscess
   b. Fistula
   c. Apical periodontitis
   d. Pulpitis

8. Which of the following is a localized collection of pus at the apex of the tooth?
   a. Periodontal abscess
   b. Fistula
   c. Apical periodontitis
   d. Pulpitis

9. Which of the following is the surgical removal of the apex of the tooth?
   a. Apicoectomy
   b. Retrofill amalgam
   c. Root amputation
   d. Obturation

10. A necrotic pulp would have which of the following responses to an electric vitality test:
    a. No response
    b. Same as the control tooth
    c. Responds to a higher electrical current than that of the control tooth
    d. Responds to a lower electrical current than that of the control tooth

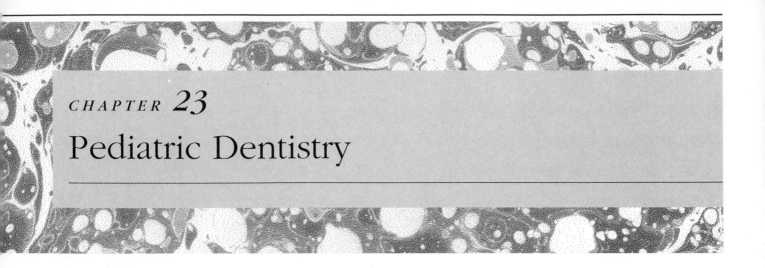

Pediatric Dentistry

KEY TERMS
Congenitally missing
Orthodontics
Pedodontics
Pulp capping
Pulpotomy
Spot-welded matrix band
Tell-show-do
Traumatic intrusion

Dentistry for children differs from dentistry for adults in three major areas: patient management, problems relating to growth and development, and restorative procedures concerned with developing dentitions. The problems relating to the emotionally and physically developing child are so unique that a separate specialty of pedodontics (children's dentistry) has been developed. **Pedodontics** predominantly deals with problems related to patient management and education, restorative procedures, and interceptive orthodontics. **Orthodontics** deals principally with problems relating to growth of the face and the development of the dentitions. However, orthodontic treatment is not limited to children.

Obviously the vast subject of dentistry for children cannot be completely discussed in the limited confines of one chapter or even an entire textbook. This chapter introduces the dental assistant to some of the most common challenges faced in this area of dentistry.

PATIENT MANAGEMENT

Virtually all successful treatment of any patient centers around how well the patient is managed. This is particu-

larly true of children. Children live in a world of their own. It is a world of limited life experiences that is greatly influenced by the child's environment and the people in it.

The success of the dental team in providing dental services for a child depends on how well the team relates to the world of the child. Both the dentist and the auxiliaries must continually nurture a positive relationship with child patients. A basic understanding and fondness for children must exist within the minds of the operating team for positive relationships to develop. Children are experts in detecting the feelings of others around them. They form opinions of others rapidly from facial expressions, tone of voice, conversational topics, and physical actions. If one is truly sincere and honest with children, they will sense it almost immediately and react positively. Conversely, if one betrays children and is dishonest and insincere, it is safe to assume that they will react negatively. Dental assistants should analyze their own feelings toward children to determine whether they possess the fundamental personality necessary in relating to children. Many experts agree that dentists and their auxiliaries who are not successful in patient management fail because they do not enjoy working with children.

Treating a child patient is much like being a parent. The operating team tries to guide and modify the child's behavior during the dental appointment. The same parental techniques that are used to modify behavior at home can be used in the dental office. Displays of fondness, firmness, fairness, honesty, sincerity, authority, and consistency are integral parts of behavior modification. However, like parents themselves, the dental team does not always succeed and may have to use premedication, at least on a temporary basis.

With the recognition that there will be some successes and failures in managing children, it is important that the operating team establish guidelines for their behavior to prevent management problems. The dentist and the staff should have a clear understanding of each person's role in patient management.

↦ **KEY POINT**
- Constant communication between the dentist and staff is essential so that the operating team is compatible in the eyes of the child who enters the dental office.

General Behavior Characteristics of Children

Children constantly undergo both physical and psychological growth. Psychological growth occurs at different rates within each individual just as physical growth varies. Psychological growth is influenced by age, environment, and other people.

Table 23-1 is a general characterization of children in various age-groups and suggested treatment modifications that may assist the dental assistant in anticipating a child's behavior.

These characteristics are by no means absolute; neither are they limited only to the age-groups stated. They may extend either way from the ages stated because of individual variability. An analysis of these characteristics may aid the dental assistant is establishing rapport with a child and developing a more relaxed conversation geared to the patient. It is hoped that a better understanding of children's behavior will contribute to more successful patient management.

Office Environment

Children are sensitive to their environment. They like bright colors and a cheery decor. Every dental office that treats children should have at least a portion of the reception room designed for the young patient. Small tables and chairs geared to children's physical size give them a sense of belonging. A variety of toys, books, and activities should be available for different age-groups to enhance this sense of belonging and to occupy the child waiting for treatment. Some dental offices have a variety of videotapes that the child can watch during treatment or to occupy waiting time. It is good to include some pictures or posters of current cartoon characters on the walls of the children's area to add familiarity to the room.

Children show a marked dislike for gloomy surroundings, unpleasant room odors (medical and otherwise), and white uniforms.

Pleasant music is as acceptable to children as it is to adult patients. Music can create a favorable mood, occupy one's mind, and mask other noises in the offices. Some offices have portable music cassette players with headphones that can help distract the child during treatment.

Table 23-1 General characterization of children in various age-groups and suggested treatment modifications

Age	Behavior	Treatment modifications
Birth to 2 yr	Not able to respond to questions Attached to parents	Communicate with caregiver about treatment or postoperative instructions Have caregiver in treatment room or hold patient in lap
2 yr	Depend on tone of voice and facial expressions to understand certain situations Startled by sudden movements or sounds	Maintain constant and upbeat verbal conversation with patient using warm facial expressions Explain changes in chair position, sounds, or activities to patient
3 yr	Obtaining independence Ask how and why questions May be willing to be treated without caregiver	Answer questions by patient honestly and sincerely If patient asks too many questions, tell patient you will answer questions after treatment is finished
4 yr	May be less cooperative May be assertive, aggressive, or resistant	Provide positive reinforcement (e.g., praise, toys, rewards)
5 yr	Accept separation from caregiver Interact socially through verbal and physical activity Interested in discussing possessions, accomplishments, and themselves	Communicate at level patient can understand but avoid baby talk Center conversation on patient and patient's recent activities and accomplishments
6 yr	Recognize authority figures other than parents and teachers; therefore patient may be more responsive to older adults Pressure and involvement with peer groups have great influence	Have child observe other well-behaved children receiving dental care
7 to 12 yr	Physically and intellectually more capable of dealing with situations that might create anxiety	Treat patient like an adult

Sound control is a factor in the office. Patients in the reception room can be readily upset by a crying child in the treatment area. Office designers should take this into account when the office is built.

Parental Management

Children have no natural fear of going to the dentist. Their fears are acquired through either the negative influence of others or their own unfavorable dental experiences. Unfortunately, many parents contribute significantly to the development of fear of dental treatment. Parents often prejudice the child against dentistry by relating their unfavorable experiences or their fears to the child at home. It is essential that parents be cautioned to let children experience dental treatment on their own without any preconceived fears passed through the family.

> **KEY POINT**
> - A typed letter can be sent to the parents of a child who will be coming to the office for the first time to assist the parent in preparing the child.

It is quite common for parents to overprepare children for their first dental visit. Although the intent may be favorable, the results are often negative. When a parent dwells on the ease of going to the dentist, the child often senses that the parent is being deceptive. Parents should be advised to minimize the significance of the visit to the dentist. Children should be informed that the dentist will look at their teeth and probably take pictures. They should be encouraged to ask the dentist what other things might be done at any appointment. The first dental appointment should be standardized, so that the parent knows what to expect. It is a sign of deceit in the mind of children if they are told that the dentist will only look at their teeth and take pictures and then the dentist gives an injection and restores a tooth. More often than not, children believe that the dentist deceived them rather than the parent. Honesty is the best policy with children. If a parent is unsure of what the dentist is going to do, children should be instructed to ask. The dentist can deal with the answer.

There is some disagreement among dentists as to whether they want the parent in the operatory during the appointment. Generally the operating team can handle a child better if the parent remains in the reception area. This practice allows children to experience dentistry on their own. It also allows the dentist and auxiliaries the opportunity to establish rapport with the patient without interference from the parent. Typically, the dental team will make the child the center of attention. If conversa-

tion is directed toward the youngster, the patient accepts directions from the dentist. If the parent is present, the child's attention is often diverted from the dentist to the parent. In addition, the child may not easily accept the dentist as an authority figure.

There are exceptions to the rule of child-parent separation. This is particularly true in children less than 3 years old and disabled children. Children who speak a different language (verbal or sign language) are also possible exceptions. This decision is made entirely by the dentist on the basis of personal experience and ability.

Dental assistants must be aware of the dentist's policies regarding managing both the parent and the child so that the parents can be informed of their role in cooperation with the dentist. Most parents are extremely willing to cooperate if they are aware of the office policy.

Timing of an appointment is sometimes a key factor in patient management. Some children can accept treatment more favorably at a certain time of day or even on certain days of the week. Parents can be helpful in setting up appointments for the child at favorable times. This may be inconvenient to parents and school officials, yet timing is of great significance in achieving success. It is often wise to schedule shorter, more frequent appointments for young children until they become accustomed to dental treatment.

Preappointment Behavior Modifications

Preappointment behavior modification is anything that is said or done to positively influence the child's behavior before treatment. Examples include viewing of videotapes or reading of books that introduce the dental office in the nonthreatening environment of the child's home or even the reception area of the dental office before the dental appointment. The child may accompany the parent to the parent's appointment for observation of a nonthreatening procedure, such as a recall maintenance appointment. A preappointment mailing (Figure 23-1) can also be used to prepare the child's parent.

Suggestions for Patient Management

Table 23-2 lists recommendations made by the American Association of Pediatric Dentistry for behavior management of child patients.

Verbal communication

1. *Dental staff communication.* The dentist and staff must be in constant communication at staff meetings and throughout the day so that there is good coordination between staff members. There should be no question as to the role each member plays in patient management.
2. *Specific positive directions.* Avoid confusing the child with inadequate directions. The directions should be positive and specific. Avoid saying "Would you like to

Dear parent:

Children who have pleasant dental appointments when they are very young are likely to have a favorable outlook toward dental care throughout life. The first appointment is very important in this attitude formation. That is the reason I am writing to you.

At our first appointment we will examine your child's teeth and gums and take any necessary x-ray films. For most children this will be an interesting and even happy occasion. All the people on our staff enjoy children and know how to work with them, but you, parents, play an important role in getting children started with a good attitude toward dental care. One of the useful things that you can do is to be completely natural and easygoing when you tell your child about the appointment with the dentist. This approach enables children to view their dental visit as an opportunity to meet some new people who want to help them stay healthy.

Your cooperation is appreciated. Remember, good general health depends partly on the development of good habits, such as sensible eating, sleeping routines, and exercise. Dental health also depends on good habits, such as proper toothbrushing, regular dental visits, and a good diet. We will have a chance to further discuss these points during your child's appointment.

Sincerely,

Figure 23-1   Letter used to assist parents in preparing children for first dental visit.

come in now, Johnny?" or "Don't you want to sit in our big chair?" (Figure 23-2). The child is given a choice with this type of direction and has to decide what to do—stay with mother or please the dentist. Directions given in a specific and positive manner prevent this dilemma. "Hi, Johnny, it's time to come in now" and "Now climb into the big chair" tell children exactly what you want and give them no choice in the matter. Most children will respond more favorably to positive directions (Figure 23-3).

3. *Child-centered treatment.* On arriving the patient must become the center of attention. All conversation should be directed toward the child. Select topics of conversation that pertain directly to the child and not someone else. A child enjoys being the center of attention. Suggested topics of conversation are clothes the child is wearing, television shows, pets, favorite toys, sports, and favorite stories. A good assistant takes time to watch some children's programs and review some popular children's stories so that conversation is easier to initiate, especially with shy children. Raise the chair to eye level during conversation so that the child does not feel dwarfed by people towering over him or her.

4. *Adjustment of language level.* Avoid baby talk to all children. It is better to adjust the vocabulary from a higher level to a lower one as needed than to assume children know nothing and talk down to them. This level is achieved as the operating team becomes more familiar with the youngster. For young children the

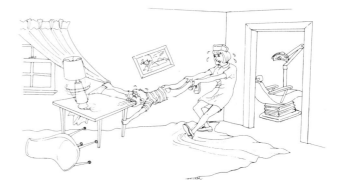

Figure 23-2   "Would you like to come in now, Johnny?"

dental assistant should explain instruments and equipment in nonthreatening words that the child can understand. Avoid words that promote fear such as hurt, shot, drill, pick, and bleeding. Substitute descriptive terms that have less unpleasantness associated with them, or none at all, such as slightly uncomfortable, mosquito bite, polisher, and cavity finder. Box 23-1 has examples of terms that can apply to the instruments and equipment in a dental treatment room.

5. *Voice tone used.* During conversation use normal voice tones. A high-pitched, singsong voice level should be avoided because a change to normal voice tone during the procedure may be interpreted by the child as a change in the relationship from friendliness

Table 23-2 American Academy of Pediatric Dentistry's Standards of Care for Behavior Management

Management type	Description	Objectives	Indications	Contraindications
1. Communicative management				
a. Tell-show-do	Explanations tailored to cognitive level, followed by demonstration, followed by actual procedure	a. Allay fears b. Shape patient's responses c. Give expectations of behavior	All patients who can communicate regardless of method of communication	None
b. Voice control	Modulation in voice volume, tone, or pace to influence and direct patient's behavior	a. Gain patient's attention b. Avert negative or avoidance behaviors c. Establish authority	Uncooperative or inattentive but communicative child	Children who are unable to understand due to age, disability, medication, or emotional immaturity
c. Positive reinforcement	Process of shaping patient's behavior through appropriately timed feedback (e.g., praise, facial expression)	a. Reinforce desired behavior	Any patient	None
d. Distraction	Diverting patient's attention from perceived unpleasant procedure	a. Decrease likelihood of unpleasant perception or threshold	Any patient	None
e. Nonverbal communication	Conveying reinforcement and guiding behavior through contact, posture, and facial expressions	a. Enhance effectiveness of other communicative management techniques b. Gain or maintain patient's attention and compliance	Any patient	None
2. Conscious sedation*	Preoperative or intraoperative administration of sedative agents	a. Reduce or eliminate anxiety b. Reduce untoward movement or reaction c. Enhance communication d. Increase tolerance for longer periods e. Aid treatment of mentally, physically, or medically compromised patient	Any ASA class I or class II patient who cannot cooperate due to lack of psychological or emotional maturity or mental, physical, or medical disability	a. Patient with minimal dental needs b. Medical contraindication to sedation

	Technique	Description	Objectives	Indications	Contraindications
3.	General anesthesia*	Use of general anesthetics (intravenous, intramuscular, inhalation) for intraoperative care	a. Provide safe, efficient, and effective dental care	Patients with certain physical, mental, or medically compromising conditions; local anesthesia is ineffective because of acute infection, allergy; extremely uncooperative, fearful, anxious, or uncommunicative child or adolescent in whom dental care cannot be deferred; extensive orofacial or dental trauma; protection of developing psyche	a. Healthy, cooperative patient with minimal dental needs b. Medical contraindication to general anesthesia
4.	Hand-over-mouth (HOM)*	Placement of hand over mouth while explaining behavioral expectations; removing hand when appropriate behavior is to be reinforced; reapplication if necessary	a. Gain child's attention for establishing communication b. Eliminate inappropriate avoidance responses c. Enhance child's self-confidence in coping during treatment d. Ensure child's safety during delivery of care	A healthy child who is able to understand and cooperate but elects to display defiant, obstreperous, or hysterical avoidance behaviors	Children who are unable to understand due to age, disability, medications, or emotional immaturity
5.	Nitrous oxide–oxygen inhalation*	Inhalation of nitrous oxide–oxygen through nasal hood	a. Reduce or eliminate anxiety b. Reduce untoward movement/reaction c. Enhance communication d. Increase tolerance for longer periods e. Aid treatment of mentally, physically, or medically compromised patient f. Reduce gagging	Fearful, anxious, or obstreperous patients; certain mentally, physically, or medically compromised patients; gag reflex is hyperactive; profound local anesthesia cannot be obtained	Chronic obstructive pulmonary diseases; severe emotional disturbances; first trimester of pregnancy; drug- or disease-induced pulmonary fibrosis
6.	Physical restraint*	Partial or complete immobilization of patient's body or portions thereof	a. Reduce or eliminate untoward movement b. Protect patient/staff from injury c. Facilitate delivery of care	Cannot cooperate due to immaturity; mental or physical disability; failure of other management techniques; safety to patient/practitioner would be at risk	Cooperative patient; those who have medical or systemic conditions contraindicating restraint

Data derived from the American Academy of Pediatric Dentistry with its permission and encouragement.
*Requires informed consent.

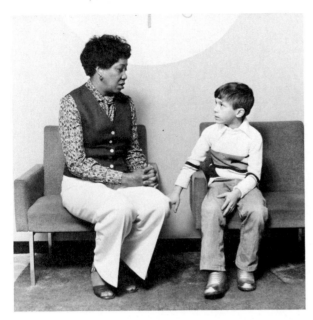

Figure 23-3   Response to positive directions.

BOX 23-1

SUGGESTED TERMS FOR INSTRUMENTS AND EQUIPMENT WHEN WORKING WITH A PEDODONTIC PATIENT

ITEM	SUGGESTED NAME
Prophylaxis angle and prophylaxis cup	Electric toothbrush
High-speed handpiece	Whistle
Saliva ejector	Mr. Thirsty
Air-water syringe	Mr. Squirt or water gun
Rubber dam	Rubber raincoat
Patient chair	Big chair
Topical fluoride	Cavity fighter
Suction	Vacuum cleaner for the mouth
Alginate	Pudding
Explorer	Tooth feeler
Anesthesia	Make the tooth sleepy
Curette	Tooth scraper

---

to seriousness. Voice tone during the procedure is an important communication device. A singsonglike "Open wide, Johnny" may not get the same result as a firm-toned "Open wide, Johnny." The tone need not be harsh or unfriendly, just firm and definite.

6. *Informing the child.* An informed child is usually less fearful. Procedures should be explained in a concise manner using nonthreatening terminology. Children experiencing the first dental appointment should be shown various nonthreatening instruments before treatment is rendered. This method of **tell-show-do** helps to allay the patient's fears of the unknown or unexpected (Figure 23-4). Before an injection tell the child that a mosquito bite will be felt. This should be done just an instant before the sensation is felt so that the child does not have an opportunity to react to the thought. Timing of this kind of information can be as influential on the child as the information itself. Care should be taken in using words that limit the procedure, such as "just" or "only." If the assistant says "Dr. Jones is only going to look at your teeth," the assistant must be sure that only that is planned. It is preferable to say "Dr. Jones will look at your teeth, and then we'll see if anything else must be done."

7. *Talkative patients.* A youngster may use talkativeness as a device to vent anxiety or as a defense mechanism to delay treatment. A patient who asks a lot of questions should be suspected of this delaying tactic. It can be halted by simply stating that it is time to go to work now, and any other questions the child wants to ask will be answered after the work has been completed. Often after treatment, previously talkative youngsters

have no further questions, but they should be given the opportunity to ask them as they were promised.

8. *Honesty.* A child patient will quickly become apprehensive and fearful if he or she is told one thing and another thing happens. It is best to be honest and sincere with the child patient to prepare the patient for the unexpected. Topical fluoride applications are one example of something new a child may experience. Although the flavors of fluoride are much improved, some children still dislike the taste. It is best to inform the patient about the purpose of the fluoride and what to expect. For example, "I'm going to give you something that will make your teeth stronger, it tastes kind of funny but you only need to have it in your mouth for a few minutes." If the dental office has several flavors, let the patient choose the flavor. For dental radiographs the assistant may say "I'm going to take a picture of your teeth by placing this film inside your mouth. Your mouth is small so the film may not feel good under your tongue but you only need to have it in for a few seconds while I run around the corner and push the button to take the picture." If the dental assistant is honest and sincere with the child patient, rapport will be established and the child gains trust in the assistant.

Nonverbal communication

1. *Facial expression.* Children are not unlike adults in that they read facial expressions and form opinions. A friendly facial expression is worth 1000 kind words. On the other hand, a firm look at the right time often achieves effective results.

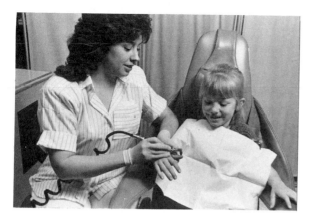

Figure 23-4 Introduction of child to dental treatment room on first visit.

2. *Touch.* By and large, young children like to be touched and see it as an expression of affection. A gentle pat, holding hands, and putting an arm around them occasionally are often well received by the youngster. A squirming child will know exactly what you mean when a firm grip is applied to an arm or leg.

3. *Eye contact.* Maintenance of eye contact during conversation enhances the sincerity of what is being said and enforces the attention being given to a child.

Appearance

1. *Uniforms.* Many children fear white uniforms because of the association with previous unfavorable medical or dental experiences. Colored uniforms help to eliminate this association. Some dentists prefer to remove clinic jackets when seeing a child patient for procedures that do not involve a water spray to further dissolve the unpleasant association.

2. *Personal hygiene.* Children, like adults, prefer neat, attractive people. They dislike people with body and breath odors, and they often say so! Attention to personal hygiene cannot be relaxed because one is treating children.

3. *Face masks.* The face covered by a surgical face mask is often a fearsome sight to the child. If it is necessary to wear one, the child should be told that you do not want to give him or her your germs. Drawing a smile on the mask can amuse the child and may relieve fear associated with the mask.

Controlling emotions

The operating team must control their negative emotions toward a child. If both the dentist and the patient are angry, the procedure is doomed to failure. It is better for the dentist to leave the room to cool off when this happens. Another appointment for the child may be necessary—with premedication if all else fails.

Praise

Youngsters thrive on praise. Reinforcement of positive behavior during the appointment should be done by offering various forms of praise. "Boy! Johnny can sure open wide, can't he, Dr. Jones?" This is an example of indirect praise that the assistant can offer during a procedure.

> **➡ KEY POINT**
> ■ Every appointment should end on a good note. There should be at least one thing that even the most unruly youngster has done during the appointment that merits praise. A few moments should be taken at the end of each appointment for some form of praise from the dentist and the assistant.

Consistency

The operating team should establish consistency in office policy, operating technique, terminology, and patient management techniques. Children respond much better to consistency. They know what to expect, and they react more predictably.

Role of Dental Assistant

The specific role of the assistant in patient management varies from one dental office to another. It is important for the dentist to clarify the role to prevent misunderstandings. Some dentists rely heavily on the assistant's involvement in handling children, whereas others prefer to minimize the assistant's role.

A typical format is to have an assistant play the predominant role in introducing the child to the office and its equipment. Establishing conversation with the youngster is an important part of this task. As the dentist enters the operatory, the assistant introduces the child to the dentist, and as the dentist establishes rapport with the child, the assistant's involvement in the conversation is gradually reduced. As the procedure progresses, the assistant should slowly aid the dentist in establishing an authority image. This is especially important if the child attempts to cling too heavily to the newly adopted mother—the assistant. The amount of verbal input the assistant should offer during a procedure is a matter of opinion. However, most dentists agree that directions to the child should be given by the dentist. Directions from two sources tend to confuse the patient and may generate problems. The assistant again plays a prominent role in directing the youngster after the procedure is finished. The dental assistant often gives postoperative instructions and dismisses the child.

This format changes somewhat for expanded-duty assistants and dental hygienists, since they assume the role of the operator. They must therefore assume a greater authority figure role.

COMMON OPERATIVE AND RESTORATIVE PROCEDURES

Dental care for the young patient involves treatment of the primary and permanent dentitions or a combination of both (the mixed dentition), depending on the age of the patient. Generally parents do not question the validity of restoring carious or fractured permanent teeth. However, parents often question the restoration of primary teeth, since the child will shed them anyway.

Restoration of the primary teeth is important for the following reasons:

1. A restoration maintains the function of the teeth in chewing, speech, and appearance.
2. A restoration helps to ensure symmetrical growth of developing jaws.
3. The primary teeth maintain space on the jaws for the permanent teeth that replace them. Primary teeth also guide the path of eruption of the permanent teeth into proper position.
4. The child should be free of discomfort and mouth odors, as is the adult patient.

The preservation of the primary teeth until they are lost by natural exfoliation (shedding) is a principal goal of operative and restorative dentistry.

Operative Dentistry

Operative dentistry techniques for children differ little from those used for adults as far as the assistant's duties are concerned. The same basic steps are used in the fabrication of composite and amalgam restorations as described in Chapters 17 and 18. Gold inlays and cohesive gold restorations are not usually done on primary teeth.

Additional features of rubber dam isolation that are beneficial in children's dentistry are that the rubber dam assists the patient in keeping the mouth open, has a quieting effect on the child, and protects the tongue and cheek.

Pulp cap

Pulp exposure caused by trauma or cavity preparation procedures indicates the need for root canal therapy. However, when small exposures of the pulp occur, the need for a root canal may be avoided by **pulp capping**. For the procedure the carious dentin is removed and a calcium hydroxide paste is applied on top of the exposed pulp. The tooth is then restored following normal restorative procedures.

Pulpotomy

Pulpotomy is a procedure that involves partial removal of the dental pulp after it has been extensively exposed.

This is in contrast to pulpectomy, which involves the complete removal of the pulp. Pulpectomy procedures are discussed in Chapter 22.

Pulpotomy procedures are usually performed on primary and young permanent teeth. Success rates drop markedly when attempts are made to treat permanent teeth of individuals past their teens. Extensive pulp exposures in older adult teeth are usually treated with a pulpectomy procedure. Pulpal circulation is reduced significantly in adult patients as a result of the constriction of the apical foramen that is a part of normal tooth development. Ample blood supply to the remaining portion of the pulp is essential to the success of a pulpotomy. Another factor in the success of a pulpotomy is the condition of the pulp at the time of treatment. Infected pulp tissue is a poorer candidate than healthier pulp tissue.

There are several different methods of performing a pulpotomy. The Formocresol method is explained below. Pulpotomy is a surgical procedure, so care must be exercised to maintain a sterile operating field as much as possible. Rubber dam isolation is indicated to prevent salivary contamination. The standard amalgam armamentarium can be used for this procedure with the following additional items:

- Formocresol
- No. 6 sterile round bur
- Zinc oxide and eugenol (ZOE) cement (IRM)

Procedure

1. Administer anesthetic, and place a rubber dam.
2. A large opening is made into the pulp chamber to expose the entire coronal portion of the pulp.
3. A No. 6 round bur in a conventional-speed handpiece or a sharp discoid spoon evacuator is used to remove this portion of the pulp to the level of the openings of the root canals (Figure 23-5, A and B).
4. The pulp chamber is irrigated, evacuated, and then dried with cotton pellets.
5. A small cotton pellet wetted with Formocresol solution is placed over the remainder of the pulp and allowed to remain for 5 minutes. This solution fixes, or mummifies, a thin layer of the remaining pulp, which stops the bleeding from the amputated pulp tissue.
6. The cotton is removed, and the pulp chamber is dried with cotton pellets.
7. A thick layer of hard-setting ZOE base material is placed over the pulp (Figure 23-5, C and D).

After completion of the pulpotomy, the final restoration, such as amalgam or a stainless steel crown, can be placed. Dentists sometimes prefer to delay placement of the final restoration until the injured pulp has an opportunity to recover from the surgical procedure. In these cases the ZOE cement is used to fill the cavity preparation completely; thus it acts as a temporary restoration.

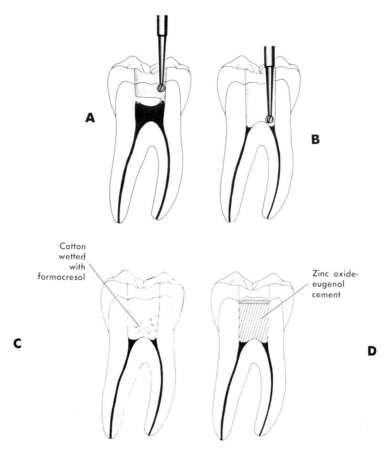

Figure 23-5 Formocresol pulpotomy. **A**, Caries removal. **B**, Removal of coronal portion of pulp. **C**, Application of Formocresol. **D**, Placement of cement.

Spot-welded matrix band

One variation that is common in the fabrication of an amalgam restoration for primary teeth is the use of a **spot-welded matrix band** for class II and VI restorations. Some dentists prefer these to the conventional matrix bands that are held in place by a matrix retainer.

The spot-welded matrix band can be made quickly as follows:

1. The matrix band material is placed around the tooth and pinched tightly with a Howe pliers or a hemostat (Figure 23-6, A). The excess length of the band (½ inch) is bent to one side to mark the proper size of the tooth.
2. The band is carried to the spot welder and welded at the bend in the band made by the pliers (Figure 23-6, B).
3. The excess band material can be cut away and the band contoured to fit the tooth (Figure 23-6, C).
4. After the band is placed around the tooth, interproximal wedges are placed as when conventional bands are used. After the insertion of the amalgam the band is removed by cutting the band on the lingual aspect and pulling it in a buccal direction with cotton pliers.

Restorative Dentistry

Elaborate cast-gold restorations are usually done only on primary teeth under special circumstances. Typically, primary teeth that are extensively destroyed because of caries or fracture are restored with temporary crowns that are cemented to the involved teeth with a permanent cementing agent. Stainless steel crowns are used on posterior teeth, and polycarbonate, preformed crowns are used on anterior teeth.

Stainless steel crowns

Stainless steel crowns can be used as interim restorations on primary teeth until they are exfoliated or on permanent teeth until a more accurately contoured cast-gold crown can be fabricated. These crowns are available in kits that contain a range of sizes for the various primary and permanent posterior teeth. The technique used in the fabrication of stainless steel crowns is given in Box 23-2.

Polycarbonate crowns

Polycarbonate crowns are fabricated for primary and permanent teeth in the same manner described in Chapter 21.

• • •

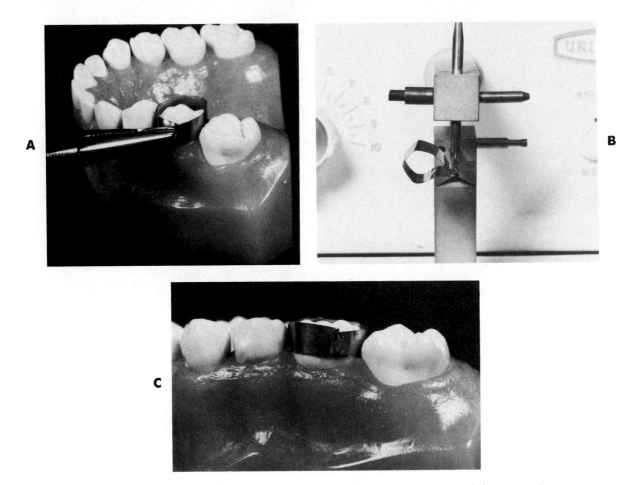

Figure 23-6 Fabrication of spot-welded matrix band. **A**, Pinching band with hemostat. **B**, Welding band. **C**, Finished band in place.

Figure 23-7 Fabrication of stainless steel crown. **A**, Trimming crown to proper length with crown-and-collar scissors. **B**, Smoothing rough edges with green stone followed by abrasive rubber wheel (Craytex). **C**, Contouring crown with contouring pliers. **D**, Longitudinal section of completed crown.

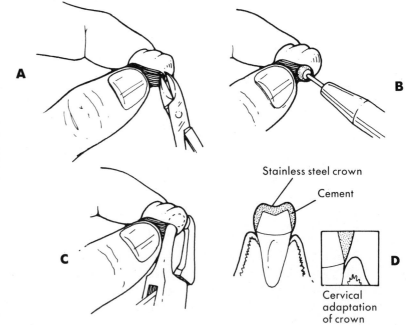

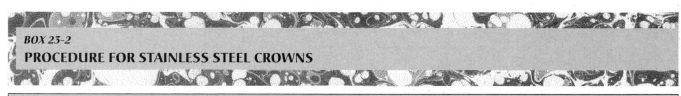

BOX 23-2
PROCEDURE FOR STAINLESS STEEL CROWNS

PROCEDURE	RATIONALE	PROCEDURE	RATIONALE
1. Tooth is prepared in way similar to that for cast-gold crown, with tapered diamond in high-speed handpiece. Entire circumference of tooth is reduced, as well as height of tooth. Caries is removed with conventional methods, and cavity medications are placed.	1. To prepare tooth and remove carious tooth structure.	4. Edges are then smoothed with a green stone, followed by polishing with rubber abrasive wheel (Figure 23-7, B).	4. To smooth rough edges created by cutting crown.
2. Proper-sized crown is selected from kit. It must fit circumference of prepared tooth and duplicate mesiodistal dimension of original crown of tooth.	2. To avoid any shifting or drifting of adjacent teeth.	5. Patient bites on articulating paper, and adjustments are made if necessary.	5. To make sure that stainless steel crown is not creating traumatic occlusion.
		6. Contouring pliers are used to bend cervical margins of crown toward tooth (Figure 23-7, C).	6. To ensure snug fit and proper cervical contour.
3. Occlusocervical height of crown is adjusted so it extends approximately 1 mm below margin of crown preparation. Crown is trimmed along cervical margin with crown-and-collar scissors (Figure 23-7, A).	3. To obtain proper fit of stainless steel crown.	7. Prepared tooth is dried thoroughly, and crown is filled with permanent cement and seated in place (Figure 23-7, D).	7. To cement stainless steel crown into place.
		8. Excess cement is removed from around tooth, and patient can be dismissed.	8. Pieces of excess cement can harbor plaque and irritate gingiva, which in turn could cause periodontal problems.

It is uncommon that a fixed bridge is used to replace a missing primary tooth. Usually a space-maintaining device is used. If several teeth are missing so that there is difficulty in speech or mastication (chewing) and significant impairment to the child's appearance, a removable partial denture can be made (Figure 23-8). This type of removable partial denture is often called a "flipper." Crown and bridge procedures are sometimes required for the restoration and replacement of permanent teeth in both the mixed and permanent dentitions.

EMERGENCY TREATMENT FOR TRAUMATIZED TEETH

Fractured Teeth

Fractured anterior teeth are common emergencies among children. The active nature of children predisposes them to this type of emergency. See Box 23-3 for appropriate treatments.

Since it is difficult for parents to assess the extent of damage done to a tooth and the surrounding tissue accurately, it is advisable for the dentist to see the patient as soon as possible. Clinical examination, documentation of the history of the accident, and radiographs are essential elements of the initial visit. Pulpal treatment and temporization are carried out as described in Box 23-3. Generally speaking, dentists prefer to delay treatment that involves further trauma to the pulp of an injured tooth for 3 to 6 months. This gives the delicate pulp tissue a greater opportunity to recover without added insult. Radiographic documentation at subsequent appointments is mandatory to determine the status of the injured teeth. Vitality tests are carried out initially to establish a basis of comparison for future tests.

After a 6-month interval, more definitive restorative procedures can be done on injured teeth with still vital pulps. Less severe fractures can be restored with composite restorations using a retention pin, acid-etch tech-

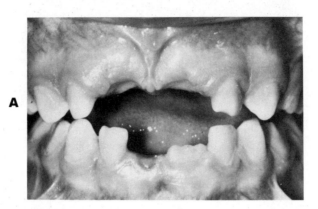

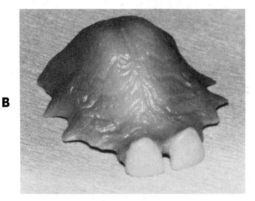

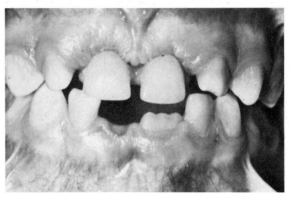

Figure 23-8 **A**, Missing primary incisors. **B**, Replaced with removable partial denture. **C**, Denture in place.

(From Law D and others: *An atlas of pedodontics*, Philadelphia, 1969, WB Saunders.)

BOX 23-3

TYPES OF PERMANENT TOOTH FRACTURES AND TREATMENT

TYPE OF FRACTURE	TREATMENT
Enamel fractures	Small fractures: smooth rough edges
	Larger fractures: place composite restoration
Enamel and dentin fractures	Cover exposed dentin with calcium hydroxide paste or glass ionomer cement
	Place composite restoration
Fractures involving pulp	Depending on clinical findings (e.g., pulp vitality, size of exposure, time elapsed since exposure), perform:
	Direct pulp cap
	Pulpotomy
	Pulpectomy (root canal)
Posterior crown fractures with pulp exposure	Stainless steel or cast metal crown
Root fractures	Reposition crown portion of tooth fragment
	Immobilize with splint for 3 to 6 months
	Root canal therapy if indicated by clinical or radiographic signs of pulp necrosis or resorption

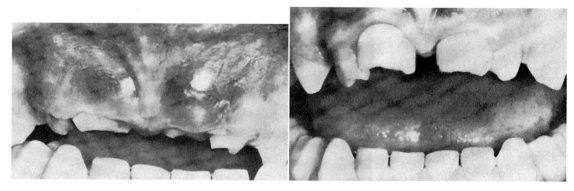

Figure 23-9   Traumatic intrusion. **A,** Intruded incisor. **B,** Reeruption. (From Law D and others: *An atlas of pedodontics,* Philadelphia, 1969, WB Saunders.)

niques, or both. More extensive fractures that require permanent crowns on still vital teeth may have to be delayed until the tooth erupts sufficiently and the apex of the root has completely developed. If the pulp has not been altered, fabrication of a permanent crown may have to be delayed until the large young pulp recedes with age. (A smaller pulp allows the dentist to prepare the tooth for the permanent crown without exposing the pulp during the preparation.) Long-term temporary crowns are used in these cases.

Traumatic Intrusion

Traumatic intrusion of primary and permanent teeth is another common injury to maxillary anterior teeth. The tooth is forcibly driven into the alveolus so that only a portion of the crown is clinically visible (Figure 23-9). Primary and permanent teeth that are intruded should be allowed to reerupt on their own. Since intruded teeth may undergo devitalization, endodontic treatment may be required later.

Intrusion of a primary tooth can present a threat to the underlying developing permanent tooth. The permanent tooth can be damaged either from the physical injury caused by the intruded primary tooth or by a developing infection in a devitalized primary tooth after the injury. There is no way in which damage to the permanent tooth can be determined for certain until it erupts. However, previously injured primary teeth should be observed so that if they become infected, endodontic treatment can be performed or the offending tooth can be extracted.

Displaced Teeth

Displaced primary teeth other than those displaced by intrusion should be repositioned by the dentist and splinted as soon as possible. Primary teeth tend to undergo root resorption more quickly after these injuries and become mobile. They should be observed for possible development of infection and removed if indicated. Permanent teeth should be repositioned as soon as possible and stabilized with a temporary splint using self-curing acrylic, wire ligatures, or orthodontic bands and arch wires. Endodontic treatment is often required in the future for these teeth.

PROSTHODONTICS FOR CHILDREN

Removable partial dentures and even complete dentures are sometimes necessary to replace missing teeth in children. The removable partial denture appliance is used to replace more than one tooth, unless the missing tooth is in the maxillary anterior region and aesthetics are greatly improved.

Children's primary teeth may be missing because of lack of development of the teeth (**congenitally missing**), developmental diseases of the teeth resulting in extraction, or premature loss of teeth caused by caries or trauma. The number of missing teeth may range from one to all of the teeth. The treatment for missing teeth varies from no treatment at all, to space-maintaining appliances, to partial dentures, to complete dentures if all the primary teeth are missing (Figure 23-10). The dentist must judge each case individually to determine the appropriate treatment plan.

PREVENTIVE DENTISTRY FOR CHILDREN

Diet control, oral hygiene procedures, and use of fluorides and pit and fissure sealants all play an important role in preventive dentistry for children (see Chapters 9 and 10). Youngsters who engage in athletic activities should be encouraged to wear protective mouth guards to help prevent traumatic injuries to oral structures.

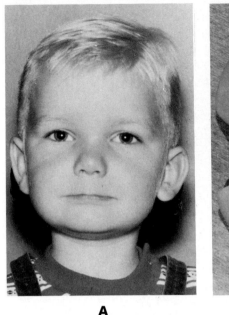
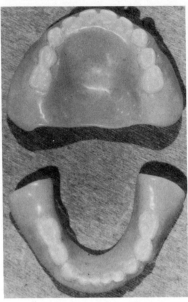
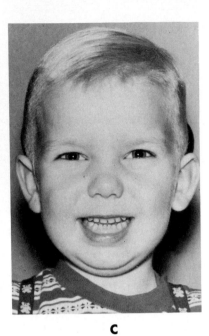

A   **B**   **C**

Figure 23-10   Replacement of all primary teeth with complete denture. **A**, Patient without denture. **B**, Complete dentures. **C**, Dentures in place.

(From Law D and others: *An atlas of pedodontics,* Philadelphia, 1969, WB Saunders.)

INTERCEPTIVE ORTHODONTICS

For a detailed discussion of interceptive orthodontics, see Chapter 24.

CHILD ABUSE AND NEGLECT

Many children each year are subjected to child abuse or neglect.* Health care professionals who identify a case of child abuse are responsible for reporting suspected abuse. The dental office can play a primary role in the identification of child abuse or neglect because orofacial injuries are common in such cases and the child's care givers are more likely to seek dental care vs. medical care.

Types of Child Abuse

The types of child abuse or neglect are as follows:
1. Physical abuse
2. Sexual abuse
3. Neglect
4. Emotional abuse

Physical abuse is nonaccidental injuries inflicted on a child. Sexual abuse can be fondling, incest, masturbation,

intercourse, rape, child pornography, or child prostitution. Physical or emotional neglect is a willful failure to provide for a child's basic needs. Physical neglect includes failure to provide food, clothing, care, and a safe environment. Emotional abuse and neglect are the failure to provide an emotionally stable environment that would allow the child to develop a sound character.

Injuries Associated With Child Abuse or Neglect

The most frequent injuries associated with child abuse or neglect are as follows:
- Fractured teeth
- Laceration of the labial frenum (forced feeding)
- Missing teeth with no obvious explanation
- Displaced teeth
- Fractures of the maxilla or mandible
- Bruised or scarred lips

If child abuse is suspected, the injury should be evaluated with certain considerations. Children who fall and bruise themselves rarely bruise in an area that is not supported by bone. Therefore bruises on the neck, earlobes, or cheeks are unlikely to be caused by falling. Multiple bruises in different stages of healing indicated by their coloration should also be suspected.

If it is suspected that the child is undergoing some form of physical abuse, examine the hands for signs of trauma. Hands are often the first line of defense for children to protect themselves from abuse. Rope marks,

---

*This discussion of child abuse is reprinted with permission from Andreason JO, Hjorting-Hansen E: Replantation of teeth. I. Radiographic and clinical study of 110 human teeth replanted after accidental loss, *Acta Odontol Scand* 24:263, 1966.

cigarette burns, bites, and immersion in hot water are some of the forms of injury that could occur to the hands of an abused child.

Lack of personal hygiene, inappropriate clothing for the weather, extensive caries, and lice are easily observable signs of neglect. A case of neglect may be confirmed by a care giver who is informed of a dental condition and who fails to take care of the problem.

Sexual abuse is more difficult to identify. Children who are subject to oral sexual abuse may display oral signs of venereal diseases such as syphilis, venereal warts, or gonorrhea. Difficulty in walking and sitting may also be a sign of sexual abuse.

Reporting Child Abuse

Health care professionals are required by law to report suspected child abuse. If child abuse is suspected, the dental office should gather as much physical information as possible to support suspicions. The following documentation is recommended:

- Intraoral radiographs
- Color photographs
- Drawings or sketches of the lesion or lesions in the chart
- Written documentation in the patient's chart
- Demographic data, such as name, age, sex, address, birth date, and care givers' names
- Primary care physician's name
- Child's and accompanying person's explanation of the injury
- Size, shape, location, color, and degree of healing of the injury

BIBLIOGRAPHY

Andreason JO, Hjorting-Hansen E: Replantation of teeth. I. Radiographic and clinical study of 110 human teeth replanted after accidental loss, *Acta Odontol Scand* 24:263, 1966.

da Fonseca MA, Idelberg J: The important role of dental hygienists in the identification of child maltreatment, *J Dent Hygiene* 57:3, 135-139, 1993.

Finn S: *Clinical pedodontics*, Philadelphia, 1957, WB Saunders.

Koch G and others: *Pedodontics: a clinical approach*, ed 2, Copenhagen, 1992, Munksgaard.

Law DB and others: *An atlas of pedodontics*, Philadelphia, 1969, WB Saunders.

McDonald RE, Avery DR: *Dentistry for the child and adolescent*, ed 6, St Louis, 1994, Mosby.

Pinkham JR and others: *Pediatric dentistry: infancy through adolescence*, ed 2, 1994, WB Saunders.

QUESTIONS—Chapter 23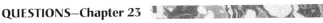

1. When a dental office sends a letter to a child's parent before the first appointment, this is an example of:
   a. Positive reinforcement
   b. Tell-show-do
   c. Nonverbal communication
   d. Preappointment behavior modification

2. When the assistant praises a child patient for cooperating, this is an example of:
   a. Positive reinforcement
   b. Tell-show-do
   c. Nonverbal communication
   d. Preappointment behavior modification

3. Which of the following procedures is performed to avoid root canal therapy in the event of a small pulpal exposure during cavity preparation:
   a. Stainless steel crown
   b. Spot-welded matrix band
   c. Pulp cap
   d. Pulpectomy

4. A deciduous tooth _____ need treatment because it will be lost eventually and be replaced by a permanent tooth.
   a. does
   b. does not

5. All the following apply to a stainless steel crown procedure *except:*
   a. The crown must extend 2 mm below the margin of the crown preparation.
   b. The crown is cemented with a permanent cement.
   c. Contouring pliers are used to bend the cervical margins of the crown.
   d. The crown must contact adjacent teeth.

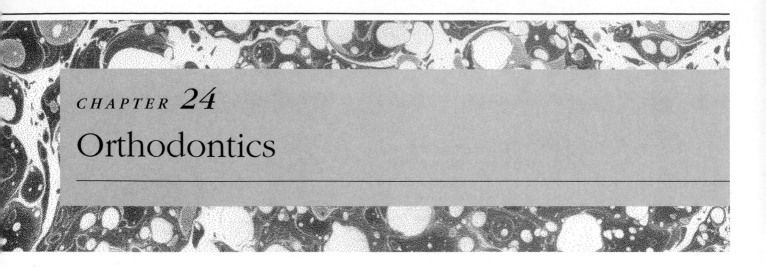

CHAPTER 24

Orthodontics

KEY TERMS

Activator
Arch wires
Bone resorption
Brackets
Buccal tubes
Buccoversion
Cephalometric radiograph
Closed coil springs
Corrective orthodontics
Crossbite
Distoversion
Elastic separators
Elastics
Exfoliation
Expansion activators
Finger springs
Fixed appliances
Functional appliances
Headgear devices
Interceptive orthodontics
Labioversion
Ligatures

Linguoversion
Malocclusion
Mesioversion
Mixed dentition stage
Occlusion
Open bite
Open coil springs
Orthodontic bands
Orthodontics
Orthodontists
Osteoblasts
Osteoclasts
Overbite
Overjet
Permanent dentition
     stage
Positioners
Primary dentition stage
Retainers
Space maintainers
Steel spring separator

Orthodontics is a specialty area of dentistry that deals with problems related to the development of the jaws, the positions of the teeth, and the oral and facial muscles that influence speech, mastication, and swallowing. Patients often seek orthodontic treatment to improve their appearance by having their teeth repositioned, whereas

orthodontists (specialists in orthodontics) concern themselves not only with a patient's appearance but also with the functional aspects of chewing, swallowing, and speech mechanisms. Although orthodontists provide treatment for complex cases, it is common practice for pedodontists and general practitioners to provide preventive and interceptive orthodontic services for their patients.

ETIOLOGY OF ORTHODONTIC PROBLEMS

The etiology, or causes, of orthodontic problems can be grouped into three basic categories—genetic influences, environmental factors, or a combination of both.

Genetic Influences

Since a child is a biological product of two adults, the child often displays characteristics unique to one or both parents. This is true of orofacial characteristics. Therefore a variety of discrepancies can occur that are genetic in origin. Some of these discrepancies are poor tooth/jaw ratio, in that a child can have teeth that do not match the size of the jaws, or poor skeletal relationship, in which the maxilla and the mandible may not grow in harmony with each other.

Environmental Factors

Environmental factors can alter the normal growth pattern, producing problems with occlusion. Environmental factors are nongenetic factors such as the following:
- Abnormal eruption of teeth
- Abnormal exfoliation of teeth
- Supernumerary teeth
- Oral habits, for example, thumb sucking, tongue thrusting, or mouth breathing

DIAGNOSIS

Diagnostic procedures identify what is wrong with a patient so that appropriate treatment can be carried out. In the field of orthodontics, diagnostic procedures are geared toward the evaluation of the teeth and the skeletal relationships of the head, as well as the surrounding orofacial soft tissues. Some of these procedures are discussed here.

Of primary concern to the dentist making an orthodontic diagnosis is the patient's occlusion. **Occlusion** is the relationship of the maxillary and mandibular teeth when they are in contact. To diagnose an orthodontic problem the orthodontist uses the characteristics of a normal occlusion as a reference. (The term *normal* implies that the occlusion does not deviate from the average patient on a statistical basis.) A general description of a normal occlusion follows.

1. Mandibular teeth are in maximum contact with the maxillary teeth throughout the entire dentition.
2. The maxillary anterior teeth should overlap the mandibular anterior teeth by approximately 1 to 2 mm (overbite). The labial surfaces of these maxillary teeth should not be more than 1 to 2 mm anterior to the mandibular anterior teeth (overjet) (Figure 24-1, *A*). There should be contact between the upper and lower anterior teeth.
3. The maxillary posterior teeth are located one cusp buccal to the mandibular posterior teeth (Figure 24-1, *B*).
4. The mesiobuccal cusp of the maxillary first permanent molar should rest in the mesiobuccal groove of the mandibular first permanent molar (Figure 24-1, *C*).
5. The cusp tip of the maxillary cuspids should rest between the mandibular cuspid and the first premolar when the teeth are brought together.
6. There should be no rotated teeth or abnormal spaces between the teeth.

Malocclusion is any deviation from normal occlusion. Malocclusion may result from the improper jaw relationships described previously, from malposed teeth, or from a combination of both, which is generally the case.

It is rare that a patient has an absolutely ideal occlusion. However, dentists generally classify a patient's occlusion as normal if the relationships just described exist to the extent that the patient has a favorable chewing mechanism, has an acceptable appearance from a dental standpoint, and has no potential for injury to other tissues present. Since normal occlusion is unique to the individual and is rarely an ideal occlusion, some dentists prefer to substitute the term *satisfactory* for normal occlusion.

Common Dental Discrepancies

A variety of dental discrepancies can be found in any case of malocclusion. Dental discrepancies are irregularities that are associated with the teeth. These discrepancies are variations in the positions of the teeth in the jaws, the number of teeth present, or the size or shape of the teeth.

Aside from the more obvious discrepancies such as supernumerary, missing, malformed, and rotated teeth, some discrepancies require further description.

Open bite   When the jaws are closed, the mandibular anterior teeth should contact the lingual surfaces of the maxillary anterior teeth. If they do not, an open bite exists (Figure 24-2). Open bites can also exist in posterior areas, but they are found more frequently in anterior areas.

Overbite   The amount of vertical overlap of the incisal edges of upper anterior teeth over the incisal edges of lower anterior teeth is called overbite. If the overlapping is excessive, it is referred to as a deep overbite. If the incisal edges of the lower anterior teeth contact the soft tissue of the palate, the patient is said to have an impinging overbite (Figure 24-3).

Crossbite   In normal occlusion the upper teeth overlap the lower teeth buccally or labially. If the opposite exists, that is, if the lower teeth overlap the upper teeth, the teeth are in crossbite (Figure 24-4). Crossbite can be limited to one or

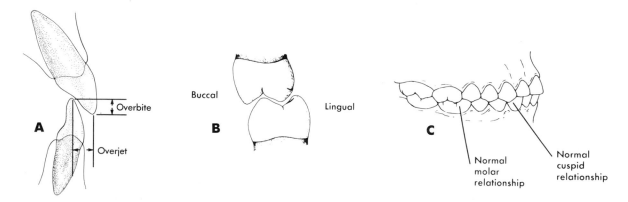

Figure 24-1   Characteristics of normal occlusion. **A,** Normal overbite and overjet. **B,** Buccolingual relationship of posterior teeth. **C,** Anteroposterior relationship of upper and lower permanent first molars and cuspids.

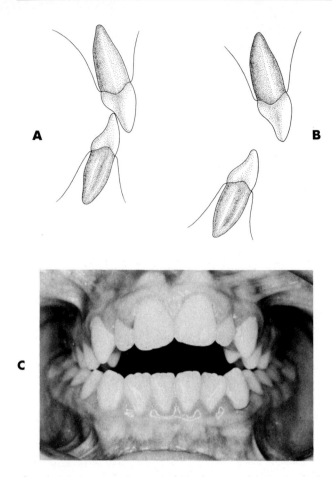

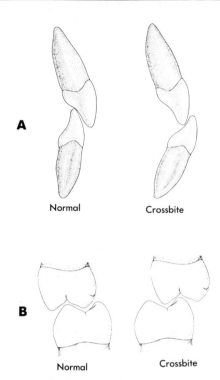

Figure 24-4   Crossbite. **A**, Anterior teeth, normal and crossbite. **B**, Posterior teeth, normal and crossbite.

Figure 24-2   Anterior open bite. **A**, Normal incisor relationship. **B**, Open bite when posterior teeth are occluded. **C**, Open bite in anterior area.

(Courtesy D.R. Balbach, DDS, Ann Arbor, Mich.)

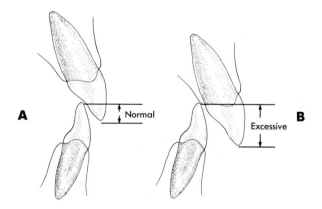

Figure 24-3   Overbite. **A**, Normal. **B**, Deep and impinging overbite.

more teeth in either the anterior or posterior regions of the dental arches.

Overjet   The horizontal distance between the incisal edges of a maxillary incisor and the mandibular incisor in an anteroposterior dimension is called overjet (Figure 24-5). If this distance is increased as a result of malposition of the incisors, the patient is described as having an excessive overjet. The common and somewhat unkind term *buckteeth* refers to an excessive overjet condition.

Tooth Positions

Common terms are used in orthodontics to describe abnormal tooth positions. This terminology adds the suffix *-version* to a root word to indicate in what direction from normal a tooth or teeth are positioned. The following are some common terms used to describe abnormal tooth positions:

Buccoversion	Buccal to normal position.
Mesioversion	Mesial to normal position.
Distoversion	Distal to normal position.
Labioversion	Labial to normal position.
Linguoversion	Lingual to normal position.

The dental assistant's understanding of the classification system and of terminology associated with the diagnosis of orthodontic conditions facilitates communication with the dentist and the patient and aids in recording information on dental records and in referral letters.

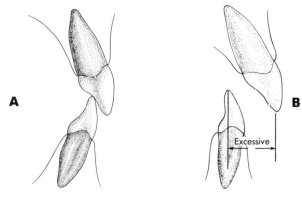

Figure 24-5   Overjet. **A**, Normal. **B**, Excessive.

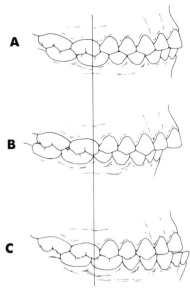

Figure 24-6   Angle's classes of malocclusion. **A**, Class I. **B**, Class II. **C**, Class III.

Angle's Classification of Malocclusion

To establish a common terminology that can be used to describe common forms of malocclusion, Edward Angle established a classification system in 1899 that is still in common use. Angle established three broad classes of malocclusion, using as a reference the relationship of the maxillary and mandibular first permanent molars when the jaws are closed. The classification system is as follows:

Class I malocclusion (Figures 24-6, *A*, and 24-7, *A*)

1. The mesiobuccal cusp of the maxillary first permanent molar rests in the mesiobuccal groove of the mandibular first permanent molar.
2. The cusp tip of the maxillary cuspid rests between the mandibular cuspid and the first premolar.
3. The jaws are in a normal relationship.
4. There is some dental discrepancy, such as malposed teeth, excessive spacing, missing teeth, open bite, overbite, crossbite, or unerupted teeth. The presence of one or more of these discrepancies differentiates between a normal occlusion and a class I malocclusion.

Class II malocclusion (Figures 24-6, *B*, and 24-7, *B*)

1. The molar relationship differs from normal in that the distobuccal cusp of the maxillary first permanent molar rests in the mesiobuccal groove of the mandibular first permanent molar.
2. The maxillary cuspid is located mesial to the mandibular cuspid.
3. The lower jaw is retruded relative to the upper jaw.
4. Dental discrepancies frequently exist. Crowding of teeth, deep overbites, tipped incisors, and overlapped maxillary lateral incisors are commonly found in this class of malocclusion.

The class II malocclusion is split into two divisions based on the relationship of the maxillary incisor teeth:

Class II, division I malocclusion
1. Jaw, molar, and cuspid relationships are as just described for the class II malocclusion.
2. The maxillary incisors are tipped in extreme labioversion (toward the lip).

Class II, division 2 malocclusion
1. Jaw, molar, and cuspid relationships are as just described for the class II malocclusion.
2. The maxillary central incisors are in a near normal position or tipped slightly in linguoversion (toward the tongue). The maxillary lateral incisors are tipped labially and mesially. They often overlap the adjacent central incisors (Figure 24-7, *C*).

Class III malocclusion (Figures 24-6, *C*, and 24-7, *D*)

1. The mesiobuccal cusp of the maxillary first permanent molar rests distal to the mandibular first permanent molar.
2. The maxillary cuspid is in an exaggerated distal relationship to the mandibular cuspid.
3. The lower jaw is protruded relative to the upper jaw.
4. Dental discrepancies can exist. Crossbites are frequently found in class III malocclusions.

Radiography

Both intraoral and extraoral radiographs are used in the diagnosis of orthodontic conditions. The following are some of the most common radiographs that are used to document the patient's condition:

1. Panoramic radiograph (Figure 24-8, *A*)
2. Cephalometric radiographs: lateral view (Figure 24-8, *B*); anteroposterior view (not shown)

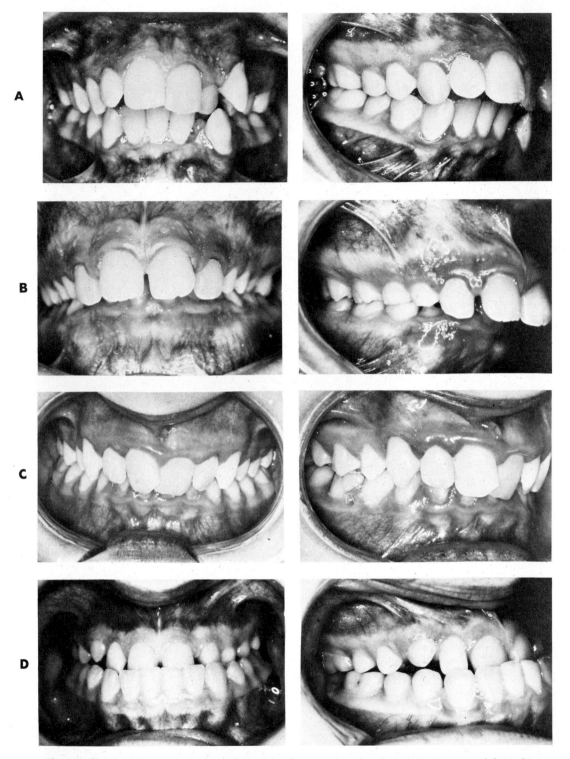

Figure 24–7   Clinical examples of Angle's classes of malocclusion (anterior and lateral views). **A**, Class I. **B**, Class II, division I. **C**, Class II, division 2. **D**, Class III.

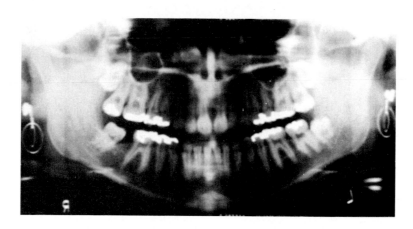

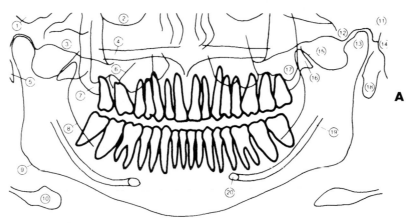

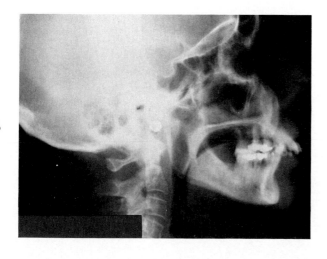

① Middle Cranial Fossa	⑪ Glenoid Fossa
② Orbit	⑫ Articular Eminence
③ Zygomatic Arch	⑬ Mandibular Condyle
④ Palate	⑭ Vertebra
⑤ Styloid Process	⑮ Coronoid Process
⑥ Septa in Maxillary Sinus	⑯ Pterygoid Plates
⑦ Maxillary Tuberosity	⑰ Maxillary Sinus
⑧ External Oblique Line	⑱ Ear Lobe
⑨ Angle of Mandible	⑲ Mandibular Canal
⑩ Hyoid Bone	⑳ Mental Foramen

Figure 24-8 **A**, Panoramic radiograph. **B**, Cephalometric radiograph (lateral view). *Continued.*

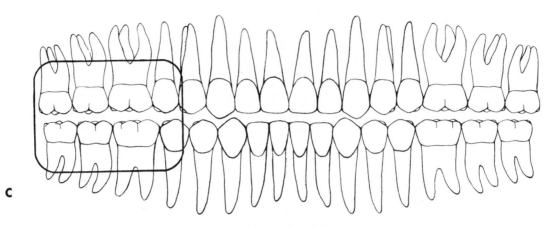

C

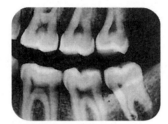

#2 Film

Molar

Figure 24-8, cont'd **C**, Bitewing radiograph technique.

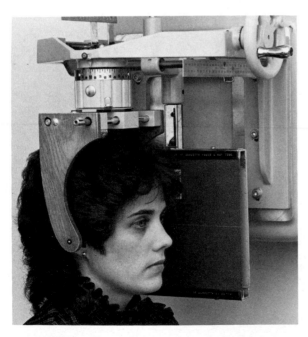

Figure 24-9 Patient positioned in cephalostat.

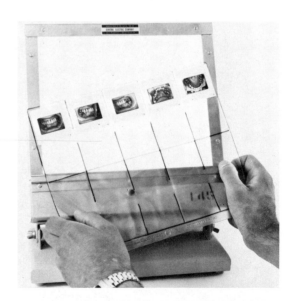

Figure 24-10 Slide holder for storage of slide photographs.

3. Bitewing radiographs (Figure 24-8, *C*)

A **cephalometric radiograph** is taken using a cephalostat. The cephalostat is a unit that holds the patient's head stationary relative to the x-ray source (Figure 24-9). This device allows the dentist to take a series of cephalometric radiographs from a standard position so that the development pattern in the skull can be compared as the patient grows or as treatment is rendered.

⊶ KEY POINT

- Radiographs can be compared over time to assess not only the growth pattern of the patient but also the effect orthodontic therapy is having on skeletal development.

Photography

Photographs are generally considered a mandatory part of the orthodontic patient record. Both intraoral and extraoral views of the patient's head are taken at the diagnostic appointment and at various intervals as treatment progresses. These photographs document the starting point in treatment and visually record the progress of treatment for both the dentist and the patient. Slide photography or photographs can be used. If slides are used, the dates that they were taken can be recorded on the slide mounts for reference (Figure 24-10). A standard photographic series that is taken includes the following:

1. Extraoral
   a. Right lateral view
   b. Front view (not smiling)
   c. Front view (smiling)
2. Intraoral
   a. Right lateral view (teeth occluded)
   b. Front view (teeth occluded)
   c. Left lateral view (teeth occluded)
   d. Maxillary occlusal view (mouth open)
   e. Mandibular occlusal view (mouth open)

Soft tissue retractors and large intraoral mirrors are used to gain access to the intraoral view that is required (Figure 24-11). The air-water syringe is used to dry the teeth just before the photograph is taken, to improve the detail in the picture. A dental assistant can hold these devices with the help of the patient while the orthodontist or another assistant operates the camera. The orthodontist can view patient photographs to analyze tooth relationships, skeletal contours, and the soft tissue configuration of a patient.

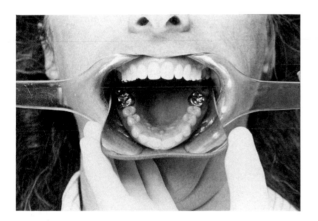

Figure 24-11 Cheek retractors and intraoral photographic mirror in use.

Study Models

A discussion of study models (Figure 24-12) is presented in Chapter 2. It should be emphasized that study models provide the dentist with a unique three-dimensional record of the patient's dentition and contour of the alveolar processes. Study models are the only diagnostic tool a dentist has that permits a view of the lingual aspect of the patient's occlusion. Like photographs, study models can be used to document the starting point of treatment and record the progress of treatment as subsequent sets of models are taken.

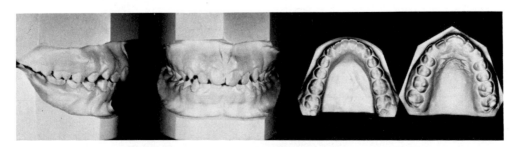

Figure 24-12 Study models.

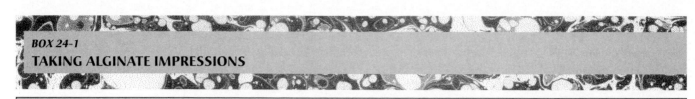

BOX 24-1
TAKING ALGINATE IMPRESSIONS

PROCEDURE	RATIONALE
1. Try each impression tray in patient's mouth. There should be 3 to 4 mm of space between inside of tray and teeth and soft tissue when tray is in place.	1. To determine appropriate size and shape of impression tray.
2. Press soft, rope-shaped utility wax onto edges of trays (see Figure 24-14, *A*). Try trays again to confirm fit.	2. To extend vertical height of impression trays and also improve patient comfort.
3. Instruct patient to rinse vigorously with mouthwash.	3. To remove thick saliva and food particles that can cause voids on surface of impression.
4. Mix alginate material with water for one impression at a time in flexible rubber bowl according to manufacturer's instructions. A wide-bladed spatula is used to press material against side of bowl. Mixing time varies between products but is typically 1 minute (see Figure 24-14, *B*).	4. To create smooth, creamy mix that is free of air bubbles.
5. Load maxillary tray with mixed material. Tray should be loaded in one large increment with wiping motion of spatula.	5. To prevent trapping air in material.
6. Wipe off excess material to level of waxed edges of tray, using a wet finger (see Figure 24-14, *C*).	6. To smooth surface of material.
7. With patient seated in upright position, use left index finger to retract patient's right cheek. Insert loaded tray into patient's mouth, and use it to push patient's left cheek out of the way (see Figure 24-14, *D*).	7. To place impression tray inside patient's mouth.

PROCEDURE	RATIONALE
8. Once tray is in patient's mouth, center it over teeth. Press posterior border of tray up against posterior border of hard palate (see Figure 24-14, *E*).	8. To center impression tray over patient's teeth and to form a seal with alginate against soft tissues in posterior area of mouth.
9. While maintaining this palatal seal, rotate anterior portion of tray upward slowly over teeth. Use your left hand to lift patient's lips and cheeks out of the way as tray is seated completely (see Figure 24-14, *F*).	9. This retraction process allows alginate material to flow upward into vestibular fold areas.
10. Pull upper lip over anterior portion of tray (see Figure 24-14, *G*). Average working time to accomplish this task is 1½ minutes. After this, material begins to set.	10. To shape anterior border of impression once tray is seated.
11. Check posterior border of tray. If necessary, excess material can be quickly wiped away with a mouth mirror. Have patient tip head downward and breathe through nose as material sets. Hold tray in place until material has completely set.	11. To be sure that excess material has not escaped from tray into patient's throat area.
12. Once material has set, remove tray by placing finger along lateral border of tray and pushing down (see Figure 24-14, *H*).	12. To break seal formed by set material so impression tray can be removed.
13. Remove tray from patient's mouth, rinse it with room temperature water, and wrap it in moist paper towel.	13. Rinsing impression removes oral fluids or debris. Impression must be kept moist to prevent evaporation of water and subsequent distortion.

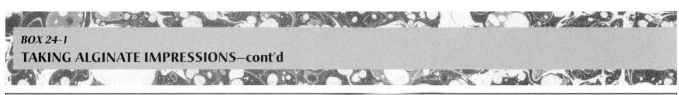

> **BOX 24-1**
> **TAKING ALGINATE IMPRESSIONS—cont'd**

PROCEDURE	RATIONALE	PROCEDURE	RATIONALE
14. Rinse patient's mouth, or have patient rinse at sink.	14. To remove residual impression material.	18. Once material has set, impression can be removed by lifting posterior border of tray upward (see Figure 24-14, *K*).	18. To break seal in order to remove impression tray.
15. Mandibular impression is taken in similar manner. In addition to instructing patient to retract lips and cheeks when tray is inserted in mouth, have patient lift tongue (see Figure 24-14, *I*).	15. Lifting tongue permits material to register impression of lingual aspect of alveolar process.	19. Rinse patient's mouth, or have patient rinse at sink.	19. To remove residual impression material.
16. Once mandibular tray is centered, press down posterior border behind last molars. Anterior portion of tray is rotated downward as lips and cheeks are retracted.	16. To form seal with alginate material and soft tissue in posterior region.	20. Impressions should be poured as soon as possible.	20. To prevent evaporation of water from impression and subsequent distortion.
17. After tray is seated, pull lower lip up over anterior portion of impression tray (see Figure 24-14, *J*).	17. To fully seat impression tray.	21. A wax bite is fabricated by instructing patient to bite into softened horseshoe-shaped piece of wax until teeth are in maximum occlusion. Allow wax to cool and then remove it from patient's mouth. It is stored with study models until it is needed during model trimming (see Figure 24-14, *L*).	21. To aid in trimming phase of study model fabrication.

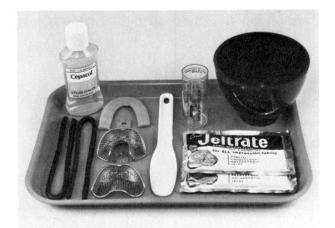

Figure 24-13 Armamentarium for alginate impression-taking.

Making study models

Since many states permit dental assistants to take impressions for study models, a description of a technique is presented here.

Materials required for impression taking
(Figure 24-13)
1. Alginate material
2. Impression trays selected to fit the size and shape of the patient's dental arches (various types are available)
3. Rope-style utility wax: used to extend the vertical height of the trays to record the shape of the alveolar processes and to increase patient comfort
4. Flexible rubber bowl with a stiff wide-bladed spatula for mixing

Impression technique. Box 24-1 and Figure 24-14 describe the technique and rationale for creating study model impressions.

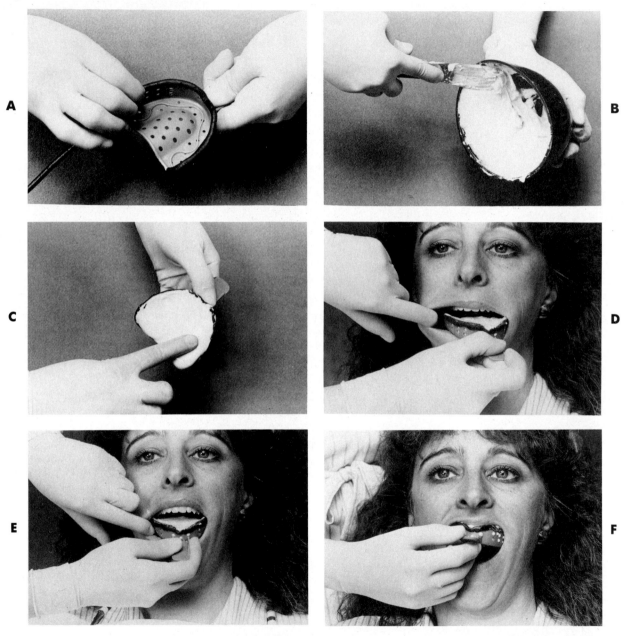

Figure 24-14   Alginate impression–taking. **A**, Bordering tray with utility wax. **B**, Mixing alginate. **C**, Smoothing surface of alginate. **D**, Inserting tray. **E**, Seating posterior border of tray. **F**, Lifting tray upward into place.

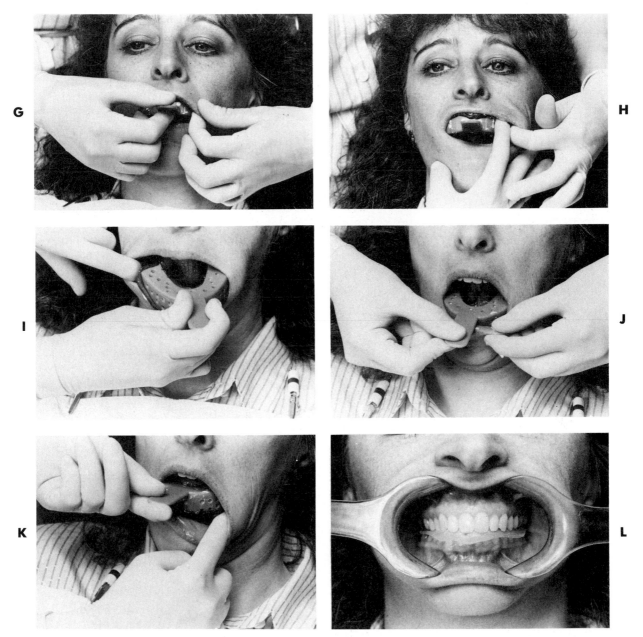

Figure 24–14, cont'd   **G**, Positioning lip over seated tray. **H**, Releasing seal when alginate has set. **I**, Inserting lower tray. **J**, Positioning lip over seated tray. **K**, Releasing seal when alginate has set. **L**, Taking wax bite.

Alginate impressions should be disinfected by immersion in an appropriate disinfectant. Figure 24-15 demonstrates disinfection of the flexible bowl, spatula, alginate impression, and wax bite.

Trimming study models

Some dental offices use specific measurement guidelines for trimming study models. Figure 24-16 describes a sample technique for trimming study models without using measurement guidelines.

Clinical Evaluation

The clinical examination of a patient provides the dentist with an opportunity to analyze the patient's skeletal and facial profile, speech, swallowing pattern, and jaw movements, as well as to examine the patient's dentition. The occlusion is classified at the examination appointment and recorded along with other clinical data.

Dentition Stage

Table 24-1 outlines the development and eruption sequence of the dentition according to age.

Primary dentition stage

The function of the primary dentition is to aid in mastication and speech, provide favorable aesthetics, and aid in guiding the eruption of the permanent teeth into proper position.

The **primary dentition stage** usually begins at 6 months of age, with the eruption of the mandibular central incisors, and ends at approximately 6 years, when the first permanent tooth erupts. The primary dentition has usually completed eruption by 24 months of age. The typical sequence* of eruption of primary teeth is central incisors, lateral incisors, first molars, canines, and second molars.

While the child is in the primary dentition stage, the permanent teeth are developing in the jaws. At approximately 6 years the onset of the mixed dentition stage is marked by the loss of a primary tooth and eruption of the first permanent molars or permanent incisors. The permanent first molars erupt just distal to the primary second molars. An important function of the primary second molars is to help to guide these permanent first molars into proper position during their eruption. If a second primary molar is lost prematurely because of dental caries, it cannot serve this important function. Then the permanent first molar can erupt out of position, and a discrepancy in the occlusion results (Figure 24-17). Such discrepancies might include shifting of the first permanent

*The mandibular member of each type of tooth usually erupts before its maxillary counterpart; for example, the mandibular central incisors erupt before the maxillary central incisors. Next the mandibular lateral incisors erupt and so on.

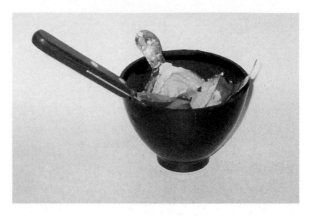

Figure 24-15 Disinfection of upper and lower alginate impressions with flexible bowl, spatula, and wax bite.

molar in a mesial direction, which can cause occlusal interferences with opposing teeth, impaction of the developing second premolar, or the eruption of the second premolar in an abnormal position (ectopic eruption). This situation emphasizes the need to preserve the primary teeth whenever possible.

Mixed dentition stage

Once the first permanent tooth erupts, the child has a dentition that is a combination of permanent and primary teeth, hence the name **mixed dentition stage**.

As the child ages and jaw growth occurs, the primary teeth are exfoliated (shed) and replaced by newly erupted permanent teeth. The **exfoliation** of the primary teeth occurs in the same sequence as the eruption of their permanent replacements. The eruption sequence of the permanent teeth usually follows the order shown in Box 24-2.

The mixed dentition is probably the most critical stage of development for the permanent occlusion. The timing of the exfoliation of a primary tooth is rather critical, especially in the posterior areas. A posterior primary tooth must be kept in place until the permanent tooth that replaces it is ready to erupt. If a posterior primary tooth is lost too soon, the teeth adjacent to the tooth can drift into the empty space (Figure 24-18). If this occurs, there is insufficient space left in the dental arch for the proper eruption of the underlying permanent tooth when it is time for it to erupt. The result is that the permanent tooth may erupt in an undesirable position (be malposed), or it may not erupt at all (be impacted) because of insufficient space in the arch. Thus a discrepancy in the occlusion results.

A similar situation can result if a primary tooth is not exfoliated just before the eruption of its permanent replacement. These "overretained" primary teeth may prevent the eruption of the underlying permanent tooth or cause it to erupt in an undesirable (ectopic) position.

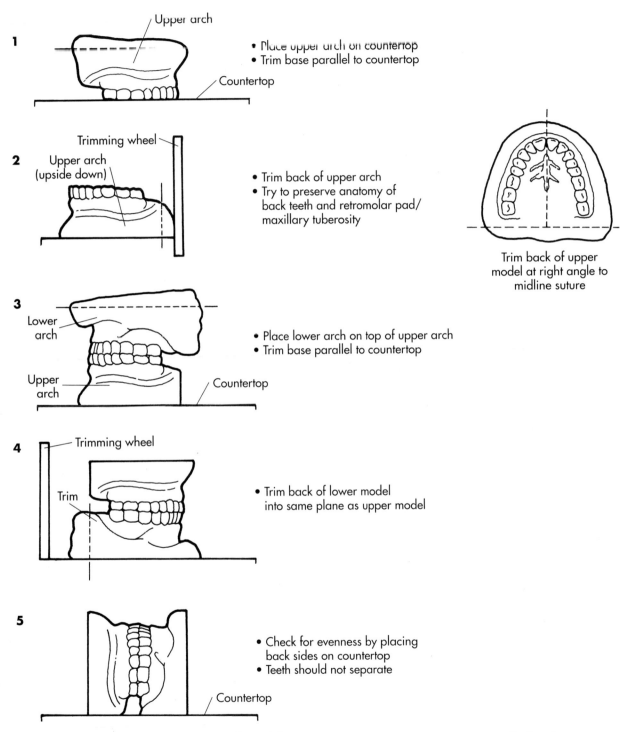

Figure 24-16 Trimming study models.

Continued.

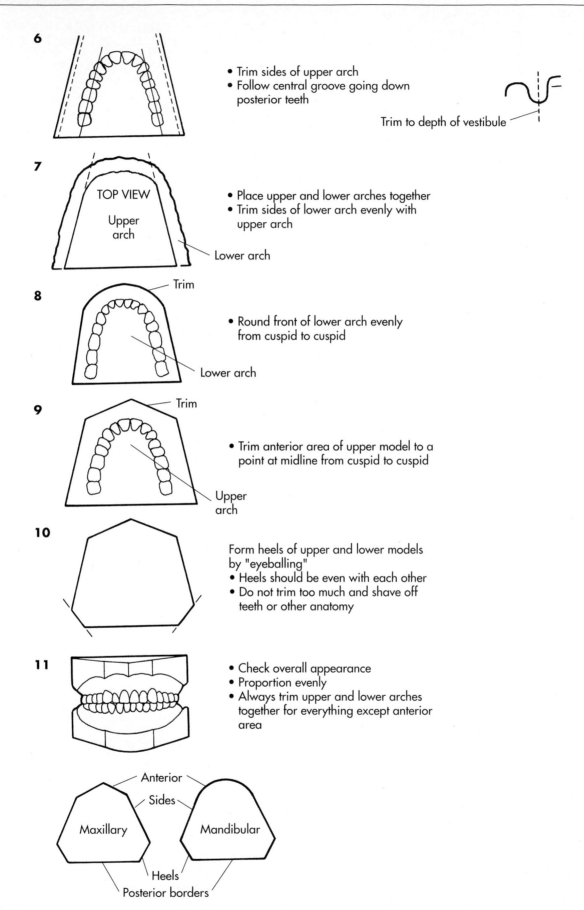

6
- Trim sides of upper arch
- Follow central groove going down posterior teeth

Trim to depth of vestibule

7
TOP VIEW
Upper arch
Lower arch
- Place upper and lower arches together
- Trim sides of lower arch evenly with upper arch

8
Trim
Lower arch
- Round front of lower arch evenly from cuspid to cuspid

9
Trim
Upper arch
- Trim anterior area of upper model to a point at midline from cuspid to cuspid

10
Form heels of upper and lower models by "eyeballing"
- Heels should be even with each other
- Do not trim too much and shave off teeth or other anatomy

11
- Check overall appearance
- Proportion evenly
- Always trim upper and lower arches together for everything except anterior area

Anterior
Sides
Maxillary
Mandibular
Heels
Posterior borders

Figure 24-16, cont'd Trimming study models.

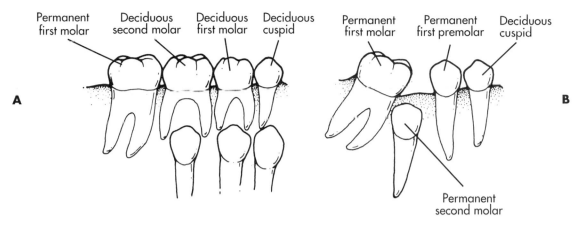

Figure 24-17 Effects of premature loss of primary second molar. **A,** Normal eruption. **B,** Loss of primary second molar results in mesial shifting of permanent first molar. This position change can prevent normal eruption of permanent second premolar.

Table 24-1 Chronology of human dentition

Tooth	Hard tissue formation begins	Amount of enamel formed at birth	Enamel completed	Eruption	Root completed
DECIDUOUS DENTITION					
Maxillary					
Central incisor	4 mo, in utero	Five sixths	1½ mo	7½ mo	1½ yr
Lateral incisor	4½ mo, in utero	Two thirds	2½ mo	9 mo	2 yr
Cuspid	5 mo, in utero	One third	9 mo	18 mo	3¼ yr
First molar	5 mo, in utero	Cusps united	6 mo	14 mo	2½ yr
Second molar	6 mo, in utero	Cusp tips still isolated	11 mo	24 mo	3 yr
Mandibular					
Central incisor	4½ mo, in utero	Three fifths	2½ mo	6 mo	1½ yr
Lateral incisor	4½ mo, in utero	Three fifths	3 mo	7 mo	1½ yr
Cuspid	5 mo, in utero	One third	9 mo	16 mo	3¼ yr
First molar	5 mo, in utero	Cusps united	5½ mo	12 mo	2¼ yr
Second molar	6 mo, in utero	Cusp tips still isolated	10 mo	20 mo	3 yr
PERMANENT DENTITION					
Maxillary					
Central incisor	3-4 mo	—	4-5 yr	7-8 yr	10 yr
Lateral incisor	10-12 mo	—	4-5 yr	8-9 yr	11 yr
Cuspid	4-5 mo	—	6-7 yr	11-12 yr	13-15 yr
First bicuspid	1½-1¾ yr	—	5-6 yr	10-11 yr	12-13 yr
Second bicuspid	2-2¼ yr	—	6-7 yr	10-12 yr	12-14 yr
First molar	At birth	Sometimes a trace	2½-3 yr	6-7 yr	9-10 yr
Second molar	2½-3 yr	—	7-8 yr	12-13 yr	14-16 yr
Third molar	7-9 yr	—	12-16 yr	17-21 yr	18-25 yr
Mandibular					
Central incisor	3-4 mo	—	4-5 yr	6-7 yr	9 yr
Lateral incisor	3-4 mo	—	4-5 yr	7-8 yr	10 yr
Cuspid	4-5 mo	—	6-7 yr	9-10 yr	12-14 yr
First bicuspid	1¾-2 yr	—	5-6 yr	10-12 yr	12-13 yr
Second bicuspid	2¼-2½ yr	—	6-7 yr	11-12 yr	13-14 yr
First molar	At birth	Sometimes a trace	2½-3 yr	6-7 yr	9-10 yr
Second molar	2½-3 yr	—	7-8 yr	11-13 yr	14-15 yr
Third molar	8-10 yr	—	12-16 yr	17-21 yr	18-25 yr

From Logan WHG, Kronfeld R: Development of the human jaws and surrounding structures from birth to the age of fifteen years, *J Am Dent Assoc* 20:379, 1933. Copyright by the American Dental Association. Reprinted by permission.

BOX 24-2
ERUPTION SEQUENCE OF PERMANENT DENTITION

PERMANENT TEETH	PRIMARY TEETH REPLACED
Mandibular first molars } Maxillary first molars }	None; erupt distal to primary teeth
Mandibular central and lateral incisors	Mandibular central and lateral incisors
Maxillary central incisors	Maxillary central incisors
Maxillary lateral incisors	Maxillary lateral incisors
Mandibular canines	Mandibular canines
Mandibular first premolars	Mandibular first molars
Maxillary first premolars	Maxillary first molars
Mandibular second premolars	Mandibular second molars
Maxillary second premolars	Maxillary second molars
Maxillary canines	Maxillary canines
Mandibular second molars } Maxillary second molars } Mandibular third molars } Maxillary third molars }	None; erupt distal to primary teeth as jaws grow

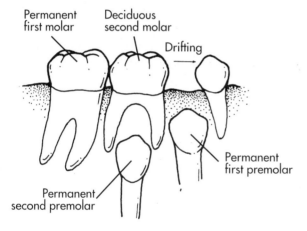

Figure 24-18 Effect of premature loss of primary first molar.

The dentist plays an important role in supervising the development of the occlusion of the child by ensuring that the timing of the exfoliation of primary teeth corresponds with the eruption of their permanent counterparts. Caries prevention and restoration of decayed primary teeth become an integral part of preservation of the primary teeth so that the transition from the primary to the permanent dentition proceeds smoothly.

Typically the mixed dentition stage ends when the child is approximately 11 or 12 years old, with the eruption of the permanent maxillary canines that replace the remaining primary canines.

Permanent dentition stage

The **permanent dentition** should be completed by 25 years of age, with the eruption of the third molars. However, in a great number of patients these teeth never erupt, since sufficient jaw space is lacking. The principal goal of dentistry is to preserve permanent teeth for a lifetime.

INTERCEPTIVE ORTHODONTICS

Interceptive orthodontics describes treatment procedures designed to intercept orthodontic problems that may worsen if left untreated. Not all orthodontic problems can be prevented. However, many can be prevented entirely or at least minimized in terms of severity through interceptive measures.

Interceptive orthodontic procedures have limitations. They do not, for example, alter skeletal disharmonies resulting from an undesirable growth pattern of the child. These procedures can be viewed as treatment techniques that assist in the development of a normal occlusion or at least in minimizing the severity of a developing malocclusion.

Some common interceptive orthodontic techniques include the use of space maintainers or the control of oral habits that could contribute to malocclusion, such as thumb sucking or tongue thrusting.

Space Maintenance

If the child loses primary teeth prematurely, the dentist must prevent adjacent teeth from drifting into the empty (edentulous) space. This is accomplished through the use of devices called **space maintainers**. These are either removable or fixed appliances that provide a brace between the teeth adjacent to the edentulous space (Figure 24-19. Space maintainers are kept in place until the eruption of the underlying permanent tooth begins. Thus they perform a function of the primary tooth had it not been lost prematurely.

When primary molars are lost on both sides of the arch, a bilateral space maintainer can be used (Figure 24-20).

Sometimes the dentist may not see a child until long after a primary tooth is lost and the adjacent teeth have drifted into the edentulous space. Space maintainers could have prevented this. After drifting has occurred, the dentist is faced with the challenge of regaining the space.

The ideal management of a child's developing occlusion is to preserve the primary teeth by vigorous caries prevention. Restoration of carious primary teeth is the second best approach to preservation of the primary teeth. If a primary tooth is lost prematurely, the third best procedure is use of space-maintainer appliances to prevent drifting and space loss. Finally, the least desirable management procedure is to regain the lost space caused by drifting.

CORRECTIVE ORTHODONTICS

Corrective orthodontic procedures are designed to reduce the severity of an existing malocclusion or to eliminate it entirely. Sometimes it is necessary to carry out both interceptive and corrective procedures simultaneously.

No attempt is made here to discuss this subject in detail, because the subject is so vast that it would require several volumes. However, it is helpful for an orthodontic assistant to know some of the principles employed in corrective orthodontics, as well as the appliances, instruments, and materials used.

Considerations Before Treatment

The ultimate goal of **corrective orthodontics** is to establish a favorable functional occlusion. Orthodontic treatment also generally improves the patient's appearance by repositioning the teeth and altering facial profiles within certain limits.

The orthodontist must have the cooperation of the patient and the patient's parents if treatment is to achieve maximum success. This is a critical factor, since corrective orthodontic treatment is often a long-term procedure that may require several years to complete. The patient's willingness to wear appliances as directed by the orthodontist and to maintain a high level of oral hygiene will help to ensure a favorable treatment outcome.

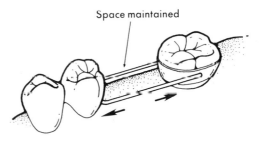

Figure 24-19   Band and loop type of space maintainer.

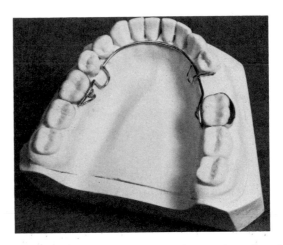

Figure 24-20   Bilateral space maintainer and regainer, loop lingual appliance.

Principles of Tooth Movement

Orthodontic appliances are devices that apply forces to a tooth or set of teeth to cause them to move to a specific position in the jaw. Orthodontic appliances can also be used to hold or retain teeth in a specific position in the dental arch. Orthodontic appliances move teeth by applying force to the crown of the tooth that is transmitted down the root to the periodontium. A tooth moves in response to force according to the following theory.

Tooth movement is a result of a remodeling process of the alveolus, or socket, in which the tooth rests. When force is applied to the tooth, some portions of the periodontal ligament are compressed, as are the capillaries in the ligament. This compression causes the bone in the area to resorb (break down) through the action of bone-removing cells called **osteoclasts**. At the same time, some areas of the periodontal ligament are stretched, which stimulates another type of cell, called **osteoblasts**, to produce new bone in these areas. As the areas of the alveolus under compression resorb, the tooth moves. The areas under tension produce new bone behind the moving tooth. Thus the alveolus is remodeled as the tooth is being moved (Figure 24-21).

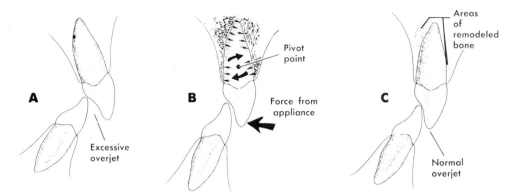

Figure 24-21 Tooth movement when tipping forces are applied to crown of tooth. **A**, Excessive overjet in anterior region. **B**, Force from orthodontic appliance causes tooth to tip lingually around imaginary pivot point. Alveolar bone is remodeled by cellular action as force is maintained. **C**, When teeth are in desired position, retainer is used to maintain position until bone remodeling is complete.

> ➡ **KEY POINT**
> ▪ **Bone resorption** occurs faster than bone formation; thus it does not take long to move a tooth in the arch. However, the bone around the tooth must be allowed to form in order to stabilize the tooth in its new position.

This is a simplified example, but the principle is the same in more complex tooth movements. The key to successful tooth movement is related to the following factors:

1. *Magnitude of force.* The optimum amount of force required to move a tooth is unique to the patient and individual tooth. Too much force can be destructive to the root of the tooth or inhibit tooth movement. Reassessment of the force applied to a tooth is a continuing concern of orthodontists.
2. *Duration of application.* The length of time force is applied influences the rate of tooth movement. Orthodontists vary in opinion about how long force should be applied to teeth.
3. *Direction of force.* Appliance design is carefully accomplished so that force can be directed properly to cause a tooth to move into the intended position.
4. *Distribution of force.* Some teeth, such as small, single-rooted teeth, move more readily in response to force than larger or multirooted teeth. In complex cases the orthodontist uses this principle to distribute forces to smaller teeth, using multirooted teeth for anchorage for the orthodontic appliance.

ORTHODONTIC APPLIANCES
Removable Appliances

Orthodontists have access to a multitude of orthodontic appliances that can reposition teeth. These appliances are generally divided into removable and fixed appliance categories.

Removable appliances can be removed and reinserted by the patient. The three categories of removable appliances are functional appliances, retainers, and positioners.

Functional Appliances

Functional appliances are generally used in the earlier phase of orthodontic treatment to make changes (both skeletal and tooth) as the patient is growing, thus minimizing the treatment that the patient will receive with fixed appliances.

There are many types of functional appliances, and which one is used depends on the needs of the patient and the preference of the dentist.

An **activator** is a functional appliance that is used to expand the upper arch, to reduce excessive overbite, to make changes in skeletal growth, and for minor tooth movement. There are several types of activators (Figure 24-22). The most commonly used activator is the Bionator. The Frankel appliance and the Bio-modulator are other activators.

Activators can also be used to expand the width of the maxillary arch. A threaded screw type of device is placed in the activator, and the patient is given a special screwdriver that is used to expand the width of the activator. When the activator is expanded, pressure is exerted on the palatal arch to create expansion of the arch. The Hamilton expansion activator, the Herbst expansion acti-

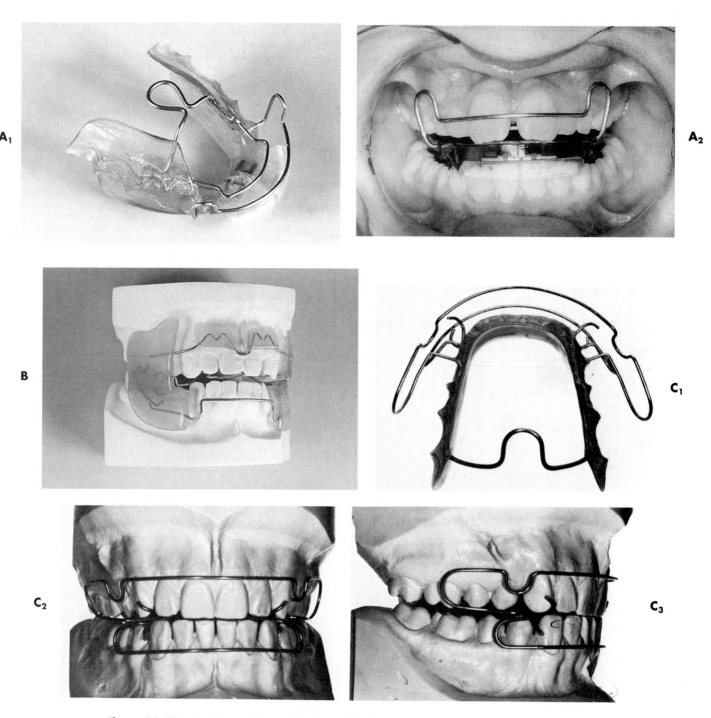

Figure 24-22 Activators. **A₁–A₂**, Bionator, **B**, Frankel appliance, **C₁–C₃**, Basic Bio-modulator.

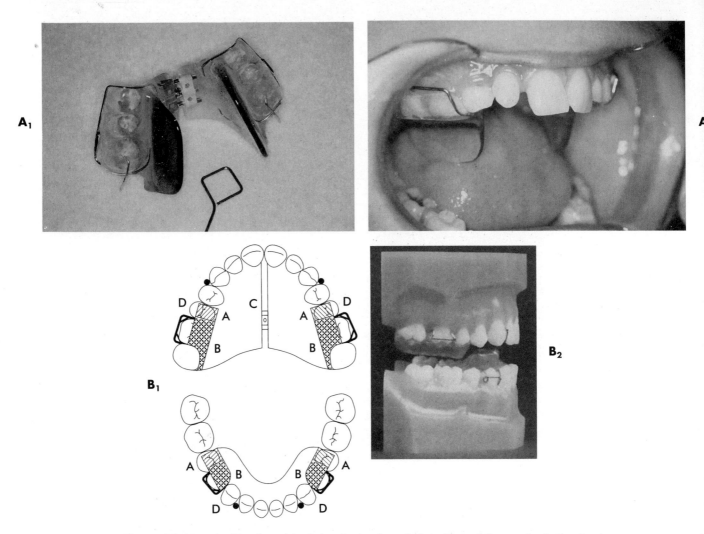

Figure 24-23 **A₁**, Hamilton bonded activator from below. Lingual flanges in dark extend toward viewer. Palatal jackscrew is partly open. **A₂**, Bonded Hamilton expansion activator on maxillary arch. Lingual guiding flanges extend toward lower arch and tongue. **B₁**, Standard twin blocks (Clark). **B₂**, Clark twin block appliances.

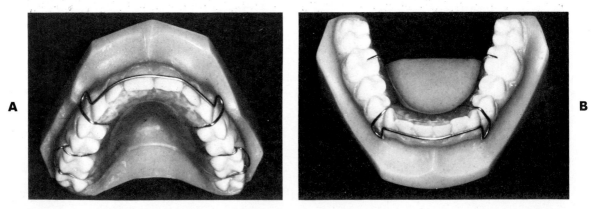

Figure 24-24 Hawley appliance (removable). **A**, Maxillary. **B**, Mandibular.

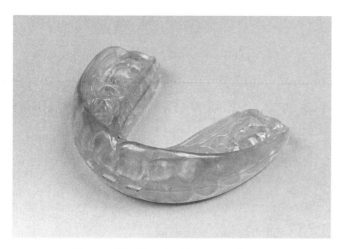

Figure 24-25   Positioner appliance.

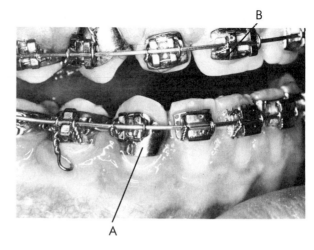

Figure 24-26   Attachments for fixed orthodontic appliances. *A,* Circumferential band. *B,* Direct bonded bracket.

vator, and the Clark expansion activator are all types of **expansion activators** (Figure 24-23).

Retainers

Retainers are usually fabricated from metal and acrylic and are used after fixed appliance treatment to hold the teeth in the desired position until the teeth become stable in the newly remodeled alveolus. The Hawley retainer (Figure 24-24) is one of the most commonly used retainers.

Positioners

Positioners (Figure 24-25) are fabricated from soft plastic and are usually used immediately after the fixed appliances are removed to maintain the alignment of the teeth and also for minor tooth positioning.

> ◆ **KEY POINT**
> ▪ Activators are usually used before fixed appliance treatment. Retainers and positioners are usually used after fixed appliance treatment.

Fixed Appliances

Fixed appliances (nonremovable) are attached to the patient's teeth with a dental cement and circumferential bands or by direct bonding (Figure 24-26). These appliances cannot be removed by the patient. Fixed appliances offer the orthodontist the advantage of more precise control over tooth movement than is possible with removable appliances. Since the patient cannot remove the appliance, treatment is less interrupted by the patient. With removable appliances, interruptions in treatment can re-

sult from the loss of the appliance or from the patient not wearing it.

Severe orthodontic cases are often treated with a variety of appliances, such as removable appliances, intraoral fixed appliances, and combination extraoral headgear appliances (Figure 24-27).

Common elements of fixed appliances

Since orthodontic appliances are tailored to the individual patient's needs, a complete description of all appliances and their variations cannot be presented within this chapter. However, some of the basic elements of some common fixed appliances will be described here.

Orthodontic bands (Figure 24-28) are circumferential stainless steel bands that are fitted to individual teeth. They serve to connect the appliance to the teeth when cemented into place. Orthodontic bands are available in a variety of sizes for each tooth in the dental arches.

Brackets (Figure 24-29) are attachments that are welded to the orthodontic bands. Brackets hold the arch wire in place and transmit the force of the arch wire to the teeth. Some brackets are designed to be bonded directly to the teeth using an acid-etch composite material, thus eliminating the need for an orthodontic band.

Arch wires (Figure 24-30) are the principal guide portions of the fixed appliance. The arch wire is attached to the brackets by wire ligatures or elastic ligatures on either the facial or lingual aspect of the teeth, depending on the task being performed by the wire. Arch wires function either to move individual teeth or to hold them in a desirable fixed position. Forces from the arch wire are transmitted to the teeth through the brackets.

Ligatures are fine wires that are used to tie, or ligate, the arch wire to the brackets. There are elastic ligatures available that can be used in conjunction with lighter-gauge arch wires.

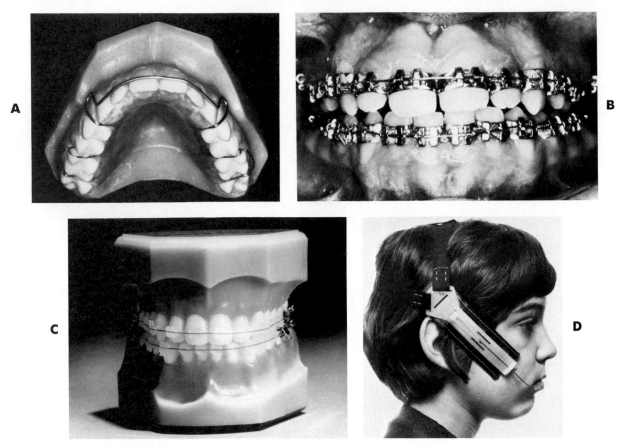

Figure 24-27   Common orthodontic appliances. **A**, Removable appliance. **B**, Circumferential band fixed appliance. **C**, Tooth-shaded, ceramic-bracket fixed appliance. **D**, Extraoral appliance.

(**C** Courtesy Unitek Corp, Monrovia, Calif.)

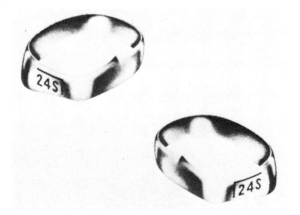

Figure 24-28   Molar bands with number code for identification.

(Courtesy Rocky Mountain Orthodontics, Denver.)

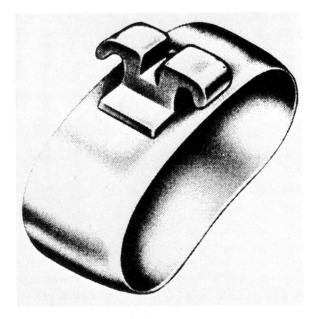

Figure 24-29   Circumferential band with edgewise style of bracket.

(Courtesy Rocky Mountain Orthodontics, Denver.)

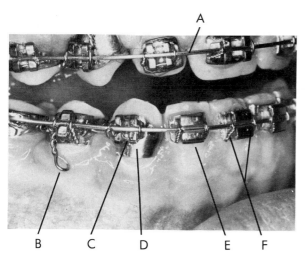

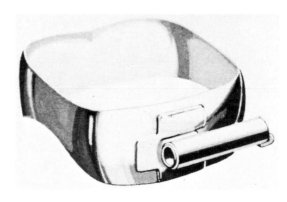

Figure 24-32   Buccal tube.

(Courtesy TP Laboratories Inc, La Porte, Ind.)

Figure 24-30   Common elements of fixed orthodontic appliance. *A,* Arch wire. *B,* Loop for elastics. *C,* Bracket. *D,* Circumferential band. *E,* Direct bonded bracket. *F,* Ligature.

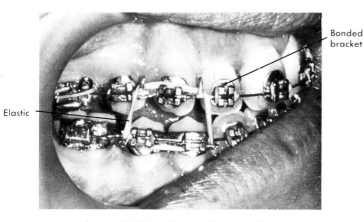

Figure 24-31   Elastics (intermaxillary).

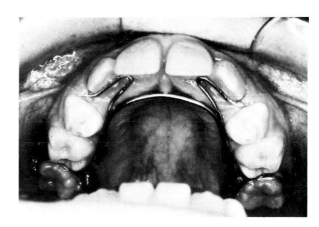

Figure 24-33   Finger springs attached to fixed appliance.

Elastics (Figure 24-31) are rubber bands that are used to exert force on teeth. Elastics are available in different lengths and thicknesses. They are frequently used to exert force between upper and lower teeth to improve occlusal relationships. Special buttons or hooks are attached to orthodontic bands and serve as connectors for the elastics.

Buccal tubes (Figure 24-32) are essentially hollow-channeled brackets that are attached to molar bands. They serve as anchors for facial arch wires.

Finger springs (Figure 24-33) are used to apply forces to individual teeth. They can be soldered to the main arch wire or used on removable appliances.

Coil springs (Figure 24-34) are attached to the arch wire. They are available in two types. **Open coil springs** are compressed between teeth and exert a pushing force on these teeth when the coil attempts to return to its normal length. **Closed coil springs** are stretched between teeth and exert a pulling force on selected teeth.

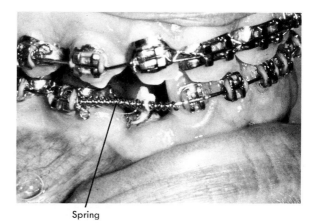

Figure 24-34   Coil spring.

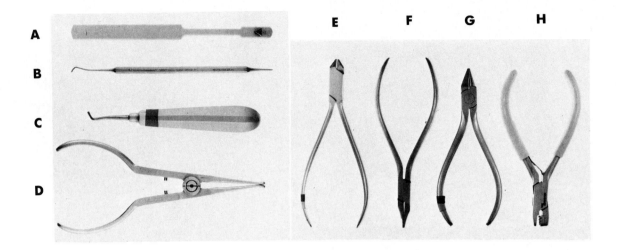

	Instrument	Principal use
A	Band seater	Seat posterior circumferential bands
B	Ligature director	Tuck twisted ends of ligature wire into embrasure areas
C	Band adaptor	Seat and adapt circumferential bands to teeth
D	Ligature-tying pliers (Coons)	Tying stainless steel ligature wires
E	Three-jaw (prong) pliers	Wire and clasp bending and adjusting
F	Tweed loop pliers	Forming loops and springs in wire
G	"Bird beak" pliers	Most common pliers for small wire and spring forming
H	De La Rosa pliers	Contouring wire loops and molar band material

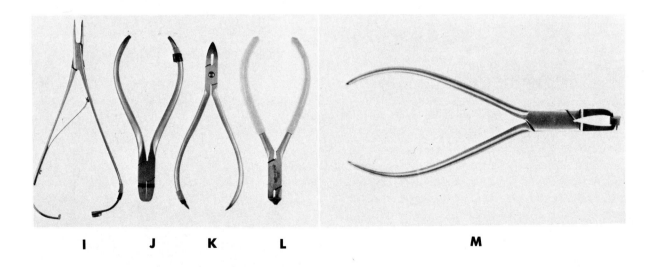

	Instrument	Principal use
I	Mathieu needle holder	Tying stainless steel ligatures and placing elastic ligatures
J	Tweed arch-bending pliers	Forming and shaping square or rectangular arch wires
K	Ligature cutter	Removing or trimming stainless steel ligatures
L	Distal-end cutter	Cutting distal ends of arch wires
M	Posterior-band removing pliers	Removing posterior circumferential bands

Figure 24–35   Common orthodontic hand instruments.

Extraoral Devices

Orthodontists can use **headgear devices** such as the one shown in Figure 24-27, *D*, either to hold teeth in a specific position or to move the maxillary molar teeth in a distal direction. Forces from these devices are transmitted to an intraoral appliance. The force to be applied to the teeth can be adjusted by altering the tension of the adjustment straps on the extraoral device.

COMMON ORTHODONTIC HAND INSTRUMENTS

Although a wide variety of hand instruments is used in orthodontic treatment, only a few of the most common ones are shown in Figure 24-35.

SPECIAL DUTIES FOR ORTHODONTIC ASSISTANT

Many states permit dental assistants to perform certain tasks that are unique to orthodontic treatment. Regardless of whether the assistant can or cannot actually perform these tasks, it is helpful for dental assistants to be familiar with the techniques described here.

Separators

Orthodontic separators are devices that are placed between the teeth to move them apart. This creates space between teeth so that orthodontic bands can be fitted properly.

Elastic separators

Elastic separators are commonly used today because they apply a constant force as the teeth move apart and are the most comfortable for the patient. Elastic separators also cause less trauma to soft tissue. Box 24-3 describes the technique for placing elastic separators with elastic separating pliers. The technique is demonstrated in Figure 24-36.

An alternative technique that can be used to place elastic separators with dental floss or tape is described in Box 24-4.

Elastic separators are removed before the orthodontic bands are placed. The scaler end of the Schure instrument is used to hook and lift the elastic separator from between the contact.

Steel spring separators

In some patients with tight contacts it is difficult to place elastic separators. In these instances a **steel spring separator** (TP brand) can be used (Figure 24-37). Box 24-5 describes how these separators are placed. Figure 24-38 shows the springs in place.

To remove steel spring separators, simply grasp either the coiled portion of the spring or its longest leg, and lift the spring in an occlusofacial direction.

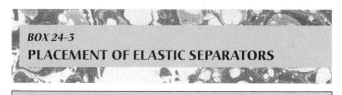

BOX 24-3
PLACEMENT OF ELASTIC SEPARATORS

PROCEDURE	RATIONALE
1. Place elastic separator on separating plier, squeeze plier handles, and stretch separator to length of approximately ½ to ¾ inch.	1. To prepare elastic separator for placement between teeth.
2. Using buccolingual sawing movement similar to that used in placement of dental floss, carefully pass cervical aspect of separator through contact area (see Figure 24-36).	2. To place elastic separator between teeth without breaking separator.
3. While cervical aspect of separator is placed under contact area, occlusal aspect is allowed to remain above contact area. Relax tension on separator, and remove separating plier. Elastic separator should completely encircle contact area.	3. Elastic separator exerts mild force between teeth and causes them to move apart over 1 to 3 weeks.

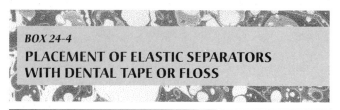

BOX 24-4
PLACEMENT OF ELASTIC SEPARATORS WITH DENTAL TAPE OR FLOSS

PROCEDURE	RATIONALE
1. Cut two strands of dental tape or floss into lengths of approximately 20 inches, and thread each strand of floss through separator.	1. Floss strands serve as handles for assistant to stretch separator while it is placed between teeth.
2. Stretch separator slightly, and using seesaw motion insert separator between teeth.	2. To place elastic separator between teeth without breaking separator.
3. Once separator completely encircles interproximal contact, pull floss out of separator.	3. To remove floss that was used to place separator between teeth.

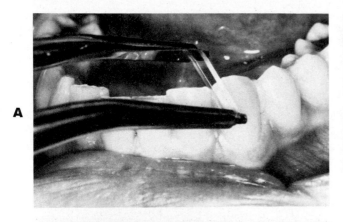

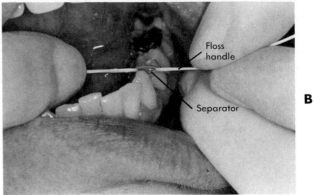

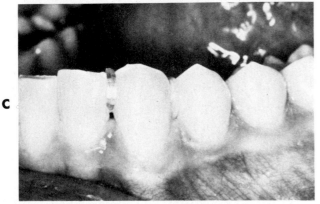

Figure 24-36 Placement of elastic separators. **A**, Use of separating pliers. **B**, Use of floss handles. **C**, Separators in place.

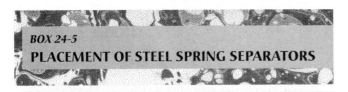

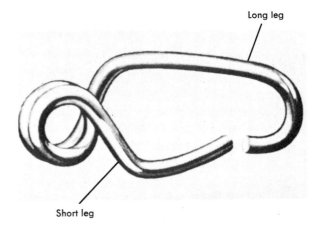

Figure 24-37 Steel separating spring.
(Courtesy TP Laboratories, Inc, La Porte, Ind.)

BOX 24-5
PLACEMENT OF STEEL SPRING SEPARATORS

PROCEDURE	RATIONALE
1. Grasp shortest leg of spring with No. 139 pliers. Place opening of spring over contact area (see Figure 24-38, *A*).	1. Steel spring separator will be placed in lingual-to-buccal direction.
2. Hook long leg of spring separator to slip under contact. Release short leg and allow it to move under contact (see Figure 24-38, *B*).	2. For correct placement of steel spring separator.
3. Use finger to push on coil of separator.	3. To check if separator is snugly wrapped around contact.

Trial Sizing of Orthodontic Bands

Orthodontic bands are available in a large assortment of sizes for each tooth in the dental arches. Most manufacturers label the bands on the mesial aspect for easy orientation and identification.

As an example a Unitek brand of band might have a code RL 36 printed on the mesial aspect of the band. This band is selected from the lower molar section of a com-

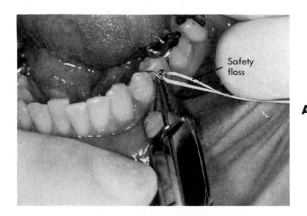

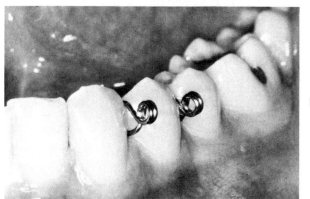

Figure 24-38 Placement of separating springs. **A**, Use of No. 139 plier. **B**, Springs in place.

plete kit of orthodontic bands. The code RL 36 simply means that it is a right lower molar band, size 36. This band could be placed on the appropriate tooth of the patient's study model to determine the approximate size range. If the band appears to be close in size, the following steps are taken to select the appropriate band:

1. Remove the elastic separators around the tooth to be banded.
2. Orient the selected band properly over the tooth with the mesial aspect toward the midline. Push the band to see if it will fit around the tooth, using finger pressure initially.
3. If the band will not fit around the tooth at all, select a larger size.
4. Once a band is selected that will move cervically on the tooth, a band pusher (seater) is used to push the band into place. The band pusher is carefully placed alternately on each corner of the band, and slight pressure is applied in a cervical direction to push the band slowly into place. The patient can assist by gently biting on the band pusher to drive the band into place a little at a time as the band pusher is moved from one corner to another (Figure 24-39).
5. A properly fitted band should fit tightly around the tooth so that it does not rock when buccal and lingual forces are applied to the band.

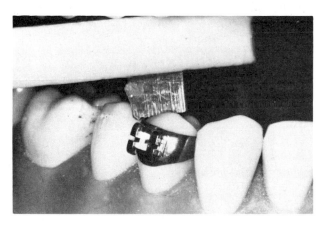

Figure 24-39 Trial sizing of orthodontic band. Band pusher is used to seat band by pushing on occlusal edges of band and on bracket.

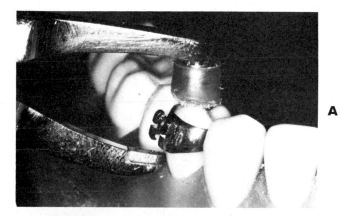

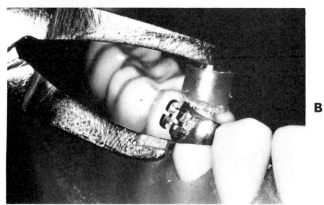

Figure 24-40 Use of band-removing pliers. **A**, Correct placement. **B**, Lifted band.

6. The band can be removed with band-removing pliers. The pointed beak of the pliers is placed on the occlusal surface on the buccal aspect of the tooth. The other hammerlike beak engages the cervical edge of the band. The pliers handles are squeezed, and the band is lifted from the tooth (Figure 24-40).

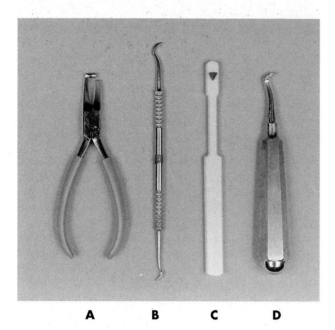

A **B** **C** **D**

Figure 24-41   Instruments used to adapt orthodontic bands. **A**, Band-removing pliers. **B**, Schure No. 349 scaler. **C**, Band biter. **D**, Band seater/adapter.

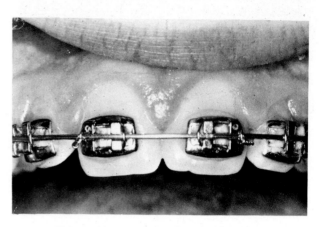

Figure 24-42   Direct bonded brackets.

7. The band is stored and identified. The dentist can make final adjustments in the adaptation of the band once all the bands have been selected. The same procedure is repeated for each tooth to be banded. Trial bands that are not selected are sterilized before they are returned to the storage container.

Cementation of Orthodontic Bands

The armamentarium for the cementation of orthodontic bands is shown in Figure 24-41.

At the band cementation appointment the steps outlined in Box 24-6 are carried out. The role of the assistant in the cementation procedure will vary according to state laws and the preference of the orthodontist.

Direct Bonding of Orthodontic Brackets

In recent years the direct bonding of orthodontic brackets (Figure 24-42) to the teeth has become popular. This technique eliminates the need for an orthodontic band in cases that are suitable for this technique. Direct bonding offers the advantage of not having bands pass between the teeth. This consumes space that could be used for tooth movement.

Special brackets are used for direct bonding. The armamentarium for direct bonding is shown in Figure 24-43. The procedure for direct bonding of brackets is described in Box 24-7.

Placement of Arch Wires

Some states permit dental assistants to place the arch wire in the attachments on the bands and ligate them in place after the orthodontist has fabricated the appropriate arch wires. The armamentarium for placement of the arch wire and ligatures is shown in Figure 24-44. Elastic or stainless steel ligatures are used to ligate the arch wire to the brackets or bands.

The decision to use either elastic or stainless steel ligatures depends on the preference of the dentist or the position of the teeth or both. Elastic ligatures can be used if the bracket and arch wire are in close alignment with each other. If the bracket is not in close alignment with the arch wire, the elastic ligature may not be able to stretch and hold the arch wire in place so a stainless steel ligature may be used.

Elastic ligature method

Small, round, elastic ligatures can be used to anchor the arch wire to the brackets. Placement of elastic ligatures is easy and frequently used. Many elastic ligatures come in a variety of colors that offer adolescent and teen patients a colorful alternative to plainer colors.

Box 24-8 describes the placement of the arch wire with the use of elastic ligatures. Figure 24-45 demonstrates the technique.

Stainless steel ligature method

Stainless steel ligatures are small preformed wires that are used to ligate the arch wire to the brackets. The method for placement of these ligatures is described in Box 24-9 and demonstrated in Figure 24-46.

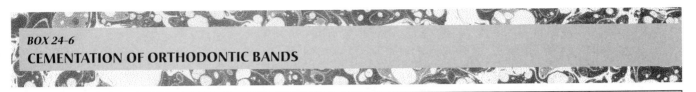

BOX 24-6
CEMENTATION OF ORTHODONTIC BANDS

PROCEDURE	RATIONALE
1. After separators are removed, teeth are polished with rubber cup and pumice.	1. To remove plaque and debris from tooth surfaces.
2. Utility wax is placed over attachments (brackets and so on).	2. To prevent cement from becoming lodged in them during cementation.
3. Some orthodontists cover occlusal aspect of band with small piece of autoclave tape during band placement.	3. This helps contain cement in band as it is carried into position on tooth.
4. Teeth to receive bands are isolated with cotton rolls.	4. To maintain dry working field.
5. Zinc phosphate cement is mixed according to technique described in Chapter 19. Final consistency should be thicker than used to cement gold restorations, although not the dough-like consistency required for cement base. Some orthodontists use a "frozen slab" technique to mix cement. Glass mixing slab is stored in a freezer and wiped dry just before mixing cement.	5. Cement should be a thick, sticky, creamlike consistency. Cold slab helps slow down set of cement so that more bands can be cemented from one mix of cement.

PROCEDURE	RATIONALE
6. Fill interior of each band completely with cement and deliver them to orthodontist on glass slab for placement on teeth. Teeth must be as dry as possible before band placement.	6. Several bands can be cemented at a time.
7. Band pusher is used on bands as previously described.	7. Band pusher is used to seat bands completely.
8. Cement is allowed to set completely before removing excess cement.	8. It is easier to remove cement in large pieces after it has hardened.
9. After cement has set, excess cement can be removed with sickle end of Schure instrument or with an ultrasonic scaler.	9. To remove excess cement.
10. Same procedure is repeated until all bands are in place.	10. To complete banding procedure.
11. After all excess cement is removed, protective wax can be removed from brackets.	11. To prepare bands for arch wire placement.

Usually wire ligatures are tied mesial to the bracket for better access. However, if a tooth is malposed and the distal end of the bracket is located further away from the arch wire than the mesial, the tie should be placed on the distal. The force applied by the ligature helps to move the tooth into alignment with the arch wire (Figure 24-47).

It is well recognized that orthodontists use a wide range of appliances, techniques, and instruments to accomplish the same task. The procedures described here should only serve as examples for the orthodontic assistant and not as the last word on how these procedures must be done.

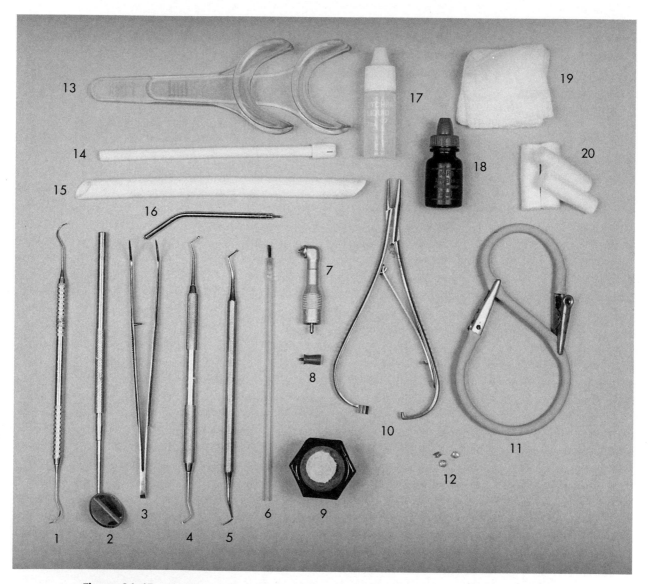

Figure 24-43   Armamentarium for bonding orthodontic brackets. *1,* Explorer; *2,* mirror; *3,* cotton pliers; *4,* spoon excavator; *5,* ball burnisher; *6,* disposable brush; *7,* prophylaxis angle; *8,* prophylaxis cup; *9,* dappen dish with flour of pumice; *10,* hemostat; *11,* napkin chain; *12,* brackets; *13,* mouth props; *14,* saliva ejector; *15,* high-volume evacuator tip; *16,* air/water tip; *17,* etching liquid; *18,* bonding material; *19,* 2 x 2–inch gauze; *20,* cotton rolls.

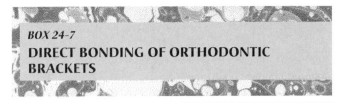

BOX 24-7

DIRECT BONDING OF ORTHODONTIC BRACKETS

PROCEDURE	RATIONALE
1. Teeth being bonded are polished with rubber cup and pumice wetted with water. Do not use prophylaxis paste because some ingredients can interfere with bonding process.	1. To remove plaque and debris from tooth surface.
2. Cotton rolls and cheek retractors are placed.	2. To isolate area, maximize visibility, and prevent moisture contamination.
3. Surfaces of teeth that receive brackets are acid etched with etching agent.	3. Acid etching creates microscopic roughness on tooth surface, which enhances bonding process.
4. Etching agent is rinsed away, and teeth are dried thoroughly and again isolated with cotton rolls.	4. Acid etch must be completely rinsed away before actual bonding of bracket to tooth.
5. Bonding agent is applied to bracket and placed on etched areas of teeth. Brackets are then positioned on teeth and held into place until bond agent is set completely.	5. Bracket must be held in place until bond agent is set; otherwise, bracket may move out of desired position.
6. Bonding agent that appears on facial surface of tooth and is not supporting bracket can be removed with Schure instrument before bond agent is completely set.	6. To remove excess bond agent.

BOX 24-8

PLACEMENT OF ARCH WIRE USING ELASTIC LIGATURES

PROCEDURE	RATIONALE
1. Insert ends of arch wire into buccal tubes that are attached to bands on last molars on both sides of arch.	1. To anchor two ends of arch wire.
2. Press arch wire into horizontal slots in brackets along entire arch.	2. To fully seat arch wire.
3. Start on anterior teeth and work toward posterior. Loop elastic over bracket using hemostat to grasp ligature. Elastic is pulled over bracket in cervical-occlusal direction (see Figure 24-25). Same procedure is continued until all brackets are ligated to arch wire.	3. To ligate arch wire to bracket.
4. Distal end cutters are used to cut off any excess arch wire that extends beyond distal ends of buccal tubes.	4. To prevent soft tissue trauma to patient from excess arch wire poking out of buccal tube.

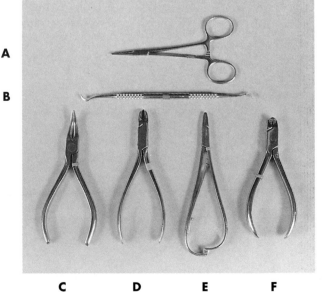

Figure 24-44 Instruments used to place wires and ligatures. **A**, Weingart utility pliers. **B**, Ligature cutter. **C**, Ligature-tying pliers. **D**, Distal end-cutting pliers. **E**, Schure No. 349 scaler. **F**, Hemostat.

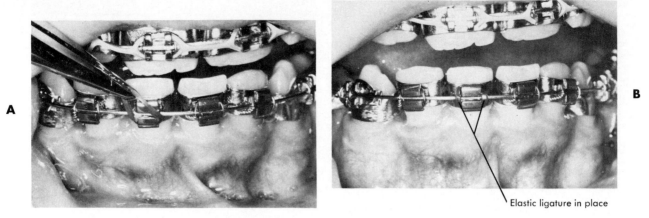

Figure 24-45 Placement of elastic ligature. **A,** Stretching elastic over bracket. **B,** Elastic in place.

Elastic ligature in place

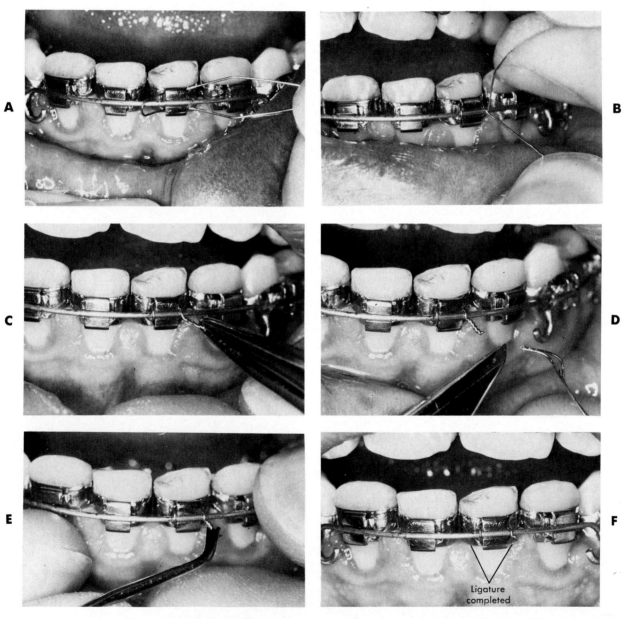

Ligature completed

Figure 24-46 Placement of stainless steel ligatures. **A,** Inserting preformed ligature wire into bracket. **B,** Initial twist of ligature over arch wire. **C,** Final twist of ligature while pulling wire with hemostat in facial direction. **D,** Cutting ligature. **E,** Tucking ligature, **F,** Completed ligature knot tucked into embrasure.

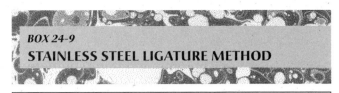

BOX 24-9
STAINLESS STEEL LIGATURE METHOD

PROCEDURE	RATIONALE
1. Insert ends of arch wire into buccal tubes attached to bands on last molars on both sides of arch.	1. To anchor two ends of arch wire.
2. Press arch wire into horizontal slots in brackets along entire arch.	2. To fully seat arch wire.
3. Starting on anterior teeth and working posteriorly, bend ligature wire to about 45-degree angle.	3. To make it easier to slide ligature wire around bracket.
4. Slide narrow preformed portion of wire in distal-to-mesial direction. Cross ends of ligature wire facial to arch wire (see Figure 24-46).	4. Crossing ends of ligature wire will hold wire in place.
5. Use hemostat to grasp crossed ligature wire, and lock beaks together. Rotate hemostat to twist ends of ligature wire together. CAUTION: Patient's eyes should be closed or protected with safety glasses while wire is twisted to prevent injury to eye from long strands of ligature wire.	5. Hemostat is used to quickly twist ligature wire.
6. All ligatures are placed in same manner and cut to length of 3 to 4 mm.	6. Before cutting, wire ligatures are long and excess needs to be removed.
7. Bend wire "pigtail" into embrasure area. Run finger over placed ligatures.	7. Bending the wire "pigtail" prevents trauma to inside of cheek and lip. Running finger over area also helps to check for sharp ends that need to be tucked in better.
8. Distal end cutters are used to cut off any excess arch wire that extends beyond distal ends of buccal tubes.	8. To prevent soft tissue trauma to patient from excess arch wire poking out of buccal tube.

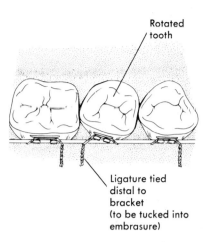

Figure 24-47 Ligature tied on end of bracket farthest from arch wire to aid in aligning malposed tooth.

BIBLIOGRAPHY

Finkbeiner BL, Johnson CS: *Mosby's comprehensive dental assisting: a clinical approach*, St Louis, 1995, Mosby.

Graber TM, Vanarsdall Jr RL: *Orthodontics: current principles and techniques*, ed 2, St Louis, 1994, Mosby.

Proffit WR: Contemporary orthodontics, ed 2, St Louis, 1993, Mosby.

QUESTIONS—Chapter 24

1. The _____ of the steel spring separator should be grasped with the No. 139 pliers to place the separator between the teeth.
   a. Long leg
   b. Short leg
   c. Coil

2. The vertical overlap of the incisal edges of upper anterior teeth over the incisal edges of lower anterior teeth is called:
   a. Overbite
   b. Overjet
   c. Crossbite
   d. Open bite

3. If the lower teeth overlap the upper teeth labially or buccally, this is called:
   a. Overbite
   b. Overjet
   c. Crossbite
   d. Open bite

4. Fine wires or elastic rings that are used to tie the arch wire to the brackets are called:
   a. Brackets
   b. Elastics
   c. Ligatures
   d. Coil springs

5. Attachments that are welded to the orthodontic bands or directly bonded to the tooth to hold the arch wire in place and transmit the force of the arch wire to the teeth are called:
   a. Brackets
   b. Elastics
   c. Ligatures
   d. Coil springs

6. Elastic separators can be placed with which of the following:
   a. Floss
   b. Elastic separating pliers
   c. Bird-beak pliers
   d. *a* and *b*
   e. *b* and *c*

7. Stainless steel ligatures are placed with which of the following instruments:
   a. Bird-beak pliers
   b. De La Rosa pliers
   c. Band pusher
   d. Hemostat

8. Which of the following is a soft plastic device used immediately after fixed appliances are removed to maintain the alignment of the teeth?
   a. Positioner
   b. Expansion activator
   c. Activator
   d. Retainer

9. A Bionator is a(n):
   a. Positioner
   b. Expansion activator
   c. Activator
   d. Retainer

10. The resorption of bone is accomplished by cells of the body called:
    a. Neurons
    b. White blood cells
    c. Osteoblasts
    d. Osteoclasts

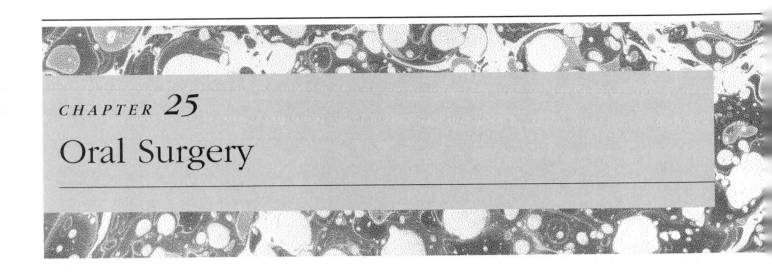

CHAPTER 25

Oral Surgery

KEY TERMS

Alveolitis

Alveoloplasty

Biopsy

Biopsy report

Bone files

Complex extraction

Dental implants

Excisional biopsy

Exfoliative cytology

Exodontia

Extraction elevators

Extraction forceps

Healing cap

Hemostat

Immediate complete
    dentures

Implant abutment

Incisional biopsy

Irrigation syringes

Lesion

Luxation

Mucoperiosteum

Needle holders

Osseointegration

Palliative therapy

Periosteal elevators

Periosteum

Prognosis

Rongeur forceps

Root picks

Routine extraction

Smear

Surgical chisel

Surgical curette

Surgical mallet

Surgical scalpel

Surgical scissors

Surgical suction tip

Suture needles

Tissue forceps

Tooth sectioning

Universal extraction
    forceps

The American Board of Oral Surgery defines oral surgery as follows: "Oral surgery is that part of dental practice which deals with diagnosis, the surgical and adjunctive treatment of the diseases, injuries, and defects of the human jaws and associated structures."

An oral surgeon is a dentist who has had extensive graduate training in surgery that involves the orofacial re-gion. The practice is limited to these tasks. As is the case with other dental specialties, oral surgery is a vast, complicated subject. This is particularly true of oral surgery because of the complex anatomy of the orofacial region and the proximity of the oral region to vital structures.

The amount of oral surgery done in a general dental practice is dictated by the interest and training of the general practitioner. Some dentists devote a great deal of their practice to surgery, whereas others prefer to refer all surgery patients to an oral surgeon.

This chapter introduces the dental assistant to some of the common surgical instruments and procedures that are most likely to be encountered in a general practice.

COMMON SURGICAL INSTRUMENTS

Scalpel

The **surgical scalpel** is a time-honored instrument used by all surgeons. Its sharp blade allows the dentist to make a precise incision into soft tissue with the least amount of trauma to the tissue.

The scalpel handle and common disposable blade styles are shown in Figure 25-1.

Surgical Curette

The **surgical curette** (Figure 25-2) is an instrument of many uses. It is scoop shaped with sharp edges, and it looks like a large spoon excavator. This design makes it an ideal instrument for scraping the interior of cavities in bone or other tissues. This curettage of such cavities is done to remove abnormal tissue or to obtain material for diagnostic purposes. The curette is also commonly used to sever the epithelial attachment of the gingiva around the tooth during the first step in tooth extraction.

Surgical curettes are available in different sizes, as shown in Figure 25-2.

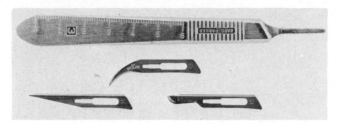

Figure 25-1 Surgical scalpel and disposable blades. *Left to right:* No. 11, No. 12B, No. 15.

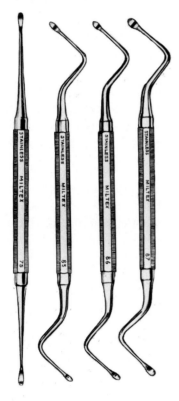

Figure 25-2 Surgical curettes.
(Courtesy Miltex Instrument Co, New York.)

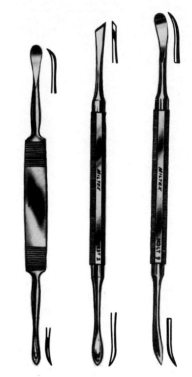

Figure 25-3 Periosteal elevators.
(Courtesy Miltex Instrument Co, New York.)

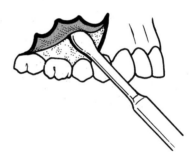

Figure 25-4 Periosteal elevator used to reflect mucoperiosteum.

Periosteal Elevator

Periosteal elevators (Figure 25-3) are varied in design, yet they all have the same basic function. They are used to separate the **periosteum** (fibrous covering of bone) from the bone surface. A secondary function of these instruments is to retract the mucoperiosteum so that access can be maintained to the underlying bone (Figure 25-4). The **mucoperiosteum** is the soft tissue covering of the jaws that consists of both the mucosa and the periosteum. The assistant is often called on to perform this retraction for the surgeon.

Surgical Mallet and Chisels

There is frequently the need for removal of some bone to facilitate removal of a tooth or to reshape the jaws. This can be accomplished with sharp **surgical chisels** tapped lightly with a **surgical mallet** (Figure 25-5).

An alternate method of removing bone is through the use of a conventional-speed straight handpiece with a surgical bur. Irrigation of the surgical site with an irrigation syringe filled with sterile saline solution is necessary to remove the loosened bone fragments. The syringe is used jointly along with the suction tip to flush and evacuate

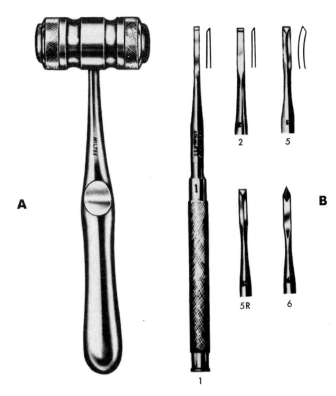

A

B

2   5

5R   6

1

Figure 25-5   **A,** Surgical mallet. **B,** Surgical chisels.
(Courtesy Miltex Instrument Co, New York.)

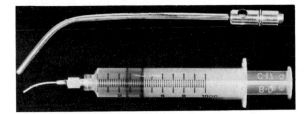

Figure 25-6   Surgical suction tip and irrigation syringe.

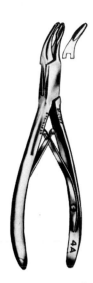

Figure 25-7   Rongeur forceps.
(Courtesy Miltex Instrument Co, New York.)

the surgical site. This procedure maintains the visibility for the operator.

> **KEY POINT**
> - If the handpiece is used for bone removal, continuous drops of saline solution should be allowed to drop from the syringe onto the bur. This prevents the bur from clogging and reduces frictional heat that can damage the remaining bone.

Suction Tips and Irrigation Syringes

Suction tips and **irrigation syringes** (Figure 25-6) are used jointly to clear the surgical site in the manner just described.

The smaller-sized suction tips are more favorable for the removal of blood from the surgical site than the larger sizes used in operative and restorative dentistry.

The suction tip should be dipped in a container of sterile saline solution periodically during a procedure to prevent it from clogging with clotted blood.

Rongeur Forceps

The **rongeur forceps** (Figure 25-7) is a nipperlike instrument that is used to trim alveolar bone. It is widely used after multiple extractions for alveoloplasty (to shape the edentulous ridge). Several styles and sizes are available.

Bone Files

Whenever an alveoloplasty is needed after the extraction of teeth or in the correction of poorly shaped edentulous ridges, the rongeur is most often used to remove the majority of the undesirable bone. **Bone files** are used to accomplish minor bone removal and to smooth the surface of the bone before wound closure.

Bone files are available in different shapes and sizes (Figure 25-8).

Extraction Elevators

Extraction elevators are leverlike instruments that are used to apply controlled force against a tooth to luxate (loosen) it in its alveolus (Figure 25-9). It is not uncom-

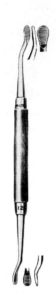

Figure 25-8 Bone file.
(Courtesy Miltex Instrument Co, New York.)

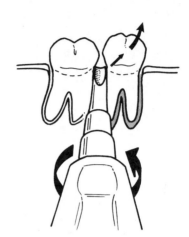

Figure 25-9 Straight elevator used to displace tooth from socket.

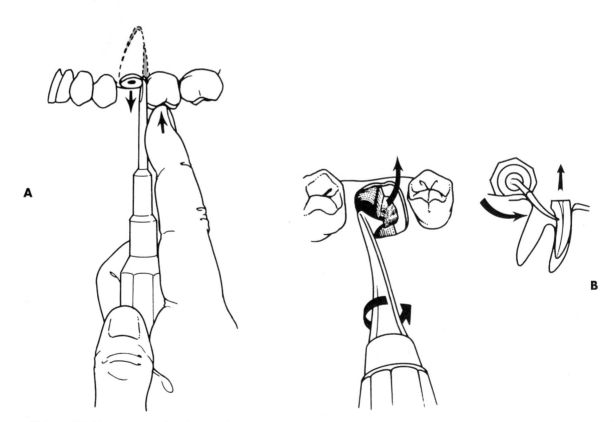

A

B

Figure 25-10 **A,** Straight elevator used as wedge to displace tooth from its socket. **B,** Triangular elevator used to retrieve root from socket.

mon for certain teeth to be completely removed with only an elevator.

Other uses of extraction elevators include the removal of residual root fragments (Figure 25-10).

Elevators are available in different styles and sizes (Figure 25-11).

Extraction Forceps

Extraction forceps are plierslike instruments that are used to grasp the tooth and deliver it from its alveolus. As with most other instruments, the individual dentist has a preference for certain forceps designs. The many choices available are divided into two basic groups. One group of forceps is designed for use on a specific group of teeth on one side of the mouth (e.g., right maxillary molars). The other group is referred to as **universal extraction forceps**. These forceps are designed for a specific group of teeth on either side of the same arch (e.g., right and left maxillary molars).

Some of the most common extraction forceps in use today are listed in Tables 25-1 and 25-2 according to their area of use.

Table 25-1 Common extraction forceps for maxillary teeth

Teeth	Forceps number	Description
Anterior	No. 1 (Figure 25-12)	Universal forceps for incisor and canine teeth
Premolars	No. 150 (Figure 25-13)	Universal forceps principally used for maxillary premolars but that can be used for incisor teeth
First and second molars	No. 18R and 18L (Figure 25-14)	Forceps specifically used for maxillary first and second molars; *R* indicates that this forceps is used on patient's right side, and *L* indicates use on left side
Third molars	No. 210 (Figure 25-15)	Universal forceps used for maxillary third molars; bayonet design assists in gaining access to third molar area

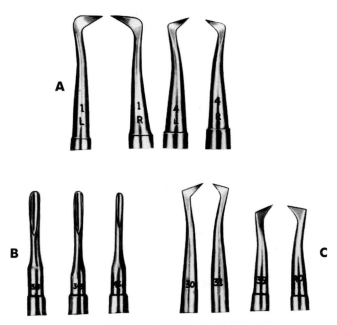

Figure 25-11   Extraction elevators.   **A,** Seldin (curved). **B,** Seldin (straight). **C,** Cryer.

(Courtesy Miltex Instrument Co, New York.)

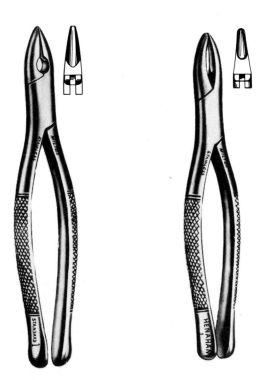

Figure 25-12   Standard No. 1 forceps for upper incisors and canines.

(Courtesy Miltex Instrument Co, New York.)

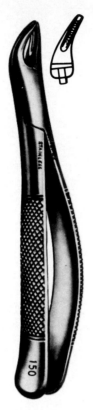

Figure 25-13   Standard No. 150 forceps used primarily for maxillary premolars.

(Courtesy Miltex Instrument Co, New York.)

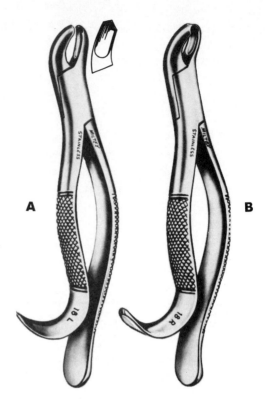

Figure 25-14   Standard No. 18R and No. 18L forceps. **A,** No. 18L for upper left first and second molars. **B,** No. 18R for upper right first and second molars.

(Courtesy Miltex Instrument Co, New York.)

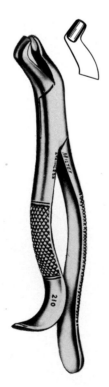

Figure 25-15   Standard No. 210 universal forceps for upper third molar.

(Courtesy Miltex Instrument Co, New York.)

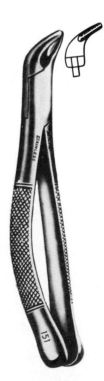

Figure 25-16   Standard No. 151 universal forceps for lower incisor, premolar, and large root fragments.

(Courtesy Miltex Instrument Co, New York.)

Table 25-2 Common extraction forceps for mandibular teeth

Teeth	Forceps number	Description
Anterior	No. 151 (Figure 25-16)	Universal forceps convenient for use on both anterior and premolar teeth; design is similar to that of No. 150, except beaks are bent at greater angle to handles for better access to lower teeth
First and second molars	No. 15 (Figure 25-17) and No. 16 (Figure 25-18)	Universal forceps designed for mandibular first and second molars; No. 16 forceps is often referred to as "cow horn" because of design of beaks; beaks of No. 16 slide into bifurcation area, which permits positive grasp of tooth; tooth is lifted somewhat from alveolus as beaks are squeezed into bifurcation area
Third molars	No. 222 (Figure 25-19)	Universal forceps that can be used on mandibular third molars; since these teeth often differ in anatomical positions because of lack of arch space, they are frequently extracted with a variety of elevators and forceps; No. 222 is generally used when tooth is in normal vertical position in dental arch

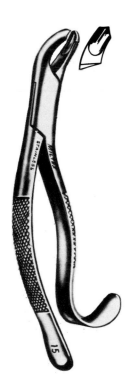

Figure 25-17 Standard No. 15 universal forceps for lower first and second molars.

(Courtesy Miltex Instrument Co, New York.)

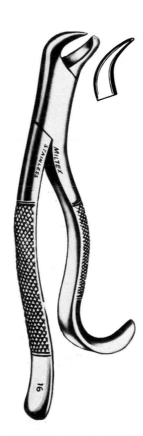

Figure 25-18 Standard No. 16 forceps used for lower first and second molars.

(Courtesy Miltex Instrument Co, New York.)

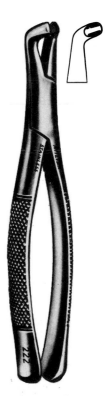

Figure 25-19 Standard No. 222 universal forceps for lower third molar.

(Courtesy Miltex Instrument Co, New York.)

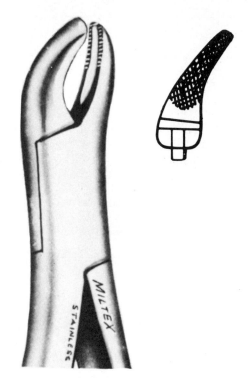

Figure 25-20   Forceps of serrated-beak design.
(Courtesy Miltex Instrument Co, New York.)

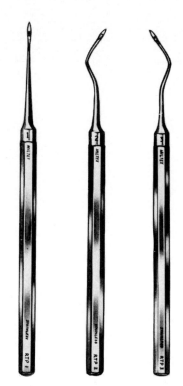

Figure 25-21   Root picks.
(Courtesy Miltex Instrument Co, New York.)

Some forceps manufacturers make forceps with both plain and serrated beaks (Figure 25-20). The style desired must be designated when these instruments are ordered.

Root Picks

Root picks (Figure 25-21) are surgical probes used to remove root fragments that may break away from the tooth during the extraction. Various shapes and sizes are available.

Surgical Scissors

A wide variety of scissors styles is available for surgical use (Figure 25-22). Many are available with smooth and serrated blades. Most of the scissors styles have handles that range in length from approximately 3½ to 6¼ inches.

Scissors are used to trim soft tissue and cut suture material. Maintaining sharpness is important for the maximum effectiveness of these instruments. **Surgical scissors** should never be used for nonsurgical tasks that would dull the cutting blades.

Tissue Forceps

An important principle of surgery is to handle soft tissue as carefully as possible to prevent trauma that may delay healing. The use of **tissue forceps** (Figure 25-23) assists the dentist in handling soft tissue with care during trim-

ming and suturing procedures. They provide a positive grasp of tissue for maximum control during these procedures.

Hemostat

The hemostat (Figure 25-24) is a multipurpose instrument. Its principal use in surgery is to clamp blood vessels that may be severed during a surgical procedure. The narrow beaks are serrated, and the handles have locks on them to hold the beaks in a closed position without force being applied by the operator.

The **hemostat** is a popular instrument used to grasp unwanted tissue that is removed during a surgical procedure. Bone and tooth fragments are conveniently removed from the surgical site with a hemostat.

Hemostats are available in a variety of sizes, with straight and curved beaks, and with different handle lengths.

Suture Needles and Holders

Surgical wounds that involve significant soft tissue incisions must be sutured to control hemorrhage and promote proper healing. Suturing is accomplished using **suture needles** attached to silk thread (Figure 25-25). The needle is guided through the tissue while it is held in the beaks of a needle holder. The needle holder is also used

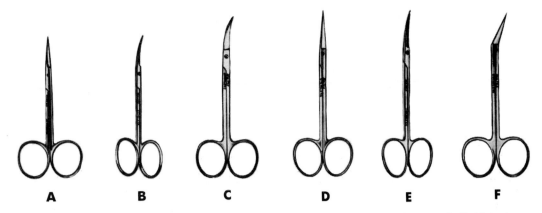

Figure 25-22   Surgical scissors.   **A**, 4-inch straight, delicate. **B**, 4-inch, curved. **C**, 4½-inch, curved sideway, delicate. **D**, 4½-inch, straight delicate. **E**, 4½-inch, curved delicate. **F**, 4½-inch, angular delicate.

(Courtesy Miltex Instrument Co, New York.)

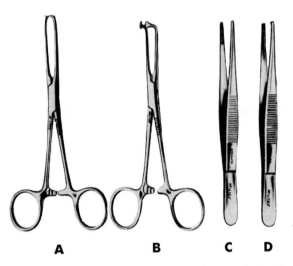

Figure 25-23   Allis tissue forceps, stainless steel, **A**, 6-inch, straight. **B**, 6-inch, angular jaws. **C**, Serrated jaws. **D**, Mouse tooth.

(Courtesy Miltex Instrument Co, New York.)

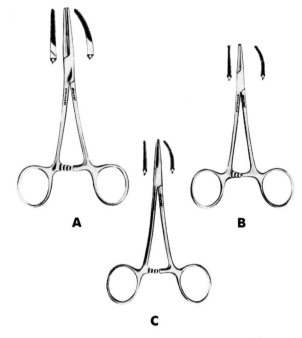

Figure 25-24   Hemostats, stainless steel.   **A**, Kelly, 5½-inch, straight and curved. **B**, Mosquito 5-inch, straight and curved. **C**, Mosquito, 5-inch, straight and curved.

(Courtesy Miltex Instrument Co, New York.)

to handle the needle and surgical thread while it is tied to secure the suture. Surgical scissors are then used to cut the silk thread to proper length.

Probably the most popular suture material used in dentistry is 3-0 black silk that is already sterilized and attached to the end of a suture needle, with the whole assembly packaged in a sterile wrap (Figure 25-26). The needle and excess suture material are discarded into a sharps container after use.

Various needle sizes are available. Intraoral suturing generally requires the use of curved-style needles (Figure 25-26).

Needle holders look and operate much like a hemostat. The beaks are straight with fine serrations. There is a groove on the serrated surface of the beaks for certain styles of suture needles.

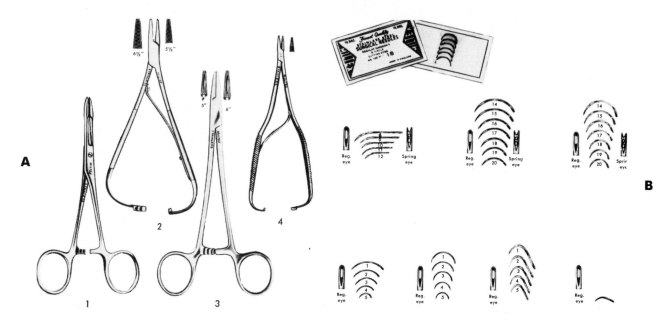

A

1

2

3

4

B

Figure 25-25   **A**, Suture needle holders, stainless steel. **B**, Resealable suture needle assortment.
(Courtesy Miltex Instrument Co, New York.)

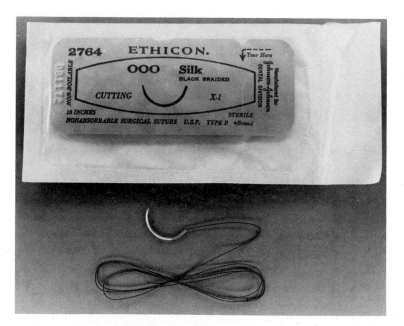

Figure 25-26   Presterilized suture material with attached needle.

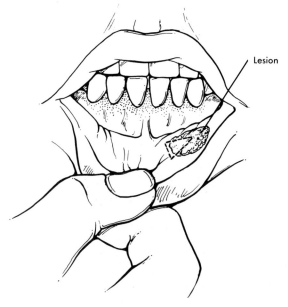

Lesion

Figure 25-27   Incisional biopsy.

ROLE OF ORAL SURGERY ASSISTANT

The oral surgery assistant performs a crucial role in oral surgical procedures. The operator may rely on the dental assistant for pretreatment, treatment, and posttreatment tasks. The following outline gives some duties the dental assistant may perform for an oral surgery procedure:

1. Pretreatment
   a. Sterilize surgical instruments.
   b. Setup treatment room.
   c. Prepare intravenous sedative equipment.
   d. Take vital signs.
   e. Confirm pretreatment medications prescribed by the dentist.
   f. Obtain informed consent from the patient.
2. Treatment
   a. Retract soft tissues.
   b. Evacuate operating field.
   c. Irrigate surgical site with sterile saline.
   d. Perform instrument transfer techniques to exchange surgical instruments.
   e. Monitor vital signs.
   f. Prepare suture material.
3. Posttreatment
   a. Provide postoperative instructions.
   b. Give patient postoperative prescriptions or medications.
   c. Dismiss patient with accompanying escort.
   d. Remove sutures if legally allowed (at a later date).

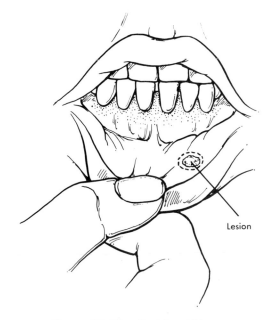

Figure 25-28   Excisional biopsy.

BIOPSY

A **biopsy** is the process of removing tissue from living patients and examining it. The information obtained from a biopsy procedure assists the dentist in arriving at a diagnosis and ultimately predicting the **prognosis** (outcome of the disease).

It is common in dentistry to remove both normal and abnormal tissue from the surgical site for purposes of comparison. The three most common biopsy procedures used in dentistry are the incisional biopsy, the excisional biopsy, and exfoliative cytology (surface scraping).

Incisional Biopsy

A localized site of abnormal tissue is referred to as a **lesion**. **Incisional biopsy** procedures involve the removal of a sample of the lesion for examination. A common method used is to cut a wedge of tissue from the lesion along with some normal adjacent tissue for comparison (Figure 25-27). The sample tissue is placed immediately in a small bottle of 10% formalin solution to preserve it. The wound is sutured, and the patient is dismissed. The tissue is sent to a pathology laboratory for analysis.

The incisional biopsy is generally used when the lesion is large or in a strategic area where complete removal of the lesion would create significant aesthetic or functional impairment. For example, biopsy of a large ulcerated lesion on the lip is done with the incisional method. Complete surgical removal of the lesion is not indicated until a final diagnosis is made, since the lesion may not be malignant and may heal in time on its own without further surgery. Complete surgical removal before a final diagnosis is made may create unnecessary alteration of the lip, caused by loss of tissue and scarring. On the other hand, if laboratory tests show the tissue is malignant, complete surgical removal is warranted.

Excisional Biopsy

Excisional biopsy involves removal of the entire lesion plus some adjacent normal tissue (Figure 25-28). This procedure is done on small lesions where complete excision (removal) would not create significant aesthetic or functional impairment. For example, a small, nonhealing sore on the buccal mucosa may be completely removed during the biopsy, since only a small volume of tissue in a nonstrategic area is being excised. Neither functional nor aesthetic impairment is involved.

Exfoliative Cytology

Another method that is helpful in diagnosing oral lesions is the nonsurgical technique of wiping or scraping the surface of the lesion to gather a sample of cells for microscopic examination. The science of examining cells that are shed (exfoliated) during the scraping process is called **exfoliative cytology**.

This procedure has limited value and is viewed as an adjunct to the surgical techniques just described. The collected cells must be placed on a glass slide and spread out for examination under the microscope. This slide setup is called a **smear**. Probably the best-known exfoliative biopsy is the Papanicolaou smear (Pap smear) that is used especially for detection of cancer of the uterine cervix.

Biopsy Report

After the tissue is removed from the patient, it is sent to a pathology laboratory for analysis. The sample tissue must be carefully handled with tissue forceps and placed immediately in a container of 10% formalin solution. There should be at least 20 times the volume of the specimen in the container to ensure proper preservation.

The specimen bottle should be labeled with the following information on a stick-on label: patient's name, patient's address, patient's age, and date of biopsy.

A short **biopsy report** (Figure 25-29) should be included with each specimen to be sent. The report should include the following information.

1. Patient's name
2. Patient's age
3. Description of lesion (size, shape, location, color, etc.)
4. History of lesion (time present, enlargement, pain, and so on)
5. Tentative diagnosis (dentist's impression of what the disease might be)

Sometimes a small sketch of the lesion is helpful to the pathologist to clarify its description and location.

The specimen bottle and biopsy report should be carefully packed and sent to the laboratory immediately. The laboratory returns a report of the pathologist's findings on completion of the analysis of the biopsy specimen.

EXODONTIA

Exodontia is the area of dental practice that deals with the removal, or extraction, of teeth. Although modern dental practice is geared toward the preservation of teeth, the fact remains that it is necessary to remove teeth under certain circumstances as a part of treatment planning.

Extractions are often thought of as the end result of severe dental caries, periodontal disease, and tooth fracture. Various studies indicate that 50% to 89% of all extractions result from these disease processes. Preventive and restorative procedures can play a major role in the reduction of this needless tooth loss. However, other circumstances may make the extraction of teeth necessary: impactions, orthodontic therapy, and involvement in surgical procedures such as treatment of neoplasms and jaw fracture. Although dentists agree that they would prefer to reduce needless loss of teeth, exodontia will always be a necessary dental service.

Since surgical procedures influence several systems of the body, it is imperative that a thorough medical-dental history be taken, as described in Chapter 3. Since most surgical procedures are irreversible, an accurate diagnosis and treatment plan are mandatory. Accurate clinical records and radiographs are essential parts of any oral surgical treatment.

Patient preparation for surgery begins with consideration for necessary premedication and medical precautions that are revealed in the health history. Once seated in the operatory, the patient must be prepared for the procedure. Dentists vary in their opinion on how a patient should be prepared for surgery. The oral cavity is a heavily contaminated surgical site. The saliva is teeming with the organisms that normally inhabit the mouth. Because of the presence of organisms in the oral cavity, some operators feel little need for much patient preparation. However, studies indicate that most patients tolerate their own organisms well but do not tolerate organisms from other sources. Therefore preparation of the patient for surgery should be geared to minimizing contamination of the mouth with organisms foreign to the patient's oral cavity.

Following are some common methods of controlling the operating field:

1. Use full-length patient drapes.
2. Wrap the patient's head with a cap or towel to cover the hair.
3. Place a sterile towel over the patient's chest on top of the drape.
4. Scrub the oronasal areas with a disinfectant soap, using a sterile 4×4-inch gauze sponge.
5. Have the patient rinse vigorously with an antiseptic mouthrinse (e.g., chlorhexidine).

In addition to patient preparation, the environment around the patient should be prepared. This includes disinfecting and sterilizing everything possible that comes in contact with the patient: light handles, evacuator tips and hose connectors, handpieces, and control switches on the chair. Surgical instruments should be kept in sterile wraps until they are set up on a sterile towel for the procedure. The surgical setup should be kept covered with a sterile towel until the procedure begins. It is recommended that the surgical team wear latex gloves, protective clothing, safety glasses, and face masks.

Dentists who perform surgical services will establish their own method of patient preparation. The assistant will be required to prepare the patient for surgery and maintain the environment for the procedure.

For purposes of discussion, extraction can be divided into three categories: routine, complex, and multiple.

Routine Extractions

It has often been said that there are no routine or simple extractions. Each extraction presents a new challenge for the dentist. The term **routine extraction** is meant to im-

YOUR LOCAL BIOPSY SERVICE

999 City Ave.

Anytown, USA 90909

Date: _____

Patient Name: John Doe

Address: 1234 Anystreet, Anytown, USA 90909

Submitted by Doctor: Toothache

Address: 6789 Anyroad, Anytown, USA 90909

Date of Birth: 7-17-53   **Occupation:** Plumber

Sex: Male   **Race:** White

History: 29-year-old white plumber with 2-month history of asymptomatic white plaque on left lateral border of tongue. He noticed it at that time and came in for an examination. It was observed for 2 weeks without a change in its appearance. An incisional biopsy was taken and was reported as mild epithelial dysplasia. The patient does not know how long it was there prior to his noticing it. The last time he saw a dentist was several years ago. He denies a history of smoking, drinking, oral habits and has had no recent changes in his activities. He cannot recall any traumatic episode or oral pain. The patient's past medical history is unremarkable. He claims there are no other lesions elsewhere on his body.

Clinical Appearance of Lesion: A 3 × 5 cm white, ragged plaque on the left lateral border of the tongue which extends onto the dorsum in one area and slightly down onto the floor of the mouth in another (see illustration). The lesion is not ulcerated in any area and feels "leathery and tough." The incisional biopsy site has healed well and cannot be identified at present. There are no local factors apparent which may have contributed to the lesion. There are no other lesions within the oral cavity or on the skin. There is no lymphadenopathy present.

Nature of Treatment: Excisional biopsy

Comments: The anterior margin is marked with one suture, the superior margin with two sutures, and the posterior margin with three sutures. One centimeter clinical margins were obtained at surgery.

Figure 25-29   Biopsy data sheet.

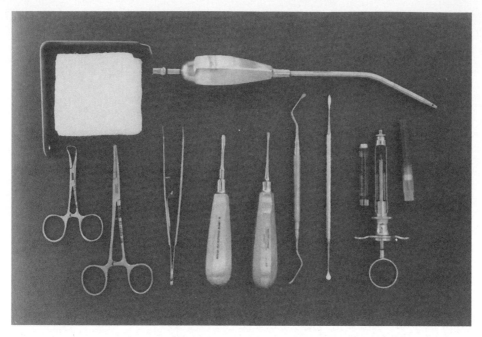

Tissue retractor
Sterile gauze
Surgical suction tip
Towel clamp
Hemostat
Cotton forceps
Straight elevator (2)
Surgical curette
Periosteal elevator
Local anesthesia setup

Figure 25-30   Armamentarium for routine extraction.

BOX 25-1

PROCEDURE FOR ROUTINE EXTRACTION

PROCEDURE	RATIONALE	PROCEDURE	RATIONALE
1. Local anesthetic is administered.	1. To anesthetize patient.	7. Suction tip is used to debride surgical site.	7. Often tooth fragments, carious tooth structure, and broken restorative material are left around open alveolus after tooth is removed. It is important to remove this debris with surgical curette so that it does not interfere with healing process.
2. Gingiva surrounding tooth to be extracted is gently probed with surgical curette.	2. To check if patient is anesthetized.		
3. Epithelial attachment is severed around tooth with surgical curette (Figure 25-31, *A*).	3. To free gingiva from tooth.		
4. Beaks of forceps are placed on tooth and seated firmly so that tips of beaks grasp tooth around cementoenamel junction (Figure 25-31, *B*).	4. To gain firm grasp on tooth.	8. After debridement, wound is covered with compress made of one or two 2 x 2–inch moistened gauze sponges. Sponges should be folded so that patient can bite down on compress to apply pressure over wound site.	8. To help control bleeding.
5. Operator moves tooth in alveolus. This is called luxation (Figure 25-31, *B* and *C*). In addition to luxation with forceps, extraction elevators are helpful in luxation of certain teeth.	5. To sever attachment of periodontal ligament around tooth and to expand size of alveolus.	9. Patient should be allowed to sit up for a few minutes while being given postoperative instructions; then patient can be dismissed.	9. Usually routine extraction sites do not require suturing.
6. After luxation, tooth is lifted from alveolus (Figure 25-31, *D*).	6. To remove tooth from bony socket.		

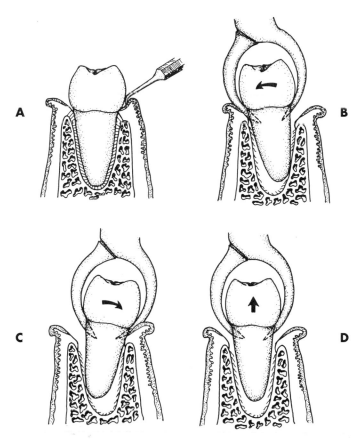

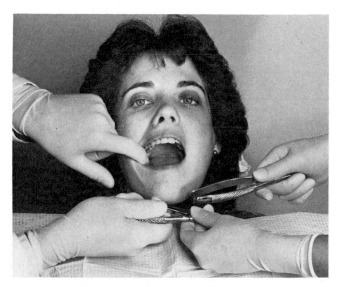

Figure 25-32 Two-handed instrument transfer.

Figure 25-31 Routine extraction sequence. **A**, Severing epithelial attachment with curette. **B**, Beaks of forceps grasp tooth at cementoenamel junction. Tooth is tipped in buccal direction. **C**, Tooth is tipped in lingual direction. **D**, Tooth is lifted from alveolus.

ply that the extraction can be done without extensive instrumentation or complication during surgery. These extractions are often referred to as forceps extractions, since they can be done with a standard forceps without removing bone or sectioning the tooth.

Armamentarium

A typical armamentarium for a routine extraction is shown in Figure 25-30.

Procedure

Box 25-1 describes the procedure for a routine extraction.

The operator must use both hands during extractions. The right hand operates the forceps while the left hand may stabilize the patient's head or jaw. The left hand may also be used to palpate the tooth while **luxation** is being done (assuming the dentist is right-handed), reflect soft tissue, or protect the teeth in the opposing arch from injury.

The assistant can deliver surgical instruments using a two-handed exchange out of the patient's line of sight. The unwanted instrument is picked up from the dentist with one hand, and the next instrument is delivered with the other (Figure 25-32). Most surgical instruments are too heavy to exchange effectively using the one-handed transfer technique. The choice of a one- or two-handed transfer is left to the operating team.

The small **surgical suction tip** should be used as needed during the extraction. It does not have to be held constantly in the surgical site during a routine extraction. However, when bleeding is present, the surgical assistant must use the suction tip aggressively to maintain optimum visibility.

The assistant should be constantly aware of the need for retraction of soft tissue during a surgical procedure. The dentist should offer some guidance in this regard so that the well-intentioned assistant does not interfere with the operator's access while trying to improve visibility.

Once the tooth is lifted from the alveolus, the assistant should take the extracted tooth in the forceps by grasping the beaks of the forceps in the palm of the hand.

It is good for the assistant to observe a patient before dismissal until it is reasonably certain the patient can stand and walk from the operatory. It is not uncommon for a patient to feel dizzy or even faint after a surgical procedure. The assistant should stand near patients, as a precautionary measure, when they first stand and walk from the operatory.

Complex Extractions

The term **complex extraction** implies that a more extensive effort is needed to extract a tooth. There is no

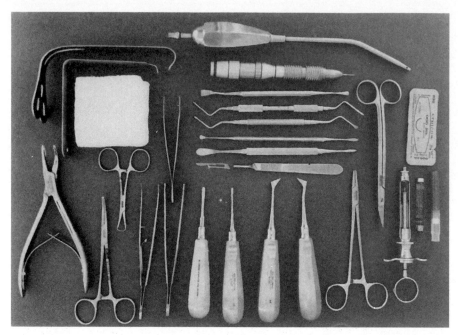

Tissue retractor (2)
2 × 2 sterile gauze
Surgical suction tip
Low-speed handpiece and bar
Bone file
Root pick
Surgical curette
Periosteal elevator (2)
Surgical scalpel blade and handle
Surgical scissors
Suture material
Needle
Rongeur
Hemostat
Towel clamp
Cotton forceps (3)
Extraction elevator (4)
Needle holder
Local anesthetic setup

Figure 25-33   Armamentarium for complicated extraction.

precise definition of a complicated extraction because extractions can be complicated for one or more reasons. Complex extractions may involve one or more of the following procedures during or after the extraction:

1. Mucoperiosteal flap retraction
2. Ostectomy (bone removal)
3. Alveoloplasty (bone shaping)
4. Tooth sectioning
5. Root recovery
6. Soft tissue resection

A classic example of a complex extraction is the removal of an impacted (unerupted) mandibular third molar. It often involves several of the procedures just mentioned.

Armamentarium

A suggested basic armamentarium for a complicated extraction is shown in Figure 25-33.

Procedure

Box 25-2 summarizes the principal steps involved in the extraction of an impacted mandibular third molar.

Multiple Extractions

The extraction of several teeth in preparation for complete or removable partial dentures presents the dentist with a special type of complicated exodontia. The operator must not only remove teeth but also surgically contour the remaining bone and soft tissue. This is necessary to provide a favorably shaped edentulous ridge on which

the denture will rest. A properly contoured ridge is essential to achieve maximum comfort and function for the denture wearer.

Armamentarium

The same basic armamentarium that was used for a single complex extraction can be used for multiple extractions. Additional extraction forceps must be added for each additional type of tooth being extracted (anterior, premolar, molar).

Procedure

Box 25-3 describes the extraction of the mandibular right premolars and molars in preparation for a complete denture.

Immediate complete dentures are dentures that are made before the removal of the anterior teeth in a patient. When the patient has the anterior teeth removed, the denture is placed over the sutured wound, and the patient is dismissed. This patient should return the next day after surgery for postoperative evaluation and cleaning of the surgical site. The immediate denture technique is described in detail in Chapter 26.

Removal of Small Root Fragments and Root Tips

Portions of the root structure of a tooth may have to be recovered separately either because the crown portion of the tooth is missing as a result of extensive caries or because the tooth is fractured during luxation by the dentist. Such root recovery is a necessary part of the extrac-

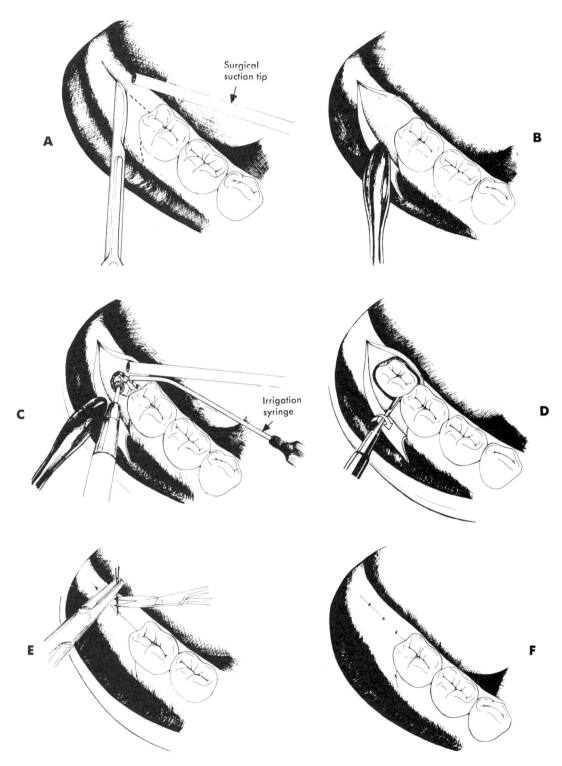

Figure 25-34 Extraction of impacted third molar with help of chairside assistant. **A,** Evacuation of incision. **B,** Retraction of both mucoperiosteal flap and cheek with periosteal elevator. **C,** Simultaneous irrigation and evacuation during bone removal. **D,** Luxation with extraction elevator. **E,** Cutting of sutures by assistant. **F,** Closed incision.

BOX 25-2
PROCEDURE FOR A COMPLICATED EXTRACTION

PROCEDURE	RATIONALE
1. Local anesthetic is administered.	1. To anesthetize patient.
2. Gingiva surrounding tooth to be extracted is gently probed with surgical curette.	2. To check if patient is anesthetized.
3. An incision is made along superior surface of alveolar ridge distal to second molar and extended down buccal aspect of ridge (Figure 25-34, A). Incision is made through both gingival mucosa and periosteum that covers underlying bone.	3. To gain access to impacted tooth.
4. **Mucoperiosteum** (combination of mucosa and periosteum) is lifted from surface of underlying bone with periosteal elevator. Assistant must constantly evacuate blood from surgical site once incision is made and flap is retracted.	4. This mucoperiosteal flap is retracted with elevator to allow operator access to bony covering over impacted tooth (Figure 25-34, B).
5. Surgical mallet and chisel or straight handpiece with surgical burs is used on bone that covers impacted tooth.	5. To remove bony covering over impacted tooth to gain access to tooth (Figure 25-34, C).
Surgical site should be irrigated with sterile saline solution and evacuated. Suction tip is held in assistant's right hand, and irrigating syringe is held in left hand.	To remove bone fragments and improve visibility. Saline solution also keeps bur from clogging and reduces frictional heat on bone.
If surgical bur in handpiece is used to remove bone, assistant must constantly drop saline solution on bur while it is cutting. Dentist retracts mucoperiosteal flap with left hand while operating handpiece with right hand.	

PROCEDURE	RATIONALE
If surgical mallet and chisel are used, assistant may be required to retract mucoperiosteal flap while operator holds chisel in one hand and surgical mallet in other. Some dentists prefer to retract flap with one hand and hold chisel in other while assistant gently taps chisel with surgical mallet.	
6. Once impacted tooth is uncovered, it can be removed by luxation and lifted from alveolus with extraction elevators (Figure 25-34, D). These are leverlike instruments that are wedged between alveolar bone and tooth being extracted. They are activated by twisting large handle so that tooth is forced in distoocclusal direction. On occasion, impacted third molar is lodged between ramus of mandible and distal surface of second molar so that there is no pathway to lift tooth from alveolus. In these cases crown of tooth may need to be divided (**tooth sectioning**; Figure 25-35) into two or more parts to allow room for luxation and removal of tooth. Sectioning is done with either mallet and chisel or surgical bur.	6. To remove tooth from bony socket.
7. After tooth is delivered from alveolus, surgical site should be irrigated, evacuated, and then examined.	7. To see that all loose debris has been removed.

BOX 25-2

PROCEDURE FOR A COMPLICATED EXTRACTION—cont'd

PROCEDURE	RATIONALE
8. In young developing third molars, dental sac still exists around tooth and should be removed from alveolus with curette.	8. To prevent future cyst formation.
9. If bony edges of opening into alveolus are sharp or rough, rongeur and bone file should be used, respectively.	9. To smooth and trim sharp or rough edges of alveolus.
10. After thorough debridement, mucoperiosteal flap is returned to its normal position over wound and sutured to undisturbed gingiva (Figure 25-34, *E* and *F*).	10. To close wound site for optimum healing.
Assistant can be of great help to dentist during suturing by retracting soft tissue, supporting suture material with left hand,	When assistant: • Retracts soft tissue, it enables operator to have optimum visibility.

PROCEDURE	RATIONALE
and cutting suture after it is tied (Figure 25-36).	• Supports suture material, it prevents suture material from dragging across patient's face • Cuts suture material, it enables operator to maintain maximum efficiency.
11. Some dentists like to give patient a cold pack to apply to face over surgical site.	11. To minimize inflammation and swelling.
12. Postoperative oral and written instructions are given, and patient should remain seated upright until comfortable to move. Patient must be instructed as to when to return for removal of sutures and postoperative evaluation.	12. To minimize risk of postoperative complications.

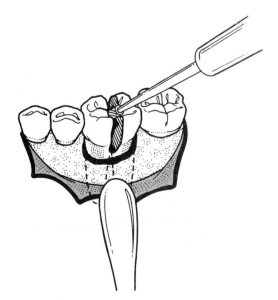

Figure 25-35   Tooth sectioning.

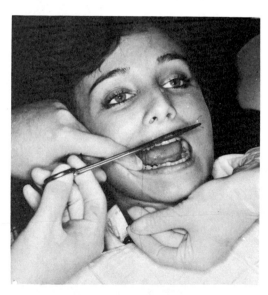

Figure 25-36   Assistant supports suture as it is drawn into surgical site.

BOX 25-3

MULTIPLE EXTRACTION PROCEDURE

PROCEDURE	RATIONALE	PROCEDURE	RATIONALE
1. Local anesthetic is administered.	1. To anesthetize patient.	6. After alveoloplasty, border of mucoperiosteal flap and remaining attached gingiva are often trimmed with surgical scissors.	6. This removes any soft tissue that may have been damaged during extraction procedure and, by eliminating excess soft tissue and provides for smoother surface of edentulous ridge.
2. Gingiva surrounding tooth to be extracted is gently probed with surgical curette.	2. To check if patient is anesthetized.		
3. Incision is made, and then mucoperiosteal flap is reflected away from teeth on buccal aspect of alveolar ridge (Figure 25-37, A and B).	3. If contouring of edentulous ridge after removal of teeth is anticipated. Contouring is almost always required to some extent.	7. Surgical site should be irrigated and evacuated before suturing.	7. To remove debris and tooth fragments.
4. Removal of teeth generally starts with most posterior tooth and moves anteriorly. Luxation of teeth is done with extraction elevators. Forceps are then used to lift teeth from their alveoli (Figure 25-37, B).	4. This gives dentist some mechanical advantage in luxation of remaining teeth.	8. Mucoperiosteal flap is repositioned and sutured to remaining attached gingiva on lingual aspect of ridge (Figure 25-37, D).	8. To close surgical site and to promote optimal healing.
		9. Moist compress of several 2 x 2-inch sterile gauze sponges is placed over surgical site, and patient is instructed to bite on compress.	9. To control postoperative bleeding.
5. After teeth have been removed and all root tips recovered (if necessary), alveolar bone is contoured with rongeur forceps and bone file (Figure 25-37, C). All sharp edges of bone are smoothed with file. This contouring of alveolar process is called an **alveoloplasty**.	5. To contour and smooth alveolar bone.	10. Patient is allowed to sit upright while postoperative instructions are given and is then escorted out of operatory. An appointment is made for postoperative evaluation and suture removal.	10. Postoperative instructions are given to minimize postoperative complications.

tion procedure. In most instances, root fragments should be removed because of the rather high potential for infection in the future.

Several techniques are used to recover root fragments. The dentist selects the technique that is suitable for the specific problem the patient presents at the time. A brief description of various root recovery methods follows.

Root-pick technique

The alveolus is rinsed and evacuated. The root pick is inserted into the periodontal ligament space and is used to gently tease out the root (Figure 25-38, A).

Forceps technique

Special root-extraction forceps are available with long, narrow beaks that are convenient for recovering root fragments of one third the root length or larger (Figure 25-38, B). Usually a mucoperiosteal flap is reflected, and buccal or labial bone is removed to gain access to the root. These forceps are often used alternately with root picks to remove the root fragment.

Elevator technique

The elevator technique (Figure 25-38, C) is a helpful method of removing roots of multirooted teeth. The teeth

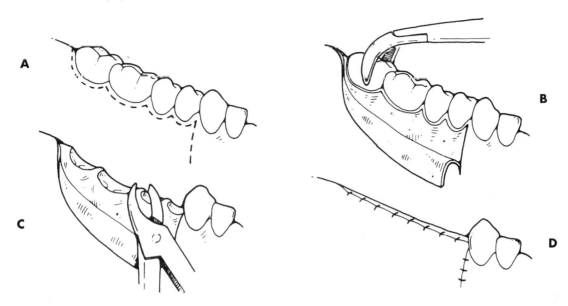

Figure 25-37   Multiple-extraction sequence. **A**, Gingival incision. **B**, Retraction of muco-periosteal flap and extraction of teeth. **C**, Alveoloplasty using rongeur. **D**, Sutured wound.

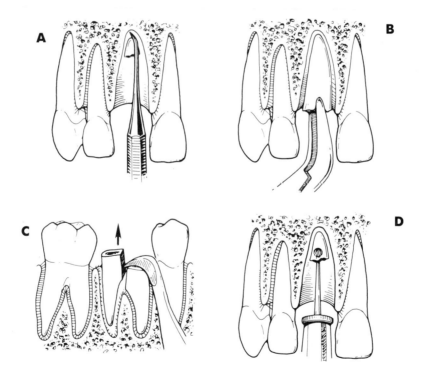

Figure 25-38   Root recovery technique. **A**, Root-pick method. **B**, Forceps method. **C**, Elevator method. **D**, Bur method.

are sectioned through the bifurcation or trifurcation of the roots with a surgical bur or chisel. An elevator is inserted in the cut area of the interdental area and twisted for luxation and elevation of the roots from the alveolus.

Bur technique

The bur technique (Figure 25-38, *D*) is helpful in the anterior and premolar areas. A straight handpiece with a No. 4 to No. 6 round bur (HP) is used to bore into the root canal of the fragment. The handpiece is tipped so that the bur locks in the canal, and the fragment is lifted from the alveolus with the handpiece. This method is usually limited to small root tips.

Postoperative Instructions

Postoperative instructions to patients are important guidelines they should follow to prevent complications and unnecessary discomfort. It is advisable to go over these instructions verbally with the patient after surgery to prevent confusion. However, the patient should be given a printed copy of the instructions to review after leaving the office. Patients tend to forget verbal instructions, especially when they are given right after surgery. The verbal instructions should be given only to emphasize the important written guidelines.

Healing of an extraction site begins with blood clot formation in the empty alveolus. This clot is the first step in the healing process. The formation and preservation of the clot in the alveolus are the principal goals of postoperative care. Anything that interferes with this process can lead to complications such as prolonged bleeding, infection, "dry socket," and delayed healing. Box 25-4 lists typical postoperative instructions and the reason for each instruction.

POSTOPERATIVE COMPLICATIONS

Careful diagnosis, treatment planning, and surgical technique can prevent many unnecessary postsurgical complications. Among the more common complications that occur after surgery are prolonged bleeding, infection, and **alveolitis,** also known as dry socket.

Prolonged Bleeding

Prolonged bleeding is the most common postoperative complication. Patients may call after removing the gauze compress and complain of continued bleeding. It is common for the saliva to contain a small quantity of blood for several hours after surgery. However, if the patient has a deep red discoloration to the saliva, a bleeding problem exists.

Prolonged bleeding should be treated initially by instructing the patient to pack a moist, folded gauze compress over the extraction site and applying biting pressure for another 20 to 30 minutes. If no gauze is available, a moistened tea bag can be used for the same purpose. If

bleeding continues after this procedure, the patient should return to the office for further treatment.

Once the patient arrives, an anesthetic is administered and the surgical wound is irrigated and inspected. A common method to control hemorrhage is to pack the alveolus with absorbable Gelfoam or oxidized cellulose (Figure 25-39). Some dentists prefer to saturate oxidized cellulose with a topical thrombin solution to enhance clotting further. These agents form a network around which blood can clot. They need not be removed, since they are absorbed by the body as healing takes place. Sutures are sometimes placed across the opening of the alveolus to hold the pack in place. The patient is instructed to bite on a new moist gauze compress for another 30 minutes. This procedure solves the majority of bleeding problems.

Alveolitis (Dry Socket)

After the extraction of a tooth from its alveolus, healing begins immediately with blood oozing into the alveolus and clotting. The clot is later replaced by scar tissue and ultimately bone as healing progresses. Unfortunately, some extraction sites do not undergo this favorable progression. The blood clot that normally fills the alveolus either does not form or forms and is lost from the alveolus. The reason for this phenomenon is still not clear. Although the exact cause is unclear, patients come in 3 or 4 days after the extraction complaining of mild to severe dull pain and a foul odor and taste. When the alveolus is inspected, the clot is found to be missing and the bone is exposed. The wound is then irritated by the oral environment.

Treatment of this condition is strictly geared to making the patient comfortable while the wound heals (Box 25-5). This is called **palliative therapy.** Healing can take from 10 to 40 days.

Armamentarium

The armamentarium for this procedure includes the following:
- Mouth mirror
- Cotton pliers
- Scissors
- Irrigation syringe
- Warm saline solution
- Iodoform gauze
- Oral evacuator tip

Systemic analgesics are often prescribed to relieve pain until the exposed bone is covered sufficiently by a layer of cells as a result of healing (granulation tissue).

Suture Removal

Suture removal (Figure 25-41) can be delegated to dental assistants where state laws permit. After the extraction site is inspected by the dentist, the assistant can remove the sutures as follows.

BOX 25-4

POSTOPERATIVE INSTRUCTIONS FOR THE SURGICAL PATIENT

INSTRUCTION	RATIONALE
1. Maintain biting pressure on gauze compress for 30 minutes. Repeat for 30 more minutes if bleeding continues.	Compression of wound is one of the best ways to stop bleeding and promote clot formation.
2. Place a cold pack on face over surgical site for the first 24 hours after surgery. This should be started as soon as possible.	Cold packs help reduce swelling in surgical area. Excessive swelling can delay healing and create aesthetic problems for patient.
3. Avoid rinsing mouth until day after surgery.	Rinsing can dislodge newly formed clot from alveolus, causing additional bleeding and delayed healing.
4. On day after surgery, *gentle* rinsing of mouth is permitted using ½ teaspoon of salt in 8-ounce drinking glass of very warm water.	Salt water is more compatible with tissue cells, since it is similar to salty nature of tissue fluid. Warmth of rinse enhances circulation to oral cavity, which promotes healing.
5. Remaining teeth should be brushed gently with soft-bristle toothbrush beginning day after surgery.	This freshens patient's mouth and removes bacterial plaque accumulation, which can increase possibility of infection.
6. Eat regular meals as soon as possible after surgery. (Soft foods may be the best immediately following surgery.) Drink lots of liquids by sipping. Do not use a straw.	Sucking on a straw can also draw clot from alveolus. Liquid consumption helps replace lost fluids during surgery and maintain favorable fluid and electrolyte balance in body.
7. Take any prescribed medication as directed.	Medications are prescribed for pain and prevention of infection in some cases.
8. If bleeding cannot be controlled, consult dentist for further instructions.	Prolonged bleeding may require additional treatment by dentist.
9. Elevate head with pillows when sleeping during first 24 hours.	This helps prevent additional bleeding and swelling.

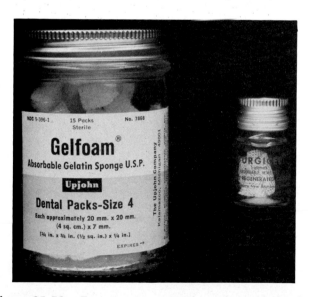

Figure 25-39   Two common materials used to pack alveolus to control hemorrhage.

BOX 25-5

PROCEDURE FOR TREATING ALVEOLITIS

PROCEDURE	RATIONALE
1. Alveolus is gently irrigated with warm saline and dried.	1. To remove accumulated debris from alveolus.
2. Narrow strip of iodoform gauze is cut to length that fills alveolus (Figure 25-40).	2. To help prevent food from becoming packed into alveolus.
3. Gauze is gently packed into alveolus.	3. Iodoform in gauze is topical antiseptic that helps prevent infection.
4. Patient is dismissed and asked to return every 1 or 2 days to have this procedure repeated.	4. Frequent recall keeps wound clean and freshens medication, which loses its effectiveness quickly.

Armamentarium

- Mouth mirror
- Cotton pliers
- Suture scissors
- 2 × 2–inch gauze

Procedure

1. Locate and account for all the sutures placed during the surgical appointment.
2. Lift each suture with the cotton pliers so that the beak of the scissors can fit under the suture material (see Figure 25-41, *A*).

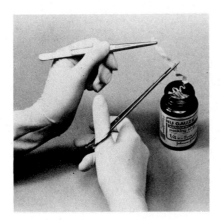

Figure 25-40   Iodoform gauze.

3. The suture should be cut as close to the tissue as possible so that a minimum of material must be pulled through the tissue (see Figure 25-41, *B*).
4. Grasp the knot of the suture and pull the suture material from the tissue (see Figure 25-41, *C*).
5. Recheck the wound to make sure all sutures have been removed.

DENTAL IMPLANTS

Dental implants are a treatment option available to patients who are missing one or more teeth. Dental implants are made out of titanium and are placed directly into the alveolar bone. Because titanium is compatible with human tissue, the implant can become fused to the bone. This phenomenon is termed **osseointegration.** Once the implant becomes osseointegrated, the dentist can fabricate a fixed or removable restoration that will be supported by the implant.

The advantage of an implant vs. a conventional fixed restoration is that adjacent teeth do not need to be prepared and restored to replace missing teeth. Implants are also indicated for edentulous patients with dentures who have bone resorption of the alveolar ridge. Dentures adhere to the patient's mouth by retention to the alveolar ridge. Without adequate ridge height, the denture may not adhere satisfactorily. Several carefully placed implants can support an entire denture.

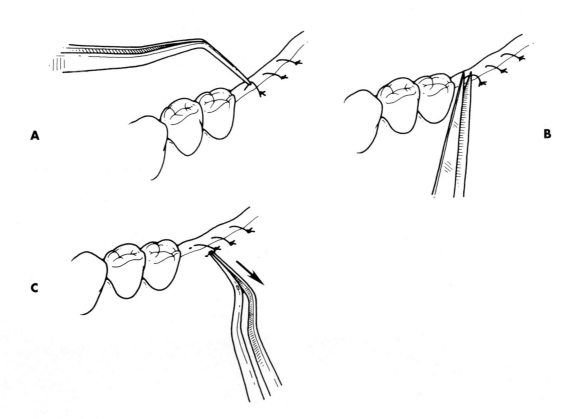

Dental implants are contraindicated when cost is a concern. Implants are quite expensive and can run into the tens of thousands of dollars for multiple tooth replacements. Poor oral hygiene is also a contraindication for implants. Dental implants must be kept meticulously clean of plaque and calculus to prevent "periimplantitis," an infection that could affect the submerged portion of the implant. Periimplantitis is analogous to periodontal disease of the teeth. Last, implants require multiple visits to the dental office and may take as long as 6 months or more to complete. Patients who do not want to commit themselves to the lengthy procedure should consider other treatment options.

Implant Placement and Restorative Procedure

Dental implants take multiple appointments over a long period. The following describes a series of appointments to place a single tooth implant.

1. *Implant placement (Figure 25-42, A and B).* An incision is made to reveal the alveolar ridge. Special burs and a slow-speed handpiece are used to prepare an opening for the placement of the implant.

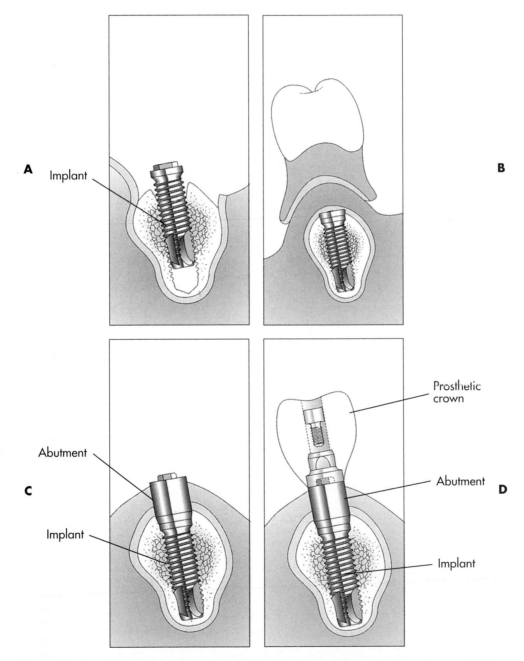

Figure 25-42   Implant procedure. **A**, Placement of implant. **B**, Osseointegration period. **C**, Placement of abutment. **D**, Prosthetic work.

Sterile saline solution is applied to the bur to prevent thermal damage to the bone. The implant is placed into the bone and either tapped or screwed into place. The wound site is sutured closed over the implant to allow for osseointegration of the implant to the bone. Complete osseointegration takes approximately 4 to 6 months.

2. *Implant uncovering (Figure 25-42, C)*. An incision is made to expose the osseointegrated implant. A **healing cap** may be placed on top of the hollow osseointegrated implant until a permanent restoration is fabricated. An alternative to a healing cap is to place an implant abutment into the implant. An **implant abutment** is a connector between the implant and the permanent restoration that will be fabricated.

3. *Restorative procedure*. Crown preparation procedures such as final impressions and bite registrations are taken and sent to a dental laboratory for fabrication of the implant restoration.

4. *Cementation procedure (Figure 25-42, D)*. The final restoration for a single tooth implant is attached to the implant abutment with a very small screw. The final restoration is tried in, and the bite is adjusted. The dentist may cover the opening above the embedded screw with a composite material.

Implant Types

The three most common types of implants are subperiosteal, transosteal, and endosteal implants (Figure 25-43). Endosteal implants are further subdivided into a plate form and a root form. Subperiosteal and transosteal im-

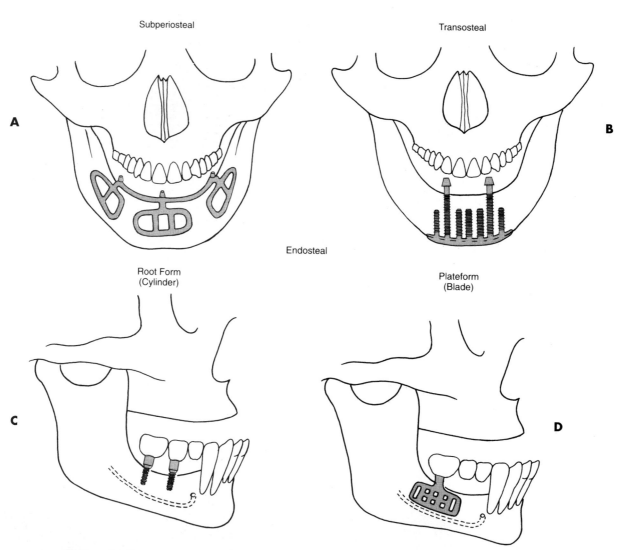

Figure 25-43 Major subgroups of dental implants. **A,** Subperiosteal. **B,** Transosteal. **C,** Endosteal root form (cylinder). **D,** Endosteal plate form (blade).

plants are used mainly for full arch denture replacement, and endosteal implants are most commonly used for partially edentulous patients.

BIBLIOGRAPHY

Andreasen JO, Andreasen FM: *Textbook and color atlas of traumatic injuries to the teeth,* ed 3, Copenhagen, 1994, Munksgaard.

Donoff RB: *Massachusetts General Hospital manual of oral and maxillofacial surgery,* ed 2, St Louis, 1992, Mosby.

Malamed SF: *Medical emergencies in the dental office,* ed 4, St Louis, 1993, Mosby.

Peterson LJ and others: *Contemporary oral and maxillofacial surgery,* ed 2, St Louis, 1993, Mosby.

Schoen MH: Frequency of tooth loss in relation to the dentist's ability to prevent the necessity of extraction, *Dent Clin North Am* 13:741, 1969.

Smith RG and others: *Dental surgery assistants' handbook,* ed 2, London, 1993, Mosby–Year Book Europe Limited.

QUESTIONS—Chapter 25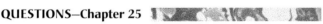

1. Which of the following instruments is used to gently tease a root fragment from the bony socket?
    a. Root pick
    b. Periosteal elevator
    c. Rongeur forceps
    d. Surgical curette

2. Which of the following instruments is used to retract the mucoperiosteum?
    a. Root pick
    b. Periosteal elevator
    c. Rongeur forceps
    d. Surgical curette

3. Which of the following instruments is used to trim alveolar bone?
    a. Root pick
    b. Periosteal elevator
    c. Rongeur forceps
    d. Surgical curette

4. The removal of an entire lesion plus the adjacent normal tissue is called an _____.
    a. Incisional biopsy
    b. Excisional biopsy
    c. Exfoliative cytology

5. When a tooth is divided into two or more parts to facilitate the removal of the tooth, this is called:
    a. Tooth sectioning
    b. Luxation
    c. Exodontia
    d. Alveoloplasty

6. Which of the following is not an appropriate postoperative instruction following a surgical extraction?
    a. Use a cold pack for the first 24 hours.
    b. Begin brushing teeth the day after the surgery.
    c. Rinse vigorously the day of the surgery.
    d. Bite on moist gauze immediately following the surgery.

7. A cow-horn extraction forceps is used for extraction of _____ teeth.
    a. Maxillary molar
    b. Anterior
    c. Mandibular molar
    d. Third molar

8. Bone removal is accomplished by all of the following *except*:
    a. Bone file
    b. Rongeur
    c. Mallet and chisel
    d. Scalpel

9. The _____ type of implant is used primarily for single tooth replacement.
    a. Endosteal
    b. Transosteal
    c. Subperiosteal

10. A patient who calls the dental office a few days after a surgical extraction complaining of pain and foul odor and taste in the mouth probably has _____.
    a. Prolonged bleeding
    b. Dry socket
    c. Loose sutures
    d. Trismus

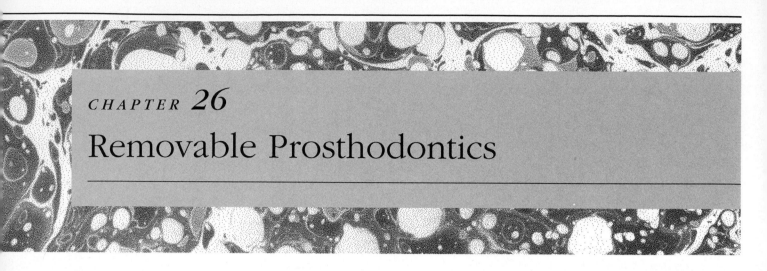

KEY TERMS
Articulator
Border molding
Centric occlusion
Denture relining
Face bow
Muscle trimming
Occlusal rims
Overdenture
Partial denture
Prosthesis
Prosthodontics
Retention clasps
Tissue conditioning

A **prosthesis** is an artificial body part. Artificial limbs, eyes, heart valves, and teeth are just a few examples of some common prosthetic devices.

In the strictest sense any dental restoration is a prosthesis. Common use of the term **prosthodontics** (prosthetics in dentistry) refers to the area of dental practice that deals with the extensive reconstruction of existing teeth and the replacement of missing teeth with various dental restorations and appliances. Generally speaking, operative restorations are not considered a part of prosthodontics. Prosthodontics is a broad term that encompasses crown and bridge procedures (fixed prosthodontics) and both complete and partial denture services (removable prosthodontics).

The use of chairside assistants in the area of removable prosthodontic services has not been as well developed as in other areas of dental practice. This is probably because

constant use of four hands during a prosthetic appointment is unnecessary. The assistant's role in prosthodontics is primarily limited to operatory preparation, laboratory duties, and preparation of impression materials. Prosthetic dentistry does not require many instrument exchanges and constant oral evacuation that are associated with other dental services.

A general understanding of denture construction will be of value to the clinical dental assistant so that appointments, surgical and restorative services, and laboratory phases can be coordinated properly.

Three common prosthetic services will be described in this chapter to provide the assistant with some of the fundamentals of prosthetic services:

- Fabrication of a removable partial denture
- Fabrication of an immediate complete denture
- A denture reline

FABRICATION OF REMOVABLE PARTIAL DENTURE: CLASS I EXAMPLE

A removable partial denture is a prosthetic device used to replace missing teeth (Figure 26-1). Since it is used to replace only a part of the dentition while some natural teeth remain, it is called a **partial denture.** The removable partial denture can and must be removed by the patient for cleaning.

A removable partial denture can be used in several edentulous situations. Box 26-1 outlines the Kennedy system of classifying these situations.

A typical appointment schedule for the fabrication of a removable partial denture is shown in Figure 26-2. As with almost all dental procedures, several methods are used to construct both partial and complete dentures. The methods to be described are only examples of common techniques currently used.

BOX 26-1

KENNEDY CLASSIFICATION SYSTEM FOR PARTIALLY EDENTULOUS CONDITIONS IN THE ORAL CAVITY

Class I: An edentulous situation in which all remaining teeth are anterior to bilateral edentulous areas

Class II: An edentulous situation in which remaining teeth of either right or left side are anterior to unilateral edentulous area

Class III: An edentulous situation in which edentulous area is bounded by teeth that are *unable* to assume total support of prosthesis; these abutments require aid of teeth that are remotely located, so that principles of cross-arch splinting and counter leverage can be used to resist lateral tilting forces

Class IV: An edentulous situation in which remaining teeth bound edentulous area posteriorly on both sides of median line

Class V: An edentulous situation in which teeth bound edentulous area anteriorly and posteriorly but where anterior abutment tooth is *not* suitable for normal abutment service

Class VI: An edentulous situation in which boundary teeth are capable of total support of required prosthesis

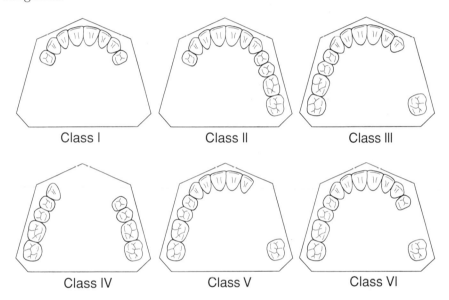

Class I   Class II   Class III

Class IV   Class V   Class VI

From Finkbeiner BL, Johnson CS: *Mosby's comprehensive dental assisting: a clinical approach,* St Louis, 1995, Mosby.

Preliminary Steps

The first step in all dental treatment is to gather all the information necessary for an accurate diagnosis and treatment planning. A complete medical-dental history, oral and radiographic examination, and study models are essential elements in achieving this goal.

A thorough dental prophylaxis should be done before examination and impression-taking for study models.

After all diagnostic information has been obtained, the dentist formulates a treatment plan and designs the partial denture on the study models. The patient returns for a case presentation, and the treatment plan is explained and fee estimates are given.

Before a partial denture is constructed, the foundation on which it will rest must be healthy and sound. Therefore the mouth must be prepared as needed to create a favorable foundation. This preparation may include operative dentistry, extensive restorative procedures, periodontal treatment, and oral surgery, depending on the condition of the individual.

An important part of mouth preparation for a partial denture is the proper contouring of the teeth where the metal framework of the partial denture rests. The occlusal surfaces of teeth that will support the framework must be contoured to hold the framework firmly in place and allow clearance between the upper and lower teeth to accommodate the thickness of the framework. The buccal and lingual contours of the abutment teeth must be favorable to allow the denture to be inserted and removed without binding and be held in place by **reten-**

Table 26-1 Typical appointment schedule for fabrication of class I removable partial denture (clasp type)

Appointment	Treatment
1	Complete oral and radiographic examination
	Dental prophylaxis
	Alginate impressions for study models
2	Case presentation; discussion of planned treatment and fee estimates
3	Mouth preparations; may require several separate appointments if periodontal or restorative treatment is required
4	Final impressions for master casts on which denture framework is made
	Occlusal registration
5	Try-in and adjustment of framework
6	Final impression of edentulous ridges on which denture base rests
	Reestablish or verify occlusal registration
	Tooth shade selection
	Delivery of denture
7	Initial denture adjustments as needed
8	Denture adjustment appointments as required

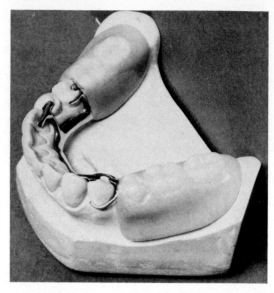

Figure 26-1   Class I removable partial denture.

tion clasps (Figure 26-1). If such contouring cannot be accomplished by minimal grinding of the enamel of these teeth, the teeth need to be recontoured by placing crown restorations on the teeth involved. This is a rather common requirement in partial denture construction. Once the mouth has been prepared, final impressions can be taken.

Procedure (Figure 26-2)
Final impressions

Once mouth preparations are complete, final impressions are taken for construction of master casts (models). These impressions must be very accurate, since the metal framework will be cast in the laboratory on a duplicate of the master cast.

1. It is recommended that the teeth be polished with a rubber cup and pumice and rinsed thoroughly with mouthwash just before the impression for greater accuracy.
2. Final impressions can be taken with any of the elastomeric impression materials (alginate, mercaptan, polyvinylsiloxane, polyether, agar hydrocolloid) prepared in the usual manner.
3. A custom acrylic tray is recommended for improved accuracy. (This can be made from the study models before the final impression appointment.)
4. Gingival retraction is not needed for these impressions. However, the syringe-tray technique offers some advantage in eliminating voids in the impression around the abutment teeth and rest areas for

the framework. The use of alginate foregoes this advantage.

5. Once the impressions are obtained, they should be poured immediately with improved stone to make the accurate master casts.
6. The impressions should be poured with the two-stage pouring technique. The impression is filled and allowed to rest upright on cotton rolls until the stone reaches its initial set (loses its glossy surface) (Figure 26-3, *A*). A new mix of stone is prepared, and the impression is inverted onto a pile of the stone on the laboratory bench (Figure 26-3, *B*). This is allowed to harden for 45 minutes before removing the impression from the stone and trimming the models.

Bite registration

A wax bite registration may be necessary to articulate the upper and lower models accurately in the laboratory.

One method is to have the patient bite into a sheet of pink baseplate wax that has been warmed in hot water and folded in half. The patient is instructed to bite down just enough to form tiny imprints in the wax.

➥ KEY POINT
- The oral evacuator and air from the air/water syringe can be used to quick-cool the wax bite (Figure 26-4).

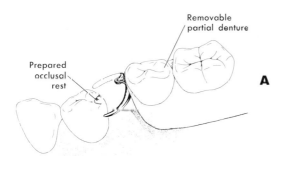

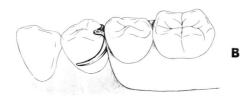

Figure 26-2 **A**, Clasp of removable partial denture and prepared abutment tooth. **B**, Clasp in place on abutment tooth.

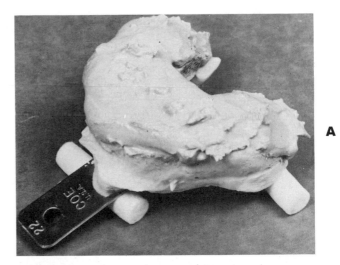

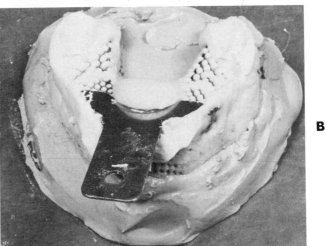

Figure 26-3 Two-stage method of pouring models. **A**, Impression is filled with improved stone and allowed to remain upright until material reaches its initial set. **B**, Filled impression is then inverted onto pile of stone to form base of model.

Jaw relationship

Some dentists may want the dental laboratory to mount the patient's diagnostic casts on an adjustable articulator that can place the casts in various jaw positions. The **articulator** represents the patient's own occlusal and biting functions (Figure 26-5, *A*). A **face bow** is used to orient the maxillary cast on the articulator (Figure 26-5, *B*).

Shade selection

If the denture is to be made entirely on the master cast without a corrected impression of the edentulous ridges, a shade is selected at this time. Conventional shade guides are used for this purpose.

The patient is dismissed, and an appointment is scheduled for the framework try-in.

Laboratory phase

1. The master casts are trimmed and sent to the laboratory along with the study models, the bite registration, the shade, and the laboratory prescription. The face bow is used to mount the master casts on an articulator.
2. The study models are used to describe the partial denture design. The dentist can sketch the design on the model and describe it in the laboratory prescription. The laboratory prescription is discussed later in this chapter.
3. The laboratory will cast the metal framework according to the dentist's design and return it to the dentist.
4. In partial denture designs that do not require an additional impression of the edentulous ridges, the entire

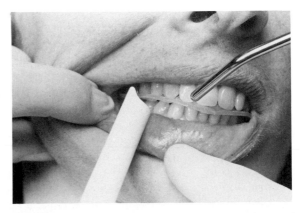

Figure 26-4 Cooling wax bite after it is reinserted in patient's mouth and teeth are closed together tightly.

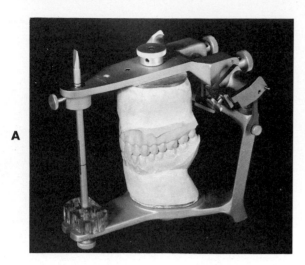
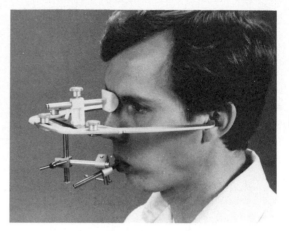

Figure 26-5 **A**, Mounting of casts on articulator. **B**, Face bow and face bow fork are assembled on patient.

(From McGivney GP, Castleberry DJ: McCracken's removable partial prosthodontics, ed 9, St Louis, 1995, Mosby.)

partial denture is fabricated and returned to the dentist for delivery to the patient.

Framework try-in

1. After the cast framework is received from the laboratory (Figure 26-6), it is fitted to the patient's mouth.
2. Adjustments are made as needed to adapt the framework to the teeth and to establish proper occlusion.

Edentulous ridge impression

In cases such as a class I partial denture design in which the denture is supported principally by the edentulous ridges, a separate impression of the ridges is helpful. This permits the dentist to contour and adapt the denture base to the edentulous areas more accurately.

1. Small acrylic "saddles" are added to the framework, using custom acrylic tray material (Figure 26-7, *A*). These saddles are used as miniature impression trays for the ridges.
2. The dentist can adjust the size of the saddles by adding softened compound around the border of the acrylic and trying it in the patient's mouth. This is called **border molding** (Figure 26-7, *B*).
3. Once the size of the saddles is established, an impression is taken of the ridge areas by coating the tissue surface of the acrylic with impression material and inserting the framework-saddle assembly in the patient's mouth. The impression materials commonly used for this purpose are elastomeric impression materials, zinc oxide and eugenol (ZOE) paste, or impression wax. The occlusion can be rechecked at this appointment.

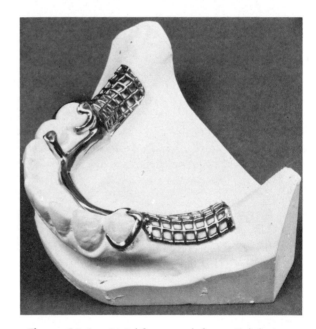

Figure 26-6 Metal framework for partial denture.

Laboratory phase

1. The impressions and master casts are returned to the laboratory along with a laboratory prescription.
2. The laboratory technician sets the denture teeth to the predetermined occlusion and fabricates the denture base with denture acrylic.

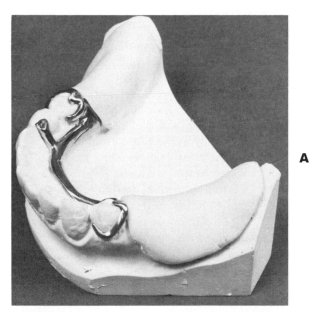

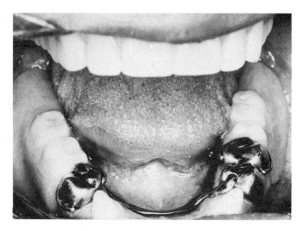

Figure 26-8   Completed removable partial denture.

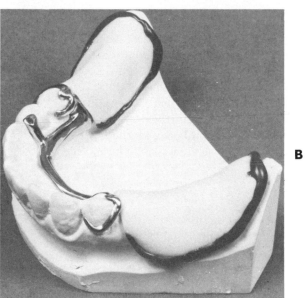

Figure 26-7   **A**, Acrylic "saddles" added to framework used to take impression of edentulous ridges. **B**, Border-molded saddles.

BOX 26-2

CARE OF REMOVABLE PARTIAL DENTURE AND COMPLETE DENTURE

1. Clean the prosthesis after eating and before going to bed.
2. A regular toothbrush and toothpaste can be used to clean the prosthesis.
3. Clean the prosthesis over a sink partially filled with water to avoid breaking the prosthesis in the event that it is accidentally dropped.
4. A denture cleaning solution can be used on any prosthesis. Soak the prosthesis once daily, followed by brushing.
5. Take the prosthesis out at night to allow the oral tissues to rest.
6. If the prosthesis is removed from the mouth for a prolonged period of time, immerse it in water to prevent dehydration and subsequent distortion.
7. Avoid using bleach or bleach solutions on a removable partial denture. The bleach can corrode the metal.

Denture delivery

1. The complete partial denture is returned from the laboratory and delivered to the patient (Figure 26-8).
2. Adjustments in fit and occlusion are made as needed at this appointment.
3. The partial denture is designed to slide on and off the remaining teeth in a specific direction. This is called the path of insertion (and removal). Patients must be instructed in the proper insertion and removal method before being dismissed.

4. Patients should be instructed in oral hygiene procedures and maintenance of the partial denture. Caries, periodontal disease, and mouth odors can develop quickly if plaque is allowed to accumulate on the partial denture framework and on the remaining natural teeth. Proper care of the removable partial denture is described in Box 26-2.
5. The patient will undergo an adjustment period to learn to speak and eat with the new appliance. The patient may experience some soreness, which could

indicate a need for an adjustment of the partial denture. Excessive salivation is common for a time after insertion of the denture. Patients are encouraged to begin using the denture on soft-textured foods until they become accustomed to the new appliance. Sticky foods, nuts, and foods with tiny seeds should be avoided, since they can be unpleasant for the denture wearer. Candies and caramels tend to stick to the acrylic denture, and seeds work under the denture base and cause discomfort.

Adjustment phase

1. Postinsertion evaluation of the patient is needed to check fit of the denture, occlusion, oral hygiene and denture maintenance, and problems encountered wearing the denture.
2. Adjustments are made on the denture as required to achieve maximum comfort and function for the patient. Patients may require several adjustment appointments to achieve this goal.

FABRICATION OF COMPLETE DENTURE (IMMEDIATE METHOD)

Patients who have all their teeth removed and replaced with complete dentures are faced with unique and difficult problems. Although some people are successful denture wearers, many are not. No denture can duplicate the comfort, efficiency, and dependability of a well-maintained, healthy, natural dentition. A common misconception regarding complete dentures is that they are a way to solve all dental problems. In truth, dentures often mark the onset of problems for many people. Dentures are prosthetic devices that replace a body part, but they do not completely restore normal function any more than does an artificial leg. Patients who are successful denture wearers simply have a greater ability to adapt to a prosthesis. They either accept or overcome the problems associated with wearing a prosthesis.

Successful denture wearing depends on several factors, including the following:

1. Jaw relationship of the patient
2. Size and shape of the edentulous ridges
3. Coordination of the patient's oral musculature
4. Attitude of the individual patient
5. Personal diet and oral habits of the individual
6. Quality of the denture construction

Prospective denture patients often comment that they have a friend or relative who wears dentures and has no problems at all. The fact is clear that people vary widely in the factors just listed. With these variables in mind, there is little reason to expect that one person should be as successful as another in wearing dentures. It is unfortunate that no one knows how well a patient will be able to function with complete dentures until after the indi-

vidual has worn them awhile. By then it is too late. The natural teeth are gone forever, and dentures are the only alternative. It is not surprising that a majority of dentists try everything possible to save natural teeth and prevent this dilemma for their dental patients. Since the emphasis on preventive and restorative dentistry and periodontal therapy has increased during the past 20 years, there has been a corresponding decline in the number of dentures made annually in the United States.

Techniques that are used to fabricate complete dentures vary widely among dentists. The following is a discussion of a common method used to construct complete dentures that will be inserted at the surgical appointment when the last remaining teeth are removed. This method is commonly called the immediate denture technique. A typical appointment schedule for this procedure is shown in Table 26-2.

Preliminary Steps

Careful diagnosis and treatment planning are just as important in the fabrication of complete dentures as they are in all other dental services. The dentist must carefully plan the needed surgery and design of the denture. The patient's health status, age, habits, jaw relationships, and jaw discrepancies are important considerations. Study models are useful aids in treatment planning for complete dentures. A thorough study of the size and shape of the remaining teeth and jaws can be made from the models to enhance the accuracy of denture design. Photographs

Table 26-2 Sample appointment schedule for fabrication of immediate complete dentures

Appointment	Treatment
1	Examination and treatment planning (includes radiographs, medical history, study model impressions, and possibly photographs)
2	Extraction of posterior teeth on one side of mouth
3	Extraction of posterior teeth on other side of mouth (Wait approximately 4 to 6 weeks until next appointment)
4	Preliminary impressions of remaining anterior teeth and edentulous ridges (alginate)
5	Final impressions of remaining teeth and edentulous ridges
6	Recording jaw relationships with occlusal rims and selecting proper shade and mold for denture teeth
7	Extraction of remaining anterior teeth and delivery of complete dentures
8	First postoperative visit (preferably on day after extractions)
9	Adjustment appointments as needed

of the patient's teeth and facial contour are also of assistance to the dentist in creating favorable aesthetics for the patient.

After treatment planning the first step in construction of an immediate denture is to remove the posterior teeth in both arches and perform the necessary alveoloplasty to shape the edentulous ridges to a favorable contour. The idea of the immediate denture is to leave the anterior teeth to preserve some aesthetics and speech quality until the dentures are ready for delivery at the surgery appointment when these remaining teeth are removed. The advantage of this technique is that patients are never completely without teeth while making the transition from natural to artificial teeth.

Construction Steps

Preliminary impressions

1. Generally, a 4- to 6-week period is required for adequate healing after the removal of the posterior teeth before alginate impressions of the partially edentulous jaws can be taken.
2. These impressions are taken with stock alginate trays.
3. Work models are made from the impressions.
4. Custom acrylic trays are then made on these work models.

Final impressions

1. The patient returns for more accurate impressions using the custom acrylic trays (Figure 26-9).
2. The borders of the tray are adjusted to the proper length with stick compound. The compound is heated with a Bunsen burner and fused to the edges (periphery) of the tray. Then the tray is dipped in warm water. The tray is inserted in the patient's mouth, and the lips, cheeks, and tongue are manipulated to form accurate lengths of the tray fingers. This is called border molding or **muscle trimming**.
3. A wash type of final impression material is made using the custom-made tray.
4. The tray is filled with the impression material, and the patient's mouth is rinsed thoroughly.
5. The tray is inserted in the mouth and removed after the material has set completely.
6. The same procedure is repeated for the opposite arch.
7. The patient is dismissed.
8. The impressions are poured in dental stone to make the master casts.

Determining jaw relationships

1. In a natural dentition the teeth determine how the lower jaw relates to the upper jaw when the mouth is closed. In the closed position with the teeth clenched together, the distance between the upper and lower jaws is determined by the length of the crowns of the posterior teeth (Figure 26-10, *A*). This distance be-

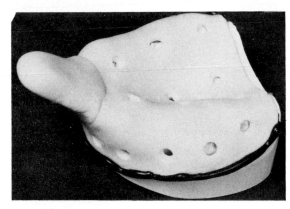

Figure 26-9 Border-molded custom acrylic impression tray used for final impression.

tween the upper and lower jaws is called vertical dimension. The natural teeth also determine how the mandible relates to the maxilla in both an anteroposterior direction and a lateral (side-to-side) position (Figure 26-10, *A* and *B*). This jaw relationship is called **centric occlusion**. In other words, centric occlusion is the normal position of the jaws when the teeth are meshed together.

2. Since the natural posterior teeth have been removed, the patient no longer has the natural guides to determine either vertical dimension or centric occlusion (Figure 26-10, *C* and *D*). The dentist must substitute artificial spacers in place of the missing teeth to determine these jaw relationships. These spacers are the wax **occlusal rims** that are mounted on temporary denture bases called baseplates (Figure 26-11). This assembly is fabricated in the laboratory on the master casts.

3. The dentist can reestablish the proper vertical dimension by adding or removing wax from the rims as needed. The occlusal rims are repeatedly tried in the patient's mouth until proper vertical dimension is established.

4. Centric occlusion can be determined by a variety of techniques that include tracing devices mounted on the occlusal rims and various manipulations of the mandible during closing exercises.

Tooth selection

1. Once jaw relationships are taken on the occlusal rims, the denture teeth must be selected. The proper shade is determined with the use of shade guides to compare with the patient's remaining natural teeth and the complexion of the facial skin. Age is a factor in shade selection, since natural teeth darken somewhat with age. A very light-shaded tooth would not look natural in an older patient's mouth. The size and shape (mold)

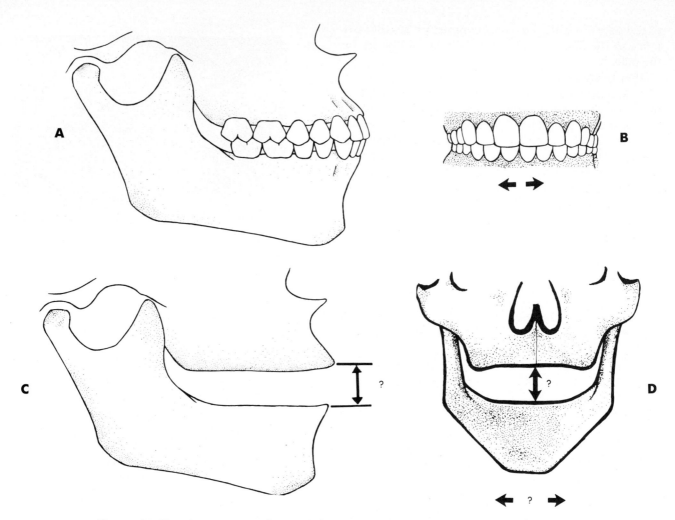

Figure 26-10 Components of vertical dimension. **A** and **B**, Natural dentition. Vertical dimension (**A**) is determined by lengths of crowns of upper and lower teeth. Centric occlusion is also determined by natural dentition. **C** and **D**, Edentulous ridges. Completely edentulous ridges or those missing only posterior teeth lose natural determination of vertical dimension and centric occlusion.

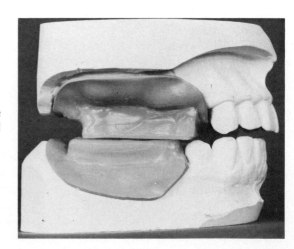

Figure 26-11 Occlusal wax rims mounted on baseplates. Excessive height exists initially so that dentist can adjust height to proper vertical dimension.

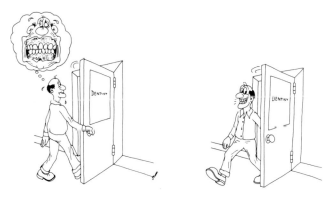

Figure 26-12

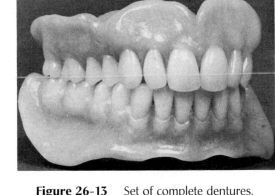

Figure 26-13 Set of complete dentures.

of the denture teeth are important in achieving natural aesthetics for the denture wearer. This can be done by comparing tooth mold guides with the remaining natural teeth if they are sufficiently intact. If these teeth are substantially destroyed by caries or fracture, the shape of the patient's face is used as a guide to selecting the proper shape of anterior teeth. There is a general correlation between the shape of the patient's face and the shape of the anterior teeth. For example, a person with a long, narrow face will have longer, more slender anterior teeth.

2. Obviously, patients are concerned about the aesthetics of their new denture, as well as with function. Creating natural-appearing complete dentures for a patient calls on the artistic skill of the dentist and the laboratory technician. Vertical dimension, shade, size, shape, and the arrangement of the teeth all play a role in aesthetics. Patients are apprehensive regarding the appearance of their dentures. The use of study models, photographs, and accurate measurements are helpful in achieving a natural-appearing denture (Figure 26-12).

3. After all measurements are taken, appointments are made for the removal of the patient's remaining teeth and the insertion of new dentures.

Laboratory phase

1. The master casts, occlusal rims, shade guide, mold, study models, and photographs are sent to the laboratory where the denture is made.

2. The finished denture will not fit the anterior portion of the dental arches precisely, since the denture is made before the teeth in this area are removed. However, this approximate fit does suffice until complete healing occurs.

Delivery of denture (Figure 26-13)

1. The remaining anterior teeth are removed, any necessary alveoloplasty is done, and sutures are placed.

2. The dentures are removed from a bath of disinfecting solution and rinsed.

3. The dentures are inserted, and adjustments are made as necessary to improve fit and the occlusion.

4. Patients should be given postsurgical instructions and asked to return the next day. Patients should not remove the dentures until then.

First Postsurgical Appointment

1. The patient is asked to return the day after surgery so that the denture can be removed and cleaned.

2. The dentist can carefully clean the surgical site.

3. Additional adjustments on the denture may be made at this time.

4. Detailed instructions on diet, eating methods, and speech exercises are given.

5. The patient returns 4 to 6 days later for suture removal.

Postinsertion Adjustments

1. The need for adjustments on a denture varies with each patient.

2. Denture adjustments may include minor alterations of the occlusion or relieving small areas of acrylic on the tissue surface of the denture base. These areas cause excessive pressure on the underlying soft tissue, resulting in denture stores.

3. Adjustments are accomplished with small grindstones and acrylic burs in the straight handpiece.

OVERDENTURES

The **overdenture** is a special complete denture that is designed to fit over roots of teeth that are retained in the jaws and treated endodontically. The crowns of these selected teeth are removed, and the roots are restored with special cast-gold posts and cores or with special prefabrication attachments (Figure 26-14).

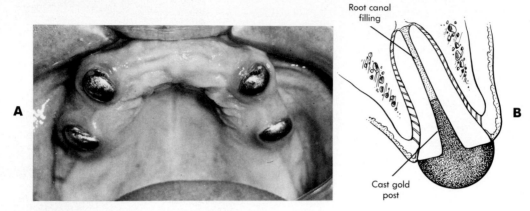

Figure 26-14   Supporting abutments for overdenture. **A,** Ideal four-abutment distribution. **B,** Roots are restored with a cast-gold post and dome-shaped core combination. (**A** from Brewer AA, Morrow RM: *Overdentures,* St Louis, 1980, Mosby.)

> **⇢ KEY POINT**
> ▪ With overdentures, the root of the tooth is retained.

Advantages

The conventional complete denture described previously rests entirely on the mucosa and is supported by the underlying bone of the dental arches. On the other hand, the overdenture is supported in part by the restored roots. This reduces the occlusal force placed on the mucosa and alveolar bone during mastication. Studies have shown that this results in less alveolar bone loss over time than with patients who wear conventional dentures.

The stability and retention of the conventional denture rely on the suction formed between the denture surface and the mucosa it contacts, as well as the shape of the alveolar ridges. If a patient has a poor ridge form, stability and retention of the denture can be difficult to achieve. Special prefabricated attachments can be inserted in the overdenture and retained roots to overcome the retention problem. Mechanical anchors offer similar retention to that associated with removable partial dentures. The Zest anchor (Figure 26-15) relies on mechanical lock of a stud located in the denture base, which inserts into a special receptacle that is cemented into the retained roots. Magnets can also used for retention (Figure 26-16).

Disadvantages

Overdentures are more costly than conventional dentures because of the endodontic treatment of any retained roots and the fabrication of retention posts or special an-chors. In addition, the patient is confronted with a greater maintenance problem, since the roots are retained. Plaque control is essential to prevent bone loss and root caries around the retained roots. Bone loss and root caries can result in loss of the overdenture and a retreat to a conventional denture for the patient.

DENTURE RELINING

After a complete or partial denture is worn for a period, it is common for the edentulous ridge to undergo a generalized reduction in size. This shrinkage results from initial healing of the ridges, and later reduction occurs in response to excessive force being placed on the dentures. Regardless of the cause of edentulous ridge reduction, the problem that results is the same—the denture no longer fits the ridge (Figure 26-17, *A*).

A technique to compensate for ridge reduction has been developed that allows the dentist to add new acrylic to the tissue surface of the denture base. This is called **denture relining.** By placing a new layer, or lining, of acrylic inside the denture, the dentist readapts the denture to the now smaller ridges, thus improving the fit without remaking the entire denture (Figure 26-17, *B*).

Two basic methods are used to reline a complete or partial denture: the chairside reline and the laboratory-processed reline. Some cases require tissue conditioning before the reline procedure.

Tissue Conditioning

Traumatization of the oral mucosa for extended periods by ill-fitting dentures can result in inflamed and enlarged tissues. The anterior segment of the maxillary arch is a common site for this phenomenon (Figure 26-18). Before

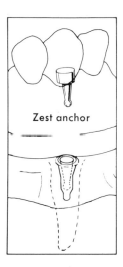

Figure 26-15   Zest intraradicular stud attachment.
(From Brewer AA, Morrow RM: *Overdentures*, St Louis, 1980, Mosby.)

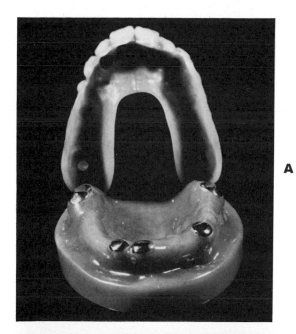

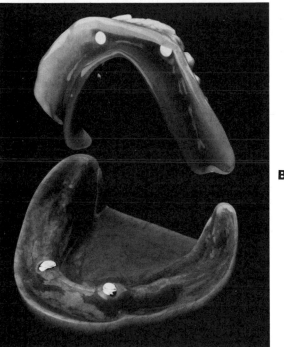

Figure 26-16   Overdentures with magnets embedded in denture base to connect with metal studs (keepers) cemented in retained roots for retention. **A,** Maxillary overdenture with open palate. **B,** Mandibular overdenture.
(Courtesy Parkell Products Inc, Farmingdale, NY.)

a reline is performed, these tissues must heal and return to normal size. A chairside procedure called **tissue conditioning** is performed several weeks before the final reline is done. The procedure is the same as the chairside reline described later with the exception of the lining material used. A soft lining material is placed in the denture and allowed to set with the denture in the patient's mouth. The excess lining material is trimmed away when the denture is removed (Figure 26-19). The patient wears this temporary soft lining while the tissue heals. In severe cases the liner must be replaced periodically as the tissue shrinks to its normal size. When the healing is complete, the permanent reline can be done. Occasionally surgery is required to remove damaged tissue before the reline procedure is accomplished.

Chairside Reline

Chairside reline is a common way of referring to a technique that allows the dentist to add a new acrylic lining to a denture as a chairside procedure without any laboratory phase. The advantage of this technique is that the entire procedure can be accomplished in one appointment, so that the patient does not have to be without a denture for any time. The disadvantage of this procedure is that the lining is generally not as durable as can be achieved with the laboratory-processed lining materials.

Preparation of denture

1. The denture to be relined is removed.
2. The tissue surface of the denture base is roughened with an acrylic grindstone.
3. The tissue surface of the denture base is cleaned for a few minutes in the ultrasonic cleaner.

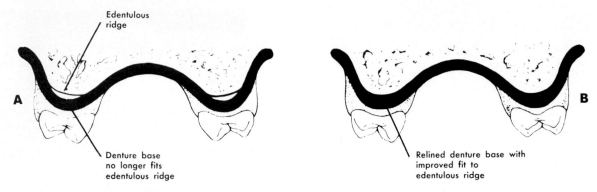

Figure 26-17 **A**, Frontal section across maxillae demonstrating poor fit of denture base to edentulous ridge. **B**, Relining denture readapts it to edentulous ridge.

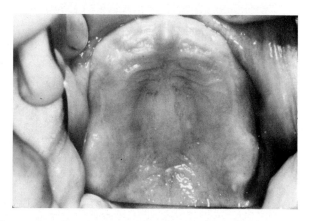

Figure 26-18 Common site of tissue irritation associated with ill-fitting denture.

(Courtesy Wayne Harvey, DDS, School of Dentistry, University of Colorado, Denver.)

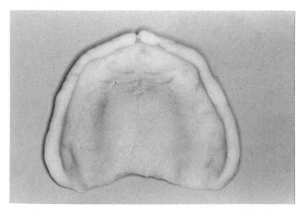

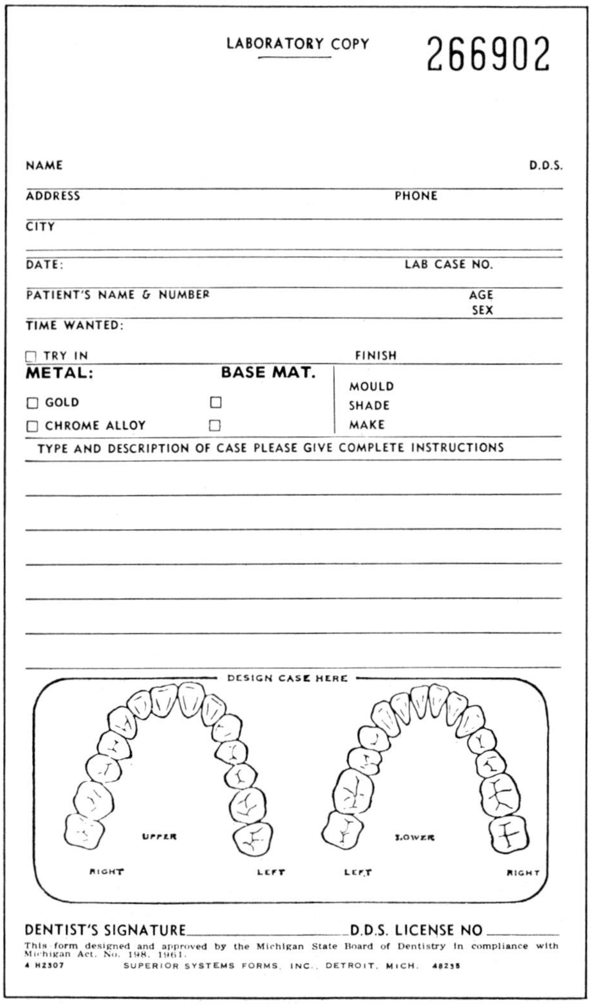

Figure 26-19 Maxillary denture with white tissue-conditioning lining in place.

(Courtesy Wayne Harvey, DDS, School of Dentistry, University of Colorado, Denver.)

LABORATORY COPY 266902

NAME D.D.S.

ADDRESS PHONE

CITY

DATE: LAB CASE NO.

PATIENT'S NAME & NUMBER AGE SEX

TIME WANTED:

☐ TRY IN FINISH

METAL: BASE MAT.

☐ GOLD ☐ MOULD

☐ CHROME ALLOY ☐ SHADE MAKE

TYPE AND DESCRIPTION OF CASE PLEASE GIVE COMPLETE INSTRUCTIONS

DESIGN CASE HERE

UPPER RIGHT LEFT

LOWER LEFT RIGHT

DENTIST'S SIGNATURE________ D.D.S. LICENSE NO ________

This form designed and approved by the Michigan State Board of Dentistry in compliance with Michigan Act. No. 198, 1961.

4 H2307 SUPERIOR SYSTEMS FORMS, INC., DETROIT, MICH. 48235

Figure 26-20 Laboratory prescription form.

(Courtesy Superior Systems Forms Inc, Detroit.)

Preparation of material

1. Several brands of self-curing acrylics are available to use as relining material. They are available also as either hard or semisoft liners.
2. The material is dispensed and mixed according to the manufacturer's instructions and added to the clean denture. The entire tissue surface of the denture base is coated with the material.

Patient preparation

1. The patient should rinse the mouth with a mouthwash to remove saliva from the tissue surface.
2. The denture is inserted and positioned properly. The patient is asked to bite gently with the teeth in proper occlusion until the material reaches its initial set. The patient should be cautioned that there may be a burning sensation from the acrylic during the initial setting time.
3. Then the denture is removed and allowed to harden completely.

Finishing of denture

1. After hardening the excess acrylic can be trimmed away and the denture polished before returning it to the patient.
2. The denture is reinserted and adjusted as needed. The patient is then dismissed.

Laboratory-Processed Reline

The laboratory-processed relining procedure involves a laboratory phase whereby the patient must part with a denture for a time. It is common to schedule the two-appointment procedure so that the patient will not have to be without teeth more than 1 day, especially in complete denture cases.

Preparation of denture

The denture is prepared in the same manner as described for the chairside procedure.

Impression

1. An impression of the edentulous ridge is made with an elastomeric impression material or a ZOE impression paste. The prepared denture is used as an impression tray for the mercaptan.
2. The impression material is dispensed and mixed in the usual manner and placed in the denture, covering the tissue surface. There should be no excess material, thus reducing the possibility of gagging the patient.
3. The denture is inserted and positioned properly. The patient is asked to close the teeth gently into occlusion until the material sets.
4. After the impression material sets, the denture is removed, and the patient is dismissed.

Laboratory phase

The denture lined with the impression is sent to the laboratory where the mercaptan is replaced with either hard or semisoft acrylic that is fused to the denture base.

Delivery of denture

1. The patient returns to receive the relined denture the day after the impression was made.
2. Adjustments are made as needed, and the patient is dismissed.
3. The immediate denture patient usually requires a reline 3 to 12 months after initial insertion of the denture. This is because of the rather dramatic reduction in ridge size during the healing process.

> **↝ KEY POINTS**
> - Denture sores indicate a need for a tissue conditioner.
> - Tissue changes that occur over time indicate a need for a denture reline if denture sores are not present.

DENTURE REPAIRS

Simple repairs to a broken denture can be done at the dental office and, depending on the extent of the damage, may not require the presence of the patient. More complex repairs such as missing teeth or complex fractures need to be sent to the dental laboratory for repairs.

LABORATORY PRESCRIPTION

The laboratory prescription is a legal authorization for a dental technician to fabricate a dental appliance, restoration, or device for a patient after all the intraoral procedures have been performed by the dentist. This document is similar to that used in prescribing medications for a patient at a pharmacy.

The prescription not only authorizes the work to be done, but also should describe in detail what the dentist wants. Figure 26-20 demonstrates a conventional form that is used. Carbon copies are essential to ensure both the dentist and the technician that communications are precise. Note the information that is included on the prescription. The assistant should use this form as a checklist to be sure all information, materials, models, and shade guide directions are included before sending the case to the laboratory. Most states require the signature and license number of the dentist on the prescription form.

BIBLIOGRAPHY

Finkbeiner BL, Johnson CS: *Mosby's comprehensive dental assisting: a clinical approach,* St Louis, 1995, Mosby.

McGivney GP, Castleberry DJ: *McCracken's removable partial prosthodontics,* ed 9, St Louis, 1995, Mosby.

Phillips RW, Moore BK: *Elements of dental materials for dental hygienists and dental assistants,* ed 5, Philadelphia, 1994, WB Saunders.

QUESTIONS–Chapter 26

1. All the following are recommended home care instructions for a removable prosthesis *except*:
   a. Take the prosthesis out at night.
   b. Scrub the prosthesis with household cleaners.
   c. Clean the prosthesis before going to bed.
   d. Place the prosthesis in water if taken out of the mouth.

2. A procedure that uses a soft lining placed on the tissue side of a denture that is used for denture sores is called:
   a. Denture relining
   b. Border molding
   c. Tissue conditioning
   d. Muscle trimming

3. A technique used to compensate for alveolar ridge reduction by adding new acrylic to the tissue surface of the denture base is called:
   a. Denture relining
   b. Border molding
   c. Tissue conditioning
   d. Muscle trimming

4. Overdentures are good because:
   a. The retained root tips help to maintain the height of the alveolar ridge.
   b. The retained root tips prevent denture sores.
   c. The overdenture requires less maintenance.
   d. Crowns can be placed over the retained roots.

5. When the patient is going to receive immediate dentures, the teeth are taken out in which order:
   a. All at once
   b. One side at a time
   c. Posterior teeth one side at a time and then anterior teeth
   d. Anterior teeth and then posterior teeth

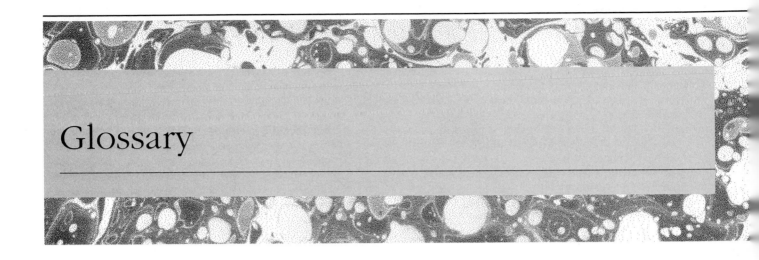

Glossary

Abrasive rubber point A device used to polish an amalgam restoration.

Abutment The teeth that support the fixed bridge at each end.

Acid etching Application of phosphoric acid to the walls and floors of the cavity preparation to dissolve the organic portion of the enamel that leaves a rough crystalline structure.

Activator A functional appliance used to reduce excessive overbite, to make changes in the skeletal growth, and for minor tooth movement.

Acute apical periodontitis Inflammation of the periodontal tissues at the apex of the tooth that comes on suddenly.

Aesthetic Pleasing to the eye.

Aesthetic crown A dental restoration that covers the crown of the tooth yet is pleasing to the eye and is most likely tooth colored.

Air-powder abrasive polisher A polishing device that sprays a solution of sodium bicarbonate and water to remove stain and plaque from the tooth surface.

Air-water syringe A device that delivers a stream of water or air and can also deliver a forceful spray of air and water. It is used to rinse the patient's mouth and also to clean and dry the working site.

All-ceramic crown A tooth-colored dental restoration made entirely from a special ceramic material.

Allergic reaction A hypersensitive response caused by sensitivity to a foreign agent.

Alveolitis The blood clot that normally fills the alveolus does not form or forms and is lost from the alveolus, which causes the painful exposure of the alveolar bone to the oral environment. Another term for alveolitis is *dry socket*.

Alveoloplasty Use of surgical instruments to shape the edentulous ridge.

Amalgam An alloy of an element or a metal with mercury as one of its components.

Amalgam carrier A hand instrument used to transport the mixed amalgam to the cavity preparation.

Amalgam carver A hand instrument used to carve the anatomical features on the occlusal aspect of an amalgam restoration.

Amalgam condenser A hand instrument with a flat surface on the working end that is used to press amalgam against the cavity walls and floors. Sometimes called a plugger.

Amalgam overhang Excess amalgam along the cervical margin.

Amalgam well A small metal dish used to hold mixed amalgam.

Amalgamator A machine that mixes the mercury and silver alloy to produce amalgam.

Ambu bag (bag-valve-mask device) A portable, self-inflating manual resuscitator used to administer cardiopulmonary resuscitation.

Angina pectoris Chest pain caused by insufficient blood supply to the heart muscle.

Apical periodontitis Inflammation of the periodontal tissues near the apex of the tooth.

Apicoectomy The surgical removal of the apex of the tooth.

Arch wires The principal guide portions of the fixed appliance. The arch wire is attached to the brackets by wire ligatures or elastic ligatures on either the facial or lingual aspect of the teeth, depending on the task being performed by the wire. Arch wires function either to move individual teeth or to hold them in a desirable fixed position.

Articulating (carbon) paper A sheet of blue or red carbon paper used to check the patient's occlusion after the placement of a restoration.

Articulating headrest A headrest that can be moved into multiple positions.

Articulator A mounting system for diagnostic casts that can position the casts in various jaw positions. The articulator represents the patient's own occlusal and biting functions.

Asepsis The avoidance of potentially pathogenic microorganisms.

Aspirate To inhale a foreign object into the airway.

Aspiration Placing negative pressure in the anesthetic cartridge by pulling back on the thumb ring to check if the needle has entered a blood vessel.

Assistant's stool The chair that the assistant uses to provide dental treatment to the patient.

Assistant's zone The part of the work circle where the dental assistant is positioned during the delivery of dental treatment; 2 to 4 o'clock position for a right-handed operator.

Asthma A condition that causes wheezing and sometimes coughing. It is brought on by constriction of the airway passages and hypersecretion of fluids in the airways.

Autochuck A special handpiece chuck used to hold and place retention pins.

Automatrix band A preformed stainless steel strip that is fabricated into a loop to fit around the prepared tooth and does not need a retainer.

Automix system A type of impression system in which hand mixing is not required.

Avulsed tooth A tooth that has been knocked out of the bony socket.

Barbed broach A thin, flexible hand instrument used to remove the pulp.

Bass method of toothbrushing A method of toothbrushing in which the toothbrush bristles are oriented in a 45-degree angle to the long axis of the tooth and a vibratory motion is used to remove plaque and debris from the teeth.

Bevel The opening of the oral evacuator tip is slightly angled to create a bevel.

Biological monitor A commercially prepared test that contains biological spores and can determine the effectiveness of a heat sterilizer.

Biopsy The surgical removal of a piece of tissue from the body for examination under the microscope.

Biopsy report A written descriptive summary of a patient's oral lesion that accompanies the actual biopsy to the pathology laboratory.

Bite registration A device used to orient upper and lower models of the teeth in the proper bite relationship during the laboratory phase of a crown fabrication.

Black's cavity classification A classification system used to code cavities according to location on the tooth.

Boiling bath Used to convert the agar hydrocolloid material from the gel stage to the sol stage.

Bone file A serrated hand instrument used for minor bone removal and to smooth the surface of the bone before wound closure.

Bone resorption The breakdown of bone by bone-removing cells called osteoclasts.

Bone surgery See Osseous surgery.

Border molding A technique used during the fabrication of a removable partial or denture. Border molding helps to adapt the border of the partial or complete denture to the patient's soft tissues.

Brackets Attachments welded to the orthodontic bands. Brackets hold the arch wire in place and transmit the force of the arch wire to the teeth.

Bridge threader A flexible plastic device used to floss under a fixed bridge to remove plaque from the interproximal surfaces.

Bruxism Tooth grinding.

Buccal tubes Hollow-channeled brackets attached to molar bands. They serve as anchors for facial arch wires.

Buccal/labial A vertical surface on the tooth that faces toward the cheek.

Buccoversion Buccal to normal position.

Bur Similar to a bit placed in a carpenter's drill. Depending on the type of bur, the dentist can remove tooth structure or polish and refine dental restorations or the teeth.

Burnisher A smooth-tipped hand instrument used to smooth the occlusal surface of the amalgam restoration.

Calculus A hard deposit formed on the tooth surface; often called tartar.

Capsule A hollow container that holds the mercury and silver alloy when the amalgam is mixed.

Cardiac arrest A condition in which the heart ceases to function.

Cardiopulmonary resuscitation (CPR) An emergency procedure used to establish an oxygen supply and blood circulation to a person who has stopped breathing and whose heart has stopped beating.

Caries Dental decay.

Cast-gold crown A substantial portion of the natural crown of the tooth is reconstructed with gold.

Cast-gold post and core A custom-made unit placed into the hollow pulp chamber and root canal to help the retention of the permanent restoration.

Cavity classification A system of classifying dental caries according to its location on the tooth surface.

Cavity liner A thin, creamlike material that lines the deepest portion of the cavity preparation.

Cavity preparation A systematic cutting of tooth structure in which any unwanted portion of the hard layers of the tooth is removed.

Cavity varnish A liquid substance that seals the open ends of the dentin tubules with a glazelike covering.

Celluloid crown forms Celluloid crown forms act as molds to reconstruct a part of or the entire crown of a prepared tooth.

Cement base A thick, doughlike material that hardens in the cavity preparation and replaces lost dentin.

Cementation appointment Gold, porcelain, and indirect composite restorations require two appointments. The first appointment is the preparation appointment, in which portions of the tooth are removed to provide a space for the restoration. The second appointment is the cementation appointment, in which the fabricated restoration is permanently cemented onto the prepared tooth.

Centric occlusion The normal position of the jaws when the teeth are meshed together.

Cephalometric radiograph A special radiograph of the entire head used by the orthodontist for diagnosis and also to evaluate and document treatment progression.

Cerebrovascular accident (CVA) A condition caused by blockage in the brain that produces insufficient blood supply to the patient.

Chemical monitor A special chemical placed on tape or sterilization wraps that turns a color when exposed to certain sterilization conditions.

Chemical vapor sterilization A heat sterilizer that uses heat, chemical vapor, and pressure to achieve sterilization. Often termed a *chemiclave*.

Chronic apical periodontitis See Granuloma.

Chuck A small screwdriver type of instrument used to replace the burs for the dental handpiece. Some handpieces have a nonremovable autochuck built into the handpiece.

Class I movements Movement of only the fingers.

Class II movements Movement of the fingers and wrist.

Class III movements Movement of the fingers, wrist, and elbow.

Class IV movements Movement of the entire arm from the shoulder.

Class V movements Movement of the entire arm and twisting of the trunk.

Cleaning The gross removal of bioburden, such as saliva or blood.

Closed coil springs Orthodontic springs that are stretched between teeth and exert a pulling force on selected teeth.

Complex extraction A more extensive effort is made to extract a tooth or teeth.

Composite resin inlay A tooth-colored restoration that is placed in class II cavity preparations.

Composite restorative material A tooth-colored resin material used to restore aesthetic areas of the mouth.

Composite syringe A device that helps to dispense the composite into the tooth preparation.

Condensation The pressing of the amalgam tightly against the cavity walls and matrix band.

Conditioner An acid solution applied to the walls and floors of the cavity preparation to prepare the tooth for the bonding process.

Congenitally missing Lack of development of the teeth.

Contouring pliers A hand instrument used to shape the matrix band to conform to the contours of a prepared tooth.

Contra-angle attachment Placed in the slow-speed handpiece setup to extend the functions of the handpiece. This type of attachment is slightly bent for easier access in the oral cavity.

Cooley peg A device used to seat a crown or bridge restoration onto the tooth preparation.

Coping material A thin sheet of plastic sometimes used for fabricating a temporary bridge with a custom acrylic material.

Corrective orthodontics Designed to reduce the severity of an existing malocclusion or to eliminate it entirely.

Cricothyrotomy An emergency procedure used to open the airway of a person who is choking. The airway is opened by cutting a small opening just below the Adam's apple.

Cross-contamination The transfer of microorganisms from one person or inanimate object to another.

Crossbite The lower teeth overlapping the upper teeth.

Crowding The dental assistant holding the instrument too close to the instrument the dentist is using before the actual instrument transfer occurs.

Cure To harden.

Curettage The removal of the delicate epithelial lining of the periodontal pocket.

Curette scalers Hand instruments with a rounded tip, a rounded back of the blade, and cutting edges along both sides of the blade. Curette scalers are used for scaling, root planing, and curettage.

Dappen dish A small glass, plastic, or rubber cup used to hold a variety of dental materials. Sometimes used to hold mixed amalgam.

Delivery corridor The primary route of instruments and materials to and from the oral cavity during a treatment procedure.

Demineralization The dissolution of minerals from the hard surfaces of the tooth caused by acid-producing bacteria.

Dental chair The chair that is used by the patient to receive dental treatment.

Dental compound A waxlike material used to stabilize the rubber dam clamp.

Dental floss A stringlike material used to remove plaque from the interproximal areas of the teeth.

Dental handpiece Similar to a carpenter's drill. The handpiece rotates cutting and polishing burs for certain types of dental procedures.

Dental implants Titanium implants placed directly into the alveolar bone and used to anchor fixed restorations or removable prostheses.

Dental operatory The primary work area in which dental treatment is performed on the patient by the dentist, assistant, and hygienist.

Dental unit The control center for the dental handpieces; often contains the oral evacuator, air-water syringe, saliva ejector, ultrasonic scaler, and fiberoptic composite light probe.

Dentifrice A dental term for toothpaste.

Dentin smear layer An organic film of debris produced by the bur rotating against the dentin surface.

Denture relining A technique used to compensate for alveolar ridge reduction by adding new acrylic to the tissue surface of the denture base.

Diagnosis Identification of a disease.

Disclosing solution A solution that will discolor plaque accumulation as stained areas on the teeth. Available in tablet form for patient home use.

Disinfection The destruction of most microorganisms but not highly resistant forms such as spores.

Disorientation The dental assistant passing an instrument to the dentist and the working end is pointed toward the wrong arch.

Disposable barrier Any impervious material, such as aluminum foil or plastic wrap, that is placed on frequently touched surfaces or equipment to prevent cross contamination.

Distal A vertical surface on the tooth that faces away from the midline.

Distal wedge procedure A surgical procedure used for deep periodontal pockets distal to the last molar.

Distoversion Distal to normal position.

Double sheer pins Two retention pins attached end to end and mounted on one plastic shank.

Draw The relationship of the cavity walls from the floor of the cavity preparation to the cavosurface margins. The walls of a cavity preparation are slightly tapered so that a rigid restoration can slide into place.

Drifting When a tooth is lost, the surrounding teeth will move out of position; usually in a tilted manner.

Dry-heat oven A heat sterilizer that uses heat to achieve sterilization.

Dual-arch tray An impression tray that takes an impression of the desired upper and lower teeth at the same time. Available for a posterior quadrant or an anterior sextant.

Dual-cure bond agent An adhesive material that can be changed to its final hardened state by light curing or by a chemical cure.

Elastic separators   A rubber device that is placed between the teeth to move them apart in preparation for the placement of an orthodontic band.

Elastics   Rubber bands that are used to exert force on teeth. Special buttons or hooks are attached to orthodontic bands and serve as connectors for the elastics.

Electric toothbrush   A toothbrush that uses electricity to simulate the brushing action of a patient using a manual toothbrush.

Electrical pulp test   A diagnostic tool that uses electrical current to stimulate nerve fibers in the pulp to test for pulp vitality.

Electrosurgery   A surgical method that uses a tiny arch of electrical current to make the incision in the gingiva.

Enamel pits and fissures   Tiny voids in the enamel that are difficult to clean because the voids are smaller than a single toothbrush bristle.

Enamel tags   Acid etching removes the organic portion of enamel, and the remaining crystalline structure forms a rough surface that is favorable for the bonding process.

Endodontic file   A hand instrument used to smooth, shape, and enlarge the root canal.

Endodontic reamer   A hand instrument used to smooth, shape, and enlarge the root canal.

Endodontic storage box   A metal compartmentalized container that holds endodontic instruments and can be heat sterilized.

Endodontics   A specialty concerned primarily with diseases of the dental pulp and periapical tissues.

Epilepsy   Uncontrolled discharges of nerve cells in the brain that cause recurrent convulsive seizures.

Etchant   A weak solution of phosphoric acid used to dissolve the organic portion of enamel to create a stronger bond between the tooth and the bonding restoration.

Etched porcelain veneers   Aesthetic porcelain facings that are placed on anterior teeth.

Ethylene oxide   A room temperature gas used to sterilize instruments and equipment.

Evacuation   The suctioning of saliva, blood, and other debris from the patient's mouth.

Excisional biopsy   The removal of an entire lesion plus some adjacent normal tissue.

Exfoliation   The shedding of primary teeth.

Exfoliative cytology   The study of tissue cells scraped from the surface of a lesion.

Exodontia   The removal or extraction of teeth.

Expansion activator   An activator also used to expand the upper arch.

Explorer   An instrument used to detect calculus, dental caries, and defective margins of restorations.

Extraction elevators   Leverlike instruments used for luxation of a tooth from its bony socket.

Extraction forceps   Plierslike instruments used to grasp the tooth and deliver it from the bony socket.

Extraoral radiographs   Dental x-rays that do not require intraoral placement of dental film.

Extrusion   Overeruption of a tooth with the occlusal surface above the occlusal plane of that arch.

Face bow   That part of the articulator that helps to orient the maxillary cast on the articulator.

Facial   A universal term for a vertical surface on the tooth that is facing toward the lips or cheek.

Field block anesthesia   The injection of a local anesthetic agent to numb larger terminal nerve branches that prevents pain impulses from the tooth to the brain.

File stops   Tiny, circular disks of silicone rubber placed on files and reamers to mark the length of the root canal.

Finger signal   The dentist bending the index finger and shifting the instrument away from the oral cavity to nonverbally communicate to the assistant readiness for the next instrument.

Finger springs   Used to apply forces to individual teeth. They can be soldered to the main arch wire or used on removable appliances.

Finishing disks   Small abrasive disks of sandpaper used to contour and polish various restorations.

Finishing stones   Rotary instruments used to smooth a composite restoration.

Fistula   A drainage tract for pus formed through the bone from a periapical abscess.

Fixed appliances   Orthodontic appliances attached to the patient's teeth with a dental cement and circumferential bands or by direct bonding.

Fixed bridge   A permanent restoration used to replace mixing teeth.

Fixed consoles   Dental cabinets that are affixed to the wall or floor of the treatment room.

Fixed prosthodontics   The area of dental practice that involves extensive restoration of teeth using a crown and bridge procedures.

Flap surgery   A surgical procedure used for deep periodontal pockets to remove the diseased lining of the periodontal pocket and also some of the adjacent marginal gingiva.

Flash   Excess material that squeezes out of the cavity preparation when the matrix strip is removed.

Floss holder   A Y-shaped floss-holding device.

Fluoride   A substance found in minerals that is caries inhibiting when ingested or used topically.

Fluorosis   A permanent staining of the teeth caused by the ingestion of fluoride over 1 ppm.

Four-handed dentistry   The delivery of dental treatment by the dentist and assistant working together at chairside.

Friction-grip bur (short shank)   A smooth-shanked bur used in the high-speed handpiece.

Fulcrum   A finger rest used by the operator to stabilize the hand.

Full crown   The natural crown of the tooth is reconstructed with gold, porcelain, or a combination of both.

Functional appliance   Generally used in the earlier phase of orthodontic treatment to make changes (both skeletal and tooth) as the patient is growing.

Galvanism   The flow of electrical current between two different metals through an electrolyte.

General anesthesia   The absence of sensation and consciousness by the administration of an anesthetic agent.

Gingival grafts   A surgical procedure that removes gingival tissue from one area of the mouth to place it in another area of the mouth that is deficient in gingiva.

Gingival pocket   A deepening of the gingival crevice or sulcus caused by the enlargement of the gingiva in gingivitis.

Gingival retraction cord A braided string inserted into the periodontal pocket surrounding the tooth to temporarily push the gingiva away from the tooth. The retraction cord allows the dentist to take an accurate impression of the cervical margins of a crown preparation.

Gingival stimulators Devices used to stimulate the circulation of blood to the soft tissues of the gingiva.

Gingivectomy The surgical removal of diseased gingival tissue.

Gingivitis Inflammation of the gingiva caused by plaque.

Gold inlay A restoration made from gold alloy that has been cast to fit a cavity preparation made by the dentist. The bulk of the restoration is contained within the confines of a tapered cavity preparation.

Gracey curette An instrument used to scale specific surfaces of the teeth.

Granuloma Inflammation of the periodontal tissues near the apex of the tooth that occurs slowly as a response to bacteria and irritants in the pulp.

Guided tissue regeneration An adjunctive effort employed during surgical flap procedures that is believed to encourage new attachment.

Gutta-percha An inert, rubberlike material used to fill and seal the root canal.

Gutta-percha plugger (condenser) A long, blunt hand instrument used to pack the gutta-percha into the root canal.

Headgear devices Extraoral device used either to hold teeth in a specific position or to move the maxillary molar teeth in a distal direction.

Healing cap A temporary covering of the hollow osseointegrated implant.

Heimlich maneuver An emergency procedure used for patients who have an airway obstruction. The choking person is grasped from behind by the rescuer. The rescuer compresses the abdomen with the arms, which are wrapped around the person who is choking.

Hemostat A multipurpose hand instrument used to clamp blood vessels, grasp unwanted tissue, and remove debris from the surgical site.

Hemostatic agent An astringent-like solution that is often placed on retraction cord to help control bleeding around a crown preparation.

High/heavy viscosity A type of impression material that is used to take an accurate replication of a tooth with a crown impression. The high/heavy viscosity material has a thick consistency. This material is often used with a low/light or medium viscosity material for a two-viscosity impression technique.

Hoe scalers Hand instruments that look similar to a gardener's hoe and are used to remove subgingival calculus.

Hyperemia An accumulation of an excessive amount of blood.

Hyperocclusion When the occlusal surface of a tooth or a restoration is raised above the occlusal plane of the teeth in the arch.

Hyperventilation Shortness of breath usually caused by anxiety.

Hypoglycemia A condition caused by lack of blood sugar.

Illumination When the operator uses the mouth mirror to shine visible light to see an area in the mouth better.

Immediate complete dentures Temporary dentures made before the removal of the anterior teeth of a patient and given to the patient immediately following the extractions.

Implant abutment A connector between the implant embedded in the bone and the fixed or removable prosthesis.

Impression trays Trays used to take a replication of the teeth and surrounding tissues.

Incident report A document that describes an accident or complication involving a patient.

Incisal A horizontal surface on the biting surface of anterior teeth.

Incisional biopsy A procedure that involves the removal of a sample of a lesion for examination.

Indirect vision When the operator uses the mouth mirror to visualize areas of the mouth.

Infection control Policies or procedures of a health facility to avoid spreading infections between patients and/or staff.

Infiltration anesthesia The injection of a local anesthetic agent to numb tiny terminal nerve branches; used to numb the tissue in the immediate area.

Informed consent A process in which the patient makes an informed decision whether to give permission for the dentist to perform an invasive procedure.

Inlay A gold, composite, or porcelain restoration fabricated at the dental laboratory. The fabricated inlay is cemented into the tooth preparation using a bond agent.

Interceptive orthodontics Treatment procedures designed to intercept orthodontic problems that may worsen if left untreated.

Interdental brushes Small straight or conical brushes inserted into a plastic or metal handle to clean interproximal areas.

Interproximal wedge A triangular, wooden or plastic wedge placed between the teeth to act as a brace to hold the matrix band tightly against the tooth.

Intraoral radiographs Dental x-ray films that require the placement of intraoral dental film packets.

Inverting/everting To tuck the rubber dam toward the gingiva to create a seal around each tooth.

Irreversible pulpitis Inflammation of the pulp that has progressed to the point at which the pulp cannot recover, even on removal of the insulating agent.

Irrigation syringe A blunt-tipped syringe used to irrigate the surgical site with sterile saline solution.

Labioversion Labial to normal position.

Latch-type bur A bur with a notch at the end of the shank. Latch-type burs are used in the slow-speed handpiece contra-angle attachment.

Lesion A localized site of abnormal tissue.

Ligatures Fine wires or elastic bands used to tie or ligate the arch wire to the brackets.

Light cure When visible light is applied to light-cured composite, the pliable composite becomes hard.

Light-activated composite systems Tooth-colored resin materials that harden by exposure to visible light.

Lingual A vertical surface on upper teeth that faces toward the tongue.

Linguoversion Lingual to normal position.

Liquid sterilant Instruments are immersed in a glutaraldehyde solution for 10 hours or more to achieve sterilization.

Local anesthesia An agent used to eliminate sensation in a limited area of the body.

Long-shank bur A bur with an elongated shank. Long-shank burs are placed in the basic slow-speed handpiece setup.

Low/light viscosity A final impression material that flows readily, thus creating an accurate impression.

Low/light viscosity impression materials A type of impression material used to take an accurate replication of a tooth with a crown impression. The low/light viscosity material has a thin consistency that allows it to be placed around the prepared tooth with a syringe. This material is often referred to as the wash.

Luxation The displacement of the tooth in the bony socket by using extraction forceps.

Magill intubation forceps A specialized instrument used to grasp objects that have accidentally fallen into the back of the patient's throat.

Malocclusion Any deviation from normal occlusion.

Malpractice Negligence that causes injury or harm to a patient.

Mandrel Used with the slow-speed handpiece to attach various polishing disks to the contra-angle attachment.

Maryland bridge A permanent restoration that replaces missing teeth with minimal tooth preparation. The bridge has one pontic supported by thin metal retainers on either side. The retainers are bonded to the abutment teeth.

Matrix band Thin strips of stainless steel sheet metal used to create a form around a prepared tooth.

Matrix strip holder A clamplike device used to hold the matrix in place after the composite has been inserted into the cavity preparation.

Matrix strips Matrix strips are made of either clear plastic or celluloid for composite restorations. The matrix strip is used to replace a missing interproximal wall or contact for composite restorations.

Mechanical pulp exposure Opening of the pulp to the oral environment by mechanical means such as improper pin placement or accidental exposure with the dental handpiece.

Medical consult form A form used to obtain recommendations from the patient's physician regarding possible contraindications to dental treatment with the patient's existing medical conditions.

Medical-dental history form Information obtained from the patient regarding the patient's health status, which is used to make treatment-planning decisions.

Medium viscosity A final impression material that has a consistency between light/low and heavy impression material; often used to add bulk to the impression tray.

Medium viscosity impression material A type of impression material used to take an accurate replication of a tooth with a crown impression. The medium viscosity material has a semithin consistency that allows it to be placed around the prepared tooth with a syringe. This material is often used with a low/light viscosity material for a two-viscosity impression technique.

Mesial A vertical surface on the tooth that faces toward the midline.

Mesioversion Mesial to normal position.

Mixed dentition stage When a child has both primary and permanent teeth in the mouth. The mixed dentition stage ends with the loss of the last deciduous tooth.

Mixing tip A mixing tip is used with an Automix impression system. The mixing tip eliminates the need for hand mixing the impression material.

Mobile cart/cabinet A movable cabinet used by the assistant to hold auxiliary items needed during the treatment procedure.

Motion economy Minimizing undesirable movements by the dental team that could cause fatigue or uncomfortable positions.

Mottling Pitting of the teeth caused by ingestion of fluoride over 1 ppm.

Mouthrinse Solution that contains medication or other solutions to control mouth odors and minimize plaque accumulation.

Mucoperiosteum The soft oral tissue covering the bone that consists of the mucosa and the periosteum.

Muscle trimming See Border molding.

Myocardial infarct (heart attack) Crushing chest pains caused by blockage of an artery supplying oxygen to the heart.

Necrosis Dead tissue.

Needle holder A hemostat-like device used to guide the suture needle through the soft tissue to close the surgical site.

Nerve block anesthesia The injection of a local anesthetic agent near a main nerve trunk.

Nonvital pulp Pulp tissue that is necrotic (dead).

Obturation Filling the root canal to eliminate space within the canal to prevent leakage.

Occlusal A horizontal surface on the biting surface of posterior teeth.

Occlusal clearance wax A thin sheet of wax used to determine if the dentist has removed enough tooth structure from the occlusal surface in onlay and crown preparations.

Occlusal equilibration A procedure performed by the dentist to eliminate discrepancies in a patient's occlusion.

Occlusal rims Wax spaces used during fabrication of a removable prosthesis to determine the jaw relationship for missing teeth.

Occlusion The relationship of the maxillary and mandibular teeth when they are in contact.

One-finger pickup The dental assistant uses the last finger of the left hand to retrieve a dental instrument from the dentist's hand.

Onlay A modification of the cast-gold or porcelain inlay in which the restoration extends over the cusps of posterior teeth to prevent fracture of the teeth when biting forces are applied.

Open bite When the jaws are closed, the mandibular anterior teeth do not contact the lingual surfaces of the maxillary anterior teeth.

Open coil springs Orthodontic springs that are compressed between teeth and exert a pushing force on these teeth when the coil attempts to return to its normal length.

Operating light The overhead light used to illuminate the patient's oral cavity for better visibility.

Operating stools The chairs the assistant and dentist use to provide dental treatment to the patient.

Operator's zone The part of the work circle where the dentist is positioned during the delivery of dental treatment; 7 to 12 o'clock position for a right-handed operator.

Opposing teeth The teeth that are located in the opposite arch of the crown preparation.

Oral evacuator   A high-volume suction used to suck out fluids and debris from the patient's mouth.

Oral evacuator tip   A metal or plastic tip inserted into the patient's mouth to pick up saliva, blood, and other debris from the delivery of dental treatment.

Oral irrigator   A device that flushes soft deposits from the surfaces of the teeth.

Orangewood stick   A device used to seat a crown or bridge restoration onto the tooth preparation.

Orthodontic bands   Circumferential stainless steel bands fitted to individual teeth. They serve to connect the appliance to the teeth when cemented into place.

Orthodontics   A specialty area of dentistry that deals with problems related to the development of the jaws, the positions of the teeth, and the oral and facial muscles that influence speech, mastication, and swallowing.

Orthodontists   Specialists in orthodontics.

Osseointegration   The fusion of a dental implant to the bone.

Osseous surgery   A surgical procedure used to remove bony defects or to augment the bony defect with a bone graft.

Osteoblasts   Bone-building cells.

Osteoclasts   Bone-removing cells.

Outline form   The overall shape of the preparation along the external surface of the enamel; sometimes called cavosurface margin.

Overbite   The amount of vertical overlap of the incisal edges of upper anterior teeth over the incisal edges of lower anterior teeth.

Overdenture   A special complete denture designed to fit over roots of teeth that are retained in the jaws and treated endodontically.

Overeruption   See Extrusion.

Overgloves   Plastic food handler–type gloves worn over treatment gloves to prevent cross-contamination.

Overjet   The horizontal overlap of the upper anterior teeth to the lower anterior teeth.

Palatal   A vertical surface on the tooth that faces toward the palate.

Palliative treatment   Treatment strictly geared to making the patient comfortable.

Palpation   The use of the examiner's sense of touch to reveal abnormalities.

Partial denture   A metal and acrylic prosthetic device used to replace missing teeth.

Paste-paste composite material   A tooth-colored resin material comprised of a base paste and catalyst paste, which when mixed together become hard because of a chemical reaction.

Pedodontics   Children's dentistry that predominantly deals with problems related to patient management and education, restorative procedures, and interceptive orthodontics.

Pellicle   A thin, noncellular, adherent layer primarily composed of protein components that forms before plaque is deposited on the tooth.

Percussion   Gentle tapping on the incisal edge or occlusal surface of a tooth to test for sensitivity.

Periapical abscess   A localized collection of pus at the apex of the tooth.

Periapical cyst   A fluid-filled cavity lined with epithelial cells at the apex of the tooth.

Periodontal disease   Inflammation of the gingiva caused by subgingival plaque; often termed *gum disease*.

Periodontal dressing   A surgical covering placed over the surgical site to protect the wound from trauma.

Periodontal file scalers   Hand instruments that resemble miniature files and can be inserted subgingivally to remove or roughen tenacious calculus.

Periodontal knives   Hand instruments used to cut, remove, and contour gingival soft tissues.

Periodontal pocket   A deepening of the gingival crevice or sulcus when the epithelial attachment migrates down the root surface because of periodontal disease.

Periodontal probe   A thin dipsticklike device used to measure the depth of the gingival crevice or sulcus.

Periodontal scaling and root planing   The removal of plaque and calculus from the tooth surface using periodontal scaling instruments.

Periodontitis   Inflammation of the periodontal structures surrounding the tooth that results in loss of alveolar bone and migration of the epithelial attachment toward the apex of the tooth.

Periodontium   The supporting tissues of the tooth including the gingiva, the alveolar bone, and the periodontal ligament.

Periosteal elevator   A hand instrument used to separate the periosteum from the bone surface and to retract the mucoperiosteum.

Periosteum   The fibrous covering of the bone.

Permanent dentition stage   When a person has only permanent teeth present in the mouth.

Pestle   A small metal device placed inside the amalgam capsule that assists in the mixing process.

Pistol grip composite syringe   A type of composite dispenser.

Pit and fissure sealants   A preventive cavity measure that is a thin plasticlike material applied to pit and fissure areas of the tooth to seal the tooth from bacteria and bacterial by-products.

Plaque   A soft adherent collection of salivary products and bacterial colonies on the teeth.

Polishing   The removal of plaque and stain with a rubber cut and slow-speed handpiece or with an air-powder abrasive polisher.

Polishing strip   Abrasive material placed on a length of plastic. The polishing strip is used to smooth and polish the interproximal areas of the composite restoration.

Pontic   The artificial tooth that replaces the missing natural tooth in a fixed bridge.

Porcelain-bonded-to-metal crown   A dental restoration that completely covers the crown of the tooth and is made of a metal substructure covered with tooth-colored porcelain.

Positioner   A soft plastic appliance used immediately after the fixed orthodontic appliances are removed.

Positive-pressure oxygen   A positive-pressure oxygen system consists of a pressurized oxygen tank, a regulator to control the flow of oxygen, and a hose and mask to deliver oxygen to the patient during CPR administration.

Preappointment behavior modification   Anything that is said or done to positively influence the child's behavior before treatment.

Premeasured amalgam capsules   The components of amalgam (mercury and silver alloy powder) are placed in a disposable mixing container by the manufacturer.

Preparation appointment   Gold, porcelain, and indirect composite restorations require two appointments. The first appointment is the preparation appointment, in which portions of the tooth are removed to provide a space for the restoration. The second appointment is the cementation appointment, in which the fabricated restoration is permanently cemented onto the prepared tooth.

Preset trays   Using a standard set of instruments for individual treatment procedures. These instruments are used only for the specific procedure and may be color coded.

Primary dentition stage   When a child has only primary teeth present in the mouth. The primary dentition stage ends with the eruption of the first permanent tooth.

Primer   A solution applied to the acid-etched or "conditioned" tooth surface that acts as a wetting agent. The primer enhances the adhesive quality of the bond agent.

Prognosis   The predicted outcome of a disease.

Programmed-setting feature   A feature found on the dental chair that allows the chair to be automatically placed in preselected positions with one touch of an activation button.

Prophy paste   An abrasive agent usually made from flour of pumice that is used to remove plaque and polish the teeth.

Prophylactic premedication   The administration of antibiotics before dental treatment for certain conditions, such as mitral valve prolapse, to prevent subacute bacterial endocarditis.

Prophylaxis   Prevention of disease by cleaning the surfaces of the teeth.

Prophylaxis angle   A metal or disposable attachment to the basic slow-speed handpiece setup that is used to polish the teeth with a brush or rubber cup.

Prosthesis   An artificial body part.

Prosthodontics   The area of dental practice that deals with the extensive reconstruction of existing teeth and the replacement of missing teeth with various dental restorations and appliances.

Pseudopocket   See Gingival pocket.

Pulp capping   A procedure that places a calcium hydroxide paste on small exposures of the pulp before restoration of the tooth in an effort to avoid the need for a root canal.

Pulp exposure   Carious invasion of the pulp.

Pulpectomy   Complete removal of the dental pulp.

Pulpitis   The inflammation of pulpal tissue.

Pulpotomy   A procedure that involves partial removal of the dental pulp after it has been extensively exposed.

Putty-wash technique   An impression technique that uses a light/low viscosity impression material and a putty type of impression material. The light/low viscosity impression material is placed over the crown preparation first; the putty is placed in the impression tray. The impression tray is seated over the crown preparation and surrounding teeth.

Radiographic view box   A "light box" used to view dental radiographs.

Radiolucency   A dark area on a dental radiograph that could indicate endodontic cysts, granulomas, and abscesses among other things.

Rapid heat transfer sterilizer   A form of a dry-heat oven that operates similar to a convection oven and can sterilize instruments quickly.

Rear delivery system   Instruments are delivered to the dentist from a unit located behind the patient.

Recapping device   A metal, plastic, or paper device that holds the cap of the needle to minimize accidental needlesticks when the cap is replaced on the needle.

Resin luting cements   A permanent cementation material that is tooth colored and can be thought of as a runny composite.

Resistance form   The internal shape of the cavity preparation.

Retainers   Usually fabricated from metal and acrylic and used after fixed orthodontic appliance treatment to hold the teeth in the desired position until the teeth become stable in the newly remodeled alveolus.

Retention clasps   That part of a removable partial denture that helps to retain the prosthesis in place by wrapping around abutment teeth.

Retention core   Teeth that have lost significant tooth structure do not have enough retention to hold a permanent restoration in place. A retention core is a buildup of material on the natural tooth to create better retention of the permanent restoration.

Retention form   The relationship that exists between different walls of the preparation.

Retention pin   A small, screw-type device placed in the dentin of a prepared tooth that has lost a considerable amount of tooth structure to help hold the amalgam restoration in place.

Retention post   Occupation of the hollow pulp chamber and root canal of the tooth for anchoring of the permanent restoration.

Retraction   To pull, hold, or press the soft tissue for a clear line of vision.

Retrofill amalgam   The sealing of the apex of the tooth with amalgam following an apicoectomy.

Reversible pulpitis   Inflammation of the pulpal tissues that clears up after the insulting agent has been removed.

Rheostat   A foot pedal that controls the rotational speed of the high- and slow-speed handpiece.

Risk management   The identification, evaluation, and correction of potential risks that could lead to patient injury.

Rongeur forceps   A nipperlike instrument used to trim alveolar bone.

Root amputation   The removal of one or more roots of a multirooted tooth.

Root canal sealer   A special cement used to obturate an endodontically treated tooth.

Root picks   Surgical probes used to remove root fragments.

Root planing   Smoothing of the root surfaces to produce a surface from which it is easy to remove plaque.

Rotary scrub method of toothbrushing   A method of toothbrushing in which the toothbrush is placed at a right angle to the tooth and circular stokes are used to clean the surfaces of the teeth.

Routine extraction   An extraction that can be done without extensive instrumentation or complication.

Rubber dam   A sheet of rubber material used to isolate single or multiple teeth from the oral environment.

Rubber dam clamps   Used to anchor the rubber dam to the teeth.

Rubber dam forceps   Used to spread the beaks of a rubber dam clamp when the clamp is placed on and removed from the anchor tooth.

Rubber dam (Young) frame   Used to support the dam on a patient's face. It maintains isolation by holding the dam out of the way.

Rubber dam lubricant   A water-based lubricant that helps to slip the septal portion of the rubber dam down between the teeth.

Rubber dam napkins   Disposable, cotton, preformed sheets that are placed under the rubber dam.

Rubber dam punch   Used to punch holes in the rubber dam so that it can be placed over the teeth.

Rubber dam stamp   The rubber dam stamp is helpful in positioning holes properly on the dam.

Saliva ejector   A device used to suck out fluids and debris from the patient's mouth. It has a weaker suction than the oral evacuator and is only used as an adjunct.

Scalers   Hand instruments used to remove local irritants from the tooth surface and to plane roughened root surfaces.

Scaling   The process of scraping adherent substances such as plaque and calculus off the surfaces of the teeth.

Selective anesthesia   A diagnostic method used to determine which teeth are the source of discomfort to the patient by placing anesthesia on the suspected tooth to see if the pain disappears, thereby detecting the involved tooth.

Semisupine position   The chair back is raised slightly from the supine position.

Shade   The combination of color and translucency of a tooth.

Shade guide   An assortment of number-coded shade samples used to match a patient's tooth coloring for an esthetic crown.

Shorting   The dental assistant holding the instrument that is to be placed in the operator's hand too closely to the middle of the handle.

Sickle scaler   An instrument with two cutting edges and a pointed toe used to scale interproximal areas.

Side delivery unit   A unit mounted on either a bracket arm or mobile cart and from which the instruments are delivered to the dentist from the side of the patient.

Sign   A measurable condition, such as blood pressure, pulse, or temperature.

Smear   The glass slide setup obtained by scraping cells from a lesion, placing the cells on a glass slide, and spreading out the cells for examination.

Solids trap   A meshlike structure that catches large debris picked up by the oral evacuator.

Space maintainer   A removable or fixed appliance used when primary teeth are lost prematurely. The space maintainer keeps an erupted tooth from drifting into an edentulous space of a future permanent tooth.

Sphygmomanometer   A device used to measure blood pressure.

Spill   How amalgam is measured. Amalgam is available in single, double, and triple spills.

Spot-welded matrix band   A custom-made matrix band that may be used for deciduous teeth.

Spreader   A long, pointed hand instrument used with lateral pressure to condense the gutta-percha points against the wall of the root canal.

Standardization   Performing dental procedures in a predictable manner.

Static zone   A nontraffic area where equipment is placed during the delivery of dental treatment; 12 to 2 o'clock position for a right-handed operator.

Statute of limitations   A law that sets a limit of time during which a lawsuit can be brought.

Steam autoclave   A heat sterilizer that uses steam, heat, and pressure to achieve sterilization.

Steel spring separators   A metal device placed between the teeth to move them apart in preparation for the placement of an orthodontic band.

Sterilization   The destruction of all forms of life.

Storage bath   A bath to store the agar hydrocolloid material once it has turned into the sol stage.

Study models   Plaster reproductions of patients' teeth and surrounding tissues.

Subacute bacterial endocarditis   A serious, life-threatening infection of the heart that can be caused by the introduction of bacteria into the bloodstream by dental procedures.

Subgingival plaque   Plaque that forms under the gum line.

Supine   To lie horizontally on the back.

Supine position   Placement of the plane of the patient's head is approximately parallel with the floor.

Supragingival plaque   Plaque that forms above the gum line.

Surgical chisel   A sharp, straight hand instrument used with a surgical mallet to remove bone.

Surgical curette   A scoop-shaped hand instrument used to sever the epithelial attachment of the gingiva around the tooth and for scraping bone or other tissues from interior cavities.

Surgical mallet   A special nylon-tipped hammer used with a surgical chisel to remove bone.

Surgical scalpel   A sharp hand instrument normally used for surgical procedures to cut tissue. For composite procedures the scalpel is used to trim excess composite along the margins of the restorations.

Surgical scissors   Sharp-bladed scissors used to trim soft tissues and cut suture material.

Surgical suction tip   A smaller-sized evacuator tip used to remove blood and other oral fluids from the surgical site.

Suture needle   A curved needle used with suture material to close the surgical site.

Symptom   Something a patient reports that he or she is experiencing, such as nausea or hearing loss.

Syncope (fainting)   A brief loss of consciousness usually caused by anxiety.

Tangling   Intertwining of the instrument the dental assistant is transferring and the instrument the dentist is holding during the exchange of instruments. Usually occurs because the transferring instrument is not parallel to the dentist's instrument.

Tell-show-do   Children experiencing the first dental appointment should be shown various nonthreatening instruments before treatment is rendered. This method helps to allay the patient's fears of the unknown or unexpected.

Tempering bath   The tempering bath is used to cool the agar hydrocolloid material in the impression tray before it is inserted in the patient's mouth.

Test cavity preparation   If all other diagnostic tests fail to determine the vitality of a highly suspected tooth, the dentist can cut a small hole in the dentin layer of the tooth without anesthesia or water coolant to see if the tooth is vital.

Three-finger pickup   The dental assistant uses the last three fingers of the left hand to retrieve a dental instrument from the dentist's hand.

Three-quarter crown A restoration that rebuilds three fourths of the crown portion of a tooth. The facial aspect of the tooth is usually left intact.

Time management The utilization of time to achieve the most tasks in the minimal amount of time.

Tipping See Drifting.

Tissue conditioning The placement of a soft, white lining material used for denture sores.

Tissue forceps Instruments that provide a positive grasp of tissue for maximum control during surgical procedures.

Tofflemire retainer A device used to hold the two ends of a universal circumferential band to form a loop that will be placed over the prepared cavity preparation.

Tofflemire retainer frame The main body of the retainer to which the vise, spindle, and adjustment knobs are attached.

Tofflemire retainer gingival aspect The openings of the guide slots on the end of the retainer, as well as the diagonal slot in the vise, are visible.

Tofflemire retainer guide slots Slots that enable matrix band loop positioning in the direction of choice.

Tofflemire retainer inner knob An adjustment knob used to slide the vise along the frame to either increase or decrease the size of the matrix band loop.

Tofflemire retainer occlusal aspect The openings of the guide slots on the end of the retainer, as well as the diagonal slot in the vise, are not visible.

Tofflemire retainer outer knob An adjustment knob used to tighten the spindle against the band in the vise.

Tofflemire retainer spindle A screwlike rod used to lock the ends of the matrix band in the vise.

Tofflemire retainer vise A clamplike device that holds the ends of the matrix band in the retainer.

Tooth sectioning Division of a tooth into two or more parts with surgical instruments to facilitate removal.

Topical anesthesia The elimination of sensation on the surface of the skin or mucosa by the application of a topical anesthetic agent.

Topical fluoride Fluoride applied to the teeth but not ingested. Available in gel and liquid forms.

Transfer zone The area where instruments and materials are transported to and from the oral cavity during the delivery of dental treatment; 4 to 7 o'clock position for a right-handed operator.

Transillumination A bright light is used to view the pulp chamber of a suspected tooth.

Transthorax delivery style Instruments are located over the patient's chest between the dentist and the assistant.

Traumatic intrusion The tooth is forcibly driven into the alveolus so that only a portion of the crown is clinically visible.

Treatment plan A carefully sequenced series of services designed to eliminate or control causative factors, repair existing damage, and create a functional, maintainable environment.

Trendelenburg position (subsupine) A position in which the patient is placed with the head below the level of the feet.

Trial-point radiograph A radiograph (x-ray) taken of an endodontically treated tooth to determine if the tip of the gutta-percha point adequately seals the apex of the tooth.

Trieger test Assessment of the psychomotor ability of the patient before and after the administration of nitrous oxide analgesia.

Trituration The mixing process of amalgam.

Twist drill A special device used to make the holes that will hold the retention pins.

Two-finger pickup The dental assistant uses the last two fingers of the left hand to retrieve a dental instrument from the dentist's hand.

Two-viscosity impression technique An impression technique that uses a thin and semithin or thick impression material to take an accurate impression of a crown preparation. The thin material is placed over the crown preparation first, the semithin or thick impression material is placed in the impression tray, and the impression tray is seated over the crown preparation and surrounding teeth.

Ultrasonic cleaner Contaminated instruments are placed in this device, which works in a manner similar to a jewelry cleaner. Detergent solution vibrates and removes debris such as blood and saliva from instruments.

Unit-dose packaging A method of dispensing gauze, cotton rolls, cotton swabs, or polishing agents in small units so that bulk packaging or storage containers are not contaminated.

Universal circumferential matrix band A preformed matrix band with two ends that must be held into a loop with a matrix retainer.

Universal curette An instrument that can be used to scale all the surfaces of the teeth.

Universal extraction forceps Extraction forceps designed to remove a specific group of teeth on either side of the same arch.

Universal precautions Assumes that all patients carry an infectious disease; therefore the same stringent infection control practices are utilized on every patient.

Universal scaler A device used by the dentist or dental hygienist to remove debris such as calculus and plaque from the tooth surfaces.

Vacuformer A machine used to soften acrylic material, which is then placed over a model of the teeth. A vacuum device in the Vacuformer can pull the softened acrylic material so it adapts closely to the model. Vacuformers are often used for temporary fabrication, bite splints, bleaching splints, and sport mouth guards.

Vasoconstrictor A drug that causes blood vessels to narrow in width, which reduces blood flow to the area injected.

Veneer A porcelain or composite facing that is applied to the facial surfaces of the anterior teeth for esthetic reasons.

Veneering Aesthetic tooth-colored facings that are placed on the anterior teeth.

Vital pulp Pulp tissue that is living.

Wash A term often used for a light/low viscosity impression material.

Work circle An imaginary circle around the patient's head that indicates the focal point of activity.

Work simplification The process of finding an easier way to do a task.

Zones of activity The working positions of both the equipment and the operating team.

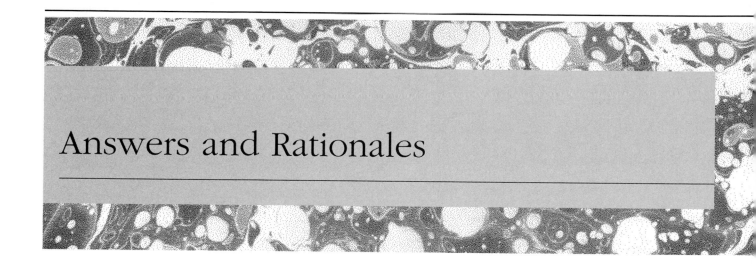

Answers and Rationales

ANSWERS AND RATIONALES—Chapter 1

1. a. The mesial surface is the surface closest to the midline.
   b. The distal surface is the surface away from the midline.
   c. *The incisal surface is the biting surface of anterior teeth.*
   d. The lingual surface is the surface closest to the tongue.
   e. The occlusal surface is the biting surface of posterior teeth.

2. a. The mesial surface is the surface closest to the midline.
   b. The distal surface is the surface away from the midline.
   c. The incisal surface is the biting surface of anterior teeth.
   d. *The lingual surface is the surface closest to the tongue.*
   e. The occlusal surface is the biting surface of posterior teeth.

3. a. *The mesial surface is the surface closest to the midline.*
   b. The distal surface is the surface away from the midline.
   c. The incisal surface is the biting surface of anterior teeth.
   d. The lingual surface is the surface closest to the tongue.
   e. The occlusal surface is the biting surface of posterior teeth.

4. a. This answer is missing information, such as mandibular or maxillary and permanent or deciduous.
   b. This answer is missing information, such as mandibular or maxillary and permanent or deciduous.
   c. This answer is missing information, such as permanent or deciduous.
   d. *The maxillary left permanent first molar is tooth #14.*
   e. The maxillary left permanent second molar is tooth #15.

5. a. This answer is missing information, such as mandibular or maxillary and permanent or deciduous.
   b. This answer is missing information, such as mandibular or maxillary and permanent or deciduous.
   c. The maxillary right permanent third molar is tooth #16.
   d. The maxillary left permanent central incisor is tooth #9.
   e. *The mandibular right permanent central incisor is tooth #8.*

6. a. The mandibular left deciduous first molar is tooth L.
   b. The maxillary right permanent second molar is tooth #2.
   c. *The mandibular left permanent first premolar is tooth #21.*
   d. The maxillary left permanent central incisor is tooth #9.
   e. The maxillary right deciduous lateral incisor is tooth D.

7. a. *The mandibular left deciduous cuspid is tooth M.*
   b. The deciduous dentition does not have third molar teeth.
   c. The mandibular left permanent second molar is tooth #18.
   d. The deciduous dentition does not have premolar teeth.
   e. The mandibular left permanent central incisor is tooth #24.

8. a. Tooth #3 is the maxillary right permanent first molar.
   b. *Tooth #6 is the maxillary right permanent cuspid.*
   c. Tooth C is the maxillary right deciduous cuspid.
   d. Tooth #11 is the maxillary left permanent cuspid.
   e. Tooth #22 is the mandibular left permanent cuspid.

9. a. *Tooth S is the mandibular right deciduous first molar.*
   b. Tooth #31 is the mandibular right permanent second molar.
   c. Tooth C is the maxillary right deciduous cuspid.
   d. Tooth #4 is the maxillary right permanent second premolar.
   e. Tooth M is the mandibular left deciduous cuspid.

Italics indicate correct answers.

10. a. This answer is missing information, such as mandibular or maxillary and permanent or deciduous.
    b. This answer is missing information, such as mandibular or maxillary and permanent or deciduous.
    c. This answer is missing information, such as permanent or deciduous.
    d. This answer is missing information, such as permanent or deciduous.
    e. *The maxillary left permanent second premolar is tooth|5.*

11. a. This answer is missing information, such as permanent or deciduous.
    b. This answer is missing information, such as permanent or deciduous.
    c. The mandibular left permanent second molar is tooth|7.
    d. The maxillary right deciduous lateral incisor is tooth B|.
    e. *The mandibular right deciduous lateral incisor is tooth B|.*

12. a. *The maxillary left permanent second molar is tooth|7.*
    b. The mandibular right permanent first molar is tooth 6|.
    c. The mandibular left deciduous lateral incisor is tooth|B.
    d. The maxillary left permanent lateral incisor is tooth|2.
    e. The mandibular right deciduous central incisor is tooth A|.

13. a. Tooth|2 is the maxillary left permanent lateral incisor.
    b. Tooth D| is the mandibular right first molar.
    c. Tooth|3 is the mandibular left permanent cuspid.
    d. *Tooth C| is the maxillary right deciduous cuspid.*
    e. Tooth|3 is the maxillary left permanent cuspid.

14. a. *Tooth 1|is the mandibular right permanent central incisor.*
    b. Tooth|5 is the maxillary left second premolar.
    c. Tooth #24 is a nonexistent number in the Zsigmondy-Palmer numbering system.
    d. Tooth #25 is a nonexistent number in the Zsigmondy-Palmer numbering system.
    e. Tooth #41 is a nonexistent number in the Zsigmondy-Palmer numbering system.

15. a. Tooth 5|is the mandibular right permanent second premolar.
    b. Tooth|7 is the maxillary left permanent second molar.
    c. *Tooth|E is the maxillary left deciduous second molar.*
    d. Tooth J is a nonexistent letter in the Zsigmondy-Palmer numbering system.
    e. Tooth D|is the maxillary right first molar.

16. a. The maxillary left permanent cuspid is tooth #23.
    b. The maxillary right deciduous first molar is tooth #54.
    c. The mandibular left deciduous second molar is tooth #75.
    d. The maxillary right permanent second molar is tooth #17.
    e. *The maxillary right permanent central incisor is tooth #11.*

17. a. The mandibular right permanent third molar is tooth #48.

b. The mandibular left permanent second molar is tooth #37.
c. The mandibular right permanent second molar is tooth #47.
d. *The mandibular left permanent lateral incisor is tooth #32.*
e. The mandibular right permanent lateral incisor is tooth #42.

18. a. *The maxillary left deciduous second molar is tooth #65.*
    b. The maxillary left permanent second molar is tooth #27.
    c. The maxillary left deciduous lateral incisor is tooth #62.
    d. The deciduous dentition does not have premolar teeth.
    e. The deciduous dentition does not have premolar teeth.

19. a. Tooth #13 is the maxillary right permanent cuspid.
    b. Tooth #17 is the maxillary right permanent second molar.
    c. Tooth #25 is the maxillary left permanent second premolar.
    d. *Tooth #27 is the maxillary left permanent second molar.*
    e. Tooth #37 is the mandibular left permanent second molar.

20. a. The FDI tooth numbering system does not have a tooth #30.
    b. Tooth #36 is the mandibular left permanent first molar.
    c. Tooth #46 is the mandibular right permanent first molar.
    d. Tooth #74 is the mandibular left deciduous first molar.
    e. *Tooth #84 is the mandibular right deciduous first molar.*

ANSWERS AND RATIONALES—Chapter 2

1. a. An explorer is part of a preset examination tray and is used to detect caries.
   b. *A hatchet is a hand cutting instrument and is not part of a preset examination tray.*
   c. Cotton pliers are part of a preset examination tray and are used for multiple purposes during the examination.
   d. A periodontal probe is part of a preset examination tray and is used to measure periodontal pockets.

2. a. *Percussion is done when the dentist taps on the teeth with a mirror handle.*
   b. Plaque disclosure is application of a disclosing agent on the patient's teeth.
   c. Study models are plaster reproductions of a patient's teeth.
   d. A biopsy is the surgical removal of a piece of tissue from the body for examination under the microscope.

3. a. The prognosis is the expected outcome from a disease, condition, or treatment.
   b. A biopsy is the surgical removal of a piece of tissue from the body for examination under the microscope.
   c. A treatment plan is formulated by the dentist after gathering diagnostic information. Treatment plans are often in written form.
   d. *The diagnosis is the identification of a disease.*

4. a. Study models are used as diagnostic aids (e.g., a model of occlusion for treatment planning).
   b. Periodontal probe readings are used to determine the periodontal status of the patient.
   c. *Pit and fissure sealants are not diagnostic aids.*
   d. Dental radiographs are used as diagnostic aids to determine the presence of caries and alveolar bone levels.

5. a. *Many standard medical-dental history forms ask the patient about dental insurance; however, the possession of dental insurance is not a diagnostic tool.*
   b. Medical-dental history forms provide important oral health information.
   c. Medical-dental history forms provide important information about general health.
   d. Medical-dental history forms are valuable legal documents.

ANSWERS AND RATIONALES—Chapter 3

1. a. *The medical history should be updated at every visit in the event that the patient has had a change in medical history that could affect dental treatment.*
   b. Patient's medical status may change suddenly and unpredictably over time; therefore it is not possible to update the medical history at a set time interval.
   c. A patient's medical status may change suddenly and unpredictably over time; therefore it is not possible to update the medical history at a set time interval.
   d. A patient's medical status may change suddenly and unpredictably over time; therefore it is not possible to update the medical history at a set time interval.

2. a. The treatment plan is a written document that outlines the proposed treatment for the patient.
   b. *An informed consent is the process by which the dentist or auxiliary has given information to the patient regarding planned treatment and the alternatives to the treatment and obtains permission from the patient.*
   c. A medical consult takes place when the dentist obtains recommendations from the patient's physician regarding possible contraindications to dental treatment with the patient's existing medical conditions.
   d. Risk management is a term used to describe the identification, evaluation, and correction of potential risks that could lead to patient injury.

3. a. It is important to respond to questions asked by patients. Saying nothing to the patient would arouse suspicion and may also elicit a negative attitude from the patient.
   b. It is unwise to make unprofessional statements or opinions about other dental health care workers. Dental professionals may be summoned to appear in court for careless remarks made about their peers.
   c. It is unwise to make unprofessional statements or opinions about other dental health care workers. Dental professionals may be summoned to appear in court for careless remarks made about their peers.

   d. *It is important not to base opinions about previous dental work or other dental health care workers from statements made solely by the patient. There are often two sides of the situation, and it is best not to form an opinion until after finding out the other side's story.*

4. a. It is best not to make statements concerning what you think may be treatment planned for the patient. If the dentist decides to perform a different procedure, the dentist will have to explain why he or she is not performing what one of the staff members suggested.
   b. It is best not to make statements concerning what you think may be treatment planned for the patient. If the dentist decides to perform a different procedure, the dentist will have to explain why he or she is not performing what one of the staff members suggested.
   c. It is best not to make statements concerning what you think may be treatment planned for the patient. If the dentist decides to perform a different procedure, the dentist will have to explain why he or she is not performing what one of the staff members suggested.
   d. *It is best to remain neutral about potential dental work to avoid contradictory statements that will need to be explained later to the patient.*

5. a. When patients ask about other dental health care professionals, it is best to try to make positive or neutral statements.
   b. It is best to avoid unprofessional statements about other dental health care workers.
   c. *Make neutral statements about other dental health care workers if you cannot think of anything positive to say.*
   d. Avoid statements that could lead to a negative opinion about other dental health care workers.

6. a. Statements like this imply incompetence and undermine the patient's confidence in the dental office.
   b. Avoid words such as "lucky," which may be taken to imply that the same complication may occur again randomly.
   c. Saying nothing would only create a sense that the office has something to hide. Patients and family members respond best when you answer their questions in an open and caring manner.
   d. *It is best to make concise statements about complications that occur during dental treatment.*

7. a. *For procedures such as extractions, the degree of pain will vary from patient to patient. Do not overemphasize or underemphasize postoperative effects that could cause surprise to the patient when they occur.*
   b. Do not overemphasize postoperative effects that may not occur.
   c. Do not underemphasize postoperative effects that could cause surprise and most likely anger to the patient when they occur.
   d. Do not underemphasize postoperative effects that could cause surprise and most likely anger to the patient when they occur.

8. a. Although this answer would be suitable, it is best to avoid contradictory statements in the dental chart.
   b. It is important to avoid entries in the chart that are possibly incorrect or misleading.
   c. Chart entries should never be altered after the fact.
   d. *Contradictory statements in the chart must be justified to demonstrate that the patient's concerns were addressed.*

9. a. Flippant or uncaring remarks to patients often result in patient dissatisfaction and potential lawsuits.
   b. Flippant or uncaring remarks to patients often result in patient dissatisfaction and potential lawsuits.
   c. *Genuine concern and patience with patients build patient rapport and may avoid potential lawsuits.*
   d. Flippant or uncaring remarks to patients often result in patient dissatisfaction and potential lawsuits.

10. a. Although this answer may be suitable, it is best to explain complications or problems to the patient in the event that another staff member inadvertently admits that the problem or complication occurred.
    b. It is best to avoid using expressions as "oops" or "uh-oh," which could alarm the patient.
    c. *It is important to communicate complications or problems with the patient in the event that another staff member inadvertently admits that the complication or problem occurred.*
    d. Although both answers are suitable, it is best to explain complications or problems to the patient in the event that another staff member inadvertently admits that the problem or complication occurred.

ANSWERS AND RATIONALES–Chapter 4

1. a. *A topical anesthetic eliminates sensation on the surface of the skin or mucosa.*
   b. A local anesthetic is an agent used to eliminate sensation in a limited area of the body.
   c. A general anesthetic produces the absence of sensation and consciousness.

2. a. Infiltration anesthesia is achieved by the injection of a local anesthetic agent to numb tiny terminal nerve branches and the tissue in the immediate area.
   b. *Nerve block anesthesia is produced by the injection of a local anesthetic agent near a main nerve trunk.*
   c. Field block anesthesia is achieved by the injection of a local anesthetic agent to numb larger terminal nerve branches, thus preventing pain impulses from the tooth to the brain.

3. a. *A vasoconstrictor narrows the blood vessels and allows the anesthetic agent to remain longer at the injection site.*
   b. An anesthetic agent without vasoconstrictor has a shorter duration of action vs. one with vasoconstrictor.

4. a. The first statement is false because the higher the gauge number, the smaller the diameter of the opening of the needle.

b. The first statement is false because the higher the gauge number, the smaller the diameter of the opening of the needle. The second statement is true—a long needle is used for the mandibular nerve block injection.
   c. *The first statement is false because the higher the gauge number, the smaller the diameter of the opening of the needle. The second statement is true—a long needle is used for the mandibular nerve block injection.*
   d. The second statement is true—a long needle is used for the mandibular nerve block injection.

5. a. The patient should be instructed to breathe through the nose and to avoid excessive laughing to prevent the escape of nitrous oxide into the immediate environment.
   b. The patient should be instructed to avoid excessive talking to prevent the escape of nitrous oxide into the immediate environment.
   c. The patient should be instructed to breathe through the nose and to avoid excessive talking and laughing to prevent the escape of nitrous oxide into the immediate environment.
   d. *If discomfort is felt by the patient while receiving nitrous oxide, 100% oxygen should be administered through the nasal hood and the patient should be instructed not to remove the nasal hood.*

6. a. *The standard regimen is amoxicillin, 3 g orally 1 hour before the appointment and 1.5 g 6 hours after the initial dose.*
   b. Amoxicillin should be taken 6 hours after the initial dose and not 6 hours after the appointment.
   c. Amoxicillin and not penicillin should be prescribed.
   d. Amoxicillin and not penicillin should be prescribed, and it should be taken 6 hours after the initial dose and not 6 hours after the appointment.

7. a. Bending, breaking, or otherwise manipulating the anesthetic needle is not recommended by the Centers for Disease Control and Prevention (CDC) to avoid inadvertent injury from unnecessary manipulation.
   b. *The anesthetic needle should not be bent; this is recommended by the Centers for Disease Control and Prevention (CDC) to avoid inadvertent injury from unnecessary manipulation.*

8. a. *The anterior superior alveolar (ASA) injection anesthetizes the cuspid and buccal tissue of the central incisor and lateral incisor on the side that is injected.*
   b. The middle superior alveolar (MSA) injection anesthetizes the first premolar, second premolar, some of the first molar, and the buccal tissue of those teeth on the side that is injected.
   c. The inferior alveolar (IA) injection or mandibular block injection anesthetizes the mandibular teeth and buccal tissue for premolars, cuspid, and incisors on the side that is injected.
   d. The nasopalatine injection anesthetizes the palatal tissue anterior to the cuspids.

ANSWERS TO LOCAL ANESTHESIA PRACTICE EXAM

Type of procedure	Type of injection	Long or short needle?
1. #2 MOD amalgam	PSA or infiltration	Short
2. #2 and 3 full gold crowns	PSA and greater palatine nerve block	Short
3. #2 and 3 O amalgams	PSA	Short
4. #5 O amalgam	MSA or infiltration	Short
5. #3 full gold crown	PSA or infiltration and greater palatine nerve block	Short
6. #4 and 5 full gold crowns	MSA and greater palatine nerve block	Short
7. #8 D composite	ASA or infiltration	Short
8. #13 full porcelain crown	MSA or infiltration and greater palatine nerve block	Short
9. #18 MOD amalgam	Inferior alveolar nerve block	Long
10. #18, 19, and 20 gold bridge	Inferior alveolar nerve block and buccal nerve block	Long
11. #19 full gold crown	Inferior alveolar nerve block and buccal nerve block	Long
12. #22 D composite	Inferior alveolar nerve block or incisive nerve block	Long for IA or short for incisive
13. #24 full gold crown	Inferior alveolar nerve block or incisive nerve block	Long for IA or short for incisive
14. #29 MO amalgam	Inferior alveolar nerve block	Long
15. #29 full gold crown	Inferior alveolar nerve block and buccal nerve block	Long
16. Scale and root plane upper right quadrant	ASA, MSA, PSA, nasopalatine and greater palatine nerve blocks	Long
17. Scale and root plane lower left quadrant	Inferior alveolar and buccal nerve block	Long
18. Scale and root plane upper anterior teeth	ASA on right and left side and nasopalatine nerve block	Short

9. a. The anterior superior alveolar (ASA) injection anesthetizes the cuspid and buccal tissue of the central and lateral incisors on the side that is injected.
   b. The middle superior alveolar (MSA) injection anesthetizes the first premolar, second premolar, and the buccal tissue of the maxillary premolars on the side that is injected.
   c. *The inferior alveolar (IA) injection or mandibular block injection anesthetizes the mandibular teeth and buccal tissue for premolars, cuspid, and incisors on the side that is injected.*
   d. The nasopalatine injection anesthetizes the palatal tissue anterior to the cuspids.

10. a. The anterior superior alveolar (ASA) injection anesthetizes the cuspid and buccal tissue of the central and lateral incisors on the side that is injected.
    b. The middle superior alveolar (MSA) injection anesthetizes the first premolar, second premolar, and the buccal tissue of the maxillary premolars on the side that is injected.
    c. The inferior alveolar (IA) injection or mandibular block injection anesthetizes the mandibular teeth and buccal tissue for premolars, cuspid, and incisors on the side that is injected.
    d. *The nasopalatine injection anesthetizes the palatal tissue anterior to the cuspids.*

ANSWERS AND RATIONALES—Chapter 5

1. a. A patient with a recent history of a heart attack has an increased risk for a second heart attack within 6 months of the initial heart attack.
   b. A patient with a recent history of a heart attack has an increased risk for a second heart attack within 6 months of the initial heart attack.
   c. *A patient who has had a heart attack should not be receiving elective dental care within 6 months of the attack.*
   d. A patient with a recent history of a heart attack has an increased risk for a second heart attack within 6 months of the initial heart attack. It is not necessary to wait 1 year.

2. a. *If the dental assistant is working alone, the patient should be told to bend over the side of the chair and cough.*
   b. The Magill intubation forceps should only be used if there are more than two people treating the patient when the emergency occurs.
   c. Seating the patient upright may cause the crown to fall farther down the patient's throat.
   d. If the dental assistant is alone with the patient during a dental emergency, the assistant should stay with the patient and summon help.

3. a. *Administration of oxygen to a hyperventilating patient may further exacerbate the condition.*
   b. It is appropriate to administer oxygen to a patient who has fainted.
   c. It is appropriate to administer oxygen to a patient experiencing asthma.

4. a. *Nausea, feelings of warmth, and dizziness are signs and symptoms of syncope.*
   b. Nausea, feelings of warmth, and dizziness are not signs and symptoms of an asthma attack.
   c. Nausea and feelings of warmth are not signs of epilepsy.
   d. Nausea and feelings of warmth are not signs of epilepsy.

5. a. A medical consultation would not have prevented this medical emergency.
   b. It is unlikely that oxygen could have been administered to this patient before the patient lost consciousness.
   c. Placing the patient in the upright position would only exacerbate the emergency.
   d. *Reviewing the medical-dental history before treatment could have revealed a prior history of anxiety or fainting.*

6. a. Activation of the emergency medical system is only necessary if the patient does not regain consciousness.
   b. The patient should never be left alone in an emergency.
   c. Oxygen and ammonia are appropriate medications to administer to a patient who has fainted; however, the patient should be placed in the supine position before the administration of any medications.
   d. *Once it has been recognized that the patient has fainted, the patient should first be placed in the supine position.*

7. a. A nondiabetic person who does not eat before a dental appointment can experience hypoglycemia.
   b. A person with diabetes who eats regularly will not experience hypoglycemia.
   c. A person with diabetes who takes his or her daily insulin but does not eat can experience hypoglycemia.
   d. *A nondiabetic person who does not eat and a person with diabetes who does not eat can experience hypoglycemia.*

8. a. A patient can experience syncope in the upright position.
   b. *It is best to place the patient in the supine position to prevent syncope.*
   c. Elevating a patient does not lower the risk of syncope.

9. a. *A patient who has aspirated an object should be placed over the side of the dental chair and told to cough.*
   b. A patient who is experiencing syncope should be placed in the supine position.
   c. A patient experiencing asthma would probably be more comfortable in the upright position.
   d. A patient experiencing angina would probably be more comfortable in the upright position.

10. a. A patient experiencing hyperventilation could place a paper bag over his or her mouth and nose to correct the emergency.
    b. *Giving a patient experiencing hyperventilation a plastic bag is not appropriate because the bag collapses on itself, which makes it difficult to correct the emergency.*
    c. A patient experiencing hyperventilation could place his or her hands cupped over mouth and nose to correct the emergency.
    d. A paper headrest cover can be used to treat a hyperventilating patient.

ANSWERS AND RATIONALES–Chapter 6

1. a. Friction-grip burs have a smooth shaft.
   b. *Latch-type burs have a small groove on the end of the instrument shaft.*
   c. Handpiece burs have a long, smooth shaft.

2. a. Prophylaxis angles are attached directly into the straight low-speed handpiece setup.
   b. *Latch-type burs are attached to the contra-angle attachment of the low-speed handpiece.*
   c. The straight low-speed handpiece uses long-shafted burs and attachments.
   d. The angle former is a hand cutting instrument.

3. a. *Mandrels are used to attach sandpaper disks and polishing devices to the handpiece.*
   b. Round burs are used in the high-speed handpiece.
   c. Rubber cups and prophy brushes are attached to the prophylaxis angle.
   d. The acrylic bur is attached to the straight low-speed handpiece.

4. a. *The high-speed handpiece has little torque or turning power.*
   b. The low-speed handpiece has high torque.

5. a. The Centers for Disease Control and Prevention recommends that high-speed handpieces should be flushed and sterilized between patients.
   b. The Centers for Disease Control and Prevention recommends that high-speed handpieces should be flushed and sterilized between patients.
   c. The Centers for Disease Control and Prevention recommends that high-speed handpieces should be flushed and sterilized between patients.
   d. *High-speed handpieces should be flushed and sterilized between patients.*

6. a. Latch-type burs are used in the low-speed handpiece.
   b. Long-shaft burs are used in the low-speed handpiece.
   c. Mandrels are used in the low-speed handpiece.
   d. *The high-speed handpiece uses friction-grip burs.*

7. a. The spoon is used to remove soft carious tooth structure.
   b. The explorer is not used to remove soft carious tooth structure.
   c. The low-speed handpiece and round bur are used to remove soft carious tooth structure.
   d. The explorer is not used to remove soft carious tooth structure.
   e. *The spoon and low-speed handpiece with round bur are used to remove soft carious dentin.*

8. a. Explorers are used to remove excess cement.
   b. *Curets and sickle scalers are used to remove calculus.*
   c. Explorers are used to detect caries.
   d. Explorers can be used to carve amalgam.

9. a. Gingival margin trimmers are used to bevel the cervical cavosurface margin in amalgam and inlay preparations.
   b. Angle formers are used to form sharp internal lines and point angles of cavity preparations.

   c. Chisels are used with a push motion to plane enamel margins.
   d. *Hoes are used with a pull motion to plane cavity walls and floors.*

10. a. *Gingival margin trimmers are used to bevel the cervical cavosurface margin in amalgam and inlay preparations.*
    b. Angle formers are used to form sharp internal lines and point angles of cavity preparations.
    c. Chisels are used with a push motion to plane enamel margins.
    d. Hoes are used with a pull motion to plane cavity walls and floors.

ANSWERS AND RATIONALES–Chapter 7

1. a. *The* Bacillus subtilis *spore test is recommended for the dry-heat oven.*
   b. The *Bacillus stearothermophilus* spore test is recommended for steam autoclaving.
   c. The *Bacillus stearothermophilus* spore test is recommended for chemical vapor sterilization.
   d. Liquid chemical sterilants do not have a test to guarantee sterilization.

2. a. One hour and 340° F are sterilization requirements for the dry-heat oven.
   b. Twenty minutes, 270° F, and 20 psi are sterilization requirements for the chemical vapor sterilizer.
   c. *Fifteen to twenty minutes, 250° F, and 15 psi are sterilization requirements for the steam autoclave.*
   d. Two hours and 320° F are sterilization requirements for the dry-heat oven.

3. a. *Universal precautions are followed by the dental staff, which assumes that all patients are infectious and the dental office must use the same stringent infection control procedures for each patient.*
   b. Cross-contamination is the spread of oral secretions and/or blood to surfaces, equipment, and instruments that are not regularly disinfected or sterilized, with gloves that have been in contact with the patient's mouth.
   c. Disinfection is a process that reduces but does not eliminate all microorganisms.
   d. Sterilization is the destruction of all forms of life including bacterial endospores.

4. a. Universal precautions are followed by the dental staff, which assumes that all patients are infectious and the dental office must use the same stringent infection control procedures for each patient.
   b. Cross-contamination is the spread of oral secretions and/or blood to surfaces, equipment, and instruments that are not regularly disinfected or sterilized, with gloves that have been in contact with the patient's mouth.
   c. Disinfection is a process that reduces but does not eliminate all microorganisms.
   d. *Sterilization is the destruction of all forms of life including bacterial endospores.*

5. a. *Steam autoclaving can cause corrosion of instruments.*
   b. A dry-heat oven does not cause corrosion of instruments.
   c. A chemical vapor sterilizer does not cause corrosion of instruments.

6. a. Iodophors do not cause corrosion of metals or damage clothing.
   b. *Chlorines can cause corrosion of metals and damage clothing.*
   c. Quaternary ammonium compounds do not cause corrosion of metals or damage clothing.
   d. Synthetic phenols do not cause corrosion of metals or damage clothing.
   e. Alcohol does not cause corrosion of metals or damage clothing.

7. a. Quaternary ammonium compounds are not acceptable for surface disinfection.
   b. Alcohol is not acceptable for surface disinfection.
   c. *Household bleach is acceptable for surface disinfection.*
   d. Two percent glutaraldehyde is acceptable for immersion disinfection but not acceptable for surface disinfection.

8. a. It is best to use a solution recommended by the manufacturer for the ultrasonic cleaner.
   b. Household bleach is corrosive to metals and should not be used in the ultrasonic cleaner.
   c. *It is best to use a solution recommended by the manufacturer for the ultrasonic cleaner.*
   d. The vibrations and the heat from the ultrasonic cleaner can cause noxious vapors from 2% glutaraldehyde.

9. a. Spraying and wiping a surface complete the cleaning step of disinfection. The surface must be sprayed and the disinfectant allowed to remain on the surface for the time recommended by the manufacturer for the disinfecting step.
   b. *The process of disinfection is a two-step process in which the surface is sprayed and wiped for the cleaning step and the surface is again sprayed with the disinfectant. The disinfectant is allowed to remain on the surface for a time recommended by the manufacturer.*
   c. The process of disinfection is a two-step process in which the surface is sprayed and wiped for the cleaning step and the surface is again sprayed with the disinfectant. The disinfectant must be allowed to remain on the surface for a time recommended by the manufacturer.
   d. The process of disinfection is a two-step process in which the surface is sprayed and wiped for the cleaning step and the surface is again sprayed with the disinfectant. The disinfectant is allowed to remain on the surface for a time recommended by the manufacturer.

10. a. Sharps should be disposed of in a puncture-proof container.
    b. Sharps should be recapped using a one-handed technique.
    c. Sharps should be recapped immediately after use.
    d. *A sharp should never be bent before being thrown away.*

ANSWERS AND RATIONALES—Chapter 8

1. a. The rubber dam clamp is used to anchor the rubber dam to the tooth.
   b. Dental floss is used to prevent accidental aspiration of the clamp.
   c. The rubber dam frame is used to support the rubber dam on the patient's face.
   d. *Inverting the rubber dam is used to prevent salivary leakage.*

2. a. A spoon excavator can be used to invert the rubber dam.
   b. A probe is not a good instrument to use to invert the rubber dam.
   c. A fishtail burnisher can be used to invert the rubber dam.
   d. A probe is not a good instrument to invert the rubber dam.
   e. *A blunt instrument such as a spoon or burnisher can be used to invert the rubber dam.*

3. a. Dental floss is used by the assistant to slip the rubber dam between the teeth.
   b. A burnisher is used to invert the rubber dam.
   c. A lubricant helps to slip the rubber dam between the teeth.
   d. A burnisher is used to invert the dam.
   e. *Dental floss and a lubricant on the rubber dam help to slip the rubber dam between the teeth.*

4. a. A cotton roll will also be needed between the teeth and the tongue.
   b. A cotton roll will also be needed in the mucobuccal fold.
   c. A Theta Dri-Angle cannot be placed in the lingual area.
   d. *A cotton roll in the mucobuccal fold and another one between teeth and tongue in the lingual area are adequate isolation for tooth #19.*

5. a. *The rubber dam clamp should be placed on the clamp tooth in a lingual to buccal direction.*
   b. The rubber dam clamp should not be placed on the clamp tooth in a buccal to lingual direction.
   c. It is best to place the rubber dam clamp onto the clamp tooth in a lingual to buccal direction.

6. a. Pulling the rubber dam off in one piece may leave pieces of the rubber dam in the interproximal areas.
   b. The interproximal rubber on the buccal aspect should be cut.
   c. *The interproximal rubber on the buccal aspect should be cut.*
   d. Cutting the interproximal rubber on the buccal and lingual aspects may leave pieces of the rubber dam in the interproximal areas.

7. a. The bow portion of the clamp is placed above the occlusal surface of the tooth.
   b. The wing portion of the rubber dam clamp aids in retraction of the rubber dam and is also used to place the rubber dam on the clamp before placing the rubber dam on the tooth.
   c. *The clamp beaks are used to engage the cervical portion of the tooth.*

8. a. An oil-based lubricant would degrade the latex material of the rubber dam.
   b. Petroleum jelly (Vaseline) is an oil-based lubricant that would degrade the latex material of the rubber dam.
   c. Cocoa butter is an oil-based lubricant that would degrade the latex material of the rubber dam.
   d. *A water-based lubricant is the best type for the rubber dam.*

9. a. Dental floss is used to slip the interproximal areas of the rubber dam between the teeth and also to ligate the rubber dam clamp.
   b. *A small piece of dental compound can be melted and shaped around the bow and clamped to stabilize the rubber dam clamp.*
   c. A small piece of rubber dam is used to anchor the rubber dam to the most anterior tooth to be isolated.
   d. A cotton roll will not stabilize the rubber dam clamp.

10. a. The medium-sized holes are generally used for the cuspids, premolars, or upper incisors.
    b. The medium-sized holes are generally used for the cuspids, premolars, or upper incisors.
    c. The second to largest hole in the rubber dam punch is generally used for the molars.
    d. *The largest hole in the rubber dam clamp is used for the clamp tooth.*

ANSWERS AND RATIONALES—Chapter 9

1. a. The ideal concentration of fluoride in the drinking water for the prevention of dental caries is 1 ppm.
   b. *The ideal concentration of fluoride in the drinking water for the prevention of dental caries is 1 ppm.*
   c. The ideal concentration of fluoride in the drinking water for the prevention of dental caries is 1 ppm.
   d. The ideal concentration of fluoride in the drinking water for the prevention of dental caries is 1 ppm.

2. a. When applying the acid etch to prepare the tooth for a pit and fissure sealant the tooth must be rinsed for a minimum of 15 to 20 seconds.
   b. *When applying the acid etch to prepare the tooth for a pit and fissure sealant the tooth must be rinsed for a minimum of 15 to 20 seconds.*
   c. When applying the acid etch to prepare the tooth for a pit and fissure sealant the tooth must be rinsed for a minimum of 15 to 20 seconds.
   d. When applying the acid etch to prepare the tooth for a pit and fissure sealant the tooth must be rinsed for a minimum of 15 to 20 seconds.

3. a. The tooth must be reetched because the contaminants from the saliva will interfere with the bonding of the sealant.
   b. The tooth must be reetched because the contaminants from the saliva will interfere with the bonding of the sealant.
   c. *The tooth must be reetched because the contaminants from the saliva will interfere with the bonding of the sealant.*
   d. The tooth must be reetched because the contaminants from the saliva will interfere with the bonding of the sealant.

4. a. When placing a pit and fissure sealant the tooth should look frosty white when dried after acid etching.
   b. When placing a pit and fissure sealant the tooth should look frosty white when dried after acid etching.
   c. *When placing a pit and fissure sealant the tooth should look frosty white when dried after acid etching.*
   d. When placing a pit and fissure sealant the tooth should look frosty white when dried after acid etching.

5. a. A daily over-the-counter fluoride rinse has been shown to decrease the caries rate by 30% to 40%; however, fluoridated drinking water decreases the caries rate by 50% to 60%.
   b. In-office fluoride treatment has been shown to decrease the caries rate by 25% to 40%; however, fluoridated drinking water decreases the caries rate by 50% to 60%.
   c. *Fluoridated drinking water offers the highest decrease in caries rate, namely, a 50% to 60% reduction.*

6. a. *Permanent discoloration of the enamel caused by too much ingestion of fluoride is called fluorosis.*
   b. Demineralization is the dissolution of the hard surfaces of the teeth by acid-producing bacteria.
   c. Dental caries is caused by plaque.
   d. Erosion is dissolution of the tooth by chemical means, such as sucking on lemons.

7. a. Plaque contains bacterial cells and other products.
   b. Supragingival plaque contains bacterial cells and other products.
   c. Subgingival plaque contains bacterial cells and other products.
   d. *The pellicle is a thin, noncellular layer produced from products in the saliva and is attached directly onto the tooth surface.*

8. a. Permanent discoloration of the enamel caused by too much ingestion of fluoride is called fluorosis.
   b. *Demineralization is the dissolution of the hard surfaces of the teeth by acid-producing bacteria.*
   c. Mottling is pitting of the enamel caused by too much fluoride ingestion.
   d. Remineralization is the uptake of minerals by the hard surfaces of the tooth.

9. a. *Actinobacillus actinomycetemcomitans* has been associated with periodontal disease but not dental decay.
   b. *Bacteroides gingivalis* has been associated with periodontal disease but not dental decay.
   c. *Streptococcus mutans has been associated with dental decay.*
   d. Spirochetes have been associated with periodontal disease but not dental decay.

10. a. The patient must be instructed not to eat, drink, or rinse for 30 minutes.
    b. Smoking is not contraindicated with fluoride treatments.
    c. *The patient must be instructed not to eat, drink, or rinse for 30 minutes.*
    d. Smoking is not contraindicated with fluoride treatments.

ANSWERS AND RATIONALES—Chapter 10

1. a. A sickle scaler has two cutting edges but has a pointed toe rather than a rounded toe. An explorer is an instrument made of fine flexible steel with a sharp point that is used to detect caries, calculus, and defective margins of restorations.
    b. *A universal curette and a Gracey curette have two cutting edges and a rounded toe.*
    c. A sickle scaler has two cutting edges but has a pointed toe rather than a rounded toe. An explorer is an instrument made of fine flexible steel with a sharp point that is used to detect caries, calculus, and defective margins of restorations.
    d. A Gracey curette and a universal curette have two cutting edges and a rounded toe.

2. a. *An ultrasonic scaler and a sonic scaler are devices that vibrate rapidly and use water coolant to remove calculus and stain from the tooth surfaces.*
    b. A universal curette is a hand instrument used to remove soft and hard deposits from the teeth. An air-powder abrasive polisher uses a solution of sodium bicarbonate and water to remove plaque and stain from the tooth.
    c. A universal curette is a hand instrument used to remove soft and hard deposits from the teeth.
    d. An air-powder abrasive polisher uses a solution of sodium bicarbonate and water to remove plaque and stain from the tooth.

3. a. The rotary scrub method of toothbrushing places the toothbrush at a right angle to the tooth and uses circular motions to brush the teeth.
    b. *The Bass method places the toothbrush at a 45-degree angle to the long axis of the tooth and uses a vibratory motion.*

4. a. Natural bristles are not recommended because the bristles have a tendency to split and abrade. Natural bristles also are less resistant to the accumulation of bacteria.
    b. Boar bristles are not recommended because the bristles have a tendency to split and abrade.
    c. Hard nylon bristles are not recommended because hard bristles can damage the gingiva and soft root surfaces.
    d. *Soft nylon bristles are the type of toothbrush bristles you should recommend to your patients.*

5. a. Snapping the floss through the contact will harm the interdental papillae.
    b. Pushing the floss up and down through the contact can harm the interdental papillae.
    c. *Seesawing the floss through the contact is the most appropriate method of placing the dental floss through the interproximal contact.*
    d. Threading the floss under the contact is possible but is time consuming and unnecessary.

6. a. *Patients should floss at least once each day.*
    b. Patients should floss at least once each day.
    c. Patients should floss at least once each day.

7. a. *A bridge threader and tufted floss can be used to clean the interproximal area of a fixed bridge.*
    b. An oral irrigator has not been proven to remove dental plaque.
    c. An oral irrigator has not been proven to remove dental plaque.
    d. A floss holder cannot be used to floss under a fixed bridge.

8. a. Although a baking soda toothpaste is effective in removing plaque with thorough toothbrushing, a fluoridated toothpaste is a better option.
    b. Although a tartar control toothpaste is effective in removing plaque and helps to control the formation of supragingival calculus, a fluoridated toothpaste is a better option.
    c. Although a hydrogen peroxide toothpaste is effective in removing plaque with thorough toothbrushing, a fluoridated toothpaste is a better option.
    d. *A patient with a high caries rate should use a fluoridated toothpaste to help control caries.*

9. a. Although a floss threader could help, it is tedious to use for each interproximal area.
    b. *A floss holder would be helpful to hold the dental floss and help the patient manipulate the floss correctly.*
    c. Although an oral irrigator is helpful in removing debris from the mouth, it has not been proven to remove dental plaque.
    d. A mouthwash is not a substitute for mechanical removal of plaque with dental floss.

10. a. Unwaxed floss will probably shred.
    b. *Waxed floss and polytetrafluoroethylene floss are helpful for patients who complain of shredding dental floss.*
    c. Tufted floss is useful for interproximal plaque removal under fixed bridges.
    d. Waxed floss and polytetrafluoroethylene floss are helpful for patients who complain of shredding dental floss.

ANSWERS AND RATIONALES—Chapter 11

1. a. Four-handed dentistry increases productivity because procedures take less time to complete.
    b. Four-handed dentistry increases efficiency because the assistant helps the dentist work quickly without moving his or her eyes away from the working area.
    c. Four-handed dentistry requires the assistant to help at chairside.
    d. *Four-handed dentistry increases productivity because procedures take less time to complete, and it increases efficiency because the assistant helps the dentist to work quickly without moving his or her eyes away from the working area.*

2. a. *It is best to have standardized operatories because this permits the dental staff to follow predictable work patterns.*
    b. Operatories that differ require the dental staff to change work patterns for each room, creating an unpredictable environment.

3. a. Class I movements involve the fingers only.
    b. Class II movements involve the fingers and wrist.
    c. *Class III movements involve the fingers, wrist, and elbow.*

d. Class IV movements involve the entire arm from the shoulder.

e. Class V movements involve the entire arm and twisting of the trunk.

4. a. Class I and II movements are preferable movements.
   b. Class II and III movements are preferable movements.
   c. Class III movements are preferable movements, whereas class IV movements should be avoided.
   d. *Class IV and V movements should be avoided.*

5. a. Using two assistants is not productive.
   b. Using two handpieces eliminates unnecessary bur changes.
   c. Using one bur simplifies the procedure and eliminates unnecessary bur changes.
   d. Using two assistants is not productive.
   e. *Using two handpieces or using only one bur eliminates the need for unnecessary bur changes.*

ANSWERS AND RATIONALES—Chapter 12

1. a. A side delivery system means that the instruments are delivered to the dentist from the side position.
   b. *A rear delivery system means that the instruments are delivered to the dentist from behind the patient.*
   c. A transthorax delivery system means that the instruments are delivered to the dentist from over the patient's chest.

2. a. A wall mount system is a fixed console used by the dentist for the delivery of instruments.
   b. *A mobile cart is a movable cart used by the assistant to hold the preset tray and adjunctive items.*
   c. An articulating headrest is located on the dental chair and moves in a variety of positions.

3. a. Doorways must be at least 32 inches wide to accommodate a disabled person.
   b. Doorways must be at least 32 inches wide to accommodate a disabled person.
   c. *Doorways must be at least 32 inches wide to accommodate a disabled person.*
   d. Doorways must be at least 32 inches wide to accommodate a disabled person.

4. a. An operator's stool should have a broad base.
   b. An operator's stool should have an adjustable seat.
   c. An operator's stool should have an adjustable back support.
   d. *The adjustable foot ring is used on an assistant's chair because the assistant sits above the dentist and the foot ring acts as a footrest.*

5. a. A foot-controlled and knee-controlled sink is the best type to use because it minimizes cross contamination.
   b. A hand-controlled sink poses a risk of cross contamination because the handles of the faucet could be handled with contaminated gloves or hands.
   c. A foot-controlled and knee-controlled sink is the best type to use because it minimizes cross contamination.
   d. *A foot-controlled and knee-controlled sink is the best type to use because it minimizes cross contamination of the sink area.*

ANSWERS AND RATIONALES—Chapter 13

1. a. The operator's zone is the 7 to 12 o'clock position.
   b. The static zone is the 12 to 2 o'clock position.
   c. The assistant's zone is the 2 to 4 o'clock position.
   d. *The transfer zone is the 4 to 7 o'clock position.*

2. a. The operator's zone is the 7 to 12 o'clock position.
   b. The static zone is the 12 to 2 o'clock position.
   c. *The assistant's zone is the 2 to 4 o'clock position.*
   d. The transfer zone is the 4 to 7 o'clock position.

3. a. The operator's zone is the 7 to 12 o'clock position.
   b. *The static zone is the 12 to 2 o'clock position.*
   c. The assistant's zone is the 2 to 4 o'clock position.
   d. The transfer zone is the 4 to 7 o'clock position.

4. a. A distance of 14 to 18 inches between the operator's nose and the patient's oral cavity should be maintained.
   b. A distance of 14 to 18 inches between the operator's nose and the patient's oral cavity should be maintained.
   c. *A distance of 14 to 18 inches between the operator's nose and the patient's oral cavity should be maintained.*
   d. A distance of 14 to 18 inches between the operator's nose and the patient's oral cavity should be maintained.

5. a. The patient is placed in the upright position when initially seated in the dental operatory.
   b. The patient is placed in the supine position for dental treatment on the maxillary arch.
   c. *The patient is placed in the semisupine position for dental treatment on the mandibular arch.*
   d. The patient is rarely placed in the subsupine position because it interferes with adequate blood flow to the body.

6. a. The patient is placed in the upright position when initially seated in the dental operatory.
   b. *The patient is placed in the supine position for dental treatment on the maxillary arch.*
   c. The patient is placed in the semisupine position for dental treatment on the mandibular arch.
   d. The patient is rarely placed in the subsupine position because it interferes with adequate blood flow to the body.

7. a. The height of the dental assistant's stool should be elevated so that the top of the assistant's head is 4 to 6 inches higher than that of the dentist during the delivery of dental treatment.
   b. *The height of the dental assistant's stool should be elevated so that the top of the assistant's head is 4 to 6 inches higher than that of the dentist during the delivery of dental treatment.*
   c. The height of the dental assistant's stool should be elevated so that the top of the assistant's head is 4 to 6 inches higher than that of the dentist during the delivery of dental treatment.
   d. The height of the dental assistant's stool should be elevated so that the top of the assistant's head is 4 to 6 inches higher than that of the dentist during the delivery of dental treatment.

8. a. The operating light should be positioned over the patient's chest when working on the maxillary arch.
   b. *The operating light should be positioned directly overhead when working on the mandibular arch.*

9. a. Placing the patient in the supine position quickly will not allow time for the patient to adjust to the change in position.
   b. *Placing the patient in the supine position with pauses in between allows time for the patient to adjust to the change in position.*
   c. The dental chair is set on a certain speed and will not allow the dental assistant to slow down the speed.

10. a. *The assistant's legs should be directed toward the head end of the dental chair.*
    b. The assistant's legs should be directed toward the head end of the dental chair.
    c. The assistant's legs should be directed toward the head end of the dental chair.

ANSWERS AND RATIONALES—Chapter 14

1. a. The bevel of the oral evacuator is held parallel to the tooth.
   b. *The bevel of the oral evacuator is held parallel to the tooth.*
   c. The bevel of the oral evacuator is held parallel to the tooth.
   d. The bevel of the oral evacuator is held parallel to the tooth.

2. a. The oral evacuator is held in the dental assistant's right hand for the right-handed operator.
   b. *The oral evacuator is held in the dental assistant's right hand for the right-handed operator.*

3. a. *The dental assistant holds the oral evacuator in the thumb-to-nose and modified pen grasp.*
   b. The dental assistant holds the oral evacuator in the thumb-to-nose and modified pen grasp.
   c. The dental assistant holds the oral evacuator in the thumb-to-nose and modified pen grasp.
   d. The dental assistant holds the oral evacuator in the thumb-to-nose and modified pen grasp.

4. a. The oral evacuator is used for retraction of soft tissue and to remove saliva and debris from the mouth.
   b. *The oral evacuator is used for retraction of soft tissue and to remove saliva and debris from the mouth.*
   c. The oral evacuator is used for retraction of soft tissue and to remove saliva and debris from the mouth.
   d. The oral evacuator is used for retraction of soft tissue and to remove saliva and debris from the mouth.

5. a. The oral evacuator is placed on the lingual aspect for an anterior facial cavity preparation.
   b. *The oral evacuator is placed on the lingual aspect for an anterior facial cavity preparation.*

ANSWERS AND RATIONALES—Chapter 15

1. a. The dental assistant uses the right hand to hold the high-volume evacuator.
   b. *The dental assistant uses the left hand to pass instruments to a right-handed dentist.*

2. a. The dental assistant uses the left hand for retraction.
   b. The dental assistant uses the left hand for instrument transfer.
   c. The dental assistant uses the left hand for operating the air-water syringe.
   d. The dental assistant uses the left hand for wiping the working end of instruments.
   e. *The dental assistant uses the right hand for holding the high-volume evacuator.*

3. a. The dental assistant should not recap an uncapped contaminated needle to minimize contact with it.
   b. *The dental assistant should not recap an uncapped contaminated needle to minimize contact with it.*

4. a. Using a recapping device is a recommended recapping method.
   b. Using the prongs of the cotton forceps is a recommended recapping method.
   c. *Holding the cap with the fingers is not recommended because it poses a risk of an accidental needle stick.*
   d. Using a scoop technique is a recommended recapping method.

5. a. *The assistant holds the tip of the air-water syringe to pass the syringe to the dentist.*
   b. The nut of the air-water syringe is too small to hold onto.
   c. The operator will be grasping the handle of the air-water syringe; therefore it would be awkward for the dental assistant to also hold the handle.
   d. The tubing is too flexible to hold to pass the air-water syringe to the dentist.

6. a. The contents of the cotton forceps will fall out if the dental assistant holds the handles of the forceps.
   b. *The dental assistant holds the beaks of nonlocking cotton forceps to pass the forceps to the dentist.*

7. a. The high-volume evacuator is usually not needed when the operator is applying a dental material.
   b. The air-water syringe is usually not needed when the operator is applying a dental material.
   c. *The dental assistant holds the mixing pad and the dental material when the dentist is applying a cement, liner, or composite material.*
   d. Cotton forceps and the air-water syringe are usually not needed when the operator is applying a dental material.

8. a. Crowding causes an awkward transfer but usually does not cause instrument tangling.
   b. Pointing the instrument toward the wrong arch will not cause instrument tangling.

c. An awkward transfer occurs when the dental assistant holds the instrument that is to be placed in the operator's hand too closely to the middle of the handle; however, it usually does not cause tangling.

d. *Tangling usually occurs when the dental assistant does not hold the transferring instrument parallel to the dentist's instrument before the transfer.*

9. a. A one-handed instrument pickup with the left hand is an appropriate method for the instrument transfer.

b. A two-handed instrument pickup is an appropriate method for the instrument transfer.

c. A one-finger instrument pickup with the left hand is an appropriate method for the instrument transfer.

d. *A four-finger instrument pickup is not an appropriate method for the instrument transfer.*

10. a. The operator uses a finger signal to alert the dental assistant that he or she is ready for the next instrument. A hand signal would cause too much unnecessary motion.

b. The operator uses a finger signal to alert the dental assistant that he or she is ready for the next instrument. A verbal signal is unnecessary.

c. *The operator uses a finger signal to alert the dental assistant that he or she is ready for the next instrument.*

d. The operator uses a finger signal to alert the dental assistant that he or she is ready for the next instrument. A foot signal would not be seen by the assistant.

ANSWERS AND RATIONALES—Chapter 16

1. a. Class I cavities are in the pit and fissure areas of teeth.

b. *Class II cavities are located on the proximal surfaces of posterior teeth.*

c. Class III cavities are on the proximal surfaces of anterior teeth that do not involve the incisal angle.

d. Class IV cavities are on the proximal surfaces of anterior teeth that require restoration of the incisal angle.

e. Class V cavities are on the cervical one third of all teeth that originate on a smooth surface.

2. a. Class I cavities are in the pit and fissure areas of teeth.

b. Class II cavities are located on the proximal surfaces of posterior teeth.

c. Class III cavities are on the proximal surfaces of anterior teeth that do not involve the incisal angle.

d. Class IV cavities are on the proximal surfaces of anterior teeth that require restoration of the incisal angle.

e. *Class V cavities are on the cervical one third of all teeth that originate on a smooth surface.*

3. a. *Class I cavities are in the pit and fissure areas of teeth.*

b. Class II cavities are located on the proximal surfaces of posterior teeth.

c. Class III cavities are on the proximal surfaces of anterior teeth that do not involve the incisal angle.

d. Class IV cavities are on the proximal surfaces of anterior teeth that require restoration of the incisal angle.

e. Class V cavities are on the cervical one third of all teeth that originate on a smooth surface.

4. a. The resistance form is the internal shape of the cavity preparation.

b. The retention form is the relationship that exists between different walls of the preparation.

c. *The outline form is the overall shape of the preparation along the external surface of the enamel.*

5. a. *Calcium hydroxide and glass ionomer are suitable materials for a cavity liner.*

b. Zinc oxide and eugenol and zinc phosphate are recommended for use as cement bases.

c. Calcium hydroxide and glass ionomer are suitable materials for a cavity liner; however, zinc oxide and eugenol cement is recommended for use as a cement base.

d. Zinc phosphate is irritating to the pulp; therefore it is not recommended for use as a cavity liner.

6. a. Calcium hydroxide and glass ionomer are cavity liners.

b. *Zinc oxide and eugenol and zinc phosphate are recommended for use as cement bases.*

c. Zinc oxide and eugenol cement is recommended for use as a cement base; however, calcium hydroxide and glass ionomer are cavity liners.

d. Zinc phosphate can be used as a cement base; however, zinc oxide and eugenol can also be used.

7. a. The cement base should be placed after the cavity liner.

b. *The correct sequence is the cavity liner and cement base followed by the varnish.*

c. The varnish is applied after the cavity liner and cement base.

d. The varnish is placed after the cement base.

8. a. Calcium hydroxide and glass ionomer are compatible with composite restorations.

b. *Varnish and zinc oxide and eugenol interfere with the hardening (setting) of the composite restoration.*

c. Calcium hydroxide and glass ionomer are compatible with composite restorations; however, varnish is not.

d. Zinc oxide and eugenol cement interferes with the hardening of the composite restoration; however, varnish is also contraindicated for composite restorations.

9. a. One layer of cavity varnish is recommended to completely seal the dentinal tubules.

b. *Two layers of cavity varnish are recommended to seal the dentinal tubules.*

c. Only two layers of cavity varnish are necessary to seal the dentinal tubules.

d. Only two layers of cavity varnish are necessary to seal the dentinal tubules.

10. a. The ratio of powder to liquid for ZOE is 1:1.

b. The ratio of powder to liquid for ZOE is 1:1.

c. *The ratio of powder to liquid for ZOE is 1:1.*

d. The ratio of powder to liquid for ZOE is 1:1.

ANSWERS AND RATIONALES—Chapter 17

1. a. Condensation is a term used to describe the pressing of the amalgam tightly against the cavity walls and matrix band.
    b. *The mixing process of amalgam using an amalgamator is called trituration.*
    c. Burnishing is the use of smooth-surface hand instruments to smooth the surface of an amalgam restoration.
    d. Carving is the use of a discoid-cleoid, half Hollenbeck, or other carving instrument to place anatomical features in the surface of an amalgam restoration.

2. a. *Condensation is a term used for the packing of the amalgam in a tooth preparation with an amalgam condenser or plugger.*
    b. The mixing process of amalgam using an amalgamator is called trituration.
    c. Burnishing is the use of smooth-surface hand instruments to smooth the surface of an amalgam restoration.
    d. Carving is the use of a discoid-cleoid, half Hollenbeck, or other carving instrument to place anatomical features in the surface of an amalgam restoration.

3. a. A discoid-cleoid and half Hollenbeck are used to carve an amalgam; however, an explorer is also used.
    b. A rubber abrasive point is used to polish an amalgam restoration.
    c. *A discoid-cleoid, half Hollenbeck, and an explorer are used to carve the amalgam restoration after it has been placed.*
    d. A rubber abrasive point is used to polish an amalgam restoration.

4. a. *An amalgamator is a device that mixes the mercury and silver alloy powder to form amalgam.*
    b. An amalgam capsule is a container that holds the mercury and silver alloy powder.
    c. An amalgam carrier is a hand instrument that is used to transport the mixed amalgam to the tooth preparation.
    d. A condenser is an instrument used to press the mixed amalgam tightly into the tooth preparation.

5. a. A matrix band is a thin strip of stainless steel sheet metal that is used to create a form around a prepared tooth.
    b. Contouring pliers are a hand instrument used to shape the matrix band to conform to the contours of a prepared tooth.
    c. *An interproximal wedge is a triangular wooden or plastic wedge that is placed between the teeth to act as a brace to hold the matrix band tightly against the tooth to prevent amalgam overhangs.*
    d. A burnisher is a smooth-surface hand instrument used to smooth the surface of an amalgam restoration.

6. a. The gingival edge of the matrix band is inserted into the Tofflemire retainer after the occlusal edge.
    b. *The occlusal edge of the matrix band must be inserted first into the Tofflemire retainer.*

7. a. *The inner knob is an adjustment knob used to slide the vise along the frame to either increase or decrease the size of the matrix band loop.*
    b. The outer knob is an adjustment knob used to tighten the spindle against the band in the vise.

    c. The spindle is a screwlike rod used to lock the ends of the matrix band in the vise.
    d. The vise is a clamplike device that holds the ends of the matrix band in the retainer.

8. a. A Tofflemire retainer and matrix band that are set up for the lower left quadrant will fit the upper right quadrant.
    b. A Tofflemire retainer and matrix band that are set up for the upper right quadrant will fit the lower left quadrant.
    c. *A Tofflemire retainer and matrix band that are set up for the lower right quadrant will also fit the upper left quadrant.*

9. a. A matrix band is not indicated for either a class I or a class V tooth preparation.
    b. *A matrix band is indicated for a class II and a class VI tooth preparation.*
    c. A matrix band is indicated for a class II and a class VI tooth preparation but not for a class I.
    d. A matrix band is indicated for a class VI and also a class II tooth preparation.

10. a. *An interproximal wedge is placed on the mesial interproximal surface only.*
    b. An interproximal wedge cannot be placed on the distal interproximal surface because there is not a tooth behind the third molar.
    c. Although an interproximal wedge can be placed on the mesial interproximal surface an interproximal wedge cannot be placed on the distal interproximal surface because there is not a tooth behind the third molar.

ANSWERS AND RATIONALES—Chapter 18

1. a. Flash is excess material that squeezes out of the cavity preparation when the matrix strip is removed.
    b. *Curing is the term used to describe the process of making a composite turn into its hardened state.*
    c. Etching is the application of phosphoric acid to the tooth preparation to dissolve the organic portion of enamel and create "enamel tags."
    d. Bonding is the use of an adhesive agent to "glue" the composite to the tooth.

2. a. If etched enamel is accidently exposed to saliva, the tooth must be reetched for 10 seconds.
    b. *If etched enamel is accidently exposed to saliva, the tooth must be reetched for 10 seconds.*
    c. If etched enamel is accidently exposed to saliva, the tooth must be reetched for 10 seconds.
    d. If etched enamel is accidently exposed to saliva, the tooth must be reetched for 10 seconds.

3. a. *The conditioner is a weak acidic solution that removes the dentin smear layer.*
    b. The primer is a wetting agent and is applied after the conditioner has removed the dentin smear layer.
    c. The bond agent is the adhesive that bonds the composite to the tooth and is applied after the conditioner and primer.
    d. The varnish is used for an amalgam restoration and is contraindicated for composite restorations.

4. a. Glass ionomer is compatible with composite materials.
    b. Calcium hydroxide is compatible with composite materials.
    c. *Zinc oxide and eugenol is contraindicated for use with composite materials because it interferes with the setting reaction of the composite.*
    d. A primer is compatible with composite materials.

5. a. *Calcium hydroxide, glass ionomer, conditioner, primer, bond agent is the correct placement of cavity medications and bonding agents in a composite restoration.*
    b. If calcium hydroxide is placed in a tooth that will be filled with composite, it is placed before the glass ionomer material.
    c. If glass ionomer material is placed in a tooth that will be filled with composite, the primer follows its placement.
    d. If calcium hydroxide is placed in a tooth that will be filled with composite, it is placed before the glass ionomer material and the primer.

6. a. The explorer has many uses but is too fragile to be used to remove excess composite from the margins of the restoration.
    b. Dental floss would not remove excess composite material from the margins of the restoration.
    c. Scissors are too bulky to be used to remove excess composite material from the margins of the restoration.
    d. *A scalpel can be used to remove excess composite material or flash from the margins of the restoration.*

7. a. Composite materials can also be used to restore class V restorations.
    b. Glass ionomer materials can also be used to restore class V restorations.
    c. It is not economically advantageous to use porcelain to restore class V restorations.
    d. *Small class V cavity preparations can be restored with glass ionomer materials or composite.*
    e. It is not economically advantageous to use porcelain to restore class V restorations.

8. a. An inlay is used to restore posterior teeth.
    b. *An aesthetic restoration that is actually a facing placed on the anterior teeth to correct crowding or tooth discoloration is called a veneer.*
    c. An onlay is used to restore posterior teeth.
    d. A core is used to build up lost tooth structure so the appropriate restoration can be placed on the tooth.

9. a. Porcelain inlays ideally require two appointments.
    b. Porcelain inlays ideally require two appointments, and CEREC system CAD/CAM inlays ideally require one appointment.
    c. *Porcelain inlays ideally require two appointments, and CEREC system CAD/CAM inlays ideally require one appointment.*
    d. CEREC system CAD/CAM inlays ideally require only one appointment.

10. a. Light-cured composites are not placed all at once in the cavity preparation because the composite shrinks when it is cured and can pull away from the tooth if placed all at once.
    b. *Light-cured composites are placed in the cavity preparation in small increments.*

ANSWERS AND RATIONALES—Chapter 19

1. a. An inlay is a restoration made from gold alloy that has been cast to fit a cavity preparation made by the dentist. The bulk of the restoration is contained within the confines of a tapered cavity preparation.
    b. *An onlay is a modification of the cast-gold inlay in which the restoration extends over the cusps of posterior teeth to prevent fracture of the teeth when biting forces are applied.*
    c. A three-quarter crown is a restoration that rebuilds three fourths of the crown portion of a tooth. The facial aspect of the tooth is usually left intact.
    d. A full crown is a reconstruction of the natural crown of the tooth.

2. a. *Alginate is used only for study models and opposing models for crown and bridge procedures.*
    b. Agar hydrocolloid is a final impression material used for crown and bridge procedures.
    c. Polyether is a final impression material used for crown and bridge procedures.
    d. Polyvinylsiloxane is a final impression material used for crown and bridge procedures.

3. a. The storage bath is used to store the agar hydrocolloid material once it has turned into the sol stage.
    b. The boiling bath is used to convert the agar hydrocolloid material from the gel stage to its sol stage.
    c. *The tempering bath is used to cool the agar hydrocolloid material in the impression tray before it is inserted in the patient's mouth.*

4. a. Polycarboxylate cements do not require a glass slab for mixing.
    b. Zinc oxide and eugenol cements do not require a glass slab for mixing.
    c. Glass ionomer cements do not require a glass slab for mixing.
    d. *Zinc phosphate cements require a glass slab for mixing.*

5. a. Polycarboxylate is an excellent permanent cement that contains some fluoride, but it is not anticariogenic.
    b. Zinc oxide and eugenol is an excellent permanent cement, but it is not anticariogenic.
    c. *Glass ionomer cements contain fluoride, which enables the cement to have anticariogenic qualities.*
    d. Zinc phosphate is an excellent permanent cement, but it is not anticariogenic.

6. a. Zinc phosphate is mixed to the correct consistency when the material strings out 1 to 1½ inches.
    b. When zinc phosphate is mixed to a doughlike stage, it is used as a base.
    c. Zinc phosphate is mixed to the correct consistency when the material strings out 1 to 1½ inches.
    d. *Zinc phosphate is mixed to the correct consistency when the material strings out 1 to 1½ inches.*

7. a. The correct ratio of powder to liquid for glass ionomer cement is 1:2.
    b. *The correct ratio of powder to liquid for glass ionomer cement is 1:2.*
    c. The correct ratio of powder to liquid for glass ionomer cement is 1:2.
    d. The correct ratio of powder to liquid for glass ionomer cement is 1:2.

8. a. An orangewood stick can be used to seat a gold restoration.
    b. A Cooley peg can be used to seat a gold restoration.
    c. A cotton roll can be used to seat a gold restoration.
    d. *A 2 × 2-inch gauze should not be used to seat a gold restoration.*

9. a. Zinc phosphate cements can be used as a permanent cement.
    b. *Zinc oxide and eugenol cements are used as a temporary cement and also as a base but not as a permanent cement.*
    c. Glass ionomer cement can be used as a permanent cement.
    d. Polycarboxylate cement can be used as a permanent cement.

10. a. Bite registration material is used to orient upper and lower models of the teeth in the proper bite relationship during the laboratory phase of a crown fabrication.
    b. Impression material is used to take an accurate replication of a tooth. The replication is used to fabricate a gold, porcelain, or porcelain and gold restoration.
    c. *Occlusal indicator wax is used to determine if the dentist has removed enough of the occlusal surface of a full crown or onlay preparation.*
    d. An orangewood stick is used to seat a crown or bridge restoration onto the tooth preparation.

ANSWERS AND RATIONALES—Chapter 20

1. a. *Porcelain is more abrasive than a natural tooth.*
    b. Porcelain is more abrasive than a natural tooth.

2. a. *Aesthetic crowns are usually placed in highly visible areas; therefore an aluminum shell temporary would be an undesirable temporary material.*
    b. A polycarbonate temporary can be used as a temporary for an aesthetic crown.
    c. A custom acrylic temporary can be used as a temporary for an aesthetic crown.
    d. A custom resin temporary can be used for an aesthetic crown.

3. a. The part of the fixed bridge that supports the fixed bridge at each end is called an abutment.
    b. A retention core is a buildup of material on the natural tooth to create better retention of the permanent restoration.
    c. *The part of the fixed bridge that is used to replace a missing tooth is called a pontic.*
    d. A retention pin is a small screwlike object that is inserted into the tooth to help the retention core stay in place.

4. a. The part of the fixed bridge that supports the fixed bridge at each end is called an abutment.
    b. *A retention core is a buildup of material on the natural tooth to create better retention of the permanent restoration.*
    c. The part of the fixed bridge that is used to replace a missing tooth is called a pontic.
    d. A retention pin is a small screwlike object that is inserted into the tooth to help the retention core stay in place.

5. a. Drifting of the tooth can occur when a tooth is lost from the dentition.
    b. Tipping of the tooth can occur when a tooth is lost from the dentition.
    c. Extrusion of the tooth can occur when a tooth is lost from the dentition.
    d. *Intrusion does not occur when a tooth is lost from the dentition.*

ANSWERS AND RATIONALES—Chapter 21

1. a. A 12B scalpel is used to incise and remove the gingiva during a gingivectomy procedure.
    b. An Orban gingival knife is used to incise and contour the gingiva during a gingivectomy procedure.
    c. A Kirkland gingival knife is used to incise and contour the gingiva during a gingivectomy procedure.
    d. *An interproximal knife (Gold knife) is used during restorative procedures to carve the interproximal area or to remove overhanging restorations.*

2. a. The dental assistant can mix the periodontal dressing during the periodontal surgery.
    b. The dental assistant can prepare the surgical sutures during the periodontal surgery.
    c. *The dental assistant cannot suture the surgical site.*
    d. The dental assistant can retract soft tissue during the periodontal surgery.

3. a. *The periodontal probe is primarily used to measure the depth of the periodontal pocket.*
    b. Although the periodontal probe can be used to measure the amount of gingival recession, the primary use is to measure periodontal pockets.
    c. Two mirror handles are used to measure mobility.
    d. Although the periodontal probe can be used to measure furcations, the primary use is to measure periodontal pockets.

4. a. A hoe scaler is not suitable for root planing because it has sharp corners that can gouge the root surface.
    b. *The curette can be used for scaling and root planing.*
    c. The 12B scalpel is used to incise and remove gingival tissue.
    d. The electrosurgery unit is used to remove gingival tissue or to cauterize blood vessels.

5. a. A gingivectomy is the surgical removal of diseased gingival tissue.
    b. Osseous surgery is a surgical procedure used to remove bony defects or to augment the bony defect with a bone graft.

c. A gingival graft is a surgical procedure that removes gingival tissue from one area of the mouth to place it in another area of the mouth that is deficient in gingiva.

d. *Flap surgery involves the removal of the lining of the periodontal pocket and some adjacent marginal gingiva.*

6. a. A gingivectomy is the surgical removal of diseased gingival tissue.

b. Osseous surgery is a surgical procedure used to remove bony defects or to augment the bony defect with a bone graft.

c. *A gingival graft is a surgical procedure that removes gingival tissue from one area of the mouth to place it in another area of the mouth that is deficient in gingiva.*

d. Flap surgery involves the removal of the lining of the periodontal pocket and some adjacent marginal gingiva.

7. a. A eugenol or noneugenol periodontal dressing should be mixed with a tongue depressor.

b. To make it easier to handle, the fingers should be lubricated before touching the periodontal dressing.

c. A eugenol or noneugenol periodontal dressing should be rolled into a rope before placing it on the surgical site.

d. *If an entire quadrant is involved in the periodontal surgery the periodontal dressing should be wrapped around the distal aspect of the last molar to help hold the dressing in place.*

8. a. Clogging can be prevented in the surgical suction tip during the periodontal surgery by periodically aspirating sterile saline solution during the procedure.

b. Tap water is not sterile and could contaminate the surgical site.

c. *Clogging can be prevented in the surgical suction tip during the periodontal surgery by periodically aspirating sterile saline solution during the procedure.*

d. The surgical suction tip has a tendency to clog with blood during periodontal surgical procedures; therefore sterile saline solution should be aspirated during the procedure.

9. a. It is normal for small pieces of the periodontal dressing to fall off. The dental office should be called only if large pieces of the dressing fall off.

b. It is normal for small pieces of the periodontal dressing to fall off. It is not necessary to put the pieces back on.

c. *It is normal for small pieces of the periodontal dressing to fall off.*

d. It is normal for small pieces of the periodontal dressing to fall off. The patient may only need to go to the dental office if large pieces of the dressing fall off.

10. a. A periodontal probe or a pocket marker can be used to outline the pocket depth before making the initial incision.

b. A pocket marker or a periodontal probe can be used to outline the pocket depth before making the initial incision.

c. A 12B scalpel is used to make the incision and remove the gingiva; it is not used to mark the pocket depth.

d. *A periodontal probe or a pocket marker can be used to outline the pocket depth before making the initial incision.*

e. A 12B scalpel is used to make the incision and remove the gingiva; it is not used to mark the pocket depth.

ANSWERS AND RATIONALES—Chapter 22

1. a. A blow to the tooth could cause either pulpal inflammation or death depending on the severity of the blow.

b. Dental caries can cause pulpal inflammation or death depending on the extent of the caries process.

c. Incomplete rinsing of acid etch could cause pulpal inflammation or pulpal death.

d. *Thumb sucking is one of the causes of malocclusion but is not a factor that could cause a tooth to need endodontic procedures.*

2. a. *RC Prep is used to lubricate the root canal during the endodontic filing procedure.*

b. Sodium hypochlorite is used to disinfect the root canal during the endodontic procedure.

c. Formocresol is used as an antimicrobial interim dressing for multiple-visit root canal treatment.

d. Root canal sealer is a cement material that is used with gutta-percha to seal the root canal.

3. a. An endodontic file is used to enlarge, smooth, and shape the root canal.

b. *A barbed broach is used to remove the pulp once the tooth has been opened.*

c. An endodontic reamer is used to enlarge, smooth, and shape the root canal.

d. An endodontic spreader is used to obturate the gutta-percha in the root canal.

4. a. *An endodontic file is used to enlarge, smooth, and shape the root canal.*

b. A barbed broach is used to remove the pulp once the tooth has been opened.

c. An endodontic plugger is used to condense the gutta-percha into the root canal, or it is heated red hot and used to remove the excess gutta-percha from the opening of the tooth.

d. An endodontic spreader is used to obturate the gutta-percha in the root canal.

5. a. If possible, an avulsed tooth should be placed back into the socket.

b. *If it is not possible to replant the tooth back into the bony socket the tooth should be stored in milk, saliva, or saline; however, water should not be used.*

c. The dentist should be seen immediately for an avulsed tooth so the tooth can be examined and stabilized.

d. A replanted avulsed tooth must be stabilized.

6. a. A necrotic pulp will have no response to an electric vitality test.

b. A tooth that is not endodontically involved would have the same response as a control tooth.

c. A tooth that has chronic pulpitis may require more electric current to react.

d. *A tooth that has pulpitis or hyperemia may require less electric current to react.*

7. a. A periodontal abscess is a localized collection of pus at the apex of the tooth.
   b. A fistula is a drainage tract for pus formed through the bone from a periapical abscess.
   c. *Apical periodontitis is inflammation of the periodontal tissues near the apex of the tooth.*
   d. Pulpitis is inflammation of the pulpal tissue.

8. a. *A periodontal abscess is a localized collection of pus at the apex of the tooth.*
   b. A fistula is a drainage tract for pus formed through the bone from a periapical abscess.
   c. Apical periodontitis is inflammation of the periodontal tissues near the apex of the tooth.
   d. Pulpitis is inflammation of the pulpal tissue.

9. a. *An apicoectomy is the surgical removal of the apex of the tooth.*
   b. A retrofill amalgam is the sealing of the apex of the tooth with amalgam following an apicoectomy.
   c. A root amputation is the removal of one or more entire roots or a multirooted tooth.
   d. Obturation is the filling of the root canal to eliminate space within the canal.

10. a. *A necrotic pulp will have no response to an electric vitality test.*
    b. A tooth that is not endodontically involved would have the same response as a control tooth.
    c. A tooth that has chronic pulpitis may require more electric current to react.
    d. A tooth that has pulpitis or hyperemia may require less electric current to react.

ANSWERS AND RATIONALES—Chapter 23

1. a. Positive reinforcement occurs when the child is praised for desired behaviors.
   b. Tell-show-do is used to show a child nonthreatening equipment and instruments before dental treatment.
   c. Nonverbal communication includes facial expressions, body language, and eye contact.
   d. *Preappointment behavior modification is anything that is said or done to influence positively the child's behavior before treatment.*

2. a. *Positive reinforcement occurs when the child is praised for desired behaviors.*
   b. Tell-show-do is used to show a child nonthreatening equipment and instruments before dental treatment.
   c. Nonverbal communication includes facial expressions, body language, and eye contact.
   d. Preappointment behavior modification is anything that is said or done to influence positively the child's behavior before treatment.

3. a. A stainless steel crown is used as an interim restoration on primary teeth until they are exfoliated, or it is used on permanent teeth until a more accurately contoured cast-gold crown can be fabricated.
   b. A spot-welded matrix band is a custom-fitted matrix band that can be used for primary teeth.

   c. *A pulp cap is performed to avoid root canal therapy in the event of a small pulpal exposure during cavity preparation.*
   d. A pulpectomy is root canal therapy.

4. a. *A deciduous tooth does need treatment even though it will be lost eventually and be replaced by a permanent tooth.*
   b. A deciduous tooth does need treatment even though it will be lost eventually and replaced by a permanent tooth.

5. a. *The stainless steel crown must extend 1 mm below the margin of the crown preparation.*
   b. A stainless steel crown is cemented with a permanent cement.
   c. Contouring pliers are used to bend the cervical margins of a stainless steel crown.
   d. A stainless steel crown must contact adjacent teeth to prevent shifting of adjacent teeth.

ANSWERS AND RATIONALES—Chapter 24

1. a. The long leg of the steel spring separator is hooked in a lingual-to-buccal direction between the interproximal contact.
   b. *The short leg of the steel spring separator should be grasped with the No. 139 pliers to place the separator between the teeth.*
   c. The coil of the steel spring separator provides the source of tension on the interproximal contact between the long and short legs.

2. a. *The vertical overlap of the incisal edges of upper anterior teeth over the incisal edges of lower anterior teeth is called overbite.*
   b. Overjet is the horizontal distance between the incisal edges of a maxillary incisor and the mandibular incisor in an anteroposterior dimension.
   c. Crossbite is the lower teeth overlapping the upper teeth.
   d. Open bite is the mandibular anterior teeth not contacting the lingual surfaces of the maxillary anterior teeth when the jaws are closed.

3. a. The vertical overlap of the incisal edges of upper anterior teeth over the incisal edges of lower anterior teeth is called overbite.
   b. Overjet is the horizontal distance between the incisal edges of a maxillary incisor and the mandibular incisor in an anteroposterior dimension.
   c. *Crossbite is the lower teeth overlapping the upper teeth.*
   d. Open bite is the mandibular anterior teeth not contacting the lingual surfaces of the maxillary anterior teeth when the jaws are closed.

4. a. Brackets are attachments that are welded to the orthodontic bands or directly bonded to the tooth to hold the arch wire in place and transmit the force of the arch wire to the teeth.
   b. Elastics are rubber bands that are used to exert forces on the teeth.

c. *Ligatures are fine wires or elastic rings that are used to tie the arch wire to the brackets.*

d. Coil springs are attached to the arch wire and are used to exert either a pushing or pulling force on selected teeth.

5. a. *Brackets are attachments that are welded to the orthodontic bands or directly bonded to the tooth to hold the arch wire in place and transmit the force of the arch wire to the teeth.*

b. Elastics are rubber bands that are used to exert forces on the teeth.

c. Ligatures are fine wires or elastic rings that are used to tie the arch wire to the brackets.

d. Coil springs are attached to the arch wire and are used to exert either a pushing or pulling force on selected teeth.

6. a. Floss can be used to place elastic separators.

b. Elastic separating pliers can be used to place elastic separators.

c. Bird-beak pliers are used for small wire and spring forming.

d. *Floss and elastic separators can be used to place elastic separators.*

e. Bird-beak pliers are used for small wire and spring forming.

7. a. Bird-beak pliers are used for small wire and spring forming.

b. De La Rosa pliers are used for contouring wire loops and molar band materials.

c. Band pushers are used to seat and adapt circumferential bands to the teeth.

d. *Stainless steel ligatures are placed with a hemostat.*

8. a. *A positioner is a soft plastic device used immediately after the fixed appliances are removed to maintain the alignment of the teeth.*

b. An expansion activator is used to expand the maxillary arch.

c. An activator is used to reduce excessive overbite, to make changes in skeletal growth, and for minor tooth movement.

d. A retainer is used after fixed appliance treatment to hold the teeth in the desired position until the teeth become stable.

9. a. A Bionator is not a positioner.

b. A Bionator is not an expansion activator.

c. *A Bionator is an activator.*

d. A Bionator is not a retainer.

10. a. A neuron is a nerve cell.

b. White blood cells are cells of the immune system.

c. An osteoblast is a bone-forming cell.

d. *An osteoclast is a cell that causes bone resorption.*

ANSWERS AND RATIONALES—Chapter 25

1. a. *A root pick is a surgical probe used to remove root fragments.*

b. A periosteal elevator is a hand instrument used to separate the periosteum from the bone surface and to retract the mucoperiosteum.

c. A rongeur forceps is a nipperlike instrument used to trim alveolar bone.

d. A surgical curette is a scoop-shaped hand instrument used to sever the epithelial attachment of the gingiva around the tooth and for scraping interior cavities of bone or other tissues.

2. a. A root pick is a surgical probe used to remove root fragments.

b. *A periosteal elevator is a hand instrument used to separate the periosteum from the bone surface and to retract the mucoperiosteum.*

c. A rongeur forceps is a nipperlike instrument used to trim alveolar bone.

d. A surgical curette is a scoop-shaped hand instrument used to sever the epithelial attachment of the gingiva around the tooth and for scraping interior cavities of bone or other tissues.

3. a. A root pick is a surgical probe used to remove root fragments.

b. A periosteal elevator is a hand instrument used to separate the periosteum from the bone surface and to retract the mucoperiosteum.

c. *A rongeur forceps is a nipperlike instrument used to trim alveolar bone.*

d. A surgical curette is a scoop-shaped hand instrument used to sever the epithelial attachment of the gingiva around the tooth and for scraping interior cavities of bone or other tissues.

4. a. An incisional biopsy is removal of only part of a lesion for examination.

b. *An excisional biopsy is the removal of an entire lesion plus the adjacent normal tissue.*

c. Exfoliative cytology is an examination of cells scraped from an oral lesion and does not require any incision.

5. a. *Tooth sectioning is division of a tooth into two or more parts to facilitate removal of the tooth.*

b. Luxation is the displacement of a tooth in the bony socket by using extraction forceps.

c. Exodontia is the removal of teeth.

d. Alveoloplasty is the use of surgical instruments to shape the edentulous ridge.

6. a. The patient should be instructed to use a cold pack for the first 24 hours to minimize inflammation and swelling.

b. The patient should be instructed to begin brushing teeth the day after the surgery.

c. *The patient should not be instructed to rinse vigorously the day of the surgery because of the risk of dislodging the blood clot.*

d. The patient should be instructed to bite on moist gauze immediately following the surgery.

7. a. Maxillary molars that are trifurcated can be extracted with an 18R or 18L extraction forceps.

b. Anterior teeth can be extracted with a No. 1 or No. 151 extraction forceps.

c. *A cow-horn extraction forceps is used for extraction of mandibular molar teeth.*

d. Maxillary third molars can be extracted with a No. 210 extraction forceps, and mandibular third molars can be extracted with a No. 222 extraction forceps.

8. a. A bone file is used to smooth and remove bone.
   b. A rongeur is used to trim alveolar bone.
   c. A mallet and chisel can be used for bone removal.
   d. *A scalpel is used to incise soft tissue.*

9. a. *The endosteal type of implant is used primarily for single tooth replacement.*
   b. The transosteal type of implant is used for full arch denture replacement.
   c. The subperiosteal type of implant is used for full arch denture replacement.

10. a. A patient with prolonged bleeding does not usually experience pain or a foul odor in the mouth.
    b. *Pain, foul odor, and a bad taste in the mouth are all symptoms of dry socket.*
    c. Loose sutures do not cause pain, foul odor, or a bad taste in the mouth.
    d. Trismus is a stiffness of the muscles of mastication usually caused by long dental procedures or local anesthetic injections.

ANSWERS AND RATIONALES—Chapter 26

1. a. It is recommended to take the prosthesis out at night to let the soft tissues rest.
   b. *It is not recommended to scrub the prosthesis with household cleaners because the cleaners are abrasive.*
   c. It is recommended to clean the prosthesis before going to bed.
   d. It is recommended to place the prosthesis in water if taken out of the mouth for prolonged periods to avoid dehydration of the prosthesis, which could lead to distortion.

2. a. Denture relining is a technique used to compensate for alveolar ridge reduction by adding new acrylic to the tissue surface of the denture base.
   b. Border molding is a technique used during the fabrication of a removable partial or complete denture. Border molding helps to adapt the border of the partial or complete denture to the patient's soft tissues.
   c. *Tissue conditioning is a procedure that uses a soft lining placed on the tissue side of a denture that is used for denture sores.*
   d. Muscle trimming is the same as border molding.

3. a. *Denture relining is a technique used to compensate for alveolar ridge reduction by adding new acrylic to the tissue surface of the denture base.*
   b. Border molding is a technique used during the fabrication of a removable partial or complete denture. Border molding helps to adapt the border of the partial or complete denture to the patient's soft tissues.
   c. Tissue conditioning is a procedure that uses a soft lining placed on the tissue side of a denture that is used for denture sores.
   d. Muscle trimming is the same as border molding.

4. a. *Overdentures are good because the retained root tips help to maintain the height of the alveolar ridge.*
   b. The retained root tips of an overdenture do not prevent denture sores.
   c. The overdenture actually requires more maintenance than a denture.
   d. Crowns are not placed over the retained roots for an overdenture.

5. a. When the patient is going to receive immediate dentures, the teeth are taken out in this order: the posterior teeth are taken out one side at a time, and then the anterior teeth are removed.
   b. When the patient is going to receive immediate dentures, the teeth are taken out in this order: the posterior teeth are taken out one side at a time, and then the anterior teeth are removed.
   c. *When the patient is going to receive immediate dentures, the teeth are taken out in this order: the posterior teeth are taken out one side at a time, and then the anterior teeth are removed.*
   d. When the patient is going to receive immediate dentures, the teeth are taken out in this order: the posterior teeth are taken out one side at a time, and then the anterior teeth are removed.

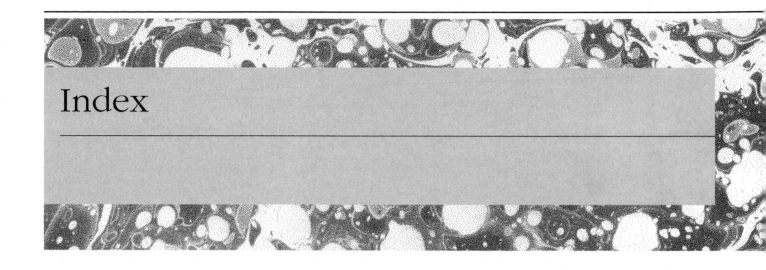

Index

A

Abdominal thrusts, airway obstruction and, 64-65
Abrasive rubber polishing points, 251
Abscess, 343, 346
    periapical, 344
    periodontal, 316
Abuse, child; *see* Child abuse and neglect
Abutments, 305-306
Acid etching, composite restorations and, 258-259
Acquired immunodeficiency syndrome (AIDS), universal precautions
       and, 98-99
Acrylic saddles, 447
Activator, 398, 401
Acute apical periodontitis, 343-344
Acute necrotizing ulcerative gingivitis (ANUG), 316
ADA; *see* American Dental Association
Adrenalin; *see* Epinephrine
Aesthetic restorations, 256-274
    bleaching and, 272, 273
    composite restorative materials for, 256-260
    porcelain, 270-273
Agar hydrocolloid impressions, 281-283, 284, 285, 293, 304
Age of patient, treatment plan and, 17
AIDS; *see* Acquired immunodeficiency syndrome
Airborne contaminants, disease transmission and, 99
Air-powder abrasive polisher, 152, 154
Air-water syringe, 184
Air-water syringe transfer, 212-213, 215
Airway obstruction, 63-68
Alginate impressions, 279, 290, 291, 388-389, 390-391
All-castable-glass restorations, 271
All-ceramic restorations, 271-273
Allergy, 74
All-porcelain restorations, 271
Aluminum shell crown method, full cast-gold crowns and, 295-296
Alveolitis, exodontia and, 436, 437
Alveoloplasty, 434
Amalgam, 237
    delivery of, 221-222
    retrofill, 361
    silver, 237

Amalgam carriers, 238, 239
Amalgam carvers, 246
Amalgam cavity preparations, 231-232, 246-251
Amalgam condensers, 239
Amalgam core, 254, 312
Amalgam overhang, 241, 254
Amalgam restorations, 237-255
   amalgam overhangs and, 254
   bonded, 251-252
   class I, 251
   class II, 246-251
   class V, 251
   class VI, 251
   instruments and supplies for, 237-246
   pin-retained, 252-254
   procedures for, 246-251
   safety precautions for, 254-256
Amalgam restorative material, 237-238
Amalgam well, 238, 239
Amalgamators, 238
Ambu bag, medical emergencies and, 58, 59
American Academy of Pediatric Dentistry's standards of care for
      behavior management, 368-369
American Board of Oral Surgery, 415
American Dental Association (ADA), 11, 29, 324-325
   sequential numbering system of, 3-5
Anesthesia
   in class II amalgam restoration, 247-248
   for class III restoration, 264
   for class IV restoration, 266
   in endodontics, 352
   field block, 40
   general, 39
     in pediatric dentistry, 369
   infiltration, 40
   in inlay cementation appointment, 293
   in inlay preparation appointment, 291
   local; *see* Local anesthesia
   nerve block, 40-41
   topical; *see* Topical anesthesia
   toxicity of, 73